SIR SYLLABUS

INTERVENTIONS IN ONCOLOGY

Charles E. Ray, Jr., M.D., *Editor*
Chief, Interventional Radiology
Denver Health Medical Center
Associate Professor of Radiology
University of Colorado Health Sciences Center
Denver, Colorado

Marshall E. Hicks, M.D., *Editor*
Professor of Radiology
Department of Interventional Radiology
The University of Texas M.D. Anderson Cancer Center
Houston, Texas

Nilesh H. Patel, M.D., FSIR, *Series Editor in Chief*
Society of Interventional Radiology
Associate Professor of Diagnostic Radiology & Nuclear Medicine
RUSH-Presbyterian - St. Luke's Medical Center
Chicago, Illinois

Published by
The Society of Interventional Radiology

NOTICE

The usage of supply items and indications and dosages of drugs in this book have been recommended in the medical literature. Products mentioned may or may not be approved by the United States Food and Drug Administration for use in the diseases and dosages for which their manufacturers recommend them. Please consult package inserts and other product information for current approved standards.

The Society of Interventional Radiology is accredited by the Accreditation Council for Continuing Medical Education to sponsor medical education for physicians.

The Society of Interventional Radiology designates this educational activity for 24 hours of category 1 of the Physicians Recognition Award of the American Medical Association.

Printed in the United States of America

10 9 8 7 6 5 4 3 2 1

ISBN 1-928625-09-6

FOREWORD

In 1991, when I was a green attending fresh out of fellowship, I answered an "any angiographer" phone call from an enlightened patient who was self-referring for embolization of his symptomatic neuroendocrine metastases to his liver. I dutifully called one of the oncologists and asked him to admit this very interesting patient. His response was "What am I, some kind of hospital whore? Why should I admit someone for you to treat him?" Thus was born the interventional oncology service, which within five years was the leading single source of revenue for the IR section, generated countless scholarly contributions, and built invaluable clinical and academic relationships with colleagues in medical oncology, radiation oncology, surgical oncology, hepatology, GI and transplant surgery, diagnostic and functional imaging, tumor biology, and engineering.

It has been predicted that by 2010, cancer will have surpassed cardiovascular diseases as the leading cause of death in the United States. Minimally invasive, image-guided therapies have a major role in the management of oncology patients and are an important part of the modern IR practice. Treating cancer involves not just high-tech regional and local therapies, but a host of ancillary procedures for venous access, palliation of obstruction, pain control, management of thromboembolic disease, and diagnosis. To participate meaningfully in the multi-disciplinary care of cancer patients, interventional radiologists need to understand fundamentals of cancer, cancer treatments, and patient care. This syllabus covers these basics, along with detailed chapters on diagnostic, therapeutic, and palliative procedures that should be part of daily practice.

Interventional oncology is a tremendous opportunity for IR, but also poses tremendous challenges. Our procedures are crude, using imaging guidance to intensify the application of non-specific drugs and energy sources that kill tissue without distinction between normal and cancerous cells. We use primitive imaging modalities that poorly discriminate tumor from non-tumor or successful tumor kill from failure. The future will bring sophisticated molecular imaging to identify malignant cells, registration of 3D imaging datasets to sculpt treatment plans, and functional imaging guidance to detect tumor kill in real-time. Interventional radiologists will need to stay on top of progress in molecular and functional imaging, image processing, and novel locoregional therapies in order to maintain their role.

My congratulations to Drs. Charles Ray, Jr. and Marshall Hicks for putting together a timely syllabus that I hope SIR members will find of practical value.

Michael C. Soulen, MD
Associate Professor of Radiology & Surgery
University of Pennsylvania

PREFACE

The Society of Interventional Radiology is proud to introduce *Interventions in Oncology*. The hard work of the coeditors, Drs. Charles Ray, Jr. and Marshall Hicks, has brought forth this new SIR syllabus. This textbook is written by the volunteer efforts of leading experts from various medical subspecialties. I am indebted to all of them for their hard work, time commitment, and devotion, without which this textbook would not exist.

This book, as well as the SIR syllabus titled *Patient Care in Interventional Radiology*, reflects the growth of our specialty. As technology and our understanding of cancer advance, so does our armamentarium of minimally invasive treatment options.

Nilesh H. Patel, MD, FSIR
Editor-in-Chief

ACKNOWLEDGMENTS

It is difficult to know where to begin in acknowledging all of the individuals instrumental in the development of this book. A special thanks to Dr. Nilesh Patel for assuming the duties not just of co-editor, but the added responsibility of editor-in-chief of the current syllabus series—his guidance proved vital. As Education Councilor of SIR, John Kaufman also provided timely and sage advice during all phases of development of this book. We would be remiss in not thanking the staff at SIR, most notably Cathy Mendelsohn, who provided tireless efforts and invaluable experience in leading us in this project. The staff at Maryland Composition, particularly Al Beringer, have also been crucial in keeping the book production timely and efficient. Our colleagues at our primary hospitals also provided assistance, either directly or indirectly, as we were involved in the development of this project—to them we owe both our debt and gratitude.

On a more personal level, patients who present to our clinics or interventional suites for care have touched us all. Certain bonds seem to develop between a patient diagnosed with cancer and their caregivers—bonds that seem to be unique in this patient population. Perhaps it is their courage expressed in the face of a daunting illness—perhaps it is the numerous times over the course of their illness that we are entitled to attempt to help them through their disease—or perhaps it is the strong ties between family and friends that develop over time. Regardless of the cause, our cancer patients provide us with our most joyous successes, and our most disheartening failures. It is for them that we continue to strive for the "magic bullet" for better and less invasive treatments; and it is to them that we dedicate this book.

Charles Ray, Jr., MD

This book is a culmination of efforts from many individuals interested in advancing the field of image-guided oncologic intervention. The combined contributions of the numerous authors will hopefully form a base upon which our subspecialty will build as the field expands and matures. I am grateful for their hard work. My co-editor, Chuck Ray, and Series Editor-in-Chief, Nilesh Patel, provided the drive and momentum necessary to achieve our goal, and were true to the task. I'd like to thank John Kaufman for his constant support and encouragement. I would especially like to express my appreciation to Cathy Mendelsohn, a very talented individual, who works mostly "behind the scenes" to ensure success. I also would like to thank Al Beringer at Maryland Composition for his patience and expertise. My gratitude also goes to those individuals who provided support for the authors or provided information for inclusion in the presented material. Finally, my sincere thanks to Bill Murphy who convinced me of the purpose and opportunity in image-guided oncologic intervention, and to Sid Wallace who paved the way for all of us.

This book represents hope for cancer patients and their families, whose lives have been forever changed. As health care providers and leaders in innovative treatments, we can work towards opening doors to new worlds of healing and health and provide hope to those who carry this burden.

Lastly, my journey into image-guided oncologic intervention has been a personal journey, as well. I would like to dedicate my contribution to my son, Graham, who, as a cancer survivor, has been my inspiration and teacher, and to my wife Kelly, whose passion for life gave us strength to endure.

Marshall Hicks, MD

CME INFORMATION

CME Essentials

The Society of Interventional Radiology (SIR) Syllabus "Interventions in Oncology" is part of a series of enduring materials planned and produced in accord with the Accreditation Council for Continuing Medical Education Essentials. It has been developed for interventional radiologists, both practicing and in training, in instructional text format.

"Interventions in Oncology" constitutes a planned activity of continuing medical education with an estimated completion time of 24 hours. The Society of Interventional Radiology designates this educational activity for a maximum of 24 category 1 credits toward the AMA Physician's Recognition Award. Topics covered for this CME activity are represented by the Table of Contents; principal faculty and their credentials can be found on pages ix–xi. An evaluation survey is provided as part of this CME activity to assess the value of these materials in meeting the educational needs of the end user.

Learning objectives addressed in this CME activity consist of the following:

1. To understand the role of interventional radiology in the diagnosis and treatment of oncology patients.
2. To review current techniques used in the interventional radiology department in the treatment of patients with cancer.
3. To understand future technologies currently undergoing evaluation that will be used by interventional radiologists in the treatment of cancer.

To become eligible for 24 hours of Category 1 CME credit, the user must submit the **original** application form, an evaluation survey and a completed quiz answer sheet, along with a $20 administrative fee. **Additional examinations, intended to be utilized by users other than the original purchaser of this syllabus, are available from the SIR office for $100. Contact the CME Administrator at 703-691-1805. All completed examinations and evaluation surveys should be mailed** to:

SIR
Attention: CME Administrator
10201 Lee Highway, Suite 500
Fairfax, VA 22030

SIR has a policy requiring disclosure of the existence of any significant financial interest or other relationship that authors have to the manufacturer(s) of any commercial product(s) discussed in any SIR-sponsored educational activity.

Each contributing author has indicated that he or she has no financial relationship with companies or organizations about whose products or services they are reporting.

SIR Syllabus XII

Interventions in Oncology

Date of Release: June 2003

Date of Next CME Review: June 2006

CONTRIBUTORS

Steven K. Arnason, M.D.
Department of Radiology
Dalhousie University
Halifax, Nova Scotia, Canada

Murray Asch, M.D., FRCPC
Assistant Professor of Medical Imaging
Department of Medical Imaging
Mount Sinai Hospital
Toronto, Ontario, Canada

Christi A. Barber, ANP
Clinical Coordinator of Pain Treatment Services
Department of Anesthesiology/Perioperative Services
SUNY Upstate Medical University
Syracuse, New York

Robert F. Berry, M.D.
Lecturer
Department of Radiology
Dalhousie University
Halifax, Nova Scotia, Canada

Richard Bihrle, M.D.
Professor of Urology
Indiana University School of Medicine
Indianapolis, Indiana

Christoph Binkert, M.D.
Assistant Professor of Radiology
Brigham and Women's Hospital
Harvard University
Boston, Massachusetts

Elias Brountzos, M.D.
Associate Professor of Radiology
Second Department of Radiology
University of Athens
Athens, Greece

Timothy W. I. Clark, M.D., MSc
Assistant Professor of Radiology and Surgery
Hospital of The University of Pennsylvania
Philadelphia, Pennsylvania

Julia T. De Sanctis, M.D.
Radiologist, Medical Center at Princeton
Princeton Radiology Associates
Kendall Park, New Jersey

Debra A. Gervais, M.D.
Director, Abdominal Intervention
Department of Radiology
Massachusetts General Hospital
Boston, Massachusetts

Sanjay Gupta, M.D.
Assistant Professor of Radiology
The University of Texas M.D. Anderson Cancer Center
Houston, Texas

Tara Hanjan, M.D.
Radiology Clinical Fellow
New York Presbyterian Hospital
College of Physicians & Surgeons of Columbia University
New York, New York

James M. Hevesi, Ph.D., FACR, FAAPM
Director of Medical Physics
Cancer Therapy and Research Center
Adjunct Professor of Radiation Oncology
The University of Texas Health Science Center at San Antonio
San Antonio, Texas

Marshall E. Hicks, M.D.
Professor of Radiology
Department of Interventional Radiology
The University of Texas M.D. Anderson Cancer Center
Houston, Texas

Syed I. Hosain, M.D.
Assistant Professor of Anesthesiology and Pain Management
Department of Anesthesiology
SUNY Upstate Medical University
Syracuse, New York

Muhammad Umar Islam, M.D.
Department of Radiology
Dalhousie University
Halifax, Nova Scotia, Canada

John Kaufman, M.D.
Professor of Radiology, Interventional Radiology, and Surgery
Dotter Interventional Institute
Oregon Health and Sciences University
Portland, Oregon

Lily Y. Kernagis, M.D.
Resident in Radiology
University of Pennsylvania
Philadelphia, Pennsylvania

George Khoriaty, M.D.
Interventional Radiologist
Department of Radiology, Diagnostic Clinic
Largo Medical Center
Largo, Florida

Bogda Koczwara, BMBS, FRACP, MBIOETHICS
Head, Department of Oncology
Flinders Medical Centre
Adelaide, Australia
Senior Lecturer
Flinders University of South Australia
Adelaide, Australia

David C. Madoff, M.D.
Assistant Professor of Radiology
Department of Interventional Radiology
The University of Texas M.D. Anderson Cancer Center
Houston, Texas

Francis J. Mangiacapra, M.D.
Assistant Professor of Radiology
SUNY Upstate Medical University
Syracuse, New York

Praveen N. Mathur, MBBS
Professor of Clinical Medicine
Division of Pulmonary, Critical Care, Allergy, and Occupational Medicine
Indiana University Medical Center
Indianapolis, Indiana

Gordon McLennan, M.D.
Assistant Professor of Radiology
Indiana University Medical Center
Indianapolis, Indiana

Donald L. Miller, M.D.
Chief, Interventional Radiology
National Naval Medical Center
Bethesda, Maryland
Professor of Radiology
F. Edward Hébèrt School of Medicine
Uniformed Services University of the Health Sciences
Bethesda, Maryland

Kenneth D. Murphy, M.D.
Associate Professor and Division Director of Interventional Radiology
SUNY Upstate Medical University
Syracuse, New York

Albert A. Nemcek, Jr., M.D.
Associate Professor of Radiology
Department of Vascular and Interventional Radiology
Northwestern University Medical School
Chicago, Illinois

Charles A. Owens, M.D.
Associate Professor of Radiology and Surgery
University of Illinois Medical Center at Chicago
Chicago, Illinois

Ketul Patel, M.D.
Assistant Clinical Instructor
Department of Anesthesiology
SUNY Upstate Medical University
Syracuse, New York

Nilesh H. Patel, M.D.
Director of Interventional Radiology
Associate Professor of Radiology
Rush-Presbyterian-St. Luke's Medical Center
Chicago, Illinois
Affiliated Radiologists, S.C.
Chicago, Illinois

Randall M. Patten, M.D.
Medical Director
Everett Radiology Medical Imaging Center
Providence Everett Medical Center
Seattle, Washington

Dheeraj K. Rajan, M.D., FRCPC
Assistant Professor of Medical Imaging
Department of Medical Imaging
University Health Network–University of Toronto
Toronto, Ontario, Canada

Charles E. Ray, Jr., M.D.
Chief, Interventional Radiology
Denver Health Medical Center
Denver, Colorado
Associate Professor of Radiology
University of Colorado Health Sciences Center
Denver, Colorado

Robert K. Ryu, M.D.
Section Chief
Interventional Radiology
Decatur Memorial Hospital
Decatur, Illinois

Kent Sato, M.D.
Interventional Radiology
Northwestern Memorial Hospital
Chicago, Illinois

Guido M. Scatorchia, M.D.
Interventional Radiology
Denver Health Medical Center
Denver, Colorado
Assistant Professor of Radiology
University of Colorado Health Sciences Center
Denver, Colorado

Michael C. Soulen, M.D.
Associate Professor of Radiology and Surgery
University of Pennsylvania
Philadelphia, Pennsylvania

Michael S. Stecker, M.D.
Assistant Professor of Radiology
Indiana University School of Medicine
Indianapolis, Indiana

Charles R. Thomas, Jr., M.D.
Vice Chairman and Associate Professor of Radiation Oncology
The University of Texas Health Science Center at San Antonio
San Antonio, Texas

John W. Thomas, M.D.
Interventional Radiologist
South Texas Radiology Group
San Antonio, Texas
Clinical Assistant Professor of Radiology
University of Texas Science Center
San Antonio, Texas

P. Sebastian Thomas, M.D.
Professor of Anesthesiology/Director of Pain Treatment Services
Department of Anesthesiology
SUNY Upstate Medical Center
Syracuse, New York

James H. Turner, M.D.
Interventional Radiology
Denver Health Medical Center
Denver, Colorado
Assistant Professor of Radiology
University of Colorado Health Sciences Center
Denver, Colorado

Jean-Nicolas Vauthey, M.D.
Professor of Surgery
Department of Surgical Oncology
The University of Texas M.D. Anderson Cancer Center
Houston, Texas

CONTENTS

CHAPTER 1

RADIOLOGICAL INTERVENTIONS: SPECIAL CONSIDERATIONS IN CANCER PATIENTS

BOGDA KOCZWARA, BM, BS, FRACP, MBIOETHICS

INTRODUCTION

Cancer constitutes one of the major health burdens of our time. It remains second only to cardiac disease as a cause of death in the United States.[1] More than half of all cases of cancer diagnosed today are in patients older than age 65 years,[2] and it is likely that with the increasing age of the world population, the prevalence of cancer will continue to rise. Direct costs of cancer care in the United States have been estimated as approximately 11% of all medical care.[3] It is likely that these costs will rise with the increased prevalence of cancer and increased complexity of cancer treatments. As cancer treatment becomes more effective, appropriate supportive care is paramount; for some patients appropriate supportive care may make a difference between cure and palliation. For others whose cancer cannot be cured, it can provide effective control of symptoms and add to their quality of life. With increased efficacy of cancer treatments, patients' survival of some cancers can be prolonged and approach that of other chronic diseases (e.g., renal failure, cardiac disease), making the need for good symptom control even more important.

In considering the overall management of cancer, two areas deserve particular attention. The first relates to the medical aspects of the malignancy, either with reference to the tumor itself or the type of treatment that has already been administered. These variables may pose specific problems that may affect further treatment. The second consideration relates to the need for careful balancing of the risks and benefits of treatment

TABLE 1-1
Glossary of Oncologic Terminology

Term	Definition
Adjuvant	Treatment given, following complete surgical removal of cancer, aiming at eradication of micrometastases and increased cure
Chemoradiotherapy	Chemotherapy and radiotherapy administered concurrently
Combined modality treatment	Treatment using more than one modality of surgery, chemotherapy, or radiotherapy
Cure	Long-term absence of cancer with return to normal life expectancy
Nadir	Lowest reading in the complete blood picture following administration of chemotherapy or the *time* when the reading is the lowest (the timing of the nadir varies with different drugs—for most, it occurs around 7–10 days after commencement of chemotherapy)
Neoadjuvant	Treatment prior to curative resection aimed at tumor shrinkage, improved resectability, and/or organ preservation
Palliation	Treatment aimed at relief of symptoms and improvement of quality of life
Performance status	Global measure of patient's fitness that correlates with outcome of treatment (as defined by a standardized scale—see Table 1-3)
Progression	Increase in tumor burden as defined by increase in tumor size and/or rise in tumor markers according to predetermined criteria
Quality of life	Multidimensional assessment of patient's physical, emotional, and social well-being (there are a number of valid scales and measurements of quality of life suitable for different cancers/circumstances)
Relapse	Regrowth of cancer following a period of remission
Remission	Temporary absence of cancer (this term is commonly used in hematologic malignancies after clearance of malignant cells from blood and bone marrow is achieved)
Response	Decrease in tumor burden as defined by decrease in tumor size and/or fall in tumor markers according to predetermined criteria
Tumor lysis syndrome	Severe electrolyte disturbance manifested by hyperkalemia, hyperphosphatemia, hypocalcemia, and hyperuricemia secondary to massive cell death after chemotherapy

in light of the overall prognosis of the malignancy. In some settings, further clinical interventions may not be appropriate and indeed may negatively affect the patient's quality of life or survival.

This chapter reviews special considerations pertaining to patients with cancer from the point of view of patient assessment and the decision-making process that must take place prior to consideration of an interventional radiologic (IR) procedure.

Table 1-1 is a glossary of terms commonly used when dealing with patients with cancer; review of these terms is recommended before readers continue with this chapter.

ASSESSMENT OF A PATIENT WITH CANCER

Prior to performance of an IR procedure, the following aspects require consideration as part of the assessment of a patient with cancer (**Table 1-2**).

Indication for Intervention

Assessment of a patient with cancer prior to any therapeutic or diagnostic intervention requires a clear understanding of the goals of the intervention and how those goals relate to the overall condition of the patient. Although it may be necessary to perform high-risk procedures in patients who are treated with the ultimate intention of cure, in those in whom cure is not possible it is important that the procedure have the lowest potential risk of compromising the patient's quality of life.

The patient's life expectancy and future treatment options may influence the type of intervention best suited in a particular setting. For example, some patients require venous access devices (VADs) for many years, whereas others may need them for only a short period of time. Patients with longer life expectancy using VADs as outpatients may have specific concerns regarding cosmetic and comfort aspects of the device, whereas those treated as inpatients may require larger

TABLE 1-2

Assessment of Patients with Cancer Prior to an Interventional Procedure

Goals of intervention	Cure versus palliation
Prognosis	Type of cancer Stage Comorbid conditions Performance status
Previous and current therapy	Immunosuppression Antibiotics Cytotoxics Surgery Radiotherapy
Coagulation	Anticoagulant treatment Need for thrombosis prophylaxis
Risk of infection	Need for antimicrobial prophylaxis
Metabolic status	Hydration Electrolyte status Renal function Nutrition Liver function

inner-diameter lumens for ease of transfusion and frequent blood tests.

Prognosis

Overall prognosis of a malignancy will affect the feasibility of achieving a specific treatment goal. In general terms, prognosis is influenced by multiple factors, including

- Type of cancer
- Stage of cancer
- Comorbid conditions
- Performance status

Among these, performance status assessment is unique to oncology. It is a relatively simple indicator of a patient's overall well-being. Despite its simplicity, it seems to correlate well with the patients' prognoses and likelihood of responding to treatment. Patients with poor performance status has cancer unlikely to respond to therapy and have limited life expectancy.[4] **Table 1-3** shows two example scales for measurement of performance status.

In addition to their impact on prognosis, stage and type of cancer may also influence the technique used to perform a given procedure or approach. For example, a different placement approach for a VAD may need to be used in a woman with chest wall tumor recurrence from her breast cancer because a subclavian approach may not be feasible, or in a patient with metastatic tumor involvement of the neck in head and neck cancer because a jugular approach may not be possible. Equally, comorbid conditions may influence the technical aspects of the intervention; for example, timing of a lengthy procedure may need to be considered in a patient with diabetes to avoid prolonged hypoglycemia, or a patient with severe pulmonary compromise may need to have a procedure performed in a semirecumbent position.

Previous and Current Therapy

Cancer treatment and supportive care therapies may influence the performance of IR procedures. Previous

TABLE 1-3

Two Commonly Used Performance Status Scales

Karnofsky Scale[4]

Description	Status
Normal; no complaints	100%
Able to carry on normal activities; minor signs or symptoms of disease	90%
Normal activity with effort	80%
Cares for self; unable to carry on normal activity or to do active work	70%
Requires occasional assistance but able to care for most of his/her needs	60%
Requires considerable assistance and frequent medical care	50%
Disabled; requires special care and assistance	40%
Severely disabled; hospitalization indicated, though death is not imminent	30%
Very sick; hospitalization necessary; active supportive treatment necessary	20%
Moribund	10%
Dead	0%
ECOG* Scale[5]	
Fully active; able to carry on all pre-disease performance without restrictions	0
Restricted in physically strenuous activity but ambulatory and able to carry out work of a light or sedentary nature	1
Ambulatory and capable of all self-care but not able to carry out any work activities; up and about > 50% of waking hours	2
Capable of only limited self-care; confined to bed or chair > 50% of waking hours	3
Completely disabled; cannot carry on any self-care; totally confined to bed or chair	4
Dead	5

**Eastern Cooperative Oncology Group*

surgery or radiotherapy may have an impact on certain anatomic considerations of the procedure, potentially making it necessary to alter the conventional approach for a given procedure. Previous chemotherapy with some agents may affect end organ function; for example, anthracyclines can cause cardiac impairment, whereas 5-fluorouracil (5-FU) can cause vasospasm.[6] Some cytotoxic agents can cause excessive toxicity when high cumulative doses are reached (e.g., anthracyclines, bleomycin); owing to this dose-related effect, they should be avoided if previously used extensively. The best known of these effects is anthracycline-induced cardiomyopathy, which varies in incidence depending on the cumulative dose given.[7] Patients with established cardiomyopathy may not tolerate large fluid loads, excessive blood loss, or large bolus injections of intravenous contrast.

Recent cytotoxic therapy may result in bone marrow suppression and a corresponding decline in the number of white blood cells and platelets, which may potentially affect immune function and blood clotting ability. Medications other than cytotoxics may affect the patient's risk of infection (antibiotics, steroids) or tolerance of analgesics (e.g., patients taking baseline narcotic analgesics will require higher doses of analgesics during the procedure).

Coagulation

Cancer increases the risk of thrombosis.[8,9] Patients with cancer who are undergoing surgery have double the risk of venous thromboembolism when compared with patients with no malignancy[9]; although not confirmed in the literature, similar risks should be expected for patients undergoing radiologic interventions. In these patients, prophylaxis using either heparin, low-molecular-weight heparin (LMWH), warfarin, or intermittent pneumatic compression devices should be considered. Some cancer treatments further increase the risk of thrombosis. For example, the risk of thrombosis in a patient whose breast cancer is treated with tamoxifen is increased regardless of whether the patient has an active malignancy or the drug is used for cancer prevention.

Patients with cancer who develop thromboembolism require treatment until free of cancer or until death. They are also at higher risk of recurrent thrombolism while taking anticoagulants.[9,10] Patients who develop recurrence while taking warfarin are often treated over the long term with LMWH, which is also used in patients with extensive malignancy-related liver disease when use of oral anticoagulants may be problematic. It is important to specifically question patients about the use of LMWH because treatment with this form of anticoagulation will not be apparent in results of standard coagulation blood screens.

Little is known about the risks of LMWH use in the setting of IR procedures, so any specific recommendations require extrapolation from quite extensive documentation of the effect of LMWH in the surgical setting. Patients taking *prophylactic* doses of LMWH can safely undergo even major surgery 12 hours after anticoagulant administration.[11] It is reasonable to assume that these patients can safely undergo many IR procedures at similar times. For instance, it would be safe to perform fine-needle aspiration biopsies or computed tomography (CT)–guided sympathectomies in patients who have received prophylactic doses of LMWH the night before their procedures (12 hours after a prophylactic dose of LMWH). The morning dose should be withheld on the day of the procedure. For patients taking *therapeutic* doses of LMWH, administration of the regular LMWH dose should be omitted for at least 24 hours to allow the anti–factor Xa activity to fall to prophylactic levels.[12] Special considerations are needed if elimination of LMWH is impaired (e.g., owing to renal dysfunction).

When a procedure must be performed urgently, a reversal of anticoagulation may be necessary. In patients undergoing anticoagulation with warfarin, reversal can be achieved by using vitamin K and fresh-frozen plasma; in patients treated with heparin or LMWH, protamine can be administered.[14] Careful consideration as to the safety of anticoagulation reversal is paramount in some patients (e.g., patients with cardiac valve replacements) because reversal may place them at extreme risk of complications. Consultation with a hematologist is helpful in these circumstances.

The timing of resumption of anticoagulation depends on the indication for anticoagulation. When the risk of thrombosis is high, administration of heparin or LMWH can be resumed after a hemorrhage-free interval of between 2 and 8 hours.[13]

Risk of Infection

Although the underlying malignancy itself can impair immune function, the risk of infection in a patient with cancer is most commonly affected by the cancer treatment.[15] Infection risk is increased, among other factors, by therapy-related loss of mucosal surfaces, placement of long-term catheters, neutropenia, and glucocorticoid use.[16,17] Risks of neutropenia can be stratified by duration and presence of comorbidities.[18] Prolonged granulocytopenia is well recognized as a risk factor for fungal infections.[19,20] Other risk factors for infection include use of broad-spectrum antibiotics, certain types of cytotoxics (high-dose cytarabine), and total body irradiation (TBI) as part of a bone marrow transplantation (BMT) conditioning regimen.[21,22] Some new immunosuppressive strategies, including T-cell deple-

TABLE 1-4
Host-Related Risk Factors for Infection in Patients with Cancer

Immunosuppression	Neutrophil dysfunction
	Cellular immune dysfunction
	Humoral dysfunction
	Age
	Immunosuppressive disease
Organ dysfunction	Mucocutaneous damage
	Renal/liver failure
	Obstruction of natural body passages
	Foreign bodies
	Asplenia
Microbial colonization	Prolonged hospitalization
Reactivation of latent infections	For example, cytomegalovirus, hepatitis, *Pneumocystis carinii* pneumonia, tuberculosis

tion as part of BMT and administration of antithymocyte globulin for aplastic anemia, also predispose to fungal infection.[23] Chemoprevention employing both oral and intravenous antibiotics is used for high-risk patients during times of high infection risk, and in some patients, antifungal prophylaxis may be needed. It is important to question patients about their prophylactic antibiotic use, particularly if use of prophylactic antibiotics is considered prior to IR procedures.

Colony-stimulating factors (G-CSF and GM-CSF) can be administered to patients who are likely to experience prolonged neutropenia as a result of cytotoxic treatment, to reduce the duration and severity of neutropenia.[24] There is less evidence for their use in a setting of established neutropenia.[25] Intravenous γ-globulin can be used in patients who are hypogammaglobulinemic.

Tables 1-4 and **1-5** list multiple risk factors for infections arising in cancer patients.

TABLE 1-5
Factors Associated with Increased Risk of Infection in a Setting of Neutropenia

- Duration of neutropenia >10 days
- Comorbidity (hypotension, altered mentation, respiratory difficulty, bleeding, dehydration, or hypercalcemia)
- Uncontrolled cancer

Metabolic Status

Adequate hydration is necessary for maintaining renal function. This is particularly important when cancer treatment is likely to result in a large burden of tumor kill, leading to a high production of tumor breakdown products. Massive cell death in some tumors (Burkitt's lymphoma, undifferentiated lymphomas, acute lymphoblastic leukemia) may result in tumor lysis syndrome and severe electrolyte disturbance, including hyperkalemia, hyperphosphatemia, hypocalcemia, and hyperuricemia. Similar electrolyte disturbances are known to occur after embolization of tumors that results in cell death.[26, 27] Uric acid nephropathy can occur as a response to treatment when a high amount of uric acid is excreted as a result of purine metabolism; this is most likely in cancers with high turnover rates (hematologic, small-cell, testicular cancers). Tumor lysis syndrome and uric acid nephropathy are best prevented with hydration, urinary alkalinization, and allopurinol, starting 48 hours before treatment. Elderly and malnourished patients may have impaired renal reserve without a significant elevation of serum creatinine; therefore, even in the setting of normal serum creatinine levels, prophylactic measures should be employed to avoid uric acid nephropathy. Patients with renal impairment may not tolerate some of the cytotoxic agents, which may result in further renal damage (cisplatin, streptozotocin) or greater toxicity (methotrexate). They are also less likely to handle large fluid loads, including bolus injections of intravenous contrast. Guidelines for prophylactic measures to avoid tumor lysis syndrome are given in **Table 1-6**.

TABLE 1-6
Management of Tumor Lysis

Phase	Protocol
Prophylaxis	Identify patients at risk: those with bulky tumors that are chemotherapy responsive (leukemia; lymphoma, especially Burkitt's)
	Hydration
	Allopurinol, 100 mg/m^2 P.O. three times a day for 48 h, then 300 mg/day
Treatment	Allopurinol, 300 mg/day
	Hydration: 3000 mL/m^2/day
	Alkalinize urine with sodium bicarbonate if hyperuricemia and azotemia are present or if patient is unable to take allopurinol
	Avoid alkalinization if hyperphosphatemia
	Monitor fluid balance

TABLE 1-7
Oncology Drugs That Require Dose Adjustments for Organ Dysfunction

Adjust for renal impairment	Adjust for liver impairment
Cisplatin	Anthracyclines
Ifosfamide	Taxanes
Methotrexate	Vincristine
Etoposide	Etoposide
Topotecan	Cyclophosphamide
Bleomycin	Methotrexate
Dacarbazine	5-fluorouracil

Some cancers predispose patients to specific metabolic abnormalities (i.e., islet cell tumors and hypoglycemia), as can cancer treatments (cisplatin and hypomagnesemia). Contrast itself may result in stimulation of pheochromocytomas to secrete vasoactive substances.[28] Consultation with a specialist and appropriate premedication are paramount for these patients.

Nutritional Status and Liver Function

Both poor nutrition and liver failure can adversely affect serum protein levels and therefore will affect the amount of unbound drug in the circulatory system. This increased concentration of unbound drug may have an impact on the toxicity of cytotoxic agents used in therapeutic interventions; it can also affect post-procedure coagulation and healing. Liver failure can also influence the body's ability to eliminate some of the cytotoxic agents used, including anthracyclines, taxanes, and some other medications, including sedatives and analgesics. Doses of cytotoxic agents used as part of IR procedures may have to be adjusted to correct for organ dysfunction (**Table 1-7**).

INFORMATION PROVISION AND COMMUNICATION

Effective communication regarding the risk and benefits of treatment is an essential component of care. When it comes to IR procedures, this includes communication with the patient and with the doctor in charge of his or her ongoing care (usually—but not always—a medical oncologist).

Communicating with the Patient

Communication with the patient is based on the principles of informed consent and includes discussion of the nature, risks, and benefits of the proposed procedure, as well as risks and benefits of alternative procedures, including no treatment. Especially in oncology, it is important to keep in mind the importance of maintaining the patient's quality of life, as many IR procedures are performed in patients whose cancer cannot be cured and in whom quality of life is the main treatment goal. Quality of life assessment is subjective by nature and is determined by the patient's perception of his or her health. It is a multidimensional feeling incorporating physical, emotional, and social measures. Therapeutic interventions may affect all these aspects of a patient's life.

Communicating with the Oncologist

Communication with the oncologist is vital to ensuring agreement on goals of the intervention and determining the potential risks that must be considered. In addition, provisions for appropriate care after the procedure must be made. In institutions where the radiologist cannot monitor the patient after the procedure, detailed instructions on how to manage patient care and how to obtain additional advice should be provided, because oncologists are often unfamiliar with post-procedure or device care.

SUMMARY

Radiologic interventions in patients with cancer require a comprehensive assessment of the patient and careful consideration of the risks and benefits of the procedure. Factors unique to oncology patients must be evaluated, and decisions regarding therapeutic benefit must be made in light of patients' prognoses and quality of life considerations. Effective communication of information about the nature, benefits, and risks of the intervention are an integral part of the treatment.

REFERENCES

1. Greenlee RT, Hill-Harmon MB, Murray T, Thun M. Cancer statistics, 2001. *CA Cancer J Clin* 2001;51:15–36.
2. Redmond K, Aapro MS, eds. *Cancer in the Elderly. A Nursing and Medical Perspective*. Elsevier Science; Amsterdam 1997.
3. Rice DP, Hodgson TA, Capell F. The economic burden of cancer, 1985; United States and California. In: Scheffler RM, Andrews NC, eds: *Cancer Care and Cost: DRGs and Beyond*. Ann Arbor, MI: Health Administration Press; 1989.
4. Karnofsky DA, et al. The use of the nitrogen mustards in the palliation treatment of carcinoma with particular reference to bronchogenic carcinoma. *Cancer* 1948;1:634–656.
5. Oleksowicz L, Bruckner H. Prophylaxis of 5-fluorouracil induced coronary vasospasm with calcium channel blockers. *Am J Med* 1988;85:750–751.

6. Oken MM, Creech RH, Tormey DC, et al. Toxicity and response criteria of the Eastern Cooperative Oncology Group. *Am J Clin Oncol* 1982;5:649–655.
7. Shan K, Lincoff M, Young JB. Anthracycline-induced cardiotoxicity. *Ann Intern Med* 1996;125:47–58.
8. Sorensen HT, Mellemkjaer L, Steffensen FH, et al. The risk of a diagnosis of cancer after primary deep venous thrombosis or pulmonary embolism. *N Engl J Med* 1998;338:1169–1173.
9. Baron JA, Gridley G, Weiderpass E, et al. Venous thromboembolism and cancer. *Lancet* 1998;351:1077–1080.
10. Hyers TM, Kessler C, Groce J. *Venous Thromboembolism and Malignancy. American Society of Clinical Oncology Fall Educational Book 1999*. Alexandria, VA: ASCO; 1999:248–250.
11. Wysowski DK, Talarico L, Bacsanyi J, Botstein P. Spinal and epidural hematoma and low-molecular-weight heparin. *N Engl J Med* 1998;338:1774–1775.
12. Levine MN, Planes A, Hirsh J, et al. The relationship between anti-factor Xa level and clinical outcome in patients receiving enoxaparine low molecular weight heparin to prevent deep vein thrombosis after hip replacement. *Thromb Haemost* 1989;62:940–944.
13. Tie M, Koczwara B. Radiology interventions in patients receiving low molecular heparin. *Australas Radiol* 2001;45(3):313–317.
14. Tollefsen DM. Disorders of hemostasis. In: Dunagan WC, Ridner ML, eds. *Manual of Medical Therapeutics*. Boston, MA: Little, Brown; 1989:338–340.
15. Lehrnbecher T, Foster C, Vazquez N, et al. Therapy induced alterations in host defense in children receiving therapy for cancer. *J Pediatr Hematol Oncol* 1997;19:399–417.
16. Freifeld AG, Pizzo PA, Walsh TJ. Infections in the cancer patient. In: *Cancer, Principles and Practice of Oncology*. 5th ed. Philadelphia, PA: Lippincott-Raven; 1997:2659–2664.
17. Berenguer J, Allende M, Lee J, et al. Pathogenesis of pulmonary aspergillosis: Granulocytopenia versus cyclosporine and methylprednisolone-induced immunosuppression. *Am J Respir Crit Care Med* 1995;152:1079–1086.
18. Talcott JA, Siegel RD, Finberg R, et al. Risk assessment in cancer patients with fever and neutropenia: a prospective, two-center validation of a prediction rule. *J Clin Oncol* 1992;10:316–322.
19. Bodey GP, Buckley M, Sathe YS, et al. Quantitative relationships between circulating leucocytes and infection in patients with leukemia. *Ann Int Med* 1966;64:328–340.
20. Bodey GP. Fungal infections complicating acute leukemia. *J Chron Dis* 1966;19:667–687.
21. Bow EJ, Shore TB, Kilpatrick MG, et al. Relationship of invasive fungal disease and high-dose cytarabine plus etoposide containing remission-induction regimens for acute myeloid leukemia. *Blood* 1991;78(suppl):55A. [Abstract]
22. Pannuti CS, Gingrich R, Pfaller MA, et al. Nosocomial pneumonia in patients having bone marrow transplant: attributable mortality and risk factors. *Cancer* 1991;69:2653–2662.
23. Weinberger M, Elattar I, Marshall D, et al. Patterns of infection in patients with aplastic anemia and the emergence of Aspergillus as a major cause of death. *Medicine* 1992;71:24–43.
24. Trillet-Lenoir V, Green J, Manegold C, et al. Recombinant granulocyte colony-stimulating factor reduces the infectious complications of cytotoxic chemotherapy. *Eur J Cancer* 1993;29A:319. [Abstract]
25. ASCO. American Society of Clinical Oncology recommendations for the use of hematopoietic colony-stimulating factors: evidence-based clinical practice guidelines. *J Clin Oncol* 1994;12:2471.
26. Burney IA. Acute tumor lysis syndrome after transcatheter chemoembolization of hepatocellular carcinoma. *South Med J* 1998;91:467–470.
27. Paye F, Farges O, Dahmane M, et al. Cytolysis following chemoembolization for hepatocellular carcinoma. *Br J Surg* 1999;86:176–180.
28. Raisanen J, Shapiro B, Glazer GM, Desai S, Sisson JC. Plasma catecholamines in pheochromocytoma: effect of urographic contrast media. *Am J Roentgenol* 1984;143:43–46.

CHAPTER 2

PRINCIPLES OF CHEMOTHERAPY

CHARLES E. RAY, JR., MD

BOGDA KOCZWARA, BM, BS, FRACP, MBIOETHICS

Anticancer agents belong to a wide variety of drug classes. Some agents have a direct effect on cell replication or protein synthesis, causing active cell destruction (cytotoxic agents). Other agents have their effects by inhibiting or stimulating the body's own hormonal activity (hormonal agents) or by affecting some other natural cellular activity (biologic response modifiers). A general understanding of drug classes, along with their effects and toxicities, is vital to any health care professional administering such medications.

Paul Ehrlich first described chemotherapy, using the term to describe medications given to treat both neoplasms and infections. Cancer drug screening was initiated after an investigator at Roswell Park Cancer Institute in Buffalo, New York, developed a rodent model that contained transplanted tumors against which the drugs could be tested. That method of testing new agents against an animal model possessing a tumor line, first described in the early 1900s, remains the standard model even today.

Historically, alkylating agents were the first agents used clinically to combat cancer. Interestingly, alkylating agents were discovered through the accidental exposure of U.S. naval personnel to mustard gas during World War II; individuals exposed to the gas were noted to have marrow and lymphoid hypoplasia. New anticancer drugs and methods of treating neoplasms represent some of the most extensively investigated areas of research in the medical field. In fact, a recent MEDLINE search using just *chemotherapy* as the search word revealed 17,584 citations—for the 6 months prior to the preparation of this manuscript.

Chemotherapeutic agents may be subclassified according to their mechanism of action and/or the source from which they are derived. This chapter focuses on the agents used most frequently in interventional radiologic (IR) practice. **Table 2-1** demonstrates the most common agents used in IR practice, classified by their mode of action.[1]

Chemotherapeutic agents are derived from a number of sources. Similar to other drug classes, many of the chemotherapeutic drugs are formulated in the laboratory and are designed specifically to interfere with a specific cell cycle or protein formation, causing cell death immediately or during cell replication. Other drugs, such as doxorubicin, are antibiotics extracted from a culture medium of the *Streptomyces* species. Still other agents, like vincristine, are derived from plant sources.

The importance of understanding the various drug classes lies in the realization that drugs belonging to the same class often have similar effects at the cellular level and similar toxicity profiles. Hence, a tumor unresponsive to an agent belonging to one drug class is unlikely to respond to another agent in the same class. Increase in efficacy is therefore more likely to be achieved by combining drugs acting through different modes of action. It is for this reason and to minimize toxicity that most multidrug regimens use drugs of various drug classes. For example, CHOP therapy is commonly used to treat non-Hodgkin's lymphoma. It consists of cyclophosphamide (an alkylating agent), hydroxydaunomycin (doxorubicin [an antitumoral antibiotic]), Oncovin (vincristine [a vinca alkyloid]), and prednisone (a steroid). Another reason to use agents from multiple drug classes is to attempt to decrease acquired drug resistance after administration of a previous agent. Although cross-resistance is poorly understood, it is likely that resistance to one drug within a specific class may lead to resistance to a separate agent in the same class.

The IR procedures that use chemotherapeutic agents vary widely. The most common procedures include chemoembolization procedures, typically of the liver; arterial chemoinfusion therapies; direct injection of agents into tumors, particularly common in head and neck cancers; and intracavitary (e.g., intraperitoneal or intrapleural) administration. Each of these clinical scenarios is discussed in detail elsewhere in this book, so clinical use of chemotherapy agents is not discussed in detail here. Rather, the purpose of this chapter is to discuss the principles of chemotherapy administration, to introduce some of the concepts of the biology involved with treatments using such agents, and to discuss some of the safety concerns with which every individual using chemotherapeutic agents should be familiar.

TABLE 2-1
Chemotherapeutic Agent Classes

Alkylating agents
- Nitrogen mustard (cyclophosphamide, chlorambucil, ifosfamide)
- Alkyl sulfonate (busulfan)
- Nitrosurea (BCNU [1,3-bis(2-chlorethyl)-1-nitrosourea], CCNU [1(2-chloroethyl)-3-(cyclohexyl)-1-nitrosourea], streptozocin)

Platinum salts
- Cisplatin
- Carboplatin

Antimetabolites
- Antifolate (methotrexate)
- Pyrimidine analogs (5-fluorouracil [5FU], gemcitabine)
- Purine analogs (mercaptopurine)

Natural products
- Plant alkaloids (vinblastine, vincristine)
- Microtubule polymer stabilizer (paclitaxel [Taxol])
- Antibiotics (bleomycin, doxorubicin [Adriamycin], mitomycin, epirubicin)
- Enzymes (asparaginase)

Hormones and hormone antagonists

Biologic agents
- Interferons
- Interleukins
- Monoclonal antibodies

Adapted from Skeel,[1] with permission.

GENERAL PRINCIPLES

Cell Biology and Division

Because most chemotherapeutic agents affect the cancer cell during either replication or protein synthesis, a review of the basics of cell biology is mandatory.

Most of the anticancer agents used in IR practice are cytotoxic—they actively cause cell destruction. In addition, most of the agents seem to have their effect by interfering with the cell's ability to form DNA, RNA, or proteins, synthetic functions that are more likely to increase during cell growth and division. Tumors that demonstrate a relatively slow growth, and therefore have few cells undergoing active replication, are less likely to be affected by cytotoxic agents. Some agents appear to have an effect *only* during DNA synthesis and, as such, are considered S phase–specific agents (**Fig. 2-1**, **Table 2-2**).[2] Other agents have a broader range of action and are considered non–phase specific agents.

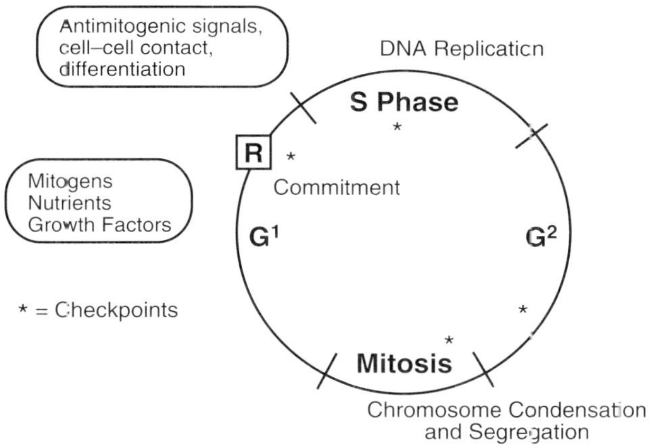

Figure 2-1. The cell cycle. Note that the S phase represents only a small portion of the cell cycle. From Cancer: Principles and Practice of Oncology, 5th edition, DeVita VT, Hellman S, Rosenberg SA, eds. Lippincott Williams & Wilkins, with permission.

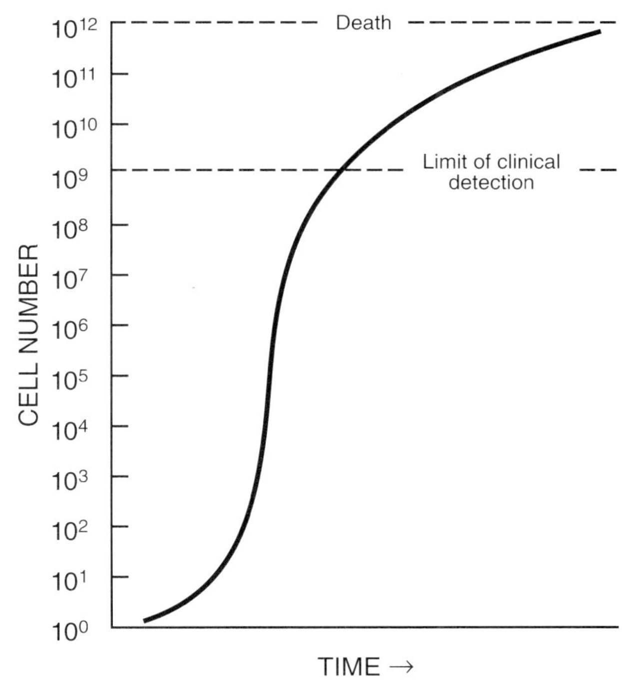

Figure 2-2. Tumor growth. Growth of tumors occurs at a slower rate once the tumor reaches a certain size. By the time the tumor is clinically detectable, the growth rate has appreciably decreased. Source: American Cancer Society's Textbook of Clinical Oncology.

Chemotherapeutic agents that are phase specific have one significant limitation. Because the chemotherapeutic agent will affect only cells undergoing active replication, the agents will have little effect on tumors with relatively low cellular turnover rates. In addition, because only a proportion of cells (those in S phase) are affected by the drug, increasing its dose of the agent administered may lead to little or no additional tumor kill. One way around this limitation is to increase the exposure time of the tumor to the agent (e.g., by obtaining constant blood levels of the agent through prolonged infusions). In this way, more cells are allowed to enter the cell-sensitive phase, thereby increasing the number of cells vulnerable to the cytotoxic effect. A second way around this limitation is to expose the tumor to multidrug regimens, particularly if each drug acts on a different cell cycle phase (**Table 2-3**).

With few exceptions, tumor growth is not exponential; rather, the growth fraction decreases exponentially as tumor size increases (so-called Gompertzian model; **Fig. 2-2**). According to the Gompertzian model, the greater tumor kill is likely to occur as the tumor gets smaller and the growth fraction increases. Furthermore, a single surviving tumor cell will lead to a treatment failure, as it will regrow into a larger tumor, given sufficient doubling time (**Fig. 2-3**). Thus, to achieve a complete tumor kill and cure, multiple treatment cycles are required with sufficient dose intensity.

Pharmacokinetics

Pharmacokinetics refers to the absorption, distribution, metabolism, and excretion of drugs. Each

TABLE 2-2
Cycles for Human Cell Replication

Cell cycle	Function	Duration, hours (representative)
G0	Resting	
G1	RNA and protein synthesis	18–30
S	DNA synthesis	16–20
G2	RNA and protein synthesis	2–10
M	Mitosis	0.5–1

Adapted from Skeel,[2] with permission.

TABLE 2-3
Benefits of Combination Chemotherapy

Prevention of resistant clones
Destruction of cells at various replication cycles
Possible synergistic effect of multiple agents
Access of agents to sanctuary sites
Drug rescue (one agent rescuing the host from the toxicity induced by a second agent)

Adapted from Skeel,[2] with permission.

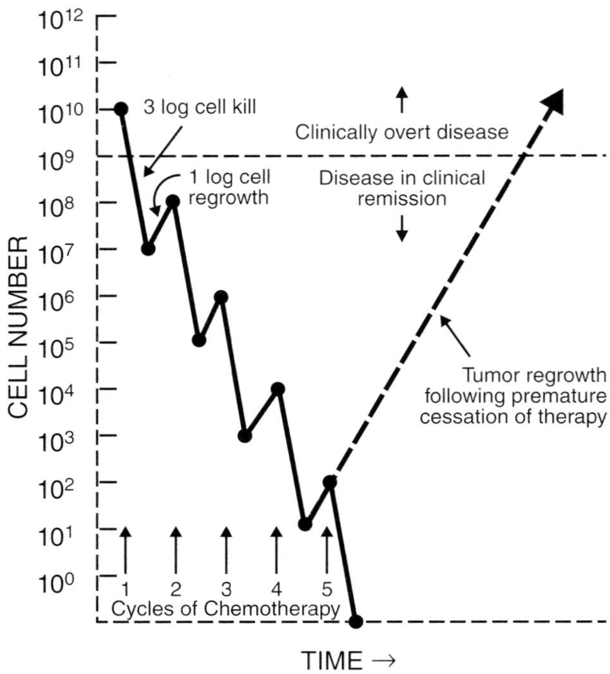

Figure 2-3. Tumor regression after cycles of chemotherapy. Each cycle of chemotherapy kills a certain proportion of the remaining cancer cells. If all the cells are not killed, the tumor will regrow to its original size, given enough time. Source: American Cancer Society's Textbook of Clinical Oncology.

chemotherapeutic agent has a distinct pharmacokinetic profile. Awareness of pharmacodynamic characteristics of specific agents is important in modifying the treatment according to specific clinical circumstances that affect pharmacodynamics. For example, doses may need to be adjusted for renal or hepatic impairment that may affect drug metabolism or excretion. In addition, pleural effusions or ascites may affect drug distribution throughout the body.

Pharmacodynamics

Pharmacodynamics refers to the prediction of likelihood of response to a given drug. Factors that may affect pharmacodynamics include prior treatment, performance status, age, concomitant medications, or comorbidities.

Drug Choice

Although it should be obvious, the primary determinant of drug choice rests with choosing a drug that has proven efficacy against a certain tumor type. This caveat holds true for direct exposure of the tumor (e.g., with intra-arterial, intracavitary, or direct injection of the agent) as well as for systemic administration of the agent. If a drug has no proven efficacy against a particular tumor when administered systemically, it will have little or no effect against the tumor when given locally. The one exception to this rule is that a drug that has marginal efficacy against a tumor when given systemically at a smaller dose may have greater efficacy when administered locally at higher doses. If, for instance, a drug is limited by its systemic dose-related toxicities, the total dose may be decreased when the drug is given locally, thereby achieving the same or better effect than when given at a lower systemic dose. This appears to be a theoretic advantage of local agent delivery, but there have been no drug regimens developed yet that take complete advantage of this local delivery effect.

Regional Chemotherapy Administration

Regional administration of chemotherapeutic agents is a common procedure for IR personnel, and in fact, it is through this procedure that many IR groups have found their niche.

Regional chemotherapy administration can be performed either by directly injecting the agent into a tumor bed or by injecting the agent into the tumor via the feeding arterial supply. The majority of the literature regarding local drug delivery deals with the latter setting. In either case, it is important to understand the clinical settings in which local drug delivery is most efficacious. The most important caveat is that the tumor undergoing treatment be limited to the area exposed to the locally delivered agent. For example, performing chemoembolization of a hepatoma would be of little benefit if the patient had extrahepatic disease, such as lung metastases. In some cases, where symptom control (e.g., pain, bleeding) is the primary goal of chemotherapy administration, local drug delivery may prove helpful in the setting of disease extension beyond the primary organ. This represents the exception rather than the rule, however.

Why does regional chemotherapy work? The relative advantage of intravascular delivery systems is given by the following formula:

$$Advantage = 1 + C/F(1 - E)$$

where C is the clearance of the drug by the body away from the target tumor, F is the blood flow through the tumor bed, and E is the extraction of the agent by the tumor.[3] Any modification of these variables will have an effect on the relative advantage of regional drug delivery. For instance, a decrease in the clearance of the drug by the tumor will concomitantly decrease the relative effect of the agent. Likewise, a decrease in the flow rate will increase the advantage conferred, because the agent will have more time to be exposed to the tumor.

CLASSES OF AGENTS

Most chemotherapeutic agents can be classified into one of several broad categories on the basis of their mechanism of action. Several of the relatively commonly used agents (e.g., hydroxyurea, procarbazine) have a unique mechanism of action and are classified under the ubiquitous heading of *miscellaneous*. The other categories, and the commonly used agents included in each category, are listed below and in **Table 2-1**. Particular attention has been given here to the agents used most frequently during IR procedures; because biologic agents and hormones are rarely if ever given during IR procedures, only short mention of them is made.

Alkylating Agents

Alkylating agents encompass a wide range of drugs that possess a positively charged electrophilic alkyl group. These positively charged electrophiles have their primary effect on DNA replication; however, they also have a secondary effect on already-formed DNA, RNA, and proteins. Because of this latter effect, at least some of the agents have a cell cycle–nonspecific effect.

Characteristics of alkylating agents that are relatively specific to this class of agent include their lipophilicity (particularly with the nitrosureas) and their carcinogenic potential. The lipophilicity of the nitrosureas makes this class of drug particularly useful in treating brain tumors because the agent can readily cross the blood–brain barrier. Any class of agent that causes cross-links or strand breaks during DNA synthesis is potentially carcinogenic.

Although carcinogenesis is a severe potential complication of treatment with alkylating agents, the exact incidence of such adverse outcomes is unknown. Administering the agents to a woman during her first trimester of pregnancy appears to increase the risk of fetal malformations. A more pressing clinical issue than carcinogenesis is the incidence of myelosuppression and immunosuppression observed with the administration of these drugs. Immunosuppression may be very severe; indeed, the immunosuppressive effects of cyclophosphamide are used to advantage in clinical practice in the treatment of vasculitis and seropositive arthropathies.

Antimetabolites

Antimetabolites represent a diverse group of agents that closely resemble naturally occurring molecules that are necessary for either cell replication or cellular function. Typically, such agents interfere with DNA or RNA synthesis by incorporating themselves into the replication cycle, leading to incorrect codes and ultimately leading to cell death. Because they have their effect predominantly during cell replication, most antimetabolites have their greatest activity during the S phase of replication. They are, therefore, cell-phase specific.

Because these agents are cell-phase specific, the agents are often given over prolonged periods of time to increase the likelihood of exposing the tumor to the agent at the appropriate cell cycle. Constant infusions, given at relatively low doses, for days at a time are common with this class of agent.

The agent 5-fluorouracil (5-FU) is commonly used in the treatment regimens of breast, gastrointestinal, and head and neck tumors. 5-FU is converted to its intracellular derivative—a deoxyribonucleoside derivative, FUDR (5-fluoro-2′ deoxyuridine), which inhibits an enzyme necessary for DNA synthesis. FUDR in turn demonstrates a very high affinity for liver tumors; 95% of FUDR is extracted from the bloodstream the first time the drug circulates through the liver. This pharmacokinetic phenomenon is termed the *first-pass effect* and is one of the reasons that FUDR is used for hepatic arterial infusion therapies.

Methotrexate, the most commonly used agent in this class, demonstrates some marrow toxicity and gastrointestinal side effects. At high doses, it can also lead to renal and/or hepatic insufficiency. To decrease the likelihood of these adverse effects, folinic acid (leucovorin), which is known to compete with methotrexate at the cellular level, can be administered following high-dose methotrexate administration (leucovorin rescue). Although fewer data are available for the alkylating class of agents, antimetabolites appear not to be carcinogenic.

Natural Products

The two major categories of these agents are alkaloids and antitumoral antibiotics. Agents belonging to this class are so named not on the basis of their mechanisms of action but rather because they are derived from plants, fungi, or bacteria.

Plant alkaloids (vincristine, vinblastine, vinorelbine) are derived from the common periwinkle (*Vinca rosacea*). They act as inhibitors of cell mitosis by disrupting cellular microtubules, which are a vital component of intracellular transport. Although relatively cell-cycle nonspecific, vinca derivatives are most active in the G1 or S phases of the cell cycle. This class of drug is used commonly in combination with other drug classes in multidrug regimens. Although hematopoietic toxicity is the main dose-limiting toxicity of vinblastine, two specific adverse effects are worth mentioning with all these plant alkaloids. They all have a severe vesicant effect and therefore must be administered only intravenously. Vincristine also demonstrates a propensity to cause peripheral neuropathy, leading to paresthesias, footdrop, and bladder or bowel neuropathies. The neurotoxicity is typically reversible with symptomatic improvement after cessation of the drug. Although neurotoxicity can occur with other vinca alkaloids, it is much less common.

Antitumoral antibiotics are derived predominantly from the soil fungus *Streptomyces*. The drugs in this class are some of the more commonly used agents in the IR suite and include doxorubicin (Adriamycin), bleomycin, and mitomycin. Originally designed as antimicrobial agents, their clinical utility was limited by their cytotoxic effects. Regardless of the species from which the antibiotics are derived, they have their effect by altering the function and synthesis of DNA and RNA. Toxicities of the antibiotic class of agent depend largely on the specific agent. Doxorubicin can cause myelosuppression, nausea and vomiting, and alopecia. In addition, however, patients who receive large cumulative doses (>350–400 mg/m^2) of doxorubicin have an increased incidence of severe cardiac toxicity. Any patient receiving cumulative doses exceeding that range should undergo periodic cardiac evaluation (e.g., nuclear medicine studies, echocardiograms). Toxicity is more likely in patients with underlying cardiac impairment.

Bleomycin, another antitumoral antibiotic, can cause pulmonary fibrosis if given over an extended period of time. Similar to the cardiac toxicity seen with doxorubicin, the pulmonary fibrosis appears to be related to the cumulative dose received (>250–450 U). In addition, a small percentage of patients receiving bleomycin will have an anaphylactoid reaction; for this reason, a test dose is often recommended.

Mitomycin is typically used in combination drug regimens. Its mechanism of action is well understood, with its major effect being to cause cross-links between complementary strands of DNA. Mitomycin seems to work best in a hypoxic environment, therefore making it a common agent used during chemoembolization procedures. The major toxicity of mitomycin is delayed bone marrow suppression, which becomes evident only weeks after administration. Because the drug has a cumulative effect on marrow stem cells, the myelosuppressive effect of mitomycin can persist for 3–6 months after ceasing drug administration. Close monitoring of marrow activity is therefore mandatory when using this agent.

Extracts of the root of a mandrake plant, *Podophyllum peltatum*, have led to the development of epipodophyllotoxins, including etoposide and related drugs. This class of drug interferes with DNA function by creating breaks in DNA. Although not routinely used in interventional radiology, these drugs play an important role in systemic treatment of cancer.

Platinum Salts

This group includes cisplatin, carboplatin, and oxaliplatin. These agents exert their cytotoxic effect by binding to DNA. Although cisplatin is effective in a variety of tumors, its main downside is its toxicity, including renal, ototoxicity, nausea and vomiting, and peripheral neuropathy, as well as problems related to the fluid load that accompanies it. Carboplatin carries a much more favorable side-effect profile but may be less efficacious in certain clinical scenarios.

Spindle inhibitors include paclitaxel (Taxol) and docetaxel. These agents interfere with cell division by action on microtubules and production of a mitotic block. They have proven efficacy in a range of tumors at a cost of moderate toxicity, including myelosuppression, nausea, and neurotoxicity. Although not currently used in interventional radiology, their relative efficacy may warrant further consideration in these applications.

Hormones, Hormone Antagonists, and Biologic Agents

Hormones, hormone antagonists, and biologic agents are a diverse group of drugs that are administered systematically for multiple primary tumor types. Although all three agent classes are important in cancer therapy, they have not been extensively investigated with IR management schedules and therefore are described only briefly here.

Hormones and hormone antagonists (e.g., tamoxifen) may have their effect either at the cellular level or by stimulating or inhibiting natural endocrine factors. These natural factors in turn lead to variations in the cancer cell growth cycle. Unlike other hormonal agents, corticosteroids appear to have a direct lytic effect on leukemic and lymphomatous cells.

Biologic agents, such as interferon or interleukin, modify the growth of tumors through regulatory proteins called cytokines. Cytokines are partially responsible in controlling the development and growth of cancer cells.

Other Agents Under Investigation

With the advancement of research in cancer, new drugs with novel modes or action are constantly being developed. Some of these agents are angiogenesis inhibitors, protein kinase inhibitors, and antibodies to tumor surface markers. Rigorous testing in phase I to III settings will be required to establish the most appropriate place for these agents in the overall anticancer armamentarium.

SAFETY ISSUES AND ADMINISTRATION OF CHEMOTHERAPEUTIC AGENTS

Administration of chemotherapeutic agents must be performed in a well-controlled, monitored environment. Although the risks arising from occasional handling of chemotherapeutic agents are not well delineated, it has been shown that individuals routinely preparing agents have significant levels of mutagenic agents in their urine.[4] Guidelines for handing cytotoxic agents have been published by the Occupational Safety and Health Administration (OSHA), the American Society of Hospital Pharmacists (ASHP), the Oncology Nursing Society (ONS), and the National Institutes of Health (NIH).[5–8] Many of the published guidelines for the handling of such agents are not applicable to the IR suite; in particular, many of the guidelines deal with preparation and reconstitution of the chemotherapeutic agents. **Table 2-4** outlines the OSHA, ASHP, ONS, and NIH guidelines as they pertain to the IR suite.

TABLE 2-4
Safety Recommendations for Chemotherapy Administration

1. If the agent is being drawn up from a vial, a sterile alcohol swab should be placed over the needle as it is withdrawn to prevent aerosolization.
2. A sterile alcohol swab should cover the needle or syringe when air is ejected from the syringe, to prevent aerosolization.
3. Nonpowdered, thick latex gloves should be worn. A long-sleeved, lint-free gown that has low permeability and elastic cuffs should also be worn. Gloves should overlap the gown cuffs.
4. A plastic-backed sheet of absorbent paper should cover the work surface.
5. All tubing and syringes should have Luer-lok fittings and should be inspected for leaks prior to use.
6. When the procedure is completed, all contaminated needles, syringes, and the protective garb should be placed in an appropriate container labeled as toxic waste.

Data from MacDonald et al.,[4] Department of Health and Human Services,[5] American Society of Hospital Pharmacists,[6] Occupational Safety and Health Administration,[7] and Oncology Nursing Society.[8]

In addition to the guidelines given in **Table 2-4**, one should always wear adequate eye protection when working with chemotherapeutic agents. Although not specifically mentioned in the guidelines, use of two sets of gloves likely provides added protection to the radiologist. Finally, one should consider setting up a second table, or at least dedicating a portion of the angiography table for chemotherapy administration, by placing additional sterile towels over the table and placing anything that comes in contact with the chemotherapeutic agent on the dedicated surface. Anything, including gauze, that comes in contact with the agent must be discarded into a chemotherapy-specific container at the end of the procedure.

SUGGESTED READINGS

DeVita VT Jr, Hellman S, Rosenberg SA, eds. *Cancer: Principles & Practice of Oncology*. 6th ed. Philadelphia, PA: Lippincott Williams & Wilkins; 2001:289–290.

Abeloff MD, Armitage JO, Lichter AS, Niederhuber JE, eds. *Clinical Oncology*. New York, NY: Churchill Livingstone; 1995:201–202.

Parkinson DR. Principles of therapy with biologic response modifiers and their role in cancer management. In: Skeel RT, ed. *Handbook of Cancer Chemotherapy*. 5th ed. Philadelphia, PA: Lippincott Williams & Wilkins; 1999:20–21.

REFERENCES

1. Skeel RT. Antineoplastic drugs and biologic response modifiers: classification, use, and toxicity of clinically useful agents. In: *Handbook of Cancer Chemotherapy*. 5th ed. Philadelphia, PA: Lippincott Williams & Wilkins; 1999:65–73.
2. Skeel RT. Biologic and pharmacologic basis of cancer chemotherapy. In: *Handbook of Cancer Chemotherapy*. 5th ed. Philadelphia, PA: Lippincott Williams & Wilkins; 1999:3–19.
3. Pentecost MJ. Principles of regional chemotherapy. In: Baum S, Pentecost MJ, eds. *Abrams' Angiography: Interventional Radiology*, volume III. Boston, MA: Little, Brown; 1997:80–84.
4. MacDonald JS, Haller DG, Mayer RJ, eds. *Manual of Oncologic Therapeutics*. 3rd ed. Philadelphia, PA: Lippincott; 1995:80–135.
5. Department of Health and Human Services. Recommended practices for personnel administering parenteral cytotoxic drugs. Recommendations for safe handling of parenteral antineoplastic drugs. Bethesda, MD: Division of Safety, National Institutes of Health; 1992: DHHS, PHS, NIH Publication No. 92–2621.
6. American Society of Hospital Pharmacists. ASHP technical assistance bulletin on handling cytotoxic drugs in hospitals. *Am J Hosp Pharm* 1985;42:131–137.
7. Occupational Safety and Health Administration. Work practice guidelines for personnel dealing with cytotoxic drugs. Washington, D.C.: U.S. Department of Labor; 1986: Publication 8–1.1.
8. Oncology Nursing Society. Safe handling of cytotoxic drugs. Pittsburgh, PA: Oncology Nursing Society; 1989.

CHAPTER 3

EMBOLIZATION: PRINCIPLES, AGENTS, AND TECHNIQUES

GEORGE KHORIATY, MD
CHARLES E. RAY, JR., MD

Embolization, the "therapeutic introduction of various substances into the circulation to occlude vessels,"[1] was first described in 1904 when Dawbarn introduced the "starvation operation for malignancy in the external carotid area." In this report, he described the preoperative injection of melted paraffin into external carotid arteries of patients with head and neck tumors.[2] In 1960, Luessenhop and Spence described the first case of intracranial arteriovenous malformation (AVM) treated by embolization using methylmethacrylate through a cutdown over the common carotid artery bifurcation.[3] The techniques did not attain widespread usage, however, until the 1970s, led by advances in imaging technology, catheter technology, and embolic agents.[4]

GENERAL PRINCIPLES OF EMBOLIZATION

The effects of embolization on a particular organ depend on the collateral flow to the organ, the clinical status of the patient, previous surgeries or interventions, concurrent disease, age of the patient, and the size and nature of the embolic material. For example, proximal embolization of the splenic artery is unlikely to cause infarction because of significant splenorenal and gastrosplenic collaterals that anastomose with the distal splenic artery. Proximal embolization of the renal artery, on the other hand, can result in infarction of the kidney secondary to a lack of significant collateral vessels. Surgical interventions, such as bowel resection, can compromise collateral flow and increase the risk of infarction from embolization. Young patients are better able to form collaterals than are the elderly. Finally, larger agents placed more proximally are less likely to infarct tissues because of peripheral collaterals, as mentioned above, whereas smaller particles and liquids that embolize to the capillary level are more likely to cause necrosis.

CLINICAL APPLICATIONS

Embolization has been used for controlling hemorrhage in the setting of trauma; hemoptysis or gastrointestinal bleeds; for the treatment of tumors either preoperatively or as the sole method of palliative control of pain, tumor growth or mass effect, paraneoplastic syndromes or bleeding; for the treatment of vascular malformations and aneurysms; and for treatment of male infertility and high-flow priapism.

Trauma

Vascular injury can result from penetrating or blunt trauma. Significant bleeding in the chest, abdomen, pelvis, retroperitoneum, or even in the extremities is not always obvious clinically, especially in the setting of blunt trauma. Diagnosis is often made by computed tomography scan, peritoneal lavage, or angiography. Death is due to blood loss in a majority of cases. Gelfoam (Upjohn Co., Kalamazoo, Michigan), polyvinyl alcohol (PVA) (Ivalon, Cook, Inc., Bloomington, Indiana), and coils have been used to control bleeding in acute arterial trauma involving the extremities, lumbar arteries, duodenal and pancreatic arteries, and renal arteries (especially after biopsy or nephrostomy tube placement).[5–8] Owing to the extensive collateral blood supply, pelvic hemorrhage may best be treated with embolization using Gelfoam or PVA without risk of infarction to the surrounding pelvic organs.

Sclafani et al. have demonstrated success in treating hemodynamically stable patients with splenic injury of all grades by placing coils in the main splenic artery proximally, thereby decreasing the splenic artery flow and pressure while preserving splenic parenchyma via gastrosplenic and splenorenal collaterals.[9–11] Embolization of liver injuries is advocated in hemodynamically stable patients with active extravasation, severe or persistent hemobilia, arteriovenous (AV) fistula, or recurrent postoperative bleeding.[12,13]

Hemoptysis

Although most acute hemoptysis is self-limited, severe hemoptysis (>500–600 mL) is life threatening because of the blood flooding the tracheobronchial tree, resulting in asphyxia. The most common causes of massive hemoptysis are cystic fibrosis in young patients and neoplasm in the elderly; less common causes include bronchiectasis and tuberculosis. The bronchial arteries are the usual culprit, although nonbronchial arteries, including intercostal, internal mammary, phrenic, lateral thoracic, and pulmonary arteries, can be alternate sources. Embolization is typically performed using 500- to 700-μm PVA particles through microcatheters placed as selectively as possible. If a spinal artery is visualized arising from the bronchial artery, embolization should be deferred or performed distal to the spinal artery origin.

OTHER USES

Embolization has also been used for controlling hemorrhage from upper and lower gastrointestinal bleeds, as well as postpartum hemorrhage. Vascular malformations can often be treated exclusively by embolization, or conversely, embolized preoperatively (as is usual for brain AVMs, for example) to decrease perioperative blood loss. Aneurysms and pseudoaneurysms, intracranial or peripheral, are often especially suited for endovascular therapy by coil embolization. Embolization has proven successful not only in controlling vaginal bleeding due to uterine fibroids but in shrinking the fibroid tumors as well. In men, success has also been demonstrated in treating varicoceles, vasogenic impotence, and high-flow priapism with embolization techniques.

GENERAL ANGIOGRAPHIC TECHNIQUES

Sheaths and Catheters

Introducer sheaths are invariably used during embolization procedures. Sheaths facilitate catheter exchanges and allow the removal of occluded catheters without loss of vascular access. Catheters are especially prone to occlusion by PVA particles or adhesives.

Most embolizations can be performed safely and efficiently by selective catheterization of the target vessel using standard tapered 4- to 7-F angiographic catheters. Nontarget embolization can be minimized by placing the catheter as selectively as possible, distal to the origin of branch vessels supplying surrounding normal tissues. This often requires a coaxial system wherein a microcatheter is introduced through the standard angiographic catheter or through a nontapered guide catheter. Microcatheters are generally 3 F or smaller and can accommodate a variety of embolic agents, including coils, particles such as PVA or Embospheres (Biosphere Medical Inc., Rockland, Massachusetts), and liquid embolic agents without significant risk of catheter occlusion. Most microcatheters track over guide wires with 0.014- to 0.018-in diameters. Some also have a floppy distal segment of catheter that can be flow directed. This is often useful in superselective catheterization, especially in tortuous vessels; flow-directed microcatheters have been especially useful in catheterizing and embolizing intracranial AVMs that can have numerous tortuous feeding arteries.

Occlusion Balloons

Balloon occlusion catheters are used during embolization procedures mainly to prevent reflux of embolic material. Double-lumen occlusion balloons are ideal for this purpose, as the second lumen can be used for embolization once the balloon is inflated. During use of liquid embolic agents such as absolute ethanol, the balloon can be inflated and contrast can be injected to determine the capacity of the vascular bed to be embolized; this estimates the volume of embolic material needed. After the balloon is deflated to allow the contrast to wash out, the occlusion balloon is reinflated and ethanol is administered through the second lumen. Prior to balloon deflation, a large syringe (e.g., 60 cc) is used to aspirate the catheter lumen to minimize reflux of ethanol into the proximal artery.

Proximal balloon occlusion also inhibits inflow, thereby preventing the passage of embolic agent into the venous circulation. This is especially useful for the treatment of large AV fistulas (AVFs). The catheter for embolization is placed distal to the occlusion balloon. The occlusion balloon is inflated, and stasis through the fistula is established until a dense coil pack is achieved prior to deflating the occlusion balloon. This decreases the risk of distal embolization of coils into the pulmonary circulation in peripheral AVFs, or into the systemic circulation in the case of pulmonary AVFs.

Digital Subtraction Angiography

High-quality fluoroscopy, including digital subtraction angiography (DSA), is especially important in embolization procedures. With DSA techniques, less contrast is used and the embolization procedure can be performed more quickly. In addition to DSA, road-mapping may allow for faster procedures, and the actual embolization, especially with particles, may be performed under road-mapping for added safety.

Embolization Agents

The choice of embolic agent depends on many factors, including the organ or lesion to be embolized, whether embolization is intended to be preoperative or as definitive therapy, whether embolization is intended to be temporary or permanent, whether proximal (large-vessel) or distal (small-vessel) embolization is desired, experience of the operator, and availability of the agent (**Table 3-1**). Embolization agents are classified as absorbable (temporary) or nonabsorbable (permanent). Temporary agents include autologous blood clot and Gelfoam; permanent agents include particulate agents (PVA, Embospheres), nonparticulate agents (coils, silk suture, detachable balloons), nonsclerosing liquids (ethiodol, cyanoacrylate), and liquid sclerosing agents (absolute ethanol, boiling contrast medium). Embolization agents can also be classified according to size with large agents, such as coils occluding medium and small arteries, and small particles or liquids occluding at the level of the smaller arterioles or capillary bed. Agents that travel to the capillary bed are more likely to cause cell death than are agents that occlude larger vessels, because the smaller agents embolize beyond potential collateral feeding vessels. Additionally, sclerosing agents such as absolute ethanol and boiling contrast cause cell death by their very nature as sclerosants. Often, the best choice is not a single agent but a combination of agents used concurrently to achieve a desired result.

Autologous Materials

Autologous skeletal muscle, fat, dura, and blood clot have all been used for embolization. Blood clot has been the most widely used, mainly for the acute treatment of hemorrhage. Blood is drawn from the patient, allowed to clot in a sterile container, and injected through the catheter into the vessel to be embolized. As an embolic agent, it is cheap and readily available; however, rapid lysis renders it unsuitable for most uses.

Gelfoam

Gelfoam (**Fig. 3-1**) is an absorbable gelatin sponge that, when introduced into a blood vessel, causes a severe panarteritis characterized by infiltration of leukocytes into all layers of the vessel wall, with disruption of the intima and elastic tissues. The panarteritis resolves within 4 months. The vessel occlusion lasts from several days to several months, with an average duration of occlusion of 3–4 months.[14]

Gelfoam is available as a sheet (sponge) or in powder form. Gelfoam sponges can be cut into small pledgets or "torpedoes," mixed with contrast media, and injected using a small 1- or 3-cc Luer-Lok syringe. Alternatively, a Gelfoam slurry can be formed by mixing Gelfoam pledgets and contrast using a three-way stopcock, then injected through a catheter to form a "cast" of the blood

TABLE 3-1
Commonly Used Embolic Agents

Agent	Particle size	Advantages	Disadvantages	Uses
Coils	2–30 mm	Easy to use; occlude large and medium size vessels; large variety of coils available	Occlude only larger vessels; collateral vessels form; may be less effective in coagulopathic patients	Trauma, varicoceles, AVFs
Gelfoam	Pledgets, slurry	Can occlude large and medium arteries; temporary		Trauma; temporary occlusion; tumors
	Powder	Temporary; distal embolization	Temporary	
PVA	50–2000 μm	Permanent; variety of sizes available	Permanent	Tumors; hemoptysis; fibroid embolizations
Embospheres	40–1200 μm	Permanent; variety of standard sizes available; unlike PVA, does not clump and is therefore less likely to occlude catheter	Permanent	Hypervascular tumors; AVMs
Silk suture	4–0 or 5–0 silk	Widely available; inexpensive	May occlude catheter; inflammatory reaction	AVMs
Lipiodol/ethiodol	Liquid	Contrast as well as embolic agent; can be mixed with chemotherapeutic agent to form emulsion		Chemoembolization of tumors
Ethanol	Liquid	Fast; permanent; sclerosant causes cell death	Occludes at the capillary level; causes cell death	AVMs; tumors; organ ablation
Adhesives	Liquid	Permanent; conform to vessel	Not widely available	AVMs
Detachable balloons	Varying sizes and shapes	Can be tested before deployment; less risk of intraprocedural migration/pulmonary embolism	May deflate and migrate; not approved for use in the United States	AVFs

AVF = arteriovenous fistula; AVM = arteriovenous malformation; PVA = polyvinyl alcohol.

A

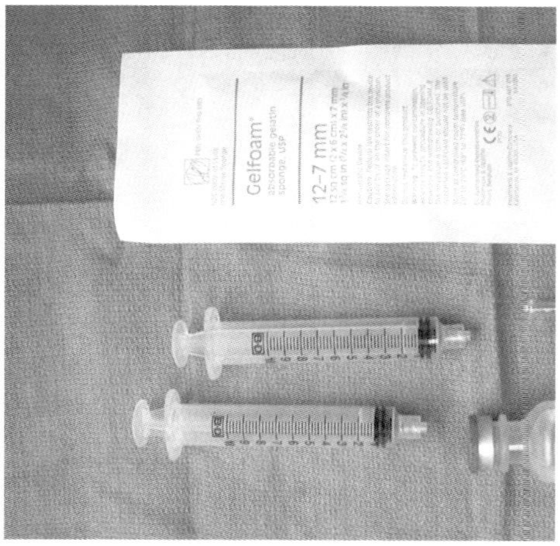

B

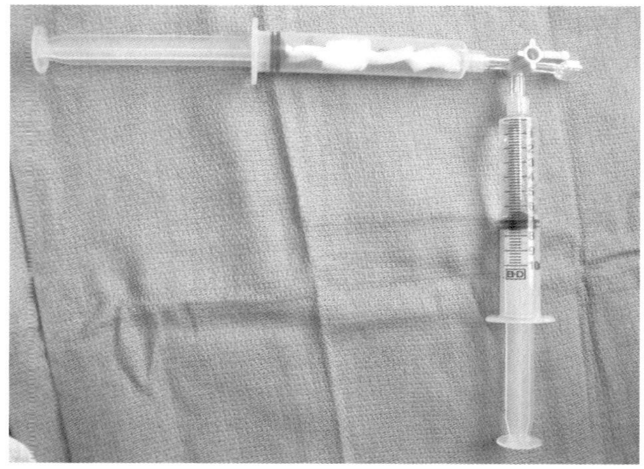

C

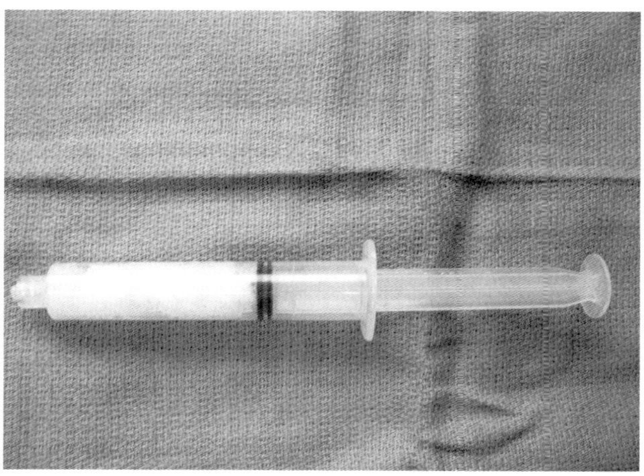

Figure 3-1. Gelfoam embolization. (A) The tools needed for Gelfoam embolization include the Gelfoam sponge, two 10-cc syringes, 5 to 10 cc of sterile water or saline, and a three-way stopcock. (B) The Gelfoam sponge is torn into quarters and backloaded into one of the 10-cc syringes. Approximately 7 cc of fluid is loaded into the second syringe, and the two syringes are connected to the three-way stopcock. (C) The fluid and Gelfoam are mixed using a to-and-fro motion from one syringe to the other. The ideal consistency of the Gelfoam slurry should approximate that of pudding, allowing a cast of the vessel into which the slurry is injected.

vessel. Gelfoam powder ranges in size from 1 to 800 μm. Gelfoam powder embolizes more distally than Gelfoam pledgets or slurry, therefore carrying a much higher risk of ischemic complications.

Polyvinyl Alcohol

PVA (**Fig. 3-2**) is produced as a sponge or block from which proper-size particles can be obtained. PVA particles can be produced from blocks, with a saw blade used to shave the surface of the block. However, PVA shavings are extremely variable in size. Therefore, most commercially available PVA is packaged as particles of various sizes (e.g., 150–250 μm, 250–300 μm), which are separated using vibrating sieves of different sizes. PVA causes vessel occlusion by initiating a fibroblast reaction, with fibrous connective tissue formation around the particles and a moderate inflammatory reaction involving the wall of the vessel. The thrombus then organizes, the arterial wall fibroses, and the inflammation subsides.[4] Vessel occlusion is typically permanent, but vessels embolized with PVA may recanalize.

The commercial availability of PVA in various standardized sizes makes it a versatile agent for a variety of uses. The larger the particle size used, the less likely the causation of ischemia or cell death secondary to preservation of collateral blood flow beyond the embolized segment. The smaller particles are useful for tumor ablation and embolization of AVMs[15,16] (**Fig. 3-3**).

Embosphere Microspheres

Embospheres are hydrophilic, nonresorbable, calibrated microspheres produced from acrylic polymer and impregnated with porcine gelatin. They are available in sizes ranging from 40 to 1200 μm. They are approved for

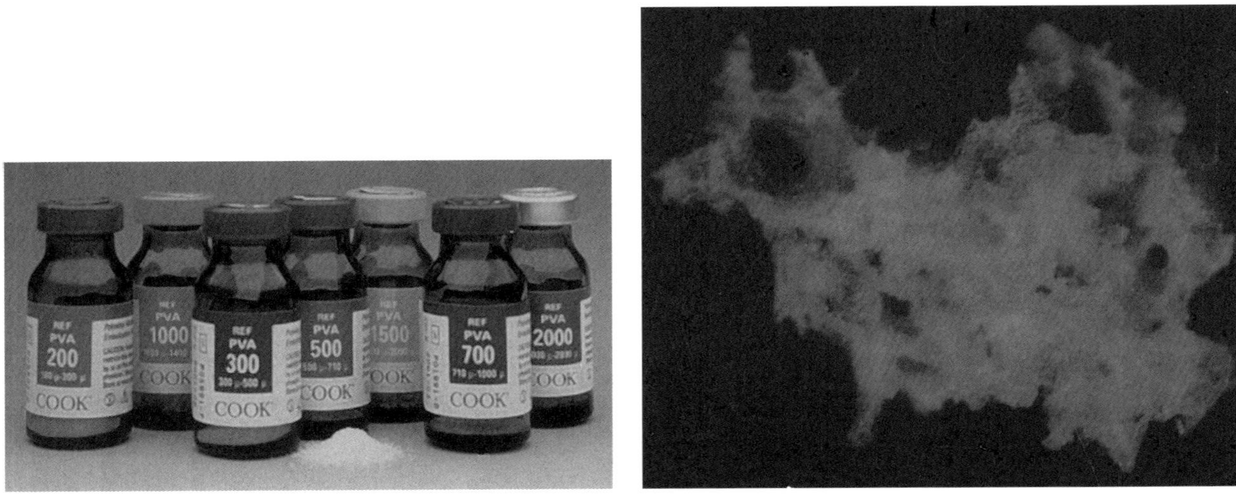

A B

Figure 3-2. Polyvinyl alcohol (PVA) embolization. (A) PVA is packaged according to the size range of the embolization particles. (B) Magnification view of a single PVA particle. Notice the irregularity of the particle; these edges cause inflammation of the surrounding vessel wall, which likely contributes to the relatively permanent vascular occlusion noted following embolization with PVA. (Photos courtesy of Cook, Inc., Bloomington, Indiana.)

embolization of hypervascular tumors and AVMs. As opposed to PVA particles, Embospheres do not form aggregates and tend to penetrate more distally than similar-size PVA particles. Therefore, larger particle sizes are generally selected than would be chosen for embolization with PVA. In addition to not forming aggregates, Embospheres can also compress 20%–30% as they pass through the delivery catheter and therefore may have less of a tendency to clump and occlude the embolization catheter.

Coils

Steel coils (**Fig. 3-4**) were introduced as embolization agents by Gianturco et al. in 1975.[17] Coils cause permanent vessel occlusion by inducing thrombosis[18]; in patients who are coagulopathic, coils may be less effective because they rely on the patient's own coagulation cascade to cause vessel occlusion. Early coils had wool strands attached to increase thrombogenicity; however, wool was found to cause a severe arteritis and was replaced with Dacron.

Coils are the equivalent of surgical ligation, occluding arteries proximally while preserving distal flow via collateral vessels. They generally do not cause complete organ infarction, with the exception of organs or tissues that have poor or no collateral vascular supply, such as the kidney. If complete organ infarction or ablation is the goal, peripheral occluding agents or sclerosing agents are employed. Because coils generally do not cause tissue infarction, they can be deployed at the origins of arteries feeding normal tissues to protect the normal tissues from nontarget embolization when peripheral occluding agents or sclerosing agents are used. An example of this would be the prophylactic embolization of the proximal gastroduodenal artery with coils to prevent reflux of chemoembolic agents during hepatic chemoembolization procedures (**Fig. 3-5**). Coils should not be used in vessels in which future catheterization or embolization is anticipated, because they will preclude future selective catheterization by effectively "burning the bridge" to the target tissue.

Platinum coils are made of a platinum wire with attached silk or synthetic fibers to increase thrombogenicity.[19] They are available in many shapes: straight, curled, and complex helix. Platinum microcoils were initially introduced and gained widespread acceptance for use in neurointerventional procedures[17] but are increasingly being used for peripheral embolizations. Platinum microcoils can be introduced through microcatheters and are delivered by placing the coil in the catheter hub and injecting the coil with a saline flush (usually for straight coils) or by advancing the coil using a coil-pusher wire. Their ability to be introduced through microcatheters makes them capable of reaching vessels that would otherwise not be accessible using standard catheter–guide wire combinations. An additional advantage to platinum coils is that platinum is extremely radiopaque, allowing even the smallest coils to be easily visualized under fluoroscopy. Detachable coils are also available that use either a mechanical or an electrical release device. Detachable coils have the advantage of being placed precisely before being deployed; in that way, if a coil is not sized properly or is malpositioned, it can be repositioned before deployment.

Silk

Silk has been used in conjunction with PVA or coils for the embolization of large AVMs, post-traumatic

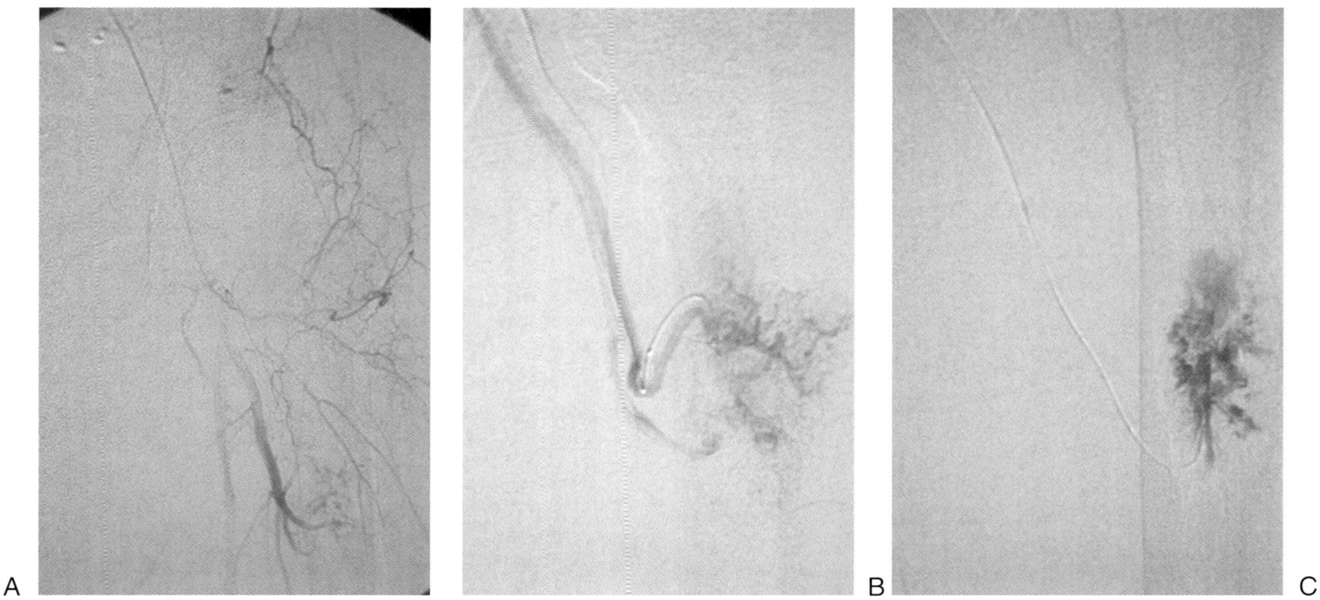

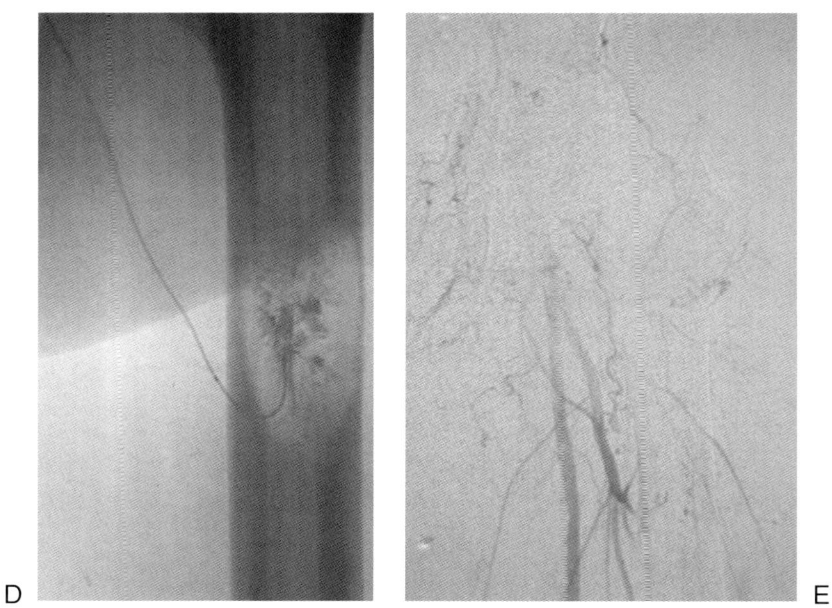

Figure 3-3. Embolization of renal cell carcinoma metastatic to the femur in a 50-year-old man with widely metastatic renal cell carcinoma. The patient had severe pain in his proximal left femur that was poorly controlled with conservative therapy. (A) Digital subtraction angiogram, before embolization, with the catheter in the profunda femoral artery (PFA). Notice the neovascularity over the proximal femur, as well as similar changes centered over the left acetabulum. (B) Digital subtraction angiogram, magnified view, with a microcatheter in one of the PFA branches supplying the femoral lesion. Again, notice the neovascularity, as well as the early draining vein. (C) Digital subtraction angiogram, magnified view, with a microcatheter in a different PFA branch. Notice the dense neovascularity at the center of the femoral lesion. (D) Unsubtracted image from the same angiogram as Figure C. (E) Final post-embolization angiogram demonstrating a near complete paucity of neovascularity in either the femoral or acetabular lesions.

AVFs, and tumor ablation.[4] Standard silk suture or ties (4–0 or 5–0) are cut into approximately 1-cm lengths, backloaded onto a 1-cc contrast-filled syringe, and injected via the catheter into the tumor. Silk streamers, composed of different numbers of silk threads, are also commercially available.

Detachable Balloons

Detachable balloons are made of latex or silicone and come in a variety of shapes and sizes. Advantages of detachable balloons are that they can be either flow directed or placed over the wire, and the effect on the vessel can be evaluated before detachment. In the case of AVFs, during the use of detachable balloons there is less intraprocedural migration and fewer instances of pulmonary embolism. However, detachable balloons may deflate over time, causing recanalization and balloon migration. Currently, detachable balloons are not approved for use in the United States.[4]

Absolute Ethanol

Absolute ethanol is a sclerosing agent that is directly toxic to the endothelium and presumably activates the clotting cascade on the dehydrated endothelial layers.[4]

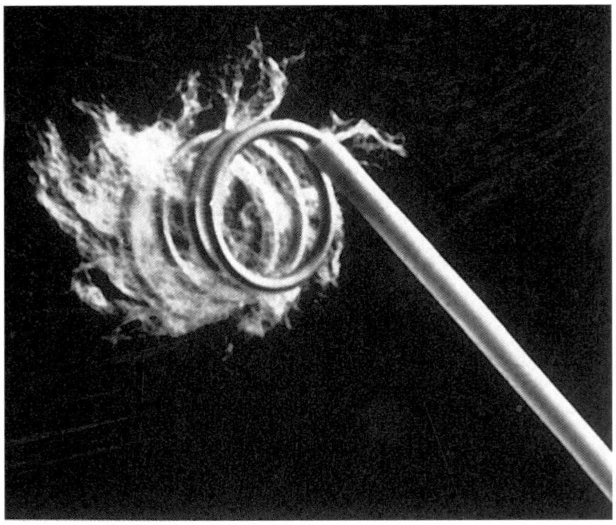

Figure 3-4. Coil embolization: The coil that has been partially deployed. Notice the Dacron fibers attached to the metal strut. It is the Dacron fibers that elicit a thrombogenic response, leading to vascular occlusion. (Photo courtesy of Cook, Inc., Bloomington, Indiana.)

The toxic effect of absolute ethanol extends beyond the blood vessels into the perivascular spaces and has been demonstrated to cause perivascular necrosis.[20] Because of this very toxic effect, embolizations performed with alcohol tend to give complete and immediate hemostasis (**Fig. 3-6**). As an embolic agent, absolute ethanol is usually delivered through balloon occlusion catheters to prevent inadvertent reflux. Alternatively, ethanol can be injected directly into the nidus of an AVM via direct percutaneous puncture.

Adhesives (Cyanoacrylate)

Cyanoacrylates (isobutyl 2-cyanoacrylate, *N*-butyl-2-cyanoacrylate) are a family of rapidly hardening adhesives. They have been used endovascularly since 1972.[21] The adhesives polymerize and harden as they come in contact with ionic media, such as blood or contrast. With variation of the technique, a focal occlusion or a "cast" of the blood vessels can be achieved. The introduction catheter must be flushed with dextrose before injection of cyanoacrylates to avoid polymerization within the catheter, and special care must be taken so as not to adhere the catheter tip to the blood vessel being embolized. Cyanoacrylates are not radiopaque and must be mixed with radiopaque material such as tantalum powder, sterile barium, or Lipiodol to make them visible during the embolization procedure.[22] They are currently approved by the U.S. Food and Drug Administration for endovascular use in the treatment of cerebral AVMs.

Iodized Oil (Lipiodol/Ethiodol)

Lipiodol is a liquid contrast agent composed of iodinated ethyl esters of fatty acids in poppyseed oil. It has been used for hysterosalpingography and lymphography for nearly 80 years. Iodized oil is used intravascularly as both a contrast agent and an embolic agent. Mixing iodized oil with doxorubicin using a three-way stopcock just prior to embolization creates a suspension that increases the intratumoral concentration and half-life of the chemotherapeutic agent, especially if followed by Gelfoam (or PVA) embolization.[23]

A 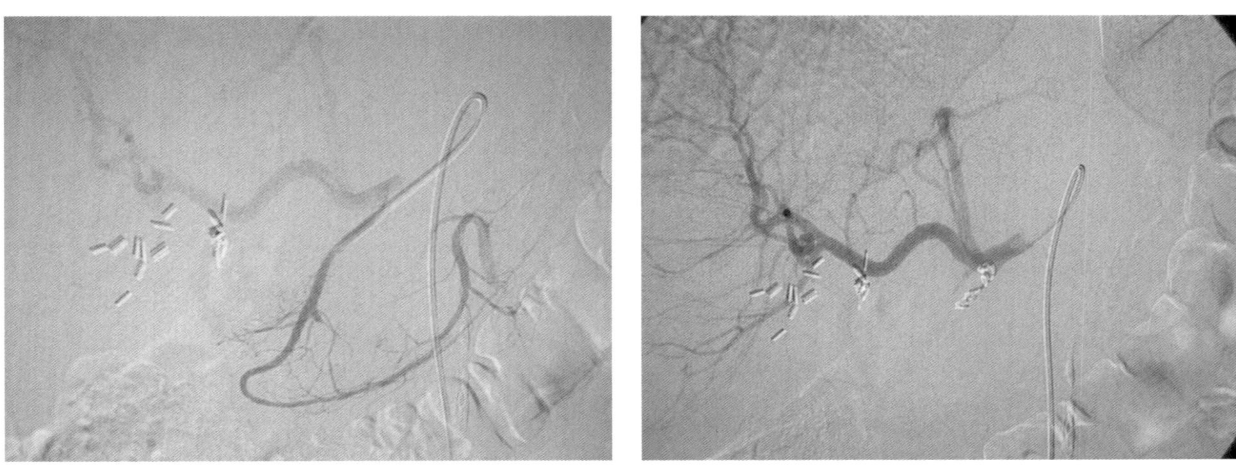 B

Figure 3-5. Prophylactic embolization of the gastroduodenal artery (GDA) in a 52-year-old man after cholecystectomy, with inoperable multifocal hepatoma. The angiogram was done preoperatively before placement of a hepatic arterial catheter for local delivery of chemotherapy. (A) Digital subtraction angiogram of a selective GDA injection. Notice the reflux of contrast into the proper hepatic artery (PHA); the PHA has a very short course before bifurcating into the right and left hepatic arteries. Because of this anatomy, a catheter could not be placed into the PHA for chemoinfusion without endangering the GDA distribution. For this reason, coil embolization of the GDA was performed. (B) Digital subtraction angiogram of the common hepatic artery after coil embolization of the GDA. Notice antegrade filling of both the right and left hepatic arteries and complete occlusion of the GDA.

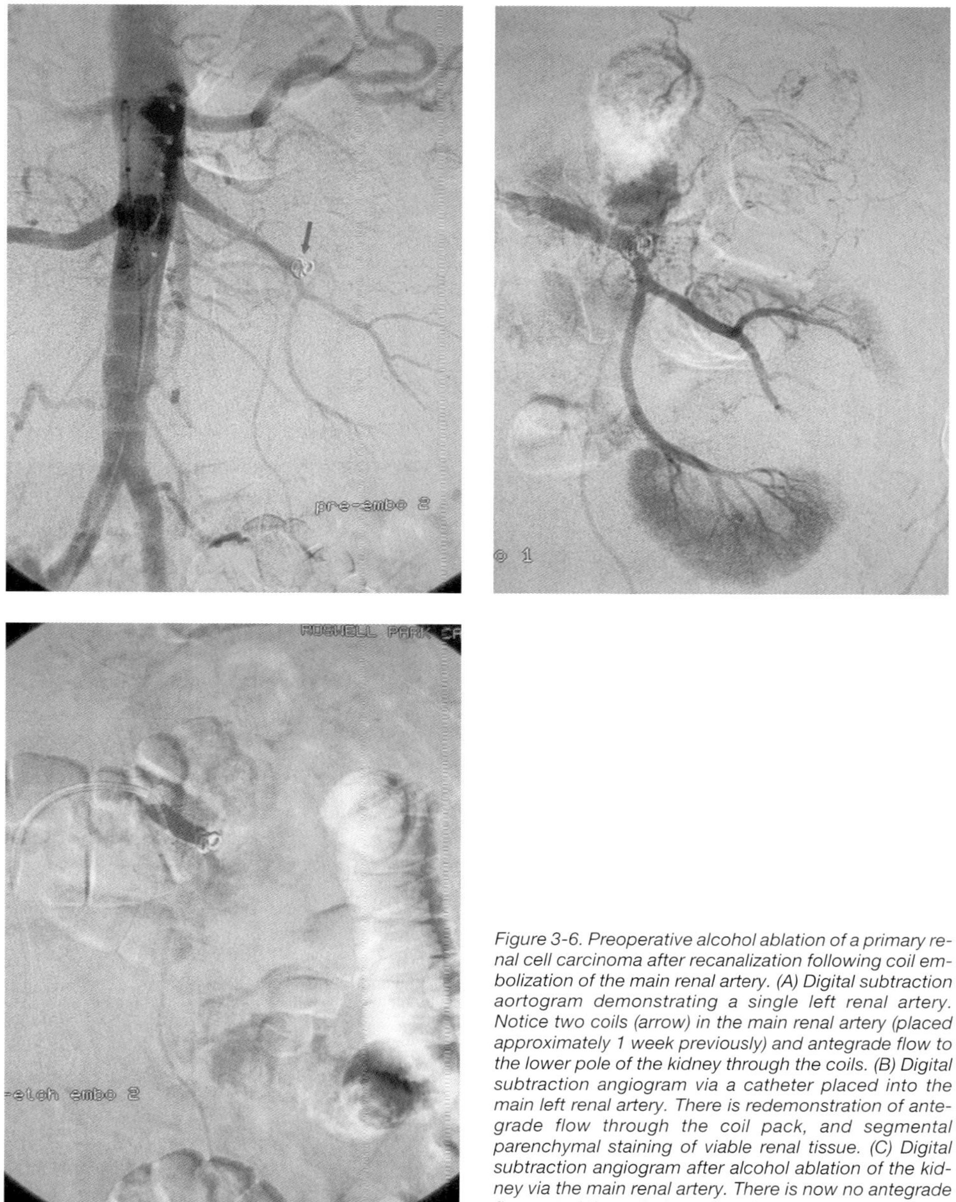

Figure 3-6. Preoperative alcohol ablation of a primary renal cell carcinoma after recanalization following coil embolization of the main renal artery. (A) Digital subtraction aortogram demonstrating a single left renal artery. Notice two coils (arrow) in the main renal artery (placed approximately 1 week previously) and antegrade flow to the lower pole of the kidney through the coils. (B) Digital subtraction angiogram via a catheter placed into the main left renal artery. There is redemonstration of antegrade flow through the coil pack, and segmental parenchymal staining of viable renal tissue. (C) Digital subtraction angiogram after alcohol ablation of the kidney via the main renal artery. There is now no antegrade flow noted through the coil packs.

ISSUES SPECIFIC TO PATIENTS WITH CANCER

Patient-specific issues often come into consideration when deciding to proceed with a palliative embolization procedure. Besides the usual risks and benefits, issues that often come into play include the possibility and availability of alternate therapies such as surgery or radiation, patient's life expectancy, and quality of life issues. All of these issues should be directly and completely addressed before consideration of the embolization procedure.

Coagulation

Patients with cancer may be either hypercoagulable or coagulopathic. As discussed previously, coils do not mechanically occlude the target vessel but rather induce thrombosis by activating the patient's own coagulation cascade. In patients who are coagulopathic, whether secondary to cancer or a separate underlying disease process, coils are less effective and generally should not be used as the sole embolic agent. If coils are used in this setting, they can be combined with other agents such as Gelfoam or PVA to cause the mechanical obstruction. In coagulopathic patients, arterial closure devices are useful in helping achieve hemostasis at the end of the procedure. The ones used most frequently in our laboratory are the VasoSeal (Datascope Corp., Montvale, New Jersey) and Perclose (Perclose, Redwood City, California) devices.

Pain Control

Patients who have a terminal illness or cancer are often receiving considerable pain medication. Their tolerance for sedatives and narcotics is often increased, and they may require significantly more medication to achieve equivalent levels of sedation and pain control. Proper cardiopulmonary monitoring using, at a minimum, pulse oximetry and cardiac and blood pressure monitoring is essential for the safe administration of conscious sedation and analgesia. A trained nurse or a physician who is not one of the operating surgeons should monitor and address the needs of the patient during the procedure.

Immunosuppression

Patients with cancer, especially after undergoing chemotherapy regimens, may be immunosuppressed secondary to bone marrow suppression. This is especially true of patients who have undergone bone marrow transplantation. Although preprocedural antibiotics are not generally indicated for routine embolization procedures, their use may be advisable in this patient population. As of this writing, however, there have been no controlled trials comparing the risks of embolization in immunosuppressed patients given preprocedural antibiotics with the risks in those not given antibiotics.

Renal Failure

The risks of contrast-induced nephropathy are well known, especially in patients with diabetes and elevated serum creatinine levels. Care should also be exercised in the cancer population because these patients may be receiving chemotherapeutic agents or antibiotics that can contribute to renal toxicity. Proper hydration before, during, and after angiographic procedures is the most important factor in reducing the risk of contrast nephropathy. Use of low-osmolar contrast media[24] and premedication with acetylcysteine[25] or fenoldopam (Corlopam; Abbott Laboratories, Abbott Park, Illinois)[26,27] have been reported to decrease risk of contrast nephropathy and may be useful in high-risk patients.

EMBOLIZATION IN PATIENTS WITH CANCER

Cancer is the second leading cause of death in the United States, responsible for over 500,000 deaths annually and having an age-adjusted death rate of 123.6 per 100,000. Additionally, cancer causes significant morbidity, with 1,266,000 hospital discharges in 1998 and an average hospital length of stay of 7.2 days.[28] The historical primary treatment modalities for cancer therapy have been surgery, radiotherapy, and systemic chemotherapy. Interventional radiologic techniques are becoming more important and common in the treatment of cancer.

As a primary treatment modality for cancer, embolization is unlikely to result in a cure. It is therefore primarily reserved for the treatment of unresectable tumors, where it can potentially lead to an improvement in quality of life through palliation of pain, control of bleeding, control or reduction in the size of primary tumors or metastases, and control of paraneoplastic syndromes.

Preoperative embolization can facilitate surgical resection by devitalizing hypervascular tumors. After preoperative embolization, both a decrease in tumor size and decrease in intraoperative blood loss and transfusion requirements have been reported.[29] Tumors that are unresectable because of their large size can potentially be made resectable by necrosing and shrinking the tumor preoperatively through embolization.[30] Preoperative embolization has been applied to a wide variety of both primary and metastatic tumors.

Systemic chemotherapy is an increasingly effective means of treating many cancers. Unfortunately, high doses of chemotherapeutic agents have cytotoxic effects on normal, rapidly proliferating cells in the body, including the skin, mucosa, and bone marrow. Systemic toxicity from chemotherapy ranges from mild nausea and vomiting to severe bone marrow suppression.[31] Local drug delivery combined with embolization can confer a therapeutic advantage by increasing local drug concentration, increasing duration of chemotherapeutic agent within the tumor (dwell time), and decreasing the systemic dose. The advantage of regional versus systemic chemotherapy is proportional to the clearance rate by the body and inversely proportional to the extraction efficiency of the drug by the tumor and blood flow through the artery infused. Thus, the greater the rate of clearance of drug from the body, the slower the blood flow supplying the tumor, and the poorer the extraction efficiency of the tumor, the greater the advantage of local drug delivery.[32] Embolization after or in combination with chemotherapeutic agents decreases the blood flow through the tumor and further increases the dwell time of the agent, thereby conferring a therapeutic advantage. An in-depth discussion on arterial interventions such as hepatic chemoembolization is given in Chapter 11.

COMPLICATIONS OF EMBOLIZATION

Although the advent of renal protection, microcatheter techniques, improved digital subtraction imaging, and a wide variety of and availability of embolic agents has improved the safety and efficacy of embolization, significant risks still exist.

Table 3-2 outlines the complications that may occur secondary to embolization procedures, and the anticipated incidence of each complication. As noted in the table, the most common complications during embolization procedures are those that may occur with any angiographic procedure.

Some complications are specific to the type of embolic agent being used during the procedure. Although very uncommon, these complications are almost always preventable with fastidious technique; the surgeon should be aware of such specific complications before attempting a procedure with the agent listed. A list of agent-specific risks is given in **Table 3-3**. Note should be made of two particular complications that may occur after an embolization procedure: post-embolization syndrome and tumor lysis syndrome.

Post-embolization Syndrome

The post-embolization syndrome consists of a constellation of findings: nausea, vomiting, leukocytosis, fever, pain, adynemia ileus, and lassitude. Some or all of the symptoms may be present, and they may be present to varying degrees. Although the exact pathogenesis of post-embolization syndrome is not understood, it likely occurs secondary to the presence of cellular breakdown products excreted into the bloodstream. The degree of symptomatology is related but not directly proportional to the amount of embolization performed; the presence of the syndrome does not appear to be related to the type of malignancy treated. Treatment is largely conservative, with treatment of symptoms indicated as they arise. Most importantly, however, the patient should be forewarned that the post-embolization syndrome could occur anywhere between 1 and 14 days after the embolization procedure. If made aware of this potential complication, patients are less likely to be bothered by the symptoms.

TABLE 3-2
Complications of Embolization

Complication	Anticipated incidence (%)
Risks of angiography	
Access-site hematoma	5
Contrast reaction	1–2
Contrast nephropathy	1–2
Vessel damage (e.g., dissection)	1–2
General risks of embolization	
Tissue ischemia or infarction	< 5
Nontarget embolization	1–2
Tumor lysis syndrome (varying degrees)	5–20
Post-embolization syndrome (varying degrees)	10–50

TABLE 3-3
Embolization Agent-Specific Risks

Agent	Specific risk
Adhesives	Catheter can become adhered to the vessel
Ethanol	Tissue necrosis
	Large doses of ethanol can have systemic cardiac or neurologic effects
Detachable balloons	Balloon may deflate and migrate
Coils	Can migrate during procedure, especially in arteriovenous fistulas without an intervening capillary bed
	Blocks larger vessels permanently, in effect "burning the bridge" for future intervention

Tumor Lysis Syndrome

Tumor lysis syndrome is another potential complication that may occur after tumor embolization. Believed to be secondary to lysis of cancer cells and concomitant efflux of cellular contents into the bloodstream (e.g., potassium, uric acid), tumor lysis can have severe systemic effects. The incidence of tumor lysis syndrome appears to be related to the amount of tumor embolized; generally speaking, the greater the volume of tumor embolized, the greater the likelihood of tumor lysis syndrome (and the more severe the complications from it). In cases in which a large tumor burden is to be embolized, prophylactic administration of allopurinol and aggressive hydration may be indicated (see Chapter 1).

CONCLUSION

Embolization is a powerful tool with a multitude of uses in both patients with cancer and those without it. Its safety and efficacy have been well documented. Familiarity with the various embolic agents, proper technique, and the potential risks of embolization therapy is of paramount importance in the safe undertaking of this procedure.

REFERENCES

1. Hensyl WR, ed. *Stedman's Medical Dictionary*. 25th ed. Baltimore, MD: Williams & Wilkins; 1990:501.
2. Dawbarn RHM. The starvation operation for malignancy in the external carotid area. *JAMA* 1904;116:792–795.
3. Luessenhop A, Spence W. Artificial embolization of cerebral arteries: report of use in a case of arteriovenous malformation. *JAMA* 1960;172:1153–1155.
4. Di Segni R, Yang AT, Qian Z, Castaneda-Zuniga WR, et al. Vascular embolotherapy: part 1. embolotherapy: agents, equipment, and techniques. In: Castaneda-Zuniga WR, ed. *Interventional Radiology*. Baltimore, MD: Williams & Wilkins; 1997:29–103.
5. Ben-Menachem Y, et al. Embolization procedures in trauma: a matter of urgency. *Semin Interv Radiol* 1985;2:107–117.
6. Sclafani SJ, Becker JA. Interventional radiology in the treatment of retroperitoneal trauma. *Urol Radiol* 1985;7:219–230.
7. Sclafani S. Angiographic control of intraperitoneal hemorrhage caused by injuries to the liver and spleen. *Semin Interv Radiol* 1985;2:138–147.
8. Panetta T, Sclafani SJ, Goldstein AS, Phillips TF, Shaftan GW. Percutaneous transcatheter embolization for arterial trauma. *J Vasc Surg* 1985;2:54–64.
9. Sclafani S. Angiographic hemostasis: its role in the salvage of the injured spleen. *Radiology* 1981;141:645–650.
10. Sclafani S, Weisberg A, Scalea TM, Phillips TF, Duncan AO. Blunt splenic injuries: nonsurgical treatment with CT, arteriography, and transcatheter arterial embolization of the splenic artery. *Radiology* 1991;181:189–196.
11. Sclafani SJ, Shaftan GW, Scalea TM, et al. Nonoperative salvage of computed tomography–diagnosed splenic injuries: utilization of angiography for triage and embolization for hemostasis. *J Trauma* 1995;39:818–827.
12. Sclafani S, Shaftan G, McAuley J. Interventional radiology in the management of hepatic trauma. *J Trauma* 1984; 24:256–262.
13. Sclafani SJ, Nayaranaswamy T, Mitchell WG. Radiologic management of traumatic hepatic artery–portal vein arteriovenous fistulae. *J Trauma* 1981;21:576–580.
14. Barth K, Strandberg J, White RJ. Long-term follow-up of transcatheter embolization with autologous clot, Oxycel, and Gelfoam in domestic swine. *Invest Radiol* 1977;12:273–280.
15. Tadavarthy S, Moller J, Amplatz K. Polyvinyl alcohol (Ivalon): a new embolic material. *Am J Roentgenol* 1975;125:609–616.
16. Chuang V, Soo C, Wallace S. Ivalon embolization in abdominal neoplasms. *Am J Roentgenol* 1981;136:729–733.
17. Gianturco C, Anderson J, Wallace S. Mechanical devices for arterial occlusion. *Am J Roentgenol* 1975;124:428–435.
18. White RI Jr, Strandberg JV, Gross GS, Barth KH. Therapeutic embolization with long-term occluding agents and their effects on embolized tissues. *Radiology* 1977;125:677–687.
19. Hilal S, et al. Synthetic fiber-coated platinum coils successfully used for the endovascular treatment of arteriovenous malformations, aneurysms and direct arteriovenous fistulas of the CNS. *Am J Neuroradiol* 1988;9:1001–1009.
20. Ekelund L, Jonsson N, Trugut H. Transcatheter obliteration of the renal artery by ethanol injection: experimental results. *Cardiovasc Interv Radiol* 1981;4:1–7.
21. Zanetti P, Sherman F. Experimental evaluation of a tissue adhesive as an agent for the treatment of aneurysms and arteriovenous anomalies. *J Neurosurg* 1972;36:72–79.
22. Goldman M, Philip P, Sarrafizadeh M. Bucrylate, a liquid tissue adhesive for transcatheter embolization. *Appl Radiol* 1984;Nov/Dec:89–94.
23. Raoul J, Heresbach D, Bretagne J. Chemoembolization of hepatocellular carcinomas: a study of the biodistribution and pharmacokinetics of doxorubicin. *Cancer* 1992;79:585–590.
24. Rudnick MR, Berns JS, Cohen RM, Goldfarb S. Contrast media-associated nephrotoxicity. *Semin Nephrol* 1997;17:15–26.
25. Tepel M, van der Giet M, Schwarzfeld C, Laufer U, Liermann D, Zidek W. Prevention of radiographic-contrast-agent-induced reductions in renal function by acetylcysteine. *N Engl J Med* 2000;343:180–184.
26. Morales PA, Hayes JV, Bailey SR. Contrast-induced nephropathy: fenoldopam, a new agent to decrease acute renal insufficiency. *Am J Cardiol* 2000; 86(suppl 8A):1.
27. Kini A, et al. Preliminary experience with a fenoldopam, a new renal vasodilator, in reducing radio-contrast nephropathy during percutaneous coronary intervention. *Am J Cardiol* 2000;86(suppl 8A):2.
28. *National Vital Statistics Report*. Atlanta, GA: Centers for Disease Control and Prevention; 1998:26.
29. Bakal CW, Cynamar J, Hakritz PS, Spragmayer S. Value of preoperative renal artery embolization in reducing blood transfusion requirements during nephrectomy for renal cell carcinoma. *J Vasc Interv Radiol* 1993;4:727–731.
30. Wallace S, Chuang VP, Swanson D, et al. Embolization of renal carcinoma. *Radiology* 1981;138:563–570.
31. Rugo HS. Cancer. In: Tierney JLM, ed. *Current Medical Diagnosis and Treatment*. Norwalk, CT: Appleton & Lange; 1995:50–79.
32. Soulen MS. Principles of regional cancer therapy. *Semin Interv Radiol* 1998;15:361–364.

CHAPTER 4

PRINCIPLES OF GENE THERAPY

JOHN W. THOMAS, MD

Initially everyone *liked* DNA. It's not that we dislike it now, but it's frightening trying to figure out what you do with all that complexity. My brain can't handle it.

James D. Watson, PhD
Cold Spring Harbor, 1999

Few areas of biologic research attract as much interest or hold as much promise as gene therapy. Gene therapy will be as revolutionary to medicine in this century as the advent of antibiotics was in the 20th century.

The first person to receive gene therapy was a 4-year-old girl with adenosine deaminase–severe combined immunodeficiency, who was treated at the National Institutes of Health (NIH) in 1990.[1] Now, more than a decade later and with 3,500 patients enrolled in 600 separate clinical trials that either are under way or have been completed worldwide (mostly in the United States), gene therapy can no longer be considered a pursuit of the basic scientist. At the time of this writing, almost 70% of the 509 U.S. gene therapy clinical trials reported to the NIH's Office of Biotechnology Activities are designed to treat cancer patients. Although no gene therapy method has entered the realm of clinical practice, a handful of clinical trials are now in phase 3, increasing the likelihood that radiologists will encounter gene therapy patients in nonacademic environments).* Radiologists who understand the tenets of this new type of therapy will be better consultants.

*For more information, see the following Web sites: (http://www4.od.nih.gov/oba/ and http://www.wiley.co.uk/wileychi/genmed/clinical/.

If the therapy is intended to affect a specific lesion, organ, or vascular segment, the gene must be delivered in such a way that it enters only the targeted cells at the level of interest. Until such a "magic bullet" is feasible, image-guided techniques will in all likelihood prevail as the means of delivery. Interventional radiologists, therefore, have the skills to be primary conveyors of many types of gene therapy.

Cystic fibrosis and sickle cell anemia commonly come to mind when one considers genetic diseases; the most common genetic disease, however, is cancer. Although cystic fibrosis and sickle cell anemia are inherited disorders, and many patients with cancer were born with chromosomal abnormalities that predisposed them to malignancy, cancer is usually an *acquired* genetic disease. Our genomes are continuously exposed to injurious agents (e.g., background cosmic radiation). We have evolved repair systems to correct these injuries, but our lifestyles may expose us to more genomic injury than can be compensated for, such as that resulting from cigarette smoking and radiation exposure.

When those acquired injuries are beyond repair, a cell usually dies either as a result of the injury or through apoptosis (programmed cell death). But a cell becomes malignant when it accumulates injuries that deregulate replication and apoptosis and bestow upon the cell the ability to survive in a milieu different from that of its origin. The genetic destabilization that results from these injuries also tends to increase the frequency of cell type variation. The genome of at least one cell in a patient with cancer has suffered this constellation of injuries.

Oncologic gene therapy strategies are designed to (1) restore the function of or replace deactivated tumor suppressor genes, (2) block the action of activated oncogenes, (3) activate the immune system against the malignancy, (4) deliver a suicide gene that kills the cell and its neighbors upon subsequent exposure to an otherwise harmless pro-drug, or (5) shut down the angiogenic ability of the tumor.

After reading this chapter, you will:

- Understand three basic strategies of current oncologic gene therapy: gene augmentation, gene blocking with antisense oligonucleotides, and gene repression with transcription factor decoys.
- Know the differences and similarities between viral oncolytic therapy and gene therapy.
- Have a gene therapy vocabulary sufficient to allow reading of gene therapy literature.
- Understand the advantages and disadvantages of several gene therapy vectors.
- Know that the principal hurdle facing gene therapy is delivery, and how interventional skills can assist in overcoming that hurdle.

WHAT IS GENE THERAPY?

Gene therapy is the introduction of recombinant genes into selective somatic cells to treat an acquired or hereditary disorder. It is a hybridization of pharmacologic therapy and bioengineering. One principal advantage of gene therapy over traditional pharmacology is the potential to achieve a local, sustained therapeutic concentration of a substance that would be toxic if administered systemically. Another is the time course of that agent. Depending on the approach used, the substance could be produced momentarily or for the remainder of the patient's life. Furthermore, the altered cells might constitutively produce the gene product, or the strategy might be that the gene product is synthesized only under specific conditions, such as in the presence of an antibiotic. Genetic manipulation of germ cells, a technique that would affect future generations and our gene pool, is currently considered inappropriate and dangerous and is not in the realm of gene therapy.

STRATEGIES OF GENE THERAPY

There are different modalities for achieving gene therapy, but most current tactics involve *gene augmentation*, whereby the desired genes are provided or inserted into the genome without removal or alteration of the host cell's original copy (**Fig. 4-1A**). Utilizing gene augmentation, one is able to either restore normal function to the cell or enhance existing gene function. For example, cells with deletion or mutation of the tumor suppressor gene *TP53* are at higher risk of malignant transformation. Inserting the wild type of that gene into tumor cells may reverse the malignant phenotype or render the tumor more susceptible to antineoplastic agents.[2, 3]

Another approach using gene augmentation is to insert a gene that codes for an enzyme that converts a nontoxic prodrug into its therapeutic form. The best known examples of the prodrug gene augmentation strategy, also known as "suicide gene therapy," is the transfer of the gene coding for herpes simplex virus thymidine kinase (HSV *tk*) into tumors followed by treatment with ganciclovir, a substrate for the HSV *tk*. Ganciclovir, for which mammalian thymidine kinase has a very low affinity, is subsequently broken down into toxic metabolites by those cells carrying the HSV *tk* transgene.[4–6] Because this technique can cause 100% tumor regression, but current gene transfer methods cause transfection of less than 10% of target cells,[7] there must be a bystander effect that treats neighboring, nontransfected cells.[8, 9]

Another promising example of prodrug gene augmentation therapy is the percutaneous injection of a

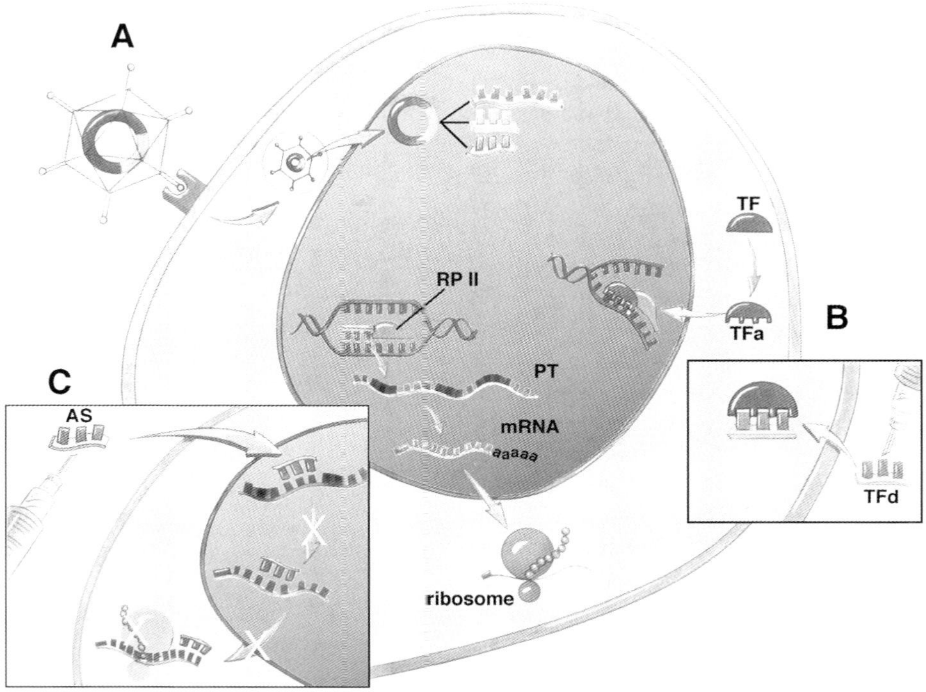

Figure 4-1. Gene therapy strategies. The basic strategies of gene augmentation and gene blocking are illustrated. (A) Gene augmentation: The gene is delivered via an expression vector. Note that the vector may convey a transgene or an oligonucleotide sequences coding for transcription factor (TF) decoys or antisense. (B) Transcription blocking by transcription factor decoy: In response to a stimulus, a transcription factor is activated. Normal: The activated TF (TFa) then enters the nucleus and binds the promoter or enhancer sequence of the gene to be transcribed. Binding of the TF allows RNA polymerase II, the enzyme responsible for transcription of DNA to RNA, to bind and commence transcription. Blocked: TF decoys (TFd) mimic the enhancer or promoter sequence, thereby binding the activated transcription factors. As shown, TF decoys may be administered via an expression vector or as a conventional pharmaceutical. (C) Translation blocking by antisense: Normal: RNA polymerase II (RP II) synthesizes the primary transcript (PT), which must be processed to yield mRNA. mRNA exits the nucleus to be translated by a ribosome. Blocked: Antisense (AS) is complementary to a portion of the primary transcript or mRNA. Antisense will bind the complementary sequence, making a portion of the RNA double-stranded and thereby preventing processing, nuclear exiting, or translation. As with TF decoys, antisense may be administered via an expression vector or as a conventional pharmaceutical. (Modified and reprinted with permission from Thomas JW, Kuo MD, Chawla M, et al. Vascular gene therapy. Radiographics 1998;18: 1373–1394.)

vector able to transfer the gene coding for cytosine deaminase into hepatic metastases from colon cancer. The patient is subsequently given oral doses of the nontoxic prodrug 5-flucytosine. This drug is deaminated to the potent chemotherapeutic agent 5-fluorouracil inside the cells that were transfected.[10]

Some types of cancer are able to escape the immune system by creating local immunosuppression. Another gene augmentation tactic is to transfer a gene coding for a substance that neutralizes this immunosuppressive effect, thereby exposing the tumor to the host immune system. The best known example of this approach is to transfer the gene coding for the cytokine interleukin-2 into a tumor with the aim of activating and propagating cytotoxic T lymphocytes and subsequent antitumor response.[11, 12] Along this same line, autologous tumor cells can be harvested, transfected with the interleukin-2 gene or another cytokine gene ex vivo, and reimplanted into the patient as a vaccine to elicit a host-wide immune response targeted against the tumor.[13, 14]

A gene therapy tactic altogether different from gene augmentation is to use the inserted genetic material, as opposed to the gene product, to block the action of an endogenous gene. Because a gene's action is manifested only after the gene has been *transcribed* (its messenger RNA [mRNA] has been synthesized using DNA as a template) and the mRNA has been *translated* (proteins have been synthesized using mRNA as a template), the action can be blocked if either process is prevented. Rather than thwart these processes nonselectively, transcription of a targeted gene can be prevented with transcription factor decoy oligonucleotides, and translation of a targeted gene's mRNA can be prevented with antisense oligonucleotides. These methods are considered briefly in the following paragraphs.

Transcription Factor Decoys

In any given cell, roughly 95% of the genetic material is quiescent at any time. When a cell must respond to an environmental change, the genes that code for the proteins needed to effect the response are transcribed. But how does a cell regulate this process? *Transcription factors* (TFs) are proteins that, in response to a stimulus, recognize and bind specific nucleotide sequences (**Fig. 4-1B**). The sequences are of two different classes known as promoters and enhancers. RNA polymerase II (the enzyme responsible for transcription) is able to bind to and initiate transcription of a gene whose promoter or enhancer has bound a TF. Repressors do just the opposite of transcription factors: they are proteins that bind to specific sequences of DNA, called operators, and prevent the binding of RNA polymerase II. The nucleotide sequence in DNA, then, codes not only for proteins but also for regulation of transcription.

A *transcription factor decoy* is an oligonucleotide sequence that mimics the promoter or enhancer region of a gene and is therefore able to compete with the genome for TF binding. Once bound to the decoy, the TF is unable to bind to the genuine promoter or enhancer, thus preventing transcription.[15] In animal models, TF decoys are being investigated as a means to restore colon cancer sensitivity to 5-fluorouracil,[16] restore estrogen receptor synthesis in estrogen receptor–negative breast cancer,[17] activate and stabilize p53 in breast cancer,[18] and inhibit the development of liver metastases by blocking gene transactivation.[19]

Antisense

As previously mentioned, only one of the two DNA strands is transcribed into mRNA during transcription. By convention, the sense DNA strand generally *is not* transcribed. The complementary DNA strand, or the antisense strand, *is* transcribed (**Fig. 4-1C**). The resultant single-stranded pre-mRNA, also known as the "primary transcript," is identical in sequence to the sense DNA strand, except for the substitution of uracil for thymine. A great deal happens to this sense pre-mRNA strand prior to translation. It is processed into its final form of mRNA through the addition of a guanosine monophosphate cap and a polyadenine tail, and the splicing out of the *introns* (noncoding sequences) residing between the *exons* (coding sequences). The mRNA must then exit the nucleus and then must be transported through the cytoplasm, recognized by a ribosome, and translated, all prior to degradation. The journey can be interrupted if even a portion of the mRNA is made double-stranded by the presence of a complementary antisense sequence. The sequence of nucleotides can be either RNA or DNA, just as long as it is complementary. The antisense strand does not have to be as long as the mRNA. In fact, a sequence of only 11–25 bases is all that is required to be both effective and specific against a targeted mRNA.[15]

The obvious genes to target for blocking in a patient with cancer are the oncogenes. Antisense to many oncogenes, including *myb*, *ras*, and *raf*, are under investigation as a possible means of treating patients with leukemia[20] and solid tumors.[21, 22] Antisense to insulin-like growth factor type I receptor has been used to treat patients with malignant astrocytoma through the induction of an immune-like response against the tumor as well as tumor cell apoptosis.[23]

Transition Factor Decoys and Antisense: Conventional Therapy or Gene Therapy?

Oligonucleotides diffuse across cell membranes, overcoming one of the major hurdles of gene delivery. These molecules act directly to compete for TFs or block translation of an mRNA transcript, so they are not prodrugs as used in gene augmentation therapy. The effective half-life of oligonucleotides is short relative to gene transfer strategies. In fact, the pharmacology of therapeutic oligonucleotides can be predictably described much like that of a conventional pharmaceutical.[24]

So why are oligonucleotides included in a gene discussion of therapy? Because instead of direct transfer of oligonucleotides to cells, the genetic sequences coding for oligonucleotides can be delivered via an expression vector, which incites synthesis of the oligonucleotide in situ. Depending on vector characteristics, the DNA can be transcribed for a limited period before degradation or can be incorporated into the host genome and thus steadily expressed. The TF decoy and antisense strategies, then, truly bridge the gap between conventional therapy and gene transfer therapy.

The gene therapy tactics of gene augmentation, antisense, and TF decoys have all been applied to combat cancer. *Targeted gene conversion* is a gene therapy approach that has yet to be employed specifically for a neoplastic disorder. This technique corrects inherited point mutations by using an RNA/DNA chimeric oligonucleotide to create a mismatched base pair with the nucleotide targeted for correction. Such an approach is being investigated as a potential cure for sickle cell disease.[25]

A developing oncologic strategy that is often included in discussions of gene therapy is the use of replication-selective viruses to destroy cancer cells. The best known example is an adenovirus, ONYX-015, that has been modified in a fashion that allows it to replicate only in cells that are deficient in p53. The modification is the deletion of the E1B 55kd gene from the viral genome. The deleted gene codes for a product that enables adenovirus to overcome the effects of mammalian cell p53, which otherwise shuts down the replication of viral DNA.

The majority of human cancers arise in cells that have lost the ability to produce competent p53. ONYX-015, therefore, should theoretically be able to replicate in and be toxic to only these p53-deficient cells. It is the virus that is being used to kill tumor cells, not a novel genetic sequence introduced via the virus. Reports indicate that intravenous, intra-arterial, intraperitoneal,[26] and intratumoral administration of ONYX-015 is safe. There is early evidence that suggests it is effective as well. To complicate matters, some investigations have shown that the effectiveness of ONYX-015 against p53-competent tumors equals[27] or exceeds[28] that against p53-deficient tumors, indicating that the selective oncolytic mechanism is not well understood.

Other replication-selective viral therapies are reovirus for the treatment of tumors with activated *Ras* pathway[29] and mutated herpes simplex virus for the treatment of glioma.[30] Although replication-selective viral oncolytic therapy may prove to be an effective antineoplastic tactic, it is not gene therapy.

THE GENE THERAPY HURDLE: DELIVERY

The problem facing gene therapists today is delivery—moving the gene from outside the patient into the target cell. The gene is first incorporated into an expression vector, which must then be deployed in a way that gets it to the cell of interest. A *vector* is the gene of interest packaged in a form that provides protection from degradation, facilitates entry into the target cell and transport into the nucleus, and ensures that transcription will occur upon arrival in the nucleus. Once the gene is delivered, many additional processes must take place for expression to occur (**Fig. 4-2**). Vector attributes determine whether or not these steps are successfully negotiated.

One way to introduce a foreign gene is to take advantage of a highly evolved organism that does just that for a living: a virus. Indeed, vectors are grouped as either viral or nonviral. Conventional viral vectors involve either replication-deficient or inactivated virus, so that each virus may infect one cell only. There is no surplus of space within a viral capsid. If the viral chromosome is to carry a new gene, an existing gene or genes must be removed. The genes that are deleted are selected so as to cripple the virus's ability to replicate but not its ability to transfect and compel expression. The two most widely used viral vectors, considered here, are retrovirus and adenovirus.

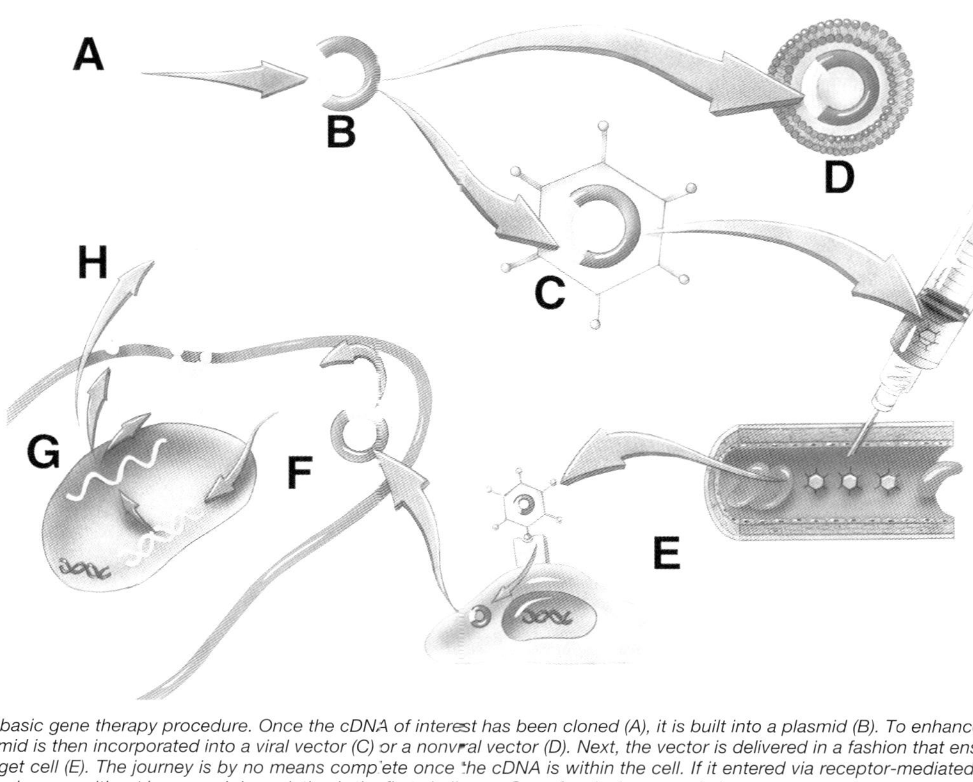

Figure 4-2. The basic gene therapy procedure. Once the cDNA of interest has been cloned (A), it is built into a plasmid (B). To enhance expression efficiency, the plasmid is then incorporated into a viral vector (C) or a nonviral vector (D). Next, the vector is delivered in a fashion that ensures approximation with the target cell (E). The journey is by no means complete once the cDNA is within the cell. If it entered via receptor-mediated endocytosis, release from the endosome without lysosomal degradation is the first challenge. Once free in the cytosol, the transgene must cross the cytoplasm, traverse the nuclear membrane, and be recognized by nuclear enzymes and transcription factors (F) to initiate transcription. The mRNA thus formed returns to the cytoplasm for translation, with subsequent production of the therapeutic product (G). The product may exhibit its action on the cell in which it was synthesized or may be secreted to have a paracrine or systemic effect (H). (Modified and reprinted with permission from Thomas JW, Kuo MD, Chawla M, et al. Vascular gene therapy. Radiographics 1998;18:1373–1394.)

Replication-Deficient Retrovirus

Retrovirus is an enveloped, double-stranded, RNA virus that enters the host cell by receptor-mediated endocytosis (**Fig. 4-3**). Once the virus is inside the cell, the RNA is converted to DNA through the actions of the enzyme reverse transcriptase. The retroviral DNA *integrates* into (assimilates genetic material from) the host genome, making it particularly ideal as a vector. Once integrated, the viral DNA will survive as long as the host cell and can be passed on to any daughter cells, ensuring expression of the desired DNA sequences for long periods.[31]

The disadvantages of retroviral vectors for oncologic gene therapy are as follows: (1) they are unable to accommodate transgenes larger than 7 kb, (2) the target cell must be actively dividing (malignant tumors ineffectively regulate replication, but the entire population of cells is not simultaneously replicating), (3) mutagenesis may occur secondary to random host-cell chromosomal incorporation, and (4) it is extremely difficult to produce high titers of virus.[31,32] In spite of these shortcomings, more gene therapy clinical trials have used retroviral vectors than any other vector. Retroviral vectors are used typically to transduce cells outside the patient; the transduced cells are subsequently administered to the patient.

Replication-Deficient Adenovirus

There are more than 50 serotypes of adenovirus; most adenoviral vectors for human gene therapy are of serotype 5 (Ad5). *Adenovirus* is a non-enveloped icosahedral double-stranded DNA virus that can infect most mammalian cell types, whether or not those cells are dividing (**Fig. 4-4**). Once inside the cell, adenoviral DNA typically resides as an independent episome within the nucleus, instead of integrating into the host genome as does a retrovirus. The likelihood of direct mutagenesis, therefore, is low with an adenovirus vector. The viral genome can be divided into early genes and late genes. The *early genes* code primarily for proteins involved in commandeering the host cell and for viral replication, and the *late genes* code primarily for structural and packaging proteins.

First-generation adenoviral vectors are rendered replication-deficient through deletion of the first early gene ($Ad5E1^-$) or both the first and third early genes ($Ad5E1^-E3^-$). An $Ad5E1^-$vector can accommodate about 7–8 kb of foreign DNA, and deleting the E3 gene makes room for an additional 2 kb. First-generation adenoviral vectors have a significant cytopathologic effect when administered in high titers.[33]

In spite of the E1 deletions, low levels of viral DNA and protein synthesis still occur and can elicit a cellular

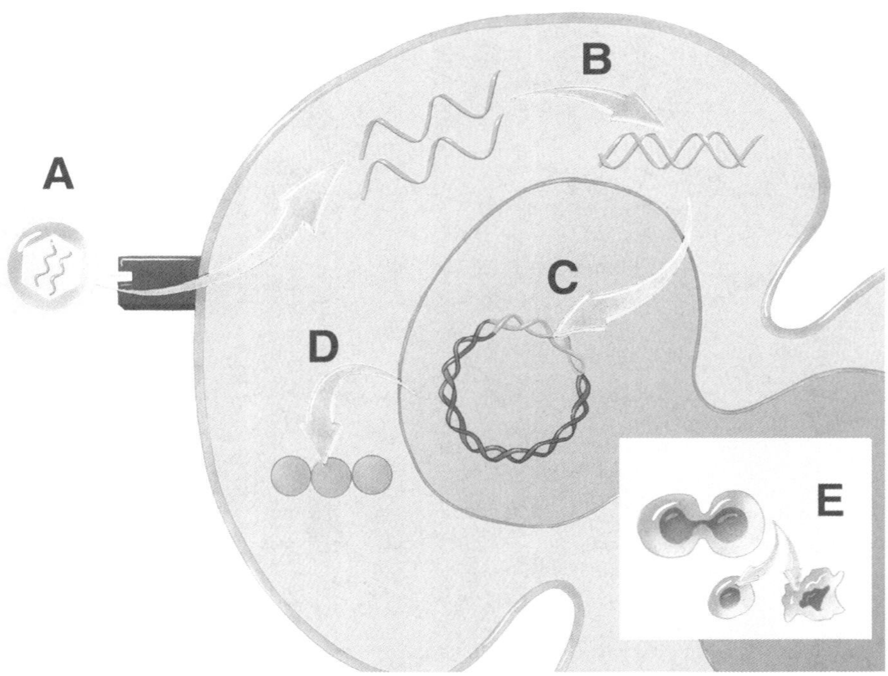

Figure 4-3. Replication-deficient retrovirus. The double-stranded RNA of the retrovirus has been engineered to carry the transgene (A). A retrovirus transfects only actively dividing cells. Once inside the cell, DNA is synthesized from the RNA template by the enzyme reverse transcriptase (B). The DNA randomly integrates into a host cell's chromosome (C), where it not only is perpetually transcribed (D) but also will be passed on to any daughter cells. One disadvantage of this random integration is the possibility of mutagenesis. The usual outcome of mutagenesis is death of the cell, although more ominous mutations, such as oncogenesis, can occur (E). (Modified and reprinted with permission from Thomas JW, Kuo MD, Chawla M, et al. Vascular gene therapy. Radiographics 1998;18:1373–1394.)

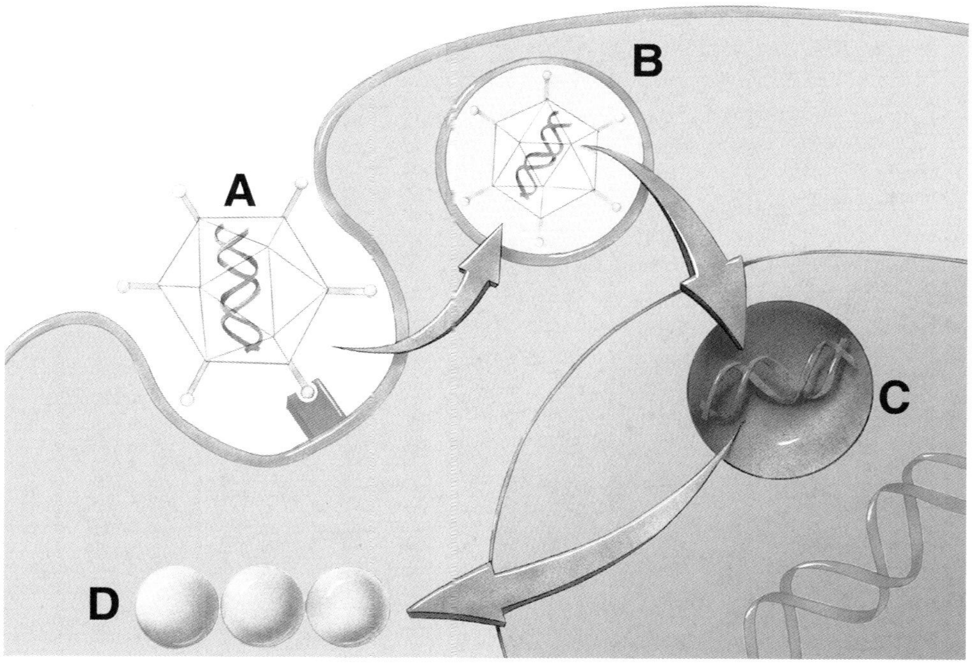

Figure 4-4. Replication-deficient adenovirus. Adenovirus can infect both dividing and nondividing cells. The linear double-stranded DNA virus, engineered to carry the transgene, enters the cell by receptor mediated endocytosis (A). Endosomal lytic proteins allow escape from the endosome, and the DNA is transported into the nucleus (B). The virus reorganizes the nuclear contents to facilitate its own reproduction (C). Key genes have been deleted from the virus, allowing it to orchestrate transcription of the transgene but not of certain elements needed for viral replication (D). The virus does not integrate, and expression is only temporary. (Modified and reprinted with permission from Thomas JW, Kuo MD, Chawla M, et al. Vascular gene therapy. Radiographics 1998;18:1373–1394.)

immune response, an effect that limits the duration of transgene expression to a few days or weeks.[34] The humoral immune response could limit the repeated use of adenoviral vectors, although repeated dosing has been found to be safe and marginally effective in clinical trials.[35, 36] Modulation or suppression of the immune system could be used as a means of extending the duration of expression.[34, 37, 38] Temporary expression can be either an advantage or a disadvantage from the standpoint of therapeutic applications, depending on the substance produced, its effect on the disorder being treated, and the acuteness or chronicity of the disorder. If the goal is to destroy target cells, temporary expression might be ideal; however, if the goal is to restore the function of a tumor suppressor gene, lifelong expression is desired.

To overcome the limitations of temporary expression and cytopathologic effect, subsequent generations of adenoviral vectors have been produced by deletions of other viral genes. Deleting more viral genes also frees up additional space for larger or more transgenes. An adenoviral vector completely devoid of viral genes might be ideal for evading the immune system, but some of the viral genes are helpful in forcing transgene expression and episome stabilization.[39] Furthermore, production of such a "gutless" vector becomes a challenge, because the functions performed by the deleted genes must be supplied in some fashion.

This production problem has been solved by the simultaneous infection of the producing cell with the vector and with large numbers of a helper virus, which provide the replication and packaging functions through sheer volume. The subsequent adenoviral vector is referred to as a *helper-dependent adenovirus* (HDAd). The genome in an HDAd must be more than 75% of the size of the native adenoviral genome. When the transgene is small, benign sequences of DNA known as "stuffer sequences" must be added to increase the size.[40] Preclinical trials of HDAd vectors have shown them to be less cytotoxic than first-generation Ad vectors,[41] able to confer expression for months to years in an immunocompetent host,[42] and effective with repeated doses using different serotypes.[43]

Adenoviral vectors are being used in most phase 3 clinical trials and are the type an interventional radiologist would most likely be asked to deliver. In spite of concerns about patient immune response and cytotoxicity, first-generation adenoviral vectors were considered very safe until the death in 1999 of an 18-year-old patient who was treated with a high-titer ($>10^{13}$ particles) dose.[44, 45] This patient's death led to reassessment of NIH oversight of gene therapy research with subsequent modifications in protocol review and adverse event reporting, but the reassessment process reaffirmed the overall safety of adenoviral vectors and the need to continue gene therapy research.[46, 47]

Other viral vectors are the herpes simplex virus, poliovirus, papillomavirus, and the unique adeno-associated virus (AAV). The last is a single-stranded DNA virus that can transfect nondividing cells, like adenovirus, and also integrates, like retrovirus. Unlike with retrovirus, however, the integration of AAV occurs into a predictable, nontoxic locus of the mammalian genome.[48] Refinement of viral vectors is an explosive field of research, including the hybridization of HDAd with the integrating machinery of AAVs, retroviruses, and transposons to produce vectors that transfect efficiently, elicit no immune response, and integrate for enduring transgene expression.[49–51]

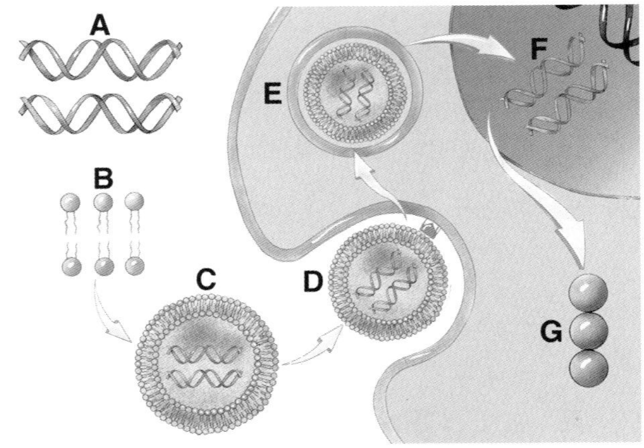

Figure 4-5. Example of a nonviral vector: cationic liposome. The genetic material (A) and lipids (B) are combined to yield a liposome (C). The liposome is delivered to the target tissue and enters by endocytosis or fusion, depending on characteristics of the liposome surface (D). Once inside the cytoplasm, the genetic material must escape the endosome, traverse the cytoplasm, and cross the nuclear membrane (E). Each of these tasks can be augmented by addition of factors to the liposome. Inside the nucleus, the DNA is transcribed (F) followed by translation in the cytoplasm (G). (Modified and reprinted with permission from Thomas JW, Kuo MD, Chawla M, et al. Vascular gene therapy. Radiographics 1998;18: 1373–1394.)

Nonviral Methods

The elegance of harnessing the viral mechanism for gene transfer is balanced by the problems inherent in using an infectious agent. The virus can be cytotoxic or may induce an immune response. The possibility of contamination with a wild type, replication-competent virus is always present. A nonviral vector can avoid these problems. Any nonviral solution must be capable of condensing the DNA into a size small enough to undergo endocytosis, allow the DNA to escape the endosome, promote transportation across the cytoplasm to the nucleus, and permit nuclear membrane penetration. These nonviral solutions range from naked DNA to complex synthetic vehicles bearing specific surface ligands and viral components (**Fig. 4-5**).

The gene within a plasmid may be applied directly to the cells of interest. A *plasmid* is a circular double strand of DNA that is transcriptionally active and can replicate autonomously from the host cell. Plasmids provide none of the protection afforded by a virus and do not pursue replication in the deliberate fashion of a virus. Hence, the transfection efficiency of a plasmid is markedly less than that of a viral vector. Plasmid transfection is most often used for ex vivo gene transfer, in which efficiency of transfection is less important.

The plasmid can be constrained within a material that facilitates cell entry. The best-known example is a *liposome*, which is a single or multilayered vesicle that can be synthesized to be neutral or negatively or positively charged and that acts as an artificial membrane. Liposomes can be used to transport macromolecules across cell membranes by receptor-mediated endocytosis. Once inside the cell, however, the plasmid remains trapped within an endosome until lysosomal fusion, which often results in destruction of the macromolecule. Cationic liposomes overcome this problem, in that they can fuse directly to the cell membrane or the wall of an endosome, releasing the DNA payload. Because a lysosome is not needed to effect release from the endosome, lysosomal degradation is avoided.[52] The addition of inactivated virus to the liposome surface can improve plasma membrane fusion.[53] Once inside the cytoplasm (a concentrated protein solution in a matrix of actin filaments, microtubules, and other structural elements), the plasmid must reach the nucleus in order to be transcribed. Its transportation to the nucleus and across the nuclear membrane is facilitated by addition of nuclear localization proteins, such as high mobility group–1, to the plasmid before liposome encapsulation.[54]

An example of a cationic liposomal vector is described by Hortobagyi et al.[55] in their report on a phase 1 clinical trial of *E1A* gene transfer to malignant cells by intrapleural or intraperitoneal injection in patients who have advanced breast or ovarian cancer with malignant pleural effusions or ascites. The adenoviral type 5 *E1A* gene product is the first to be expressed in a cell after infection. The product, a transcription factor, is responsible for activating transcription of other viral genes as well as reorganizing expression of the host cell's genome so that viral genes are transcribed more efficiently. The *E1A* product has been shown to repress the *HER2/neu* promoter in human cancer cells. *HER2/neu* encodes for a transmembrane growth factor receptor. Cells that overexpress *HER2/neu* often have constitutive signaling in the absence of ligand, resulting in unregulated cell growth and a cancer that is more aggressive than one without overexpression of *HER2/neu*.[56] The *HER-2/neu*-overexpressing tumor cells demonstrated downregulation of *HER-2/neu* expression, increased apoptosis, and reduced DNA replication after E1A gene transfer.[56]

Liposomes are arguably the best known nonviral vectors, but other synthetic approaches are under investigation. For example, Medina-Kauwe et al.[57] synthesized proteins from the adenoviral capsid and condensed them with DNA and the targeting ligand heregulin to create a vector specific for HER2-positive carcinoma. One can envision a specific vector for treating breast or ovarian malignancy through the combination of this vector with the AdE1A transgene.

Current nonviral vectors do not integrate with the host genome, reducing any possibility of mutagenesis. Although non-integration results in temporary expression, as with the adenoviral vectors, there should be little or no immune response to prevent repeated treatments, and there is no question of possible contamination with wild-type virus. Transfection efficiencies of nonviral vectors are lower than with viral vectors, but the lines between viral and nonviral vectors will likely continue to blur as the field of vector design progresses. Combining favorable elements from various types of viral and nonviral vectors will produce hybrid vectors customized to the condition being treated.

VECTOR DELIVERY

As previously stated, the major hurdle to using gene transfer for therapy is delivery of the transgene. This discussion has so far considered the vectors, which assist in moving the transgene from outside of the cell to an effective intracellular location. How is the vector brought to the cell? There are two broad approaches: (1) expose cells to the vector in a controlled setting outside the patient and then return them to the patient (ex vivo delivery) or (2) administer the vector to the patient directly (in vivo delivery).

Cell-Mediated, Ex Vivo Gene Delivery

In the cell-mediated approach, autologous cells are harvested surgically or by core biopsy from the patient and grown in culture (**Fig. 4-6**). The cells might be from the patient's cancer or could be nonmalignant cells, such as fibroblasts, that are simply chosen to serve as autologous vectors. The harvested cells are subsequently transfected with the appropriate recombinant DNA and then reimplanted into the patient. Nonautologous cells can be used, but they must be reintroduced in a manner that evades the immune system. The cells are typically reimplanted into a subcutaneous location with the aim of eliciting a hostwide response, such as an immune response.[13, 14, 23] If those cells must be delivered to the actual tumor site to achieve a paracrine or bystander effect, image-guided injection or intravascular methods may be required, calling on the skills of interventional radiology.[58]

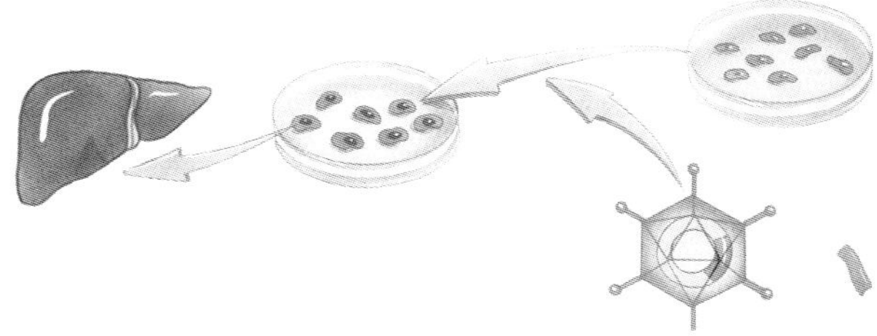

Figure 4-6. Ex-vivo gene transfer: Cells harvested from the patient are cultured, transfected, and reimplanted. The reimplantation site is the liver in this example. (Modified and reprinted with permission from Thomas JW, Kuo MD, Chawla M, et al. Vascular gene therapy. Radiographics 1998;18:1373–1394.)

The primary advantage of the ex vivo method is that it allows reliable evaluation of gene expression of the target cell prior to reimplantation. The major disadvantages of this technique are the requisites for obtaining syngeneic cell lines and time delay from harvesting of cells, through the quantification of transfection efficiencies, to reimplantation.

Direct Gene Transfer: In Vivo Gene Delivery

Direct gene transfer entails the in vivo delivery of recombinant DNA to the cells of interest. This technique is faster and simpler than ex vivo gene delivery but comes at the price of less precise cell-specific transfection. Current human gene therapy protocols utilize an assortment of in vivo vector delivery methods, including inhalation, percutaneous injection, endoscopic delivery, intravascular infusion, and open surgical technique.[59] The widespread clinical application of gene therapy will likely depend on noninvasive or minimally invasive vector delivery methods.

Noninvasive methods of delivery, such as oral administration, intravenous infusion, and intramuscular and subcutaneous injections, depend on the development of targeting methods that drive the vector specifically toward the malignancy. This targeting is being attempted through vector modifications that make them tumor specific.[60] Minimally invasive methods of delivery, such as image-guided percutaneous injection and catheter-based intravascular infusion, must suffice until specific targeting methods become a reality.

Percutaneous Injection

Because of the relatively low efficiency of in vivo transfection with current vectors, percutaneous injection of vector into the tumor or tissues adjacent to tumor can be therapeutic only if the transgene product can move from cell to cell (*paracrine effect*) or triggers a response in adjacent cells that is either lethal or therapeutic (*bystander effect*). Furthermore, distribution of a vector away from the injection site occurs not just by simple diffusion, as with percutaneous alcohol injection, but also depends on vector traits and cell receptor levels. For example, a retrovirus can come into contact with any number of cells but will enter a cell only if the retroviral surface glycoproteins bind to specific receptors on the cell's outer membrane. Not only does the specificity of the interaction determine the tissue tropism of the virus, but the number of available cell receptors versus the number of vector particles injected in part determines how far away from the injection site the virus distributes. This characteristic makes injection of gene therapy vectors fundamentally different from that of other agents that interventional radiologists typically inject into patients. From a technique standpoint, this characteristic is generally in our favor, as it means there is probably little reason to attempt to distribute the vector in tiny aliquots throughout the tumor; it is best to simply inject the vector suspension into the target and let the vector distribute itself through receptor saturation (**Fig. 4-7**). Vector distribution after percutaneous injection, however, is a poorly understood area that warrants further investigation.

Intravascular Infusion

When percutaneous injection of vector is impractical, such as in the presence of widespread liver metastases, or when the vector target is the endothelium, intra-arterial infusion may afford an ideal delivery route. In clinical trials, adenoviral vectors, replication-selective adenovirus, and autologous cells have been delivered safely via the hepatic artery to the liver.[45, 58, 61]

There are potential advantages to targeting the endothelial cells recruited by the tumor rather than the malignant cells. First, no tumor can grow beyond a microscopic size without the ability to induce neovascularization. The endothelial cells of these neovessels are not in themselves malignant and do not share the same genetic instability as the cancer they support; therefore, therapy targeted against the endothelial cells is much less likely to select out a resistant cell line.[62] Second, a large number of tumor cells, between 5 and 50, depend on each endothelial cell; the effect of therapy aimed at the endothelial cell is therefore amplified.

Another distinct and interesting advantage of directing therapy toward endothelial cells is that interventional radiologists have direct access to these cells via angiographic catheters. A vector can be infused into the lumen or a specialized catheter can be used to deliver the vector to a specific segment of vessel. Such specialized catheters range in complexity from simple hydrogel-coated balloon angioplasty catheters to devices that isolate the vessel wall from the lumen to permit prolonged contact between vector suspension and the endothelium.[63]

CONCLUSION

The use of genes to combat disease may eventually be considered just another treatment modality. Ashanthi De Silva is the young girl who was the first human to wade forth into the post–gene therapy era. Having survived what can be considered a discrete step in the evolution of our species, she is now a teenager. Although there has been a death attributable to gene

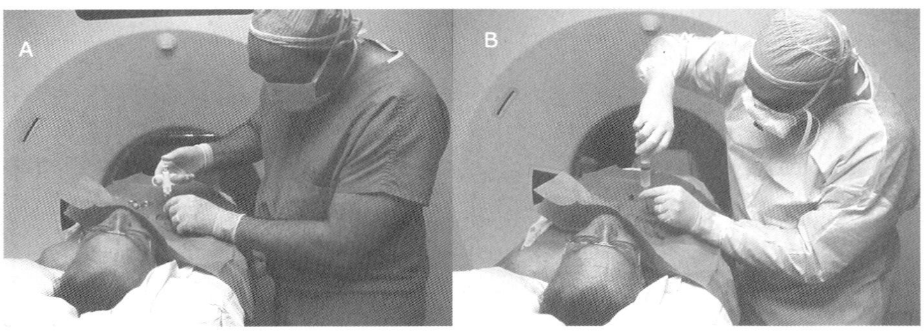

Figure 4-7. Interventional radiologist turned gene therapist: Percutaneous injection of a vector solution can be very similar to current interventional techniques. In this example, a patient enrolled in a trial of TP53 gene transfer via adenoviral vector as adjunctive treatment of non-small cell lung cancer has a core biopsy of the lesion followed by injection of the vector. Between the computerized tomography (CT) guided biopsy (A) and the injection (B), the operator has put on a protective gown and mask. Negative-pressure ventilation in this CT room helps prevent escape of vector. The biopsy was performed coaxially, and the guide needle was used to administer the vector suspension.

therapy, the results of U.S. phase 1 clinical trials have uniformly shown that gene therapy is safe.[46, 59]

Achieving efficacy is the next obstacle. Many elaborate and elegant multigene vectors have been created, but the principal problem that needs solving remains gene delivery. Until vectors are created that are so cell type–specific they can simply be taken like routine drugs, minimally invasive methods to optimize exposure of vectors to the target cells are needed. Interventional radiologists will likely play a critical role in this exciting new field. You should get involved with the gene therapy trials in your local area. Make sure the investigators understand your capabilities of image-guided delivery. Combining the forces of gene therapists and interventional radiologists may lead to the breakthrough needed to make oncologic gene therapy a clinical reality.

REFERENCES

1. Blaese RM, Culver KW, Miller AD, et al. T lymphocyte-directed gene therapy for ADA-SCID: initial trial results after 4 years. *Science* 1995;270:475–480.
2. Merritt JA, Roth JA, Logothetis CJ. Clinical evaluation of adenoviral-mediated p53 gene transfer: review of INGN 201 studies. *Semin Oncol* 2001;28:105–114.
3. Swisher SG, Roth JA, Nemunaitis J, et al. Adenovirus-mediated p53 gene transfer in advanced non-small-cell lung cancer. *J Natl Cancer Inst* 1999;91:763–771.
4. Oldfield EH, Ram Z, Culver KW, et al. Gene therapy for the treatment of brain tumors using intra-tumoral transduction with the thymidine kinase gene and intravenous ganciclovir. *Hum Gene Ther* 1993;4:39–69
5. Ram Z, Culver KW, Oshiro EM, et al. Therapy of malignant brain tumors by intratumoral implantation of retroviral vector-producing cells. *Nat Med* 1997;3:1354–1361.
6. Sandmair AM, Loimas S, Puranen P, et al. Thymidine kinase gene therapy for human malignant glioma, using replication-deficient retroviruses or adenoviruses. *Hum Gene Ther* 2000;11:2197–2205.
7. Puumalainen AM, Vapalahti M, Agrawal RS, et al. Beta-galactosidase gene transfer to human malignant glioma in vivo using replication-deficient retroviruses and adenoviruses. *Hum Gene Ther* 1998;9:1769–1774.
8. Floeth FW, Shand N, Bojar H, et al. Local inflammation and devascularization—in vivo mechanisms of the "bystander effect" in VPC-mediated HSV-Tk/GCV gene therapy for human malignant glioma. *Cancer Gene Ther* 2001;8:843–851.
9. Freeman SM, Abboud CN, Whartenby KA, et al. The "bystander effect": tumor regression when a fraction of the tumor mass is genetically modified. *Cancer Res* 1993;53:5274–5283.
10. Crystal RG, Hirschowitz E, Lieberman M, et al. Phase I study of direct administration of a replication deficient adenovirus vector containing the *E. coli* cytosine deaminase gene to metastatic colon carcinoma of the liver in association with the oral administration of the pro-drug 5-fluorocytosine. *Hum Gene Ther* 1997;8:985–1001.
11. Belldegrun A, Tso CL, Zisman A, et al. Interleukin 2 gene therapy for prostate cancer: phase I clinical trial and basic biology. *Hum Gene Ther* 2001 12:883–892.
12. Hoffman DM, Figlin RA. Intratumoral interleukin 2 for renal-cell carcinoma by direct gene transfer of a plasmid DNA/DMRIE/DOPE lipid complex. *World J Urol* 2000;18:152–156.
13. Wittig B, Marten A, Dorbic T, et al. Therapeutic vaccination against metastatic carcinoma by expression-modulated and immunomodified autologous tumor cells: a first clinical phase I/II trial. *Hum Gene Ther* 2001;12:267–278.
14. Golumbek PT, Lazenby AJ, Levitsky HI, et al. Treatment of established renal cancer by tumor cells engineered to secrete interleukin-4. *Science* 1991;254:713–716.
15. Helene C, Toulme JJ. Specific regulation of gene expression by antisense, sense and antigene nucleic acids. *Biochim Biophys Acta* 1990;1049:99–125.
16. Obama K, Kanai M, Kawai Y, et al. Role of retinoblastoma protein and E2F-1 transcription factor in the acquisition of 5-fluorouracil resistance by colon cancer cells. *Int J Oncol* 2002;21:309–314.
17. Penolazzi L, Lambertini E, Aguiari G, et al. Cis element 'decoy' against the upstream promoter of the human estrogen receptor gene. *Biochim Biophys Acta* 2000;1492:560–567.
18. Lee YN, Park YG, Choi YH, et al. CRE-transcription factor decoy oligonucleotide inhibition of MCF-7 breast cancer cells: cross-talk with p53 signaling pathway. *Biochemistry* 2000;39:4863–4868.
19. Kawamura I, Morishita R, Tsujimoto S, et al. Intravenous injection of oligodeoxynucleotides to the NF-kappaB binding site inhibits hepatic metastasis of M5076 reticulosarcoma in mice. *Gene Ther* 2001;8:905–912.
20. Gewirtz AM. Myb targeted therapeutics for the treatment of human malignancies. *Oncogene* 1999;18:3056–3062.
21. O'Dwyer PJ, Stevenson JP, Gallagher M, et al. c-raf-1 depletion and tumor responses in patients treated with the c-raf-1 antisense oligodeoxynucleotide ISIS 5132 (CGP 69846A). *Clin Cancer Res* 1999;5:3977–3982.
22. Cunningham CC, Holmlund JT, Geary RS, et al. A Phase I trial of H-*ras* antisense oligonucleotide ISIS 2503 administered as a continuous intravenous infusion in patients with advanced carcinoma. *Cancer* 2001;92:1265–1271.
23. Andrews DW, Resnicoff M, Flanders AE, et al. Results of a pilot study involving the use of an antisense oligodeoxynucleotide directed against the insulin-like growth factor type I receptor in malignant astrocytomas. *J Clin Oncol* 2001;19:2189–2200.
24. Diasio RB, Zhang R. Pharmacology of therapeutic oligonucleotides. *Antisense Nucleic Acid Drug Dev* 1997;7:239–243.
25. Cole-Strauss A, Yoon K, Xiang Y, et al. Correction of the mutation responsible for sickle cell anemia by an RNA-DNA oligonucleotide. *Science* 1996;273:1386–1389.
26. Vasey PA, Shulman LN, Campos S, et al. Phase I trial of intraperitoneal injection of the E1B-55-kd-gene-deleted adenovirus ONYX-015 (dl1520) given on days 1 through 5 every 3 weeks in patients with recurrent/refractory epithelial ovarian cancer. *J Clin Oncol* 2002;20:1562–1569.
27. Petit T, Davidson KK, Cerna C, et al. Efficient induction of apoptosis by ONYX-015 adenovirus in human colon cancer cell lines regardless of p53 status. *Anticancer Drugs* 2002;13:47–50.
28. Geoerger B, Grill J, Opolon P, et al. Oncolytic activity of the E1B-55 kDa-deleted adenovirus ONYX-015 is independent of cellular p53 status in human malignant glioma xenografts. *Cancer Res* 2002;62:764–772.
29. Norman KL, Coffey MC, Hirasawa K, et al. Reovirus oncolysis of human breast cancer. *Hum Gene Ther* 2002;13:641–652.
30. Mineta T, Rabkin SD, Yazaki T, et al. Attenuated multi-mutated herpes simplex virus-1 for the treatment of malignant gliomas. *Nat Med* 1995;1:938–943.
31. Varmus H. Retroviruses. *Science* 1988;240:1427–1435.
32. Donahue RE, Kessler SW, Bodine D, et al. Helper virus induced T cell lymphoma in nonhuman primates after retroviral mediated gene transfer. *J Exp Med* 1992;176:1125–1135.
33. Prince GA, Porter DD, Jenson AB, et al. Pathogenesis of adenovirus type 5 pneumonia in cotton rats (*Sigmodon hispidus*). *J Virol* 1993;67:101–111.
34. Yang Y, Nunes FA, Berencsi K, et al. Cellular immunity to viral antigens

limits E1-deleted adenoviruses for gene therapy. *Proc Natl Acad Sci U S A* 1994;91:4407–4411.
35. Herman JR, Adler HL, Aguilar-Cordova E, et al. In situ gene therapy for adenocarcinoma of the prostate: a phase I clinical trial. *Hum Gene Ther* 1999;10:1239–1249.
36. Zabner J, Ramsey BW, Meeker DP, et al. Repeat administration of an adenovirus vector encoding cystic fibrosis transmembrane conductance regulator to the nasal epithelium of patients with cystic fibrosis. *J Clin Invest* 1996;97:1504–1511.
37. Ilan Y, Prakash R, Davidson A, et al. Oral tolerization to adenoviral antigens permits long-term gene expression using recombinant adenoviral vectors. *J Clin Invest* 1997;99:1098–1106.
38. Dedieu JF, Vigne E, Torrent C, et al. Long-term gene delivery into the livers of immunocompetent mice with E1/E4-defective adenoviruses. *J Virol* 1997;71:4626–4637.
39. Lieber A, He CY, Kay MA. Adenoviral preterminal protein stabilizes mini-adenoviral genomes in vitro and in vivo. *Nat Biotechnol* 1997;15:1383–1387.
40. Parks RJ, Graham FL. A helper-dependent system for adenovirus vector production helps define a lower limit for efficient DNA packaging. *J Virol* 1997;71:3293–3298.
41. O'Neal WK, Zhou H, Morral N, et al. Toxicity associated with repeated administration of first-generation adenovirus vectors does not occur with a helper-dependent vector. *Mol Med* 2000;6:179–195.
42. Schiedner G, Morral N, Parks RJ, et al. Genomic DNA transfer with a high-capacity adenovirus vector results in improved in vivo gene expression and decreased toxicity. *Nat Genet* 1998;18:180–183.
43. Morral N, O'Neal W, Rice K, et al. Administration of helper-dependent adenoviral vectors and sequential delivery of different vector serotype for long-term liver-directed gene transfer in baboons. *Proc Natl Acad Sci U S A* 1999;96:12816–12821.
44. Marshall E. Gene therapy death prompts review of adenovirus vector. *Science* 1999;286:2244–2245.
45. Raper SE, Yudkoff M, Chirmule N, et al. A pilot study of in vivo liver-directed gene transfer with an adenoviral vector in partial ornithine transcarbamylase deficiency. *Hum Gene Ther* 2002;13:163–175.
46. Harvey BG, Maroni J, O'Donoghue KA, et al. Safety of local delivery of low- and intermediate-dose adenovirus gene transfer vectors to individuals with a spectrum of morbid conditions. *Hum Gene Ther* 2002;13:15–63.
47. Crystal RG, Harvey BG, Wisnivesky JP, et al. Analysis of risk factors for local delivery of low- and intermediate-dose adenovirus gene transfer vectors to individuals with a spectrum of comorbid conditions. *Hum Gene Ther* 2002;13:65–100.
48. Teramoto S, Bartlett JS, McCarty D, et al. Factors influencing adeno-associated virus-mediated gene transfer to human cystic fibrosis airway epithelial cells: comparison with adenovirus vectors. *J Virol* 1998;72:8904–8912.
49. Soifer H, Higo C, Kazazian HH, Jr, et al. Stable integration of transgenes delivered by a retrotransposon-adenovirus hybrid vector. *Hum Gene Ther* 2001;12:1417–1428.
50. Ehrhardt A, Kay MA. A new adenoviral helper-dependent vector results in long-term therapeutic levels of human coagulation factor IX at low doses in vivo. *Blood* 2002;99:3923–3930.
51. Bilbao G, Feng M, Rancourt C, et al. Adenoviral/retroviral vector chimeras: a novel strategy to achieve high-efficiency stable transduction in vivo. *FASEB J* 1997;11:624–634.
52. Felgner PL, Ringold GM. Cationic liposome-mediated transfection. *Nature* 1989;337:387–388.
53. Kunisawa J, Nakagawa S, Mayumi T. Pharmacotherapy by intracellular delivery of drugs using fusogenic liposomes: application to vaccine development. *Adv Drug Deliv Rev* 2001;52:177–186.
54. Kaneda Y, Iwai K, Uchida T. Increased expression of DNA cointroduced with nuclear protein in adult rat liver. *Science* 1989;243:375–378.
55. Hortobagyi GN, Ueno NT, Xia W, et al. Cationic liposome-mediated E1A gene transfer to human breast and ovarian cancer cells and its biologic effects: a phase I clinical trial. *J Clin Oncol* 2001;19:3422–3433.
56. Gusterson BA, Gelber RD, Goldhirsch A, et al. Prognostic importance of c-*erb*B-2 expression in breast cancer. International (Ludwig) Breast Cancer Study Group. *J Clin Oncol* 1992;10:1049–1056.
57. Medina-Kauwe LK, Maguire M, Kasahara N, Kedes L. Nonviral gene delivery to human breast cancer cells by targeted Ad5 penton proteins. *Gene Ther* 2001;8:1753–1761.
58. Lohr M, Hummel F, Faulmann G, et al. Microencapsulated, CYP2B1-transfected cells activating ifosfamide at the site of the tumor: the magic bullets of the 21st century. *Cancer Chemother Pharmacol* 2002;49 (suppl 1):S21-S24.
59. Ross G, Erickson R, Knorr D, et al. Gene therapy in the United States: a five-year status report. *Hum Gene Ther* 1996;7:1781–1790.
60. Gollan TJ, Green MR. Selective targeting and inducible destruction of human cancer cells by retroviruses with envelope proteins bearing short peptide ligands. *J Virol* 2002;76:3564–3569.
61. Habib NA, Sarraf CE, Mitry RR, et al. E1B-deleted adenovirus (dl1520) gene therapy for patients with primary and secondary liver tumors. *Hum Gene Ther* 2001;12:219–226.
62. Boehm T, Folkman J, Browder T, O'Reilly MS. Antiangiogenic therapy of experimental cancer does not induce acquired drug resistance. *Nature* 1997;390:404–407.
63. Thomas JW, Kuo MD, Chawla M, et al. Vascular gene therapy. *Radiographics* 1998;18:1373–1394.

CHAPTER 5

REGIONAL PAIN IN THE CANCER PATIENT: INTERVENTIONAL IMAGE-GUIDED PAIN TREATMENT MODALITIES

P. SEBASTIAN THOMAS, MD

SYED I. HOSAIN, MD

KETUL PATEL, MD

CHRISTI A BARBER, ANP

INTRODUCTION

Approximately 75% to 80% of the more than 1 million people diagnosed with cancer each year experience debilitating pain. This pain affects the patients, their families, and their caregivers. The pain may arise from the cancer itself or from the various treatment modalities being applied. It is important to remember that a cancer patient may also experience pain that is completely unrelated to the cancer. As with all pain treatment, the initial step is a thorough assessment that includes a detailed history, physical examination, psychosocial assessment, and diagnostic evaluation.

A very clear and concise guide to the appropriate continuum of pain management for cancer pain is available in *Reference Guide for Clinicians: Management of Cancer Pain: Adults*, published by the U.S. Department of Health and Human Services.[1] A synopsis of this pathway is shown in **Table 5-1**.

For the purpose of this chapter, we focus on five nerve blocks performed with the aid of radiography for the treatment of regional cancer pain. Three primary regions of cancer pain syndromes are the autonomic nervous system, the central nervous system, and the peripheral nervous system. Autonomic nerve blocks include the celiac plexus nerve block, ganglion impar nerve block, and superior hypogastric plexus nerve block. Central nerve blocks include the trigeminal nerve block and glossopharyngeal nerve block. Peripheral nerve blocks include the brachial plexus nerve block and

TABLE 5-1
Management of Cancer Pain in Adults

Step 1. Assessment
Step 2. Diagnosis of cancer pain
Step 3. Initiate the World Health Organization's analgesic ladder
Add as indicated:
- Palliative therapies
  - Radiation therapy
  - Nerve blocks
  - Surgery
  - Antineoplastic therapy
- Adjuvant drugs
- Psychosocial interventions
- Physical modalities

Step 4. Reassessment - if pain persists, then repeat palliative therapies or consider other etiologies and treatments such as
- Unacceptable side effects
- Diffuse bone pain
- Neuropathic pain - peripheral neuropathies, plexopathies, spinal cord compression
  - Adjuvant drugs
  - Options titrated to effect
  - Radiation therapy
  - Spinal opioids with local anesthetics
  - Neurolytic procedures
- Movement related pain
  - Surgical or physical stabilization of affected part
  - Nerve blocks
  - Neuroablative surgery and neurolytic procedure

cervical plexus nerve block. These are examples of specific blocks that may be performed to mediate the pain of each of these three nervous systems.

Radiography is generally not needed as a guide for peripheral nerve blocks, unless tumor growth or surgery grossly distorts the region. In that case, radiography may be needed to locate the precise area of the nerve to be blocked. Because they so rarely require radiography, peripheral nerve blocks are not discussed further in this chapter.

AUTONOMIC NERVOUS SYSTEM

Celiac Plexus Block

Treatment of intractable, intolerable cancer pain arising from the abdominal organs may be treated effectively by the performance of a computed tomography (CT)–guided celiac plexus block. Like any other invasive procedure, this block is performed only in the patient for whom the standard pain management continuum has failed to garner appreciable, lasting relief of pain.[2–4]

Although celiac plexus blockade is employed most commonly for the treatment of pain due to pancreatic cancer, it may also be used for neoplasm of the liver, gallbladder, abdominal viscera, stomach, small bowel, large bowel to the splenic flexure, omentum, biliary tract, spleen, adrenal glands, and kidneys. Pain originating in the autonomic plexuses responds better to opioids than pain due to invasion of a somatic nerve plexus, but the patient usually experiences unrelenting colicky, cramping, dull aching pain that eventually breaks through pharmacological treatment. Once the diagnosis of an abdominal cancer has been made and conservative treatments have failed, the decision is made to attempt a celiac plexus block.

As with all nerve blocks, a diagnostic celiac plexus block should be performed first. This preliminary block is essential both to confirm the actual location of the source of pain and to temporarily eliminate the pain. Profound, short-term relief of the pain experienced is the primary indication for the progression to a CT-guided neurolytic block of the celiac plexus.

Anatomy

The celiac plexus is located anterolateral to the celiac artery and anterior to the aorta. The largest of the three plexuses of the sympathetic nervous system, the celiac plexus innervates the abdominal organs.[5]

Approach and Positioning

The approach chosen depends on the presence and size of a bulky tumor, which would alter normal anatomy and the ability of the patient to maintain positioning on the abdomen. Various approaches are the transaortic, the anterior, and direction of the needle more toward T11 and T12 to provide access to the splanchnic nerves. Most commonly, the patient is placed in the prone position with a pillow under the abdomen (**Fig. 5-1**). The prone position is used for the purpose of this discussion.

Landmarks

With the use of the CT scanner, a lateral scout film is obtained to identify the body of L1. Axial sections are obtained at the level of L1, 0.5 cm cephalad and 0.5 cm caudad, made at the level marked with the CT scanner (**Figs. 5-2 and 5-3**). Once the axial view is completed, the following measurements can be made: *measurement 1,* from the scanner's midline to the needle inser-

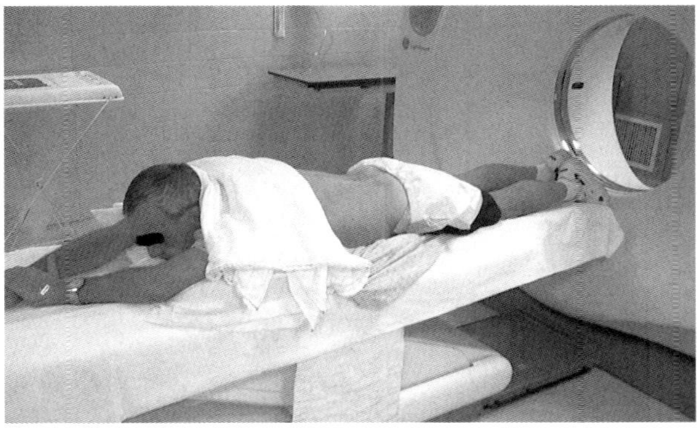

Figure 5-1. Celiac plexus block: Patient in the prone position with pillows under the abdomen.

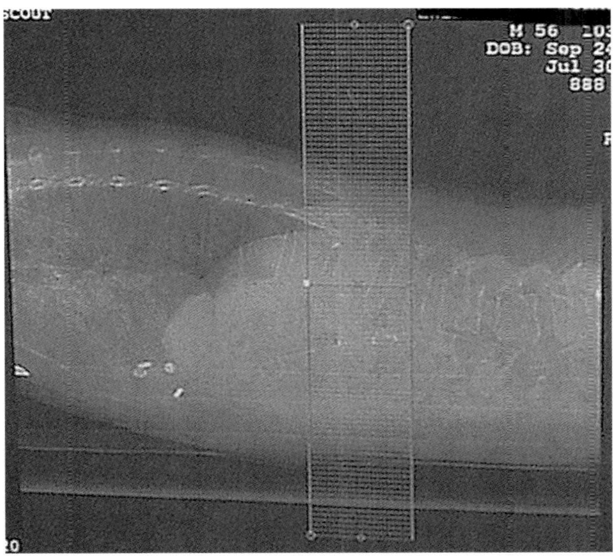

Figure 5-2. Celiac plexus block: Computed tomography scan showing location of the axial slices to be obtained.

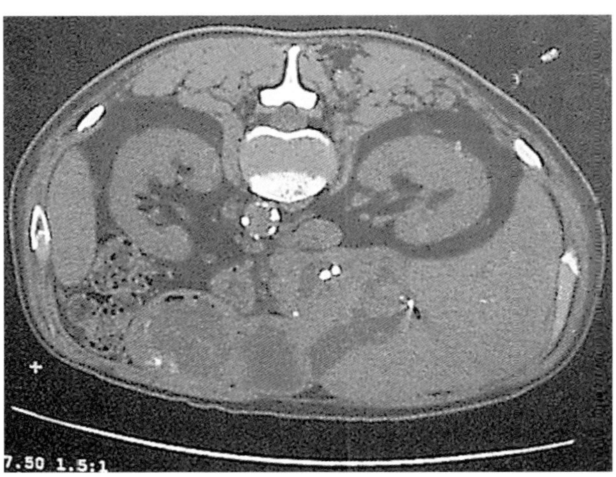

Figure 5-3. Celiac plexus block: Selected axial image.

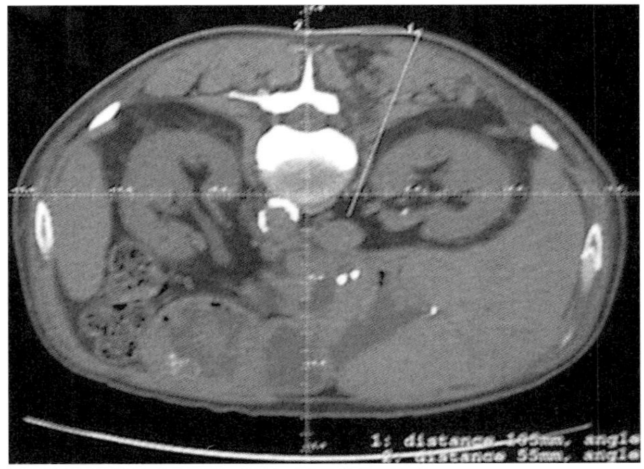

Figure 5-4. Celiac plexus block: Measurements for anticipated path and position of the needle.

tion point; *measurement 2,* from the depth from the needle insertion point to the anterior portion of the vertebral body; and *measurement 3,* of the angle between these lines (**Fig. 5-4**). The CT scanner projects external position marks via laser (**Fig. 5-5**), which denote the scanner's midline and the level of the appropriate transverse section. These landmarks are then marked on the skin with indelible marker.[6, 7]

Procedure

The skin is prepared with an antiseptic solution and draped in routine fashion. With 1% lidocaine, wheals are

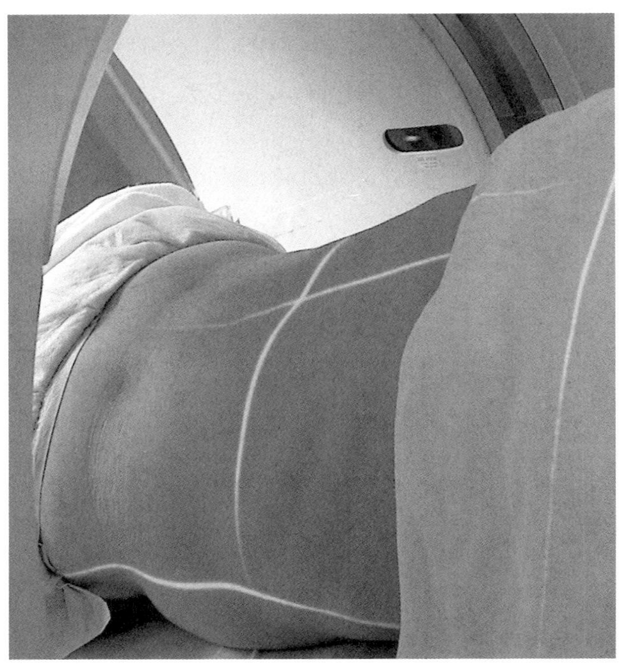

Figure 5-5. Celiac plexus block: External projection via laser.

raised at the distance from the mark derived from measurement 1. A 22-gauge, 6-inch needle is inserted at an angle of 45 degrees to the body of L1. It is then repositioned to the predetermined angle needed (measurement 3) to bypass the vertebra and is inserted to the depth determined from measurement 2 (**Fig. 5-6**). A lateral scout film is taken to determine the location of the tip of the needle. An axial section is then obtained to determine final position of the needle tip (**Fig. 5-7**). After results of aspiration for blood or cerebrospinal fluid (CSF) are found to be negative, a 2–3-mL test dose is injected. This injectate may include radiopaque contrast dye to confirm spread of the injectate as well as the position of the needle.[8–10]

Agents

The local anesthetics most commonly employed in both diagnostic and neurolytic blocks are 2% lidocaine and 0.25%–0.75% bupivacaine. Neurolysis is obtained with the use of 6% phenol or absolute alcohol mixed with local anesthetic to provide a 50%–100% solution of the alcohol. The precision of the CT scanner allows the use of less injectate than with other techniques. A total volume of 30–40 mL, evenly divided between two needles, is needed for bilateral block, and of 15–20 mL for a unilateral block. Alcohol may cause pain upon injection.

A

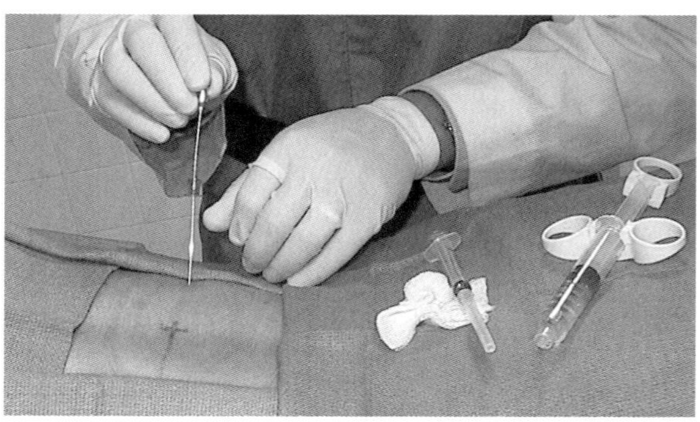

B

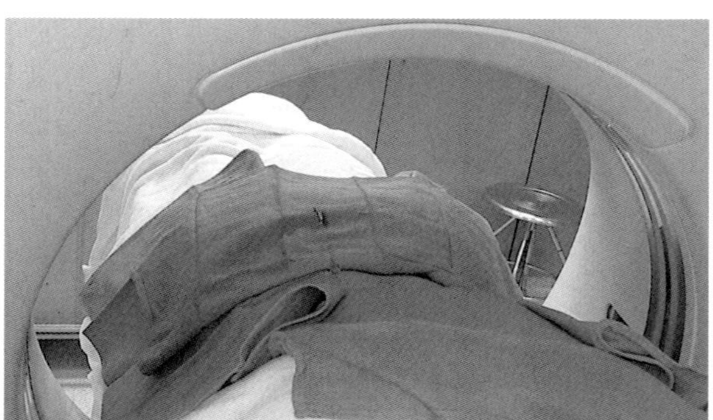

Figure 5-6. (A and B) Celiac plexus block: Insertion of the needle.

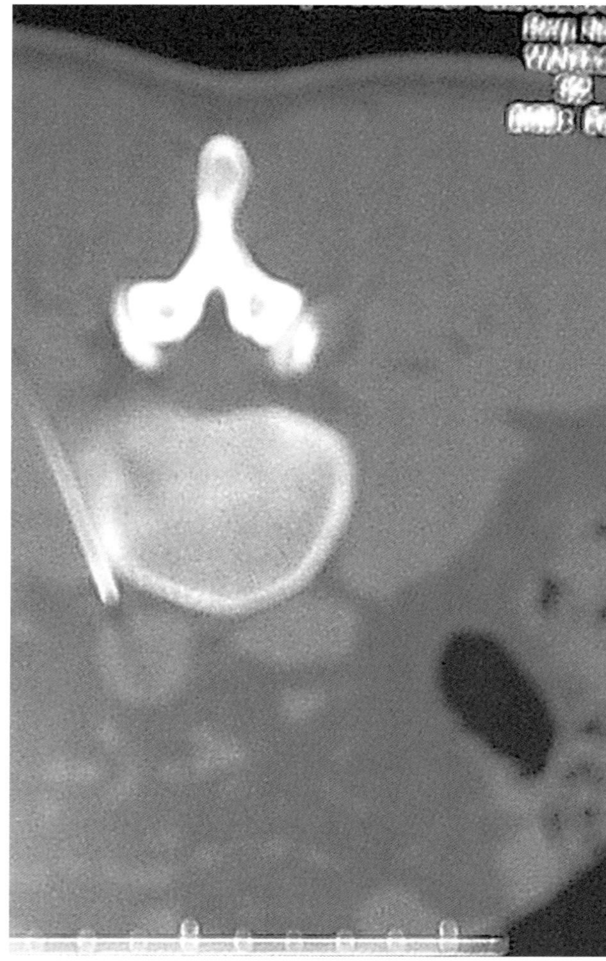

Figure 5-7. Celiac plexus block: Axial image showing final position of the needle tip.

This pain may last beyond the duration of the injection and causes nonselective nervous system tissue damage. This effect may last up to 6 months before nerve regeneration occurs.[11]

Complications

Potential complications arising from celiac plexus block are direct damage during placement of the needle, sympathetic nerve blockade, and damage to any of the surrounding structures by the neurolytic agent itself. Manifestations of these complications include a decrease in blood pressure, pain with injection, diarrhea, excessive bleeding due to puncture of blood vessels, injection into the aorta or inferior vena cava, total spinal paralysis, injury to the kidney or bowel, and possible sexual dysfunction. The celiac plexus block may be repeated within 2–3 months if necessary as the disease progresses.

Ganglion Impar Block

The perineal area may be a source of severe pain in patients with neoplasms of the pelvic organs. In some of these patients, there may be a sympathetic nervous system component to this pain. Sympathetic pain arising in the perineum or anal area is typically described as a vague pain in the perineal area. The pain is often burning in character and may be accompanied by a sense of urgency in the bladder or the rectum. In the past, attempts to treat perineal pain tended to focus on its somatic component. Some of the treatments were destructive of somatic nerve fibers. A new approach developed in the early part of the last decade involves neurolysis of at least one of the sympathetic pathways from the perineum.[12–14] Block of the ganglion impar was first described by Plancarte and colleagues.[15]

Anatomy

The *ganglion impar* is the terminal ganglion of the two lumbar sympathetic chains. The ganglion is a solitary retroperitoneal structure lying at the junction of the lower end of the sacrum and the coccyx. It contains predominantly sympathetic fibers.

Technique and Agents

A modified 22-gauge spinal needle is used to perform the block. The stylet is removed from the needle. The needle is then bent 45 degrees along the axis at a point about 3–4 cm from the tip. This modification allows the needle to be inserted in front of the coccyx and to conform to the curvature of the coccyx so as to reach the coccygeosacral junction. The patient is placed in the lateral decubitus position or the prone position. The area of the natal cleft is carefully cleaned. The anococcygeal ligament and the overlying skin are infiltrated with 1% lidocaine. The specially modified needle is inserted through the anococcygeal ligament in the midline. The concavity of the needle should face posteriorly. The needle is inserted until the tip is just in front of the junction of the coccyx and the sacrum. The needle position is confirmed by injection of 1–2 mL of water-soluble contrast agent (**Fig. 5-8**). The dye should form a smooth contour resembling an apostrophe. Then, 4 mL of local anesthetic, either 0.25% bupivacaine or 1% lidocaine, is injected; 4 mL of 10% aqueous phenol may be injected for neurolysis of the ganglion.

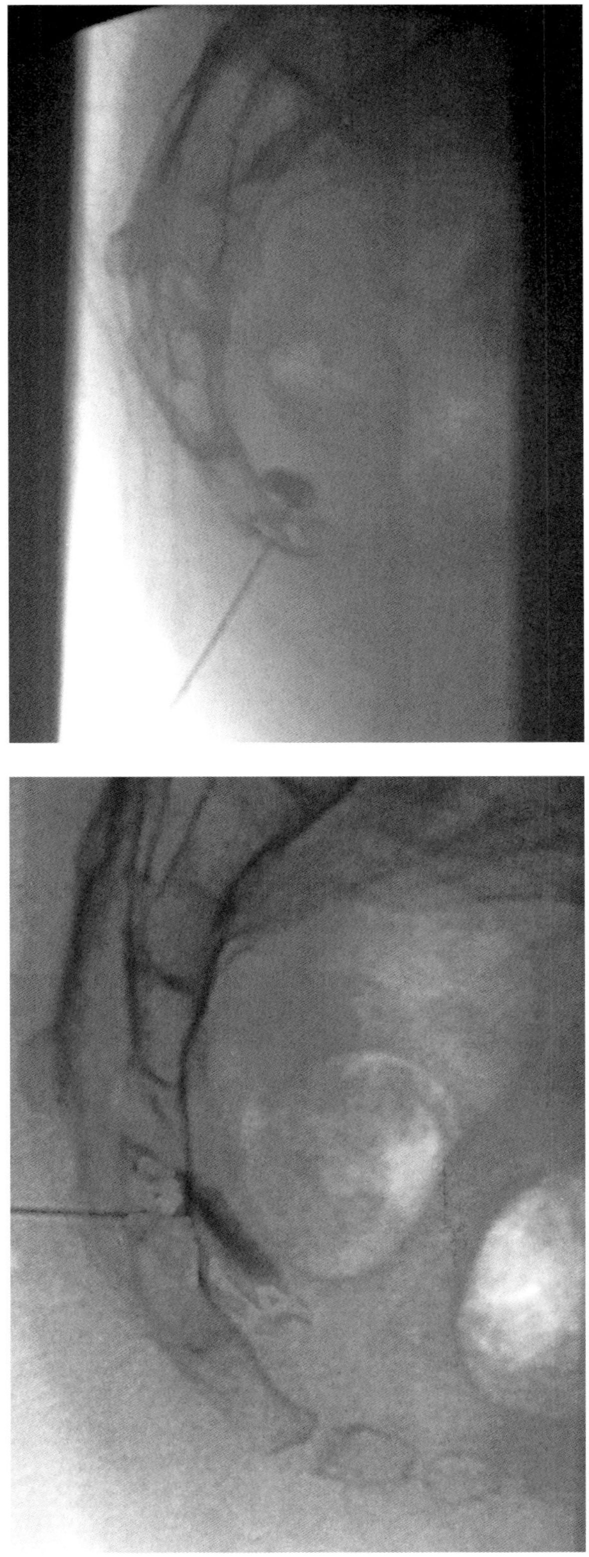

A

B

Figure 5-8. (A and B) Ganglion impar block: Fluoroscopic images showing the classic appearance of the dye as it is injected.

Complications

Possible complications and difficulties associated with ganglion impar block include caudal injection, which results in epidural or spinal anesthesia.

Perforation of the rectum and preinstall injection are also possible.[15]

Superior Hypogastric Plexus Block

The blockade of autonomic nerve pathways was applied widely in the treatment of several chronic pain syndromes. The advantages of not interrupting the motor and somatic pathways and the low risk of neuronal formation helped popularize these techniques. The superior hypogastric plexus forms part of a chain of autonomic plexuses from the cardiac plexus to the ganglion impar. Plancarte and colleagues[15] first described a percutaneous technique for neurolysis of the superior hypogastric plexus in 1990. They treated 28 patients with intractable pain secondary to pelvic neoplasms and reported a 70% reduction in pain.

Anatomy

The superior hypogastric plexus lies in front of the bifurcation of the aorta and overlies the left iliac vein. The plexus is at the anterior border of the lowest lumbar vertebra, the fifth lumbar vertebra, and the promontory, or uppermost portion, of the sacrum. The superior hypogastric plexus is a retroperitoneal structure that may also be referred to as the *presacral nerve*. This description implies that the plexus consists of one single nerve overlying the sacrum, which is not the case. The superior hypogastric plexus is made up by the termination of the two lumbar sympathetic chains. The plexus also receives some parasympathetic fibers from the pelvic organs, although many of these fibers may bypass it. The superior hypogastric plexus gives off two nerves inferiorly, which are referred to as the *inferior hypogastric nerves*. These two nerves go on to form the inferior hypogastric plexus, which lies on either side of the rectum and the lower part of the bladder. Because of its anatomic position, the inferior hypogastric plexus is not amenable to surgical ablation or percutaneous neurolysis.

Indications

Neoplasm of the pelvic organs associated with intractable pain is the indication for blockade and subsequent neurolysis of the superior hypogastric plexus. Conservative measures must be tried and must have failed to relieve the patient's pain before one resorts to neurolysis of any plexus in the body. Other invasive measures used to fight cancer pain include implantation of intrathecal and epidural opiate delivery systems. These techniques may be especially useful in patients in whom the neoplasm has spread beyond the territory innervated by the superior hypogastric plexus. Such spread is not uncommon in female patients with gynecological neoplasm.[16]

Technique

The technique of superior hypogastric plexus block involves placing a needle into a narrow window between the transverse process of the L5 vertebra and the anterior rim of the ilium. Intravenous access should be established before this block is attempted, because of the proximity of vascular structures and the spinal nerve roots and their meninges. This block should not be attempted without the aid of fluoroscopy or CT scanning.

The patient is positioned on the procedure table in the prone position. Pillows or padding are placed under the patient's pelvis. Enough padding is required to flatten the normal lumbar lordosis. The skin of the lumbosacral area is widely cleaned on both sides of the midline and then draped with sterile towels. The posterior superior iliac crests are identified on either side of the midline, and a line is drawn through the most apical part of the crests. This line corresponds approximately to the L4–L5 interspace (**Fig. 5-9**). The line is confirmed fluoroscopically, and a point approximately 5–7 cm from the midline is marked on either side; these are the entry points for the needles. Wheals are raised with lidocaine, and subcutaneous infiltration is performed.

The needles are inserted one at a time at an angle of 45 degrees to the coronal plane. Each needle should also point caudad approximately 30–40 degrees toward the anterolateral edge of the inferior part of the L5 vertebra.

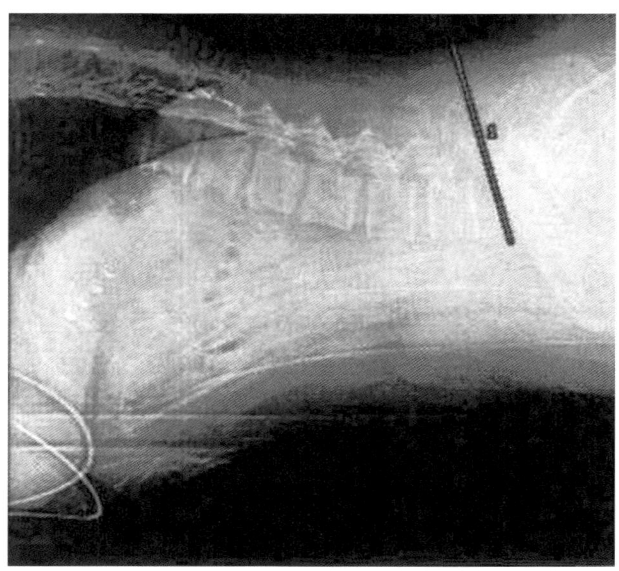

Figure 5-9. Superior hypogastric plexus block: Scout film showing marker denoting appropriate needle route.

The transverse process of L5 may be encountered superficially, in which case the needle should be directed slightly more caudad. The iliac crest may also necessitate a more medial starting point for the needle. The position of the needle should be confirmed frequently by biplane fluoroscopy (**Fig. 5-10**). Anteroposterior and lateral images will help to guide needle positioning. The needle should be gradually walked off the anterolateral aspect of the L5 vertebra and then advanced about 1 cm farther so as to penetrate the anterior fascial boundary of the psoas muscle. Injection of neurolytic agent into the psoas muscle could have devastating consequences because of the lumbar plexus. The use of a depth marker attached to the needle may facilitate judgment as to how much farther the needle should be inserted after it makes contact with the vertebral body.

When the position of the needle appears satisfactory on biplane views, the position is confirmed by the injection of water-soluble contrast agent; a volume of 2–5 mL on each side is sufficient (**Fig. 5-11A**). In the anteroposterior view, the contrast agent forms a patch confined to the paramedian aspect of the vertebral column. A sharp linear outline implies injection into the psoas muscle. In the lateral view, a smooth contour forms just anterior to the body of L5 and part of S1.[8, 17–22] **Figure 5-12** illustrates the final position of the needle when the procedure is performed with CT guidance.

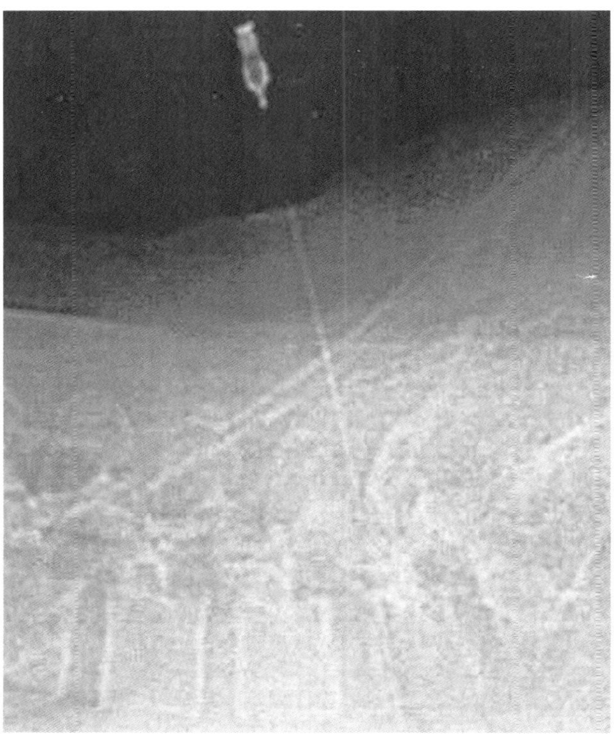

Figure 5-10. Superior hypogastric plexus block: Scout film showing needle position.

A

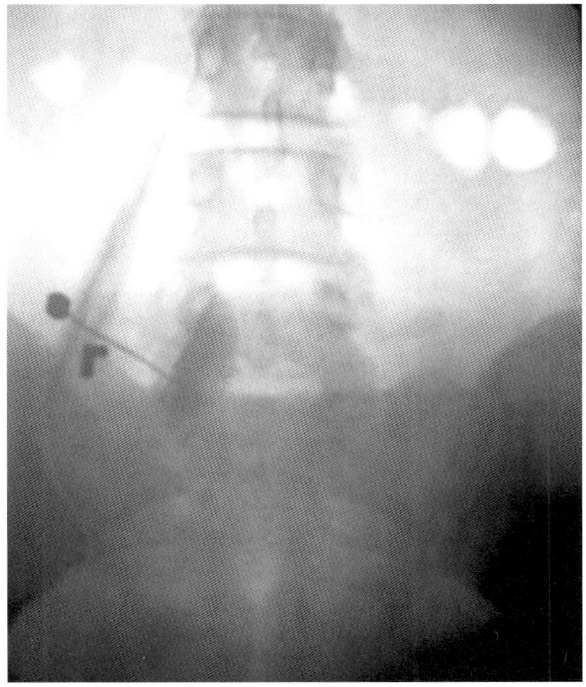

B

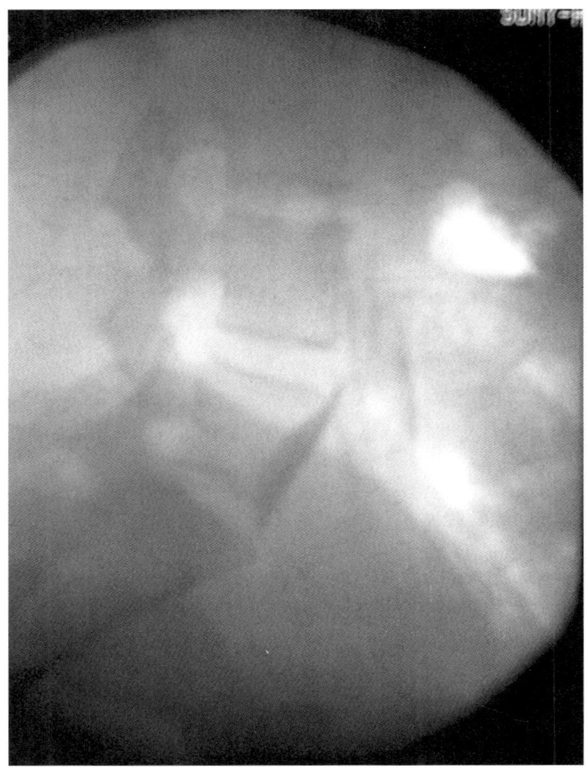

Figure 5-11. (A and B) Superior hypogastric plexus block: Fluoroscopic images showing needle position and the classic appearance of the dye as it is injected.

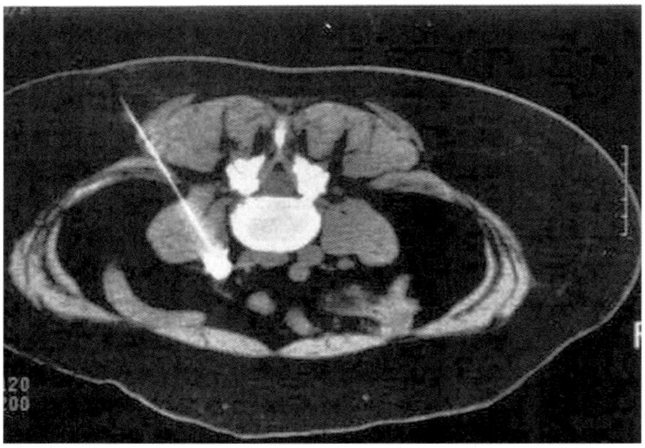

Figure 5-12. Superior hypogastric plexus block: Computed tomography scan with dye confirming the final needle position.

Agents

For diagnostic blockade prior to neurolysis, 8–10 mL of 0.25% bupivacaine or 1% lidocaine is satisfactory on each side. For neurolysis, an aqueous solution of 10% phenol, 8–10 mL on each side, is used.

Complications

The complications of superior hypogastric plexus block are somatic nerve trauma, intravascular injection, intrathecal and epidural injection, trauma to the ureters, intramuscular injection, and intraperitoneal injection.[23]

CENTRAL NERVOUS SYSTEM

Trigeminal Nerve Block

If facial pain arises from the diagnosis of tumor invasion into the trigeminal ganglion, the pain may respond well to a trigeminal nerve block. Because the anatomy of the trigeminal ganglion is quite complex and adjacent structures are in very close proximity, the use of fluoroscopy is highly recommended.

Anatomy

The trigeminal ganglion is located within Meckel's cave,[6] within the apex of the petrous bone. The structures lying in close proximity are the internal carotid artery, the posterior cavernous sinus (which contains the third, fourth, fifth, and sixth cranial nerves), the temporal lobe, the arch of the zygoma, and a fold of dura contained within Meckel's cave that contains CSF. It is obvious that any damage to these structures would be detrimental. **Figure 5-13** illustrates the location of the foramen ovale.

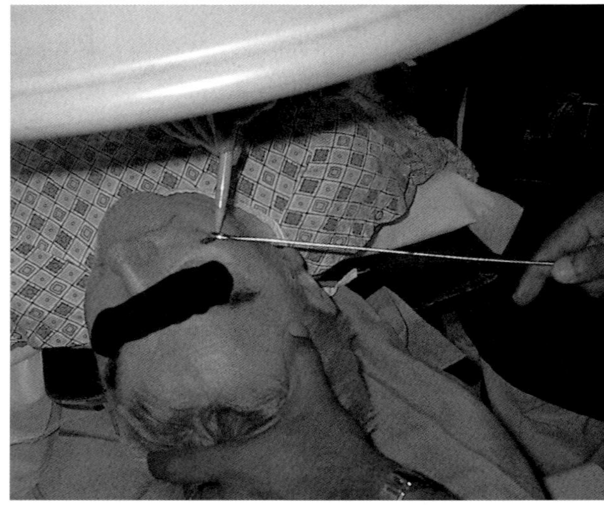

Figure 5-13. Trigeminal nerve block: External marker showing foramen ovale.

Technique

The patient is placed supine on the fluoroscopy table. Scout films should be obtained in the modified Water's view and in the submentovertex view to ensure correct location of the foramen ovale (**Fig. 5-14**). The needle will enter in the cheek above the second molar. A 22-gauge, 8-cm needle is inserted in line with the pupil and toward the midpoint of the zygomatic arch (**Fig. 5-15**). Viewing of the fluoroscopic images commonly shows that the needle must be redirected more laterally

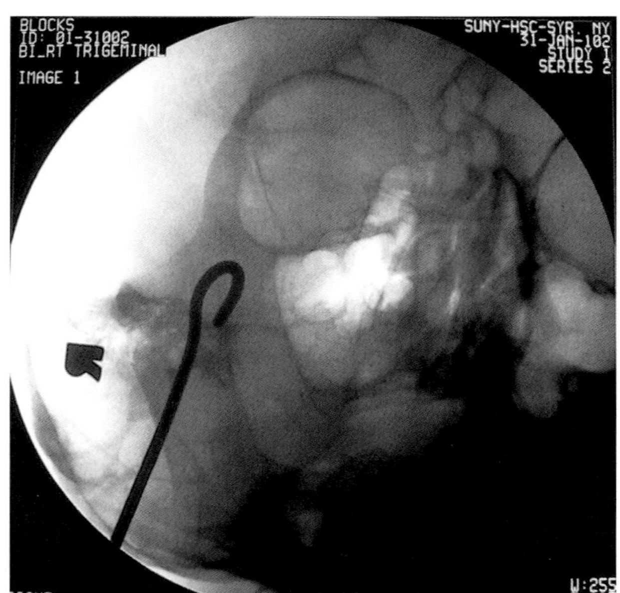

Figure 5-14. Trigeminal nerve block: Fluoroscopic image showing correct positioning of the external marker.

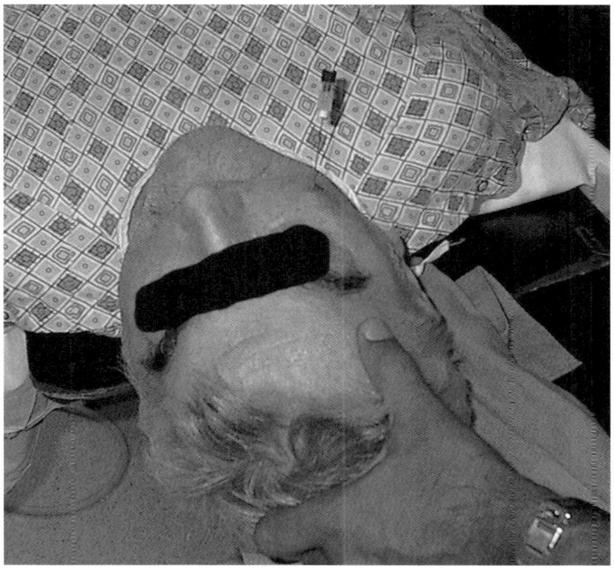

Figure 5-15. Trigeminal nerve block: Placement of the needle.

and less cephalad. Paresthesias may be elicited and are useful in judging the depth of the needle as it is passed into Meckel's cave (**Fig. 5-16**). Aspiration for CSF and blood should be performed to rule out misplacement of the needle. For a diagnostic trigeminal block, 0.25% bupivacaine is most commonly employed. If the patient's pain is reduced or eradicated, the appropriate effect will be achieved by the therapeutic block. A neurolytic agent such as alcohol or phenol may be injected to achieve a nerve block of much longer duration.[8, 24, 25]

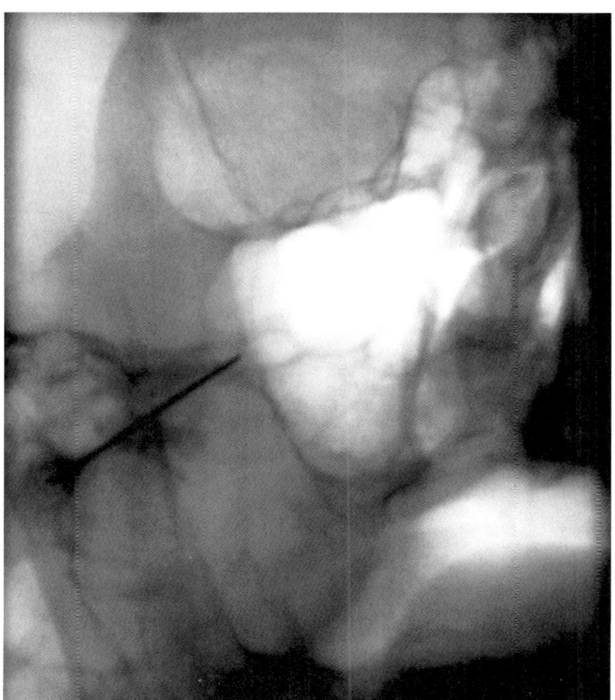

Figure 5-16. Trigeminal nerve block: Image showing needle in the foramen ovale.

Complications

As mentioned previously, the close proximity of the internal carotid artery, cranial nerves, and CSF to the superior hypogastric plexus requires precise placement of the needle and the injectate. Any misplacement of injectate intravascularly or intrathecally could necessitate cardiorespiratory support. Damage to the cranial nerves might cause unconsciousness. Misapplication of the neurolytic agents could result in anesthesia dolorosa. Other complications are trigeminal motor weakness, keratitis, and corneal ulceration.

Glossopharyngeal Nerve Block

Pain described as sharp and burning in the oropharynx and radiating to one or both ears may be an indication of pharyngeal or laryngeal cancer. The CT-guided glossopharyngeal block is an important tool in the armamentarium of pain specialists. Depending on the results of a diagnostic block of the glossopharyngeal nerve, either a neurolytic block or surgical decompression is performed to relieve the patient's pain.[26, 27]

Anatomy

The glossopharyngeal nerve comes through the jugular foramen along with the vagus nerve, the internal jugular vein, and the spinal accessory nerve. It lies along the posterior and medial aspect of the styloid process, lateral to the internal carotid artery. The glossopharyngeal nerve innervates the posterior third of the tongue, oropharynx, epiglottis, fauces, and pharynx. As with the trigeminal nerve block, the close proximity of these structures suggests that radiologic guidance would serve to ensure a safer and more effective glossopharyngeal nerve block.[28]

Technique

The patient lies supine on the table with the head tilted so that the affected side is up. The area of needle placement is midway along a line drawn from the angle of the mandible to the mastoid process. The patient is moved into the CT scanner, and this midpoint is localized (**Fig. 5-17**). A scout film is then taken to define the glossopharyngeal nerve—specifically, its position in relation to the styloid process. A blunt, beveled, 22-gauge needle is then placed at a distance halfway to the nerve.

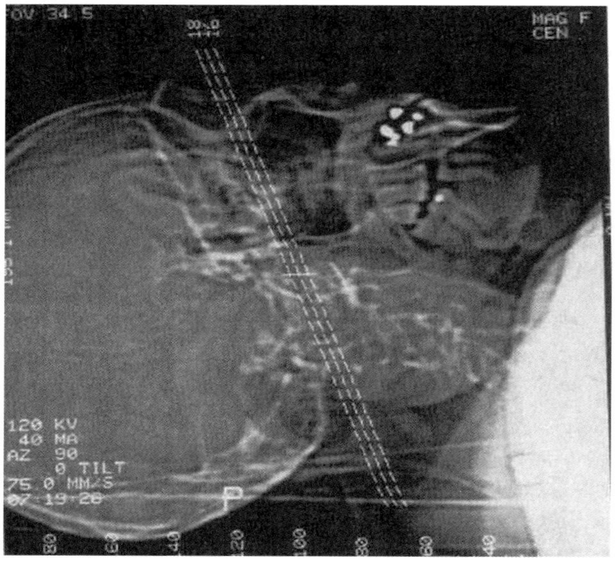

Figure 5-17. Glossopharyngeal nerve block: Selected axial cuts.

CT scanning is repeated to guide the direction and depth of the needle (1–3 cm from the skin) as well as its proximity and posterior relation to the styloid process (**Fig. 5-18**). Radiopaque dye is then injected to determine spread of the injectate; then the anesthetic agent is injected until the patient reports the desired relief. The amount injected is usually 0.5 to 1 mL.[29]

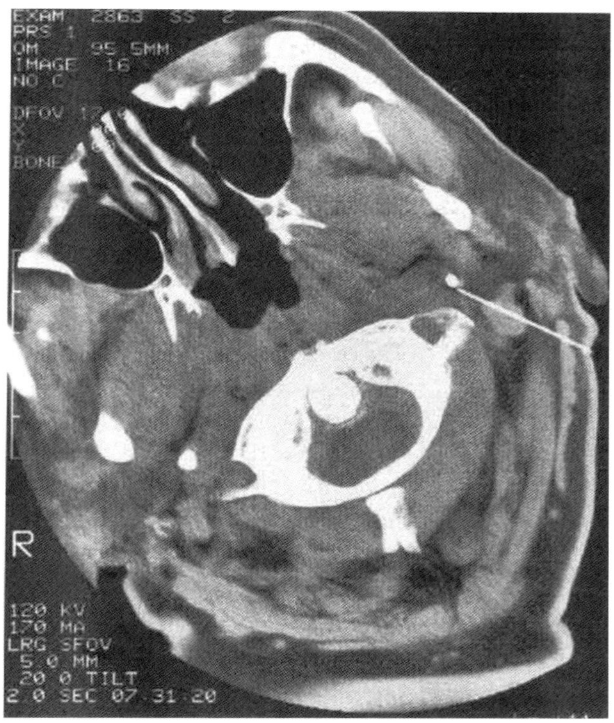

Figure 5-18. Glossopharyngeal nerve block: Final needle position near the styloid process.

Complications

Expected effects of glossopharyngeal nerve block that should be explained to the patient before the procedure are probable hoarseness and decreases in blood pressure and heart rate. Because of the latter two effects, bilateral procedures would pose too great a risk to the patient and should not be performed. Intravascular injection and tissue necrosis may occur with more frequency if the procedure is performed without CT guidance. The CT guidance allows for the use of far less injectate, which in turn decreases the potential for adverse effects.

REFERENCES

1. U. S. Department of Health and Human Services, Public Health Services, Agency for Health Care Policy and Research Executive Office Center Suite 501, 2101 East Jefferson Street, Rockville Maryland, 20850. *Reference Guide for Clinicians: Management of Cancer Pain: Adults*.
2. Bridenbaugh LD, Moore DC, Campbell DD. Management of upper abdominal cancer pain treatment with celiac plexus block with alcohol. *JAMA* 1964;190:877–880.
3. Brown DL. A retrospective analysis of neurolytic celiac plexus block for nonpancreatic intra-abdominal cancer pain. *Reg Anesth* 1989;14:63.
4. Brown DL, Bulley TK, Uiel EL. Neurolytic celiac plexus block for pancreatic cancer pain. *Anesth Analg* 1987;66:869–873.
5. Filshie J, Golding S, Robbie DS, et al. Unilateral computerized tomography guided celiac plexus block: A technique for pain relief. *Anesthesia* 1983;38:498–503.
6. Gray H. *Anatomy, Descriptive and Surgical*. 15th ed. New York: Bounty Books; 1977.
7. Hegedus V. Relief of pancreatic pain by radiography-guided block. *Am J Roentgenol* 1979;133:1101–1103.
8. Thomas PS. *Image-Guided Pain Management*. Philadelphia: Lippincott-Raven; 1997.
9. Raj PP. *Practical Management of Pain*. 2nd ed. St Louis: Mosby Year Book; 1992.
10. Thompson GE, Moore DC, Bridenbaugh LD, Artin RY. Abdominal pain and alcoholic celiac plexus nerve block. *Anesth Analg* 1977;56:1–5.
11. Jones J, Gough D. Coeliac plexus block with alcohol for relief of upper abdominal pain due to cancer. *Ann R Coll Surg Engl* 1977;59:46–49.
12. Patt RB, Reddy SK, Black RG. Neural blockade for abdominopelvic pain of oncologic origin. *Int Anesthesiol Clin* 1998;36:87–104.
13. Rigor BM Sr. Pelvic cancer pain. *J Surg Oncol* 2000;75:280–300.
14. Yeo SN, Chong JL. A case report on the treatment of intractable anal pain from metastatic carcinoma of the cervix. *Ann Acad Med Singapore* 2001;30:632–635.
15. Plancarte R, Amescua C, Pratt RB, et al. Presacral blockade of the ganglion of Walther (ganglion impar). *Anesthesiology* 1990;73:A751.
16. Plancarte R, DeLeon-Casasola OA, El-Helaly M, Allende S, Lema MJ. Neurolytic superior hypogastric plexus block for chronic pelvic pain associated with cancer. *Reg Anesth* 1997;22:562–568.
17. DeLeon-Casasola OA, Kent E, Lema MJ. Neurolytic superior hypogastric plexus block for chronic pelvic pain associated with cancer. *Pain* 1993;54;145–151.
18. Orlandini G. Selection of patients undergoing neurolytic superior hypogastric plexus block. *Pain*1994;56:121;discussion 122.
19. Cariati M, DeMartini G, Pretolesi F, Roy MT. CT-guided superior hypogastric plexus block. *J Comput Assist Tomogr* 2002;26:428–431.
20. Chan WS, Peh WC, Ng KF, Tsui SL, Yang JC. Computed tomography scan-guided neurolytic superior hypogastric block complicated by

somatic nerve damage in a severely kyphoscoliotic patient. *Anesthesiology* 1997;86:1429–1430.

21. Kanazi CE, Perkins FM, Thakur R, Dorson E. New technique for superior hypogastric plexus block. *Reg Anesth Pain Med* 1999;24:473–476.
22. DeLeon-Casasola OA, Plancarte-Sanchez R, Patt RB, Lema MJ. Superior hypogastric plexus block using a single needle and computed tomography guidance. *Reg Anesth* 1993;18:63.
23. Stevens DS, Balatbat GR, Lee FM. Coaxial imaging technique for superior hypogastric plexus block. *Reg Anesth Pain Med* 2000;25:643–647.
24. Bonica JJ, Buckley FP, Moricca G, Murphy TM. Gasserian ganglion block in neurolytic blockade and hypophysectomy. In: Bonica JJ, Loesser JD Chapman CR, Fordyce WE, eds. *The Management of Pain*, 2nd ed. Malvern, Pa: Lea & Febiger; 1990.
25. Warwick R, Williams PL, eds. The Trigeminal Nerve in Neurology. Gray's Anatomy, 35th ed. Edinburgh: Longman Group; 1978.
26. Murphy TM. Somatic blockade of head and neck. In: Cousins MJ, Bridenbaugh PO, eds. Neural Blockade in Clinical Anesthesia and Management of Pain, 2nd ed. Philadelphia: JB Lippincott; 1988:533–558.
27. Waldman SD, Wilson WL, Kreps RD. Superior hypogastric plexus block using a single needle and computed tomography guidance: description of a modified technique. *Reg Anesth* 1991;16:286–287.
28. Bonica JJ. Local anesthesia and regional blocks. In: Wall PD, Melzack R, eds. *Textbook of Pain*. London: Churchill Livingstone; 1984.
29. Fagius J, Wallin BG, Sundlof G, Nerhed C, Englesson S. Sympathetic outflow in man after anaesthesia of the glossopharyngeal and vagus nerves. *Brain* 1985;108:423–438.

CHAPTER 6

PERTINENT PATIENT MANAGEMENT ISSUES

FRANCIS J. MANGIACAPRA, MD
KENNETH D. MURPHY, MD

INTRODUCTION

Interventional radiologists play an important role in the diagnosis and treatment of patients with cancer. However, such patients usually present with a complex set of medical problems, whether from their underlying disease or from the consequences of the treatments that they are receiving. These problems may require special attention from any provider of medical care to patients with cancer. The interventional radiologist should understand these issues and should serve as a front-line provider of the care given these patients to help minimize potential complications. This chapter discusses some of the issues that must be addressed in the total care of the patient with cancer.

NAUSEA AND VOMITING

Nausea and vomiting constitute a common symptom in the oncologic patient population. Nausea and vomiting can result from the malignant disease, medications, or procedures associated with a patient's clinical state.[1, 2] The possible consequences of not controlling the nausea and vomiting induced by cancer treatment are medical complications such as malnutrition, electrolyte abnormalities, delay in treatment for the primary problem, and a diminished quality of life. The results of vomiting include fatigue, muscle strain, esophageal tears, gastric herniation, dental erosions, aspiration, and purpura. Electrolyte abnormalities occur from losses of sodium and potassium that accompany the loss of gastric acid. Finally, the fear and discomfort engendered by these sequelae lead to an aversion to food, which compounds the problem of malnutrition.

The drugs given to patients with cancer may cause nausea, especially opiates prescribed for pain relief. This issue may be problematic, in the sense that it is a complex circle to break: the patient with pain may require higher doses of narcotics, which may induce or worsen nausea, resulting in a different form of discomfort. In addition to opiates, chemotherapy (especially regimens containing cisplatin) may induce nausea. Patients undergoing tumor embolization procedures such as hepatic chemoembolization may have nausea related to postembolization syndrome[3]; however, the effect of the chemotherapy agent itself should always be considered.

It is important not to neglect the treatment of nausea. Initial patient therapy for postprocedure nausea may be managed with oral prochlorperazine [Compazine]; however, patients may not tolerate oral medications, and rectal suppositories may be more effective. Effecting serotonin or 5-hydroxytryptamine type 3 (5-HT3) antagonism through the type 3 serotonin receptor is an important approach in controlling chemotherapy-induced emesis. Agents such as ondansetron (Zofran), which are selective type 3 serotonin receptor antagonists, are more effective than prochlorperazine in controlling chemotherapy-induced nausea. Certain procedures, such as hepatic chemoembolization, require aggressive antiemetic treatment. At our institution, we use ondansetron, 4 to 8 mg intravenously (IV) as a premedication for the procedure and then 4 to 8 mg IV every 8 hours as needed until discharge the next day. We also give an outpatient prescription for nausea control to use as needed.

PAIN MANAGEMENT

Pain in the patient with cancer can be multifactorial. The patient may have pain related directly to the tumor and its mass effect as well as to capsular distention or adjacent compression of organs. If there is metastatic disease with bony involvement, the patient may experience chronic bone pain. The interventional radiologist should be concerned about positioning such a patient for procedures to minimize the distress from the procedure. Positioning is also important with respect to patients with bone metastasis, who are susceptible to pathologic fractures.

Patients who are receiving long-term opiate therapy for pain control may have a higher threshold for pain medications. For most interventional procedures, sedation and analgesia with intravenous midazolam [Versed] (1–2 mg IV) and fentanyl (25–50 μg IV) may be adequate; however, a particular patient's tolerance to narcotics may necessitate higher doses to achieve comfort. As with any procedure performed with the use of moderate sedation, preprocedural assessment of the patient is important to evaluate the anticipated analgesic needs and the potential risks of higher levels of analgesia. Continuous monitoring of the patient during and after the procedure is necessary to ensure safety and comfort.

Because most of the sedative and analgesic agents given during the procedure are short acting, postprocedure analgesia should address both the procedural pain and any chronic pain issues. Patients receiving opiates should be asked about their bowel habits, because constipation is a common problem with opiate administration. At our institution, the hospital pain service is usually consulted, especially after tumor embolization, to provide patients with patient-controlled anesthesia (PCA) intravenous pumps. Also, use of nonsteroidal anti-inflammatory drugs (NSAIDs) (e.g., Toradol), especially those supposed to cause fewer gastrointestinal side effects, may help control postembolization pain.

VENOUS ACCESS

Interventional radiologists are increasingly seeing patients for placement of venous access devices, whether peripherally inserted central catheters (PICCs), subcutaneous ports, or tunneled central venous catheters. The interventional radiologist not only must be skilled in the placement of these devices but also must be able to manage problems associated with them and to treat the complications that arise from their use. Patients also must receive education about the proper care of these devices, to reduce the incidence of device-related complications.

The patient should be assessed for any potential problems in obtaining central venous access. In patients who have undergone chemotherapy through peripheral access, it may be difficult to place PICCs. A PICC may be a useful route for chemotherapy, and its placement under ultrasound guidance enables some patients with difficult superficial veins to obtain longer-term central venous access. Devices that have already been placed in the subclavian vein, or that are still placed there, may occlude central venous vessels.

Placement of subcutaneous chest ports in the interventional radiology suite is as effective as placement of such devices in the conventional operating room.[4] An added benefit of performing the placement in the interventional suite is the superior image guidance available during puncture and insertion of the catheter. Also, it may be easier to schedule port insertions for the interventional radiology suite, in most cases on the next day, than for most operating rooms, with their full schedules.

The preferred site for venous access, whether for a port or a tunneled central venous catheter, is the internal jugular vein (IJV).[5] Using the right IJV avoids possible injury to the thoracic duct.[6] However, choice of the most appropriate site must include consideration of the location of the tumor and of prior surgical procedures. This issue is especially important for patients with breast or lung cancer, in whom local irradiation may also impede wound healing. At our institution, all patients who will receive tunneled or completely subcutaneous devices receive preprocedural antibiotics; we usually use cefazolin 1 gm IV or, for the patient with penicillin allergy, clindamycin 600 mg IV. After placement of a chest or arm port, the patient is usually discharged with a prescription for dicloxacillin, 250 mg qid × 5 days. Our patients receive a follow-up appointment with an interventional radiologist about 1 week after placement of subcutaneous devices, to ensure that incisions are well healed without evidence of infection. This issue is especially important for patients with cancer, who may be immunocompromised; many patients may also have delayed wound healing secondary to chemotherapy and malnutrition.

Finally, knowing what the venous access device is to be used for is also important in the planning stage. Occasionally, we have observed patients whose ports were used for chemotherapy and then as access for total parenteral nutrition; one such patient experienced a port infection, which required explantation of the port, subsequent wound packing, and antibiotic therapy until the site healed.

ANTIBIOTICS

Antibiotic coverage for interventional procedures is especially important in patients with cancer, who may be immunocompromised or may soon start therapy that will reduce their ability to fight infection. Antibiotics should be administered within 2 hours of the procedure. The choice of antibiotics should be made with respect to the pathogen likely to be encountered.[7] For most percutaneous procedures in which a stent or central line is being placed, coverage for *Staphylococcus* species with cefazolin may be adequate. Patients with a true penicillin allergy may require clindamycin IV. Patients with gastrointestinal malignancies that result in biliary obstruction require coverage for gram-negative flora with third-generation cephalosporins or fluoroquinolones such as levofloxacin.

TUMOR FEVER

Fever is an increase in the body temperature above the daily variation of lower temperatures in the morning and higher temperatures in the afternoon. Fever can be indicative of acute or chronic disease. In oncologic patients, the presence of fever has to be evaluated in the context of the underlying disease. Even in this patient population, the majority of fevers are caused by infectious agents; however, in some solid tumors, fever is a sign or a presenting feature.

Fever arising solely as a manifestation of malignancy is termed *neoplastic fever*. The mechanism of neoplastic fever involves pyrogenic cytokines produced by host macrophages in response to tumor or, in some circumstances, by the tumor itself. The pyrogenic cytokines are tumor necrosis factor, interleukins 1 and 6, and interferon. The cytokines stimulate production of prostaglandins, which enter the circulation and induce changes at the hypothalamic thermoregulatory center, resulting in fever. Examples of known malignant cells that produce pyrogenic cytokines are renal cell carcinoma, lymphomas, and acute and chronic myelogenous leukemias.

Tumor fever must be a consideration for the interventional radiologist managing a patient with cancer. Fever may result in delay or cancellation of an interventional radiology procedure or may serve as a marker of a procedural complication. For example, it is not uncommon for patients to have low-grade fever after hepatic chemoembolization. The fever may be due in part to embolization-induced tumor necrosis and release of tumor necrosis factor, although infectious causes must always be considered and sought in the context of clinical presentation.

In general, antipyretics reduce fever regardless of its cause; some studies also suggest that tumor fever is preferentially reduced by NSAIDs.[8] On the basis of small studies, the use of naproxen, an NSAID, has been proposed as a useful test to discriminate between neoplastic fever and infectious fever. The mechanism of this agent's pathway and its inhibition of tumor fever remain undescribed. Other studies suggest that naproxen effectively reduces fever of both tumor and infectious causes. Larger studies are necessary to validate the "naproxen test" as a marker for fever.[9]

THROMBOCYTOPENIA

Patients presenting for interventional radiology procedures may be thrombocytopenic because of either chemotherapy or an underlying disease state. For most venous procedures, such as subcutaneous port placement, a platelet count of about 50,000 cells/dL is usually acceptable. PICCs may be placed under ultrasound guidance in patients with platelet counts as low as 15,000 to 20,000 cells/dL. Patients who need platelet transfusion prior to interventional procedures may require leukodepleted irradiated platelets. Planning with the hospital blood bank, hematologist, oncologist, or all three may be necessary to achieve a safe platelet count for the procedure.

The interventional radiologist should also be aware of iatrogenic causes of thrombocytopenia, especially if the patient is undergoing heparin therapy. In this case, fastidious attention to medications given before and after the procedure is necessary.

PSYCHOLOGICAL STATE OF THE PATIENT

In addition to all of the complexity of cancer treatment regimens, the patient with cancer may have been diagnosed with cancer only recently and so has not yet accepted the condition. Such a patient has probably encountered many different specialists, all telling him or her about new procedures and drugs. The patient may be suffering from anxiety about lack of information or may be unable to cope with the effects of the cancer diagnosis on relationships with family and friends. Patients may also feel a major financial disruption because of the illness.

Cancer centers and community hospitals alike usually have multidisciplinary groups to offer psychosocial services and maintain staff awareness of these issues in patient care. Support groups for patients with specific types of cancer may help patients address similar concerns or experiences. The goal is to improve the psychological well-being and quality of life of all patients with cancer.[10, 11]

REFERENCES

1. Andrews PLR, Sanger GJ. The problem of emesis in anti-cancer therapy: an introduction. In: *Emesis in Anti-Cancer Therapy—Mechanisms and Treatment*. London, New York: Chapman and Hall; 1993.
2. Berger AM, Clark-Snow RA. Adverse effects of treatment. In: *Cancer: Principles and Practice of Oncology, 5th Edition*. Philadelphia: Lippincott-Raven; 1997;2705–2714.
3. Leung DA, Goin JE, Sickles C, Raskay BJ, Soulin MC. Determinants of postembolization syndrome after hepatic chemoembolization. *J Vasc Interv Radiol* 2001;12:321–326.
4. Funaki B, Szymski GX, Hackworth CA, et al. Radiologic placement of subcutaneous infusion chest ports for long-term central venous access. *Am J Roentgenol* 1997;169:1431–1434.
5. Gordon AC, Saliken JC, Johns D, Owen R, Gray RR. US-guided puncture of the internal jugular vein: complications and anatomic considerations. *J Vasc Interv Radiol* 1998;9:333–338.
6. Kwon SS, Falk A, Mitty HA. Thoracic duct injury associated with left internal jugular vein catheterization: anatomic considerations. *J Vasc Interv Radiol* 2002;13:337–339.
7. McDermott VG, Schuster MG, Smith TP. Antibiotic prophylaxis in vascular and interventional radiology. *Am J Roentgenol* 1997;169:31–38.
8. Dinarello CA, Bunn PA. Fever. *Semin Oncol* 1997;24:288–298.
9. Johnson M. Neoplastic fever. *Palliat Med* 1998;12:208–209.
10. Holland JC. Improving the human side of cancer care: psycho-oncology's contribution. *Cancer J* 2001;7:458–471.
11. Holland JC. History of Psycho-oncology: overcoming attitudinal and conceptual barriers. *Psychosom Med* 2002;64:206–221.

CHAPTER 7

DIAGNOSTIC DILEMMAS: ALGORITHMS FOR NON-INVASIVE IMAGING OF HEPATIC MASSES

RANDALL M. PATTEN, MD

The differential diagnosis of a hepatic mass is broad, encompassing both primary and secondary hepatic malignancies and benign lesions as well as non-tumorous masses that may mimic liver tumors. The task of distinguishing among the possible causes and tumor types should prompt a systematic evaluation that relies on both clinical information and diagnostic imaging. Clinical information and non-invasive imaging can certainly narrow the differential diagnosis and may at times provide a definitive answer. The diagnosis, however, may be difficult or nonspecific without histopathologic confirmation, and ultimately percutaneous or open biopsy may be required. The purposes of this chapter are (1) to give a broad overview of clinical data and non-invasive imaging that may be helpful in narrowing the differential diagnosis of a hepatic mass and (2) to provide some specific recommendations for the work-up of several of the more common hepatic lesions.

Common benign hepatic tumors include cysts and hemangiomas; common malignant tumors are metastases and hepatocellular carcinoma (HCC). Less common hepatic tumors include focal nodular hyperplasia (FNH), adenoma, fibrolamellar HCC, intrahepatic cholangiocarcinoma, lymphoma, sarcoma, and hepatoblastoma in children. Occasionally, a non-tumorous mass, such as focal fat-sparing, abscess, or hematoma, may simulate a liver tumor. In the patient with cirrhosis, regenerating nodules and hepatic fibrosis can be difficult to distinguish from tumors.

Metastases are far more common than primary hepatic malignancies. Hence, in a patient with a hepatic mass of unknown cause, the presence of a known extrahepatic malignancy is probably the single most useful fact that the clinician can supply. Additional clinical information includes the age and sex of the patient. In adults younger than 40 years, metastases, fibrolamellar HCC, FNH, and hepatic adenoma account for a majority of hepatic lesions; in those older than 50 years, metastases, hemangioma, HCC, cholangiocarcinoma, and angiosarcoma predominate.[1]

Hemangioendothelioma and hemangiomas account for most hepatic masses in infants younger than 6 months; hemangioblastoma is seen in children younger than 3 years. Hepatic masses in older children and adolescents tend to be HCC or undifferentiated sarcoma. Knowledge of the patient's gender also can be helpful, because primary hepatic malignancies seem to be more common in men and benign lesions tend to occur more frequently in women.[2]

Clinical information provides a useful initial guide to formulating a differential diagnosis, but noninvasive imaging tests are necessary to differentiate further among the likely possibilities. Computed tomography (CT) tends to be the workhorse of hepatic diagnostic imaging, but ultrasound imaging (US), magnetic resonance imaging (MRI), nuclear scintigraphy, and angiography can offer additional diagnostic clues. These modalities may show whether a lesion is single or multiple and can provide information about its location and morphologic and functional characteristics. Determination of the need for and feasibility of surgical resection also are questions that may be answered noninvasively.

Imaging evaluation of a known hepatic mass usually begins with CT. Modern CT scanning for screening and staging of hepatic tumors uses dynamic volumetric scanning techniques performed during the mechanical power injection of an iodinated intravenous contrast agent. Typically, the liver is scanned during a single breath-hold by the patient, with 5-mm slice collimation, a pitch of 1–2, during a rapid bolus (2–4 mL/s) of 120–150 mL of a nonionic contrast agent. This examination may be performed as a single-phase contrast-enhanced CT (CECT) or as a dual-phase (biphasic) examination. During the single-phase CECT examination, the liver is imaged during the peak of parenchymal enhancement (portal venous phase), beginning approximately 60 seconds after initiation of the injection of contrast agent. Most hepatic tumors are identified during this phase because they appear hypodense relative to the enhanced normal liver.

Biphasic CT examination scans the liver twice (during both the arterial and portal venous phases of contrast enhancement) after injection of a single bolus of contrast agent and can be accomplished because of the rapid scanning times provided by helical CT.[3–6] Some liver tumors receive their blood supply from the hepatic artery, whereas the normal hepatic parenchyma receives 80% of its blood supply from the portal vein. Thus, certain liver tumors (especially hypervascular tumors) are strongly enhanced during the arterial phase of contrast medium enhancement (20 seconds after the start of injection) and appear hyperdense relative to the normal liver. Because of rapid washout of the contrast agent, these lesions may not be apparent on standard portal venous phase images (appearing isodense to enhanced hepatic parenchyma).

Benign cavernous hemangiomas are common lesions that show a characteristic peripheral nodular enhancement and delayed "fill-in" during CECT. Focal nodular hyperplasia may demonstrate an enhancing central scar on delayed imaging. After the initial single-phase or biphasic CECT scan, delayed images taken at 5–10 minutes may show this characteristic pattern and provide a definitive diagnosis. Biphasic CT scanning is considered the modality of choice for scanning suspected HCC and can also detect the complications of hemoperitoneum and vascular invasion.[7,8]

Noncontrast-enhanced CT (NCECT) is rarely necessary in the characterization of hepatic masses but may occasionally be useful in the setting of diffuse liver disease, such as hemochromatosis or cirrhosis, or when subtle calcifications are suspected. In these situations, NCECT may be combined with the biphasic CECT (triple-phase CT).

US is commonly used in general screening for right upper quadrant abdominal pain and hepatic metastases; the modality may therefore be the first one to demonstrate a hepatic mass. High-resolution transducers and color-flow Doppler evaluation have improved the ability of US to detect and characterize hepatic lesions. Small cavernous hemangiomas have a suggestive US appearance that is hyperechoic with no identifiable Doppler flow and occasional enhanced through transmission. Target lesions (with hyperechoic center and hypoechoic rim) are more likely to be malignant than benign. Development of US contrast agents further may improve the detectability and characterization of lesions. Its noninvasive character makes US an optimal modality for relatively inexpensive and timely follow-up of suspected or equivocal hepatic lesions.

MRI can readily detect hepatic masses and may be the primary imaging modality for diagnosis, especially in patients who have an allergy to iodinated contrast agents. In many cases, however, MRI is still used in a limited role in the abdomen. A typical indication for MRI may be the patient who has a lesion judged to be indeterminate for malignancy on an alternative modality imaging examination. Alternatively, MRI may be the test of choice in a patient who has known or suspected liver disease (e.g., chronic hepatitis, cirrhosis, or hemochromatosis) with an associated high risk of HCC. MRI techniques have been reported to be at least as good as dynamic CECT, and MRI has certain advantages over CT in terms of diagnostic sensitivity and specificity.[9] Optimal MRI evaluation consists of both T1- and T2-weighted imaging plus multiphase dynamic scanning with gadolinium-chelate intravenous contrast media. Additional MRI pulse sequences and techniques, including gradient-recalled-echo imaging, chemical shift imaging, and fat suppression, may be helpful in providing information about tissue characterization.

Other MRI contrast media are being investigated. Mangafodipir-trisodium (Mn-DPDP) may be useful in the characterization of questionable lesions.[10] Mn-DPDP is a hepatobiliary agent that is taken up by lesions that contain hepatocytes (such as HCC), resulting in increased signal intensity of the lesion on T1-weighted images. Intravenous administration of superparamagnetic iron oxide (SPIO) also increases the sensitivity and specificity of MRI.[11] SPIO is cleared by the reticuloendothelial system and therefore may be helpful to detect and characterize HCC and FNH on T2-weighted sequences, since HCC contains no Kupffer cells while FNH does. The role of MRI contrast agents, such as Gd-ethoxybenzyl (EOB)-DTPA and Gd-benzoxypropionictetra-acetate (BOPTA), is under investigation and yet to be determined.[12,13]

Nuclear scintigraphy has a limited role to play in the diagnostic evaluation of hepatic masses. Standard liver-spleen scans with technetium Tc99m sulfur colloid are of limited value because scintigraphic defects are nonspecific. However, uptake of isotope in FNH (containing active Kupffer cells) may distinguish this entity from other hepatic masses. Scans performed with technetium-labeled red blood cells may confirm hemangioma with a high degree of specificity, provided that the lesion is large enough (usually <3 cm).

Angiography may provide diagnostic characterization of various tumors, including hemangiomas, hepatomas, and FNH, and may also provide a vascular "road map" for surgical planning. Angiography is essential for CT arterial portography, which most likely remains the most sensitive method of preoperative detection of liver metastases.[14] Flow-related artifacts limit the specificity of this examination, however, which is limited to patients who are potential candidates for surgical resection of tumor.

The American College of Radiology has developed appropriateness criteria for the use of diagnostic imaging in the characterization of liver lesions.[15] These criteria, summarized in **Tables 7-1 and 7-2**, are the recommendations from an expert panel of gastrointestinal imaging specialists for the appropriate use of imaging modalities in diagnosis. The modalities of US, CT, MRI, nuclear scintigraphy, and angiography are rated on an appropriateness scale of 1 (least appropriate) to 9 (most appropriate) for various categories of liver lesions.

Many small lesions (<1 cm) may be detected incidentally on screening CT or US examinations and may be difficult to characterize. Although most of these lesions are benign, follow-up imaging is recommended. For larger lesions (cysts and hemangiomas) that appear typically benign on screening CT or US and that are found in patients who have no known history of or clinical suspicion for malignancy, no further imaging work-up is necessary. However, for the finding of such a lesion in a patient with a history of known malignancy, follow-up US or CT (same test with which the lesion was detected initially) is suggested, even though the mass shows typically benign characteristics. For lesions that appear typically malignant on screening CT or US, no additional imaging is necessary, and percutaneous biopsy is recommended.

For patients who have an otherwise normal liver but in whom a mass is detected and judged to be indeterminate for malignancy, additional diagnostic imaging is appropriate. MRI (appropriateness rating [AR] = 8) is a more appropriate imaging modality for this category than CECT (AR = 6), but in most practices in which the lesion is initially detected by US, CECT is the next examination performed for lesion characterization. If the lesion was initially detected on CT scanning and its identity is indeterminate, MRI is the next modality used. For liver lesions that remain indeterminate for malignancy despite extensive diagnostic imaging, percutaneous biopsy is essential.

Finally, characterization of liver lesions in patients with cirrhosis is best performed with MRI. MRI is the most appropriate modality to differentiate among regenerating nodules, dysplastic nodules, and HCC and may be used to monitor suspect lesions to detect any change in size or appearance.[16,17]

Table 7-1
Imaging Recommendations for Common Benign Hepatic Masses

Imaging modality	Hemangioma	Focal nodular hyperplasia	Hepatic adenoma
Ultrasound imaging	AR = 8 Hyperechoic, well-defined, faint acoustic enhancement. If imaging findings are classic and there is no history of primary malignancy, probably no need for additional imaging.	AR = 6 Well-demarcated hyperechoic homogeneous mass with central scar. Color Doppler US shows hypervascularity with radiating vessels.	AR = 6 Nonspecific. Typically shows large hyperechoic heterogeneous mass with central necrosis or hemorrhage. Color Doppler US shows hypervascularity with peripheral vessels and occasional intratumoral volume.
Computed tomography	AR = 6 NCECT shows well-defined, low-density mass with calcification in 10%–20%. CECT shows globular peripheral enhancement with delayed "fill-in."	AR = 6 NCECT shows homogeneous hypodense mass with low-density central scar apparent in 1/3 of cases. CECT shows hyperdense mass and low-density central scar on arterial-phase images. CECT shows isodense mass on portal venous phase images. Delayed images show late enhancement of central scar.	AR = 6 NCECT shows heterogeneous hypodense mass due to presence of fat and glycogen. Occasionally, hemorrhage may cause areas of hyperdensity. If lesions are small, biphasic CECT shows rapid enhancement and rapid washout. Larger lesions have a nonspecific appearance.
Magnetic resonance imaging	AR = 4 T1WI: variable appearance. T2WI : marked hyperintensity of lesion with bright signal persisting on long TR/TE sequences. Gd-DTPA–enhanced images show nodular peripheral enhancement with delayed "fill-in."	AR = 8 T1WI show isointense mass with hypointense central scar. T2WI show mass to be slightly hyperintense to isointense. Gd-DTPA–enhanced images show early enhancement of mass and and late enhancement of central scar.	AR = 8 T1WI show heterogeneous mass with hyperintense regions (hemorrhage and fat) and hypointense regions (necrosis). Fibrous capsule in 1/3. T2WI show mass to be heterogeneously hyperintense. Adenomas may take up SPIO, resulting in decreased signal intensity on T2WI.
Nuclear scintigraphy	AR = 4 Focal defect on hepatobiliary and sulfur colloid scans. Tagged red blood cell scans show defect in early stages with delayed "fill-in."	AR = 6 Normal tracer uptake on sulfur colloid scans in 50% of cases. Hot spots in 10% of cases related to increase in number of Kupffer cells in lesion.	AR = 6 Sulfur colloid scans show a defect in 80% of cases. Hepatobiliary scans show uptake but no excretion because of the lack of bile ductules.

AR = American College of Radiology appropriateness rating[15]; CECT = contrast-enhanced computed tomography; Gd-DTPA = gadolinium diethylenetriaminepentaacetic acid; NCECT = non–contrast-enhanced computed tomography; T1WI = T1-weighted images; T2WI = T2-weighted images; US = ultrasound imaging.

Table 7-2
Imaging Recommendations for Common Malignant Hepatic Masses

Imaging modality	Hepatocellular carcinoma	Fibrolamellar carcinoma
Magnetic resonance imaging	AR = 8 T1WI: variable appearance, depending on amounts of fat and fibrosis, and dominant histologic pattern. Low-signal-intensity capsule identified. T2WI: typically hyperintense. On gadolinium- and Md-DPDP-enhanced images, typically hyperintense with vascular invasion identified.	AR = 8 T1WI: hypointense or isointense mass with hypointense central scar. T2WI: isointense or slightly hyperintense mass with hypointense central scar.
Computed tomography	AR = 6 Variable appearance depending on tumor size. Capsule usually identified. NCECT shows nonspecific mass appearance. Biphasic CECT shows arterial enhancement (especially in tumors < 3 cm).	AR = 6 NCECT shows hypodense mass with well-defined contour. Central low-density scar or necrosis and hemorrhage. CECT shows hypervascular, hyperdense mass. May show invasion of portal vein.
Ultrasound imaging	AR = 4 Variable appearance. Frequently hyperechoic, especially if fatty change. Color Doppler US may show hypervascularity or vascular invasion/thrombus.	AR = 5 Large hyperechoic, homogeneous mass. May demonstrate calcification as hyperechoic foci with acoustic shadowing.
Nuclear scintigraphy	AR = 4 Defect on sulfur colloid scan. Also, may show typical findings of cirrhosis with hepatomegaly, heterogeneous hepatic uptake, and colloid shift to spleen and bone marrow. Uptake by tumor in hepatobiliary scans (50% of cases) because of biliary production by tumor. Gallium uptake avid.	AR = 5 Defect on sulfur colloid scan. Gallium uptake avid. May show early uptake and late defect on tagged red blood cell scan secondary to hypervascularity.

AR = American College of Radiology appropriateness rating[15]; CECT = contrast-enhanced computed tomography; NCECT = non–contrast-enhanced computed tomography; T1WI = T1-weighted images; T2WI = T2-weighted images; US = ultrasound imaging.

REFERENCES

1. Ros PR, Taylor HM. Malignant tumors of the liver. In: Gore RM, Levine MS, eds. *Textbook of Gastrointestinal Radiology*. 2nd ed. Philadelphia: WB Saunders; 2000:523–1168.
2. Taylor HM, Ros PR. Hepatic imaging: an overview. *Radiol Clin N Am* 1998 36:237–245.
3. Bluemke DA, Soyer P, Fishman E. Helical (spiral) CT of the liver. *Radiol Clin N Am* 1995;33:863–885.
4. Baron RL, Oliver JH III, Dodd GD III, et al. Hepatocellular carcinoma: evaluation with biphasic, contrast-enhanced helical CT. *Radiology* 1996;199:505–511.
5. Oliver JH III, Baron RL, Federle MP, et al. Detecting hepatocellular carcinoma: value of unenhanced or arterial phase CT imaging or both used in conjunction with conventional portal venous phase contrast-enhanced CT imaging. *Am J Roentgenol* 1996;167:71–77.
6. Kanematsu M, Oliver JH III, Baron RL, et al. Hepatocellular carcinoma: the role of biphasic contrast-enhanced CT versus CT during arterial portography. *Radiology* 1997;205:75–80.
7. Freeny PC, Baron RL, Teefey SA. Hepatocellular carcinoma: reduced frequency of typical findings with dynamic contrast-enhanced CT in a non-Asian population. *Radiology* 1992;182:143–148.
8. Matsui O, Kadoya M. Diagnosis and staging of hepatocellular carcinoma. In: Meyers MA, ed. *Neoplasms of the Digestive Tract: Imaging, Staging and Management*. Philadelphia: Lippincott-Raven;1998:333–346.
9. Martin DR, Semelka RC. Imaging of benign and malignant focal liver lesions. *Magn Reson Imaging Clin N Am* 2001;9:785–802.
10. Murakami T, Baron RL, Peterson MS, et al. Hepatocellular carcinoma:

MR imaging with mangofodipir sodium (MnDPDP). *Radiology* 1996;200:69–77.

11. Yamamoto H, Yamashita Y, Yoshimatsu S, et al. Hepatocellular carcinoma in cirrhotic livers: detection with unenhanced and iron-oxide-enhanced MR imaging. *Radiology* 1995;195:106–112.
12. Caudana R, Morano G, Pirovano GP, et al. Focal malignant lesions: MR imaging enhanced with gadolinium benzyloxypropionictetra-acetate (BOPTA)—preliminary results of phase II application. *Radiology* 1996;199:513–520.
13. Vogl TJ, Kummel S, Hammerstingl R, et al. Liver tumors: comparison of MR imaging with Gd-EOB-DTPA and Gd-DTPA. *Radiology* 1996;200: 59–67.
14. Soyer P, Levesque M, Elias D, et al. Preoperative assessment of resectability of hepatic metastases from colonic carcinoma: CT portography vs sonography and dynamic CT. *Am J Roentgenol* 1992;159: 741–744.
15. Saini S, Ralls PW, Balfe DM, et al. Liver lesion characterization. American College of Radiology. ACR Appropriateness Criteria. *Radiology* 2000;215(suppl):193–199.
16. Murakami T, Kim T, Nakamura H, et al. Hepatitis, cirrhosis and hepatoma. *J Magn Reson Imaging* 1998;8:346–358.
17. Mitchell DG, Rubin R, Siegelman ES, et al. Hepatocellular carcinoma within siderotic regenerative nodules: appearance as a nodule within a nodule on MR images. *Radiology* 1991;178:101–103.

CHAPTER 8

PERCUTANEOUS IMAGE-GUIDED BIOPSY: REVIEW OF AND EMPHASIS ON SPECIAL APPROACHES

DEBRA A. GERVAIS, MD

INTRODUCTION

In current practice, image-guided percutaneous biopsy plays a central role in disease management for many patients with cancer. Chemotherapy protocols, whether they are standard or clinical trials, require tissue diagnosis for patient enrollment. Percutaneous biopsy may be an aid not only in diagnosing a cancer but in staging as well. For example, results from biopsy of an adrenal lesion in a patient with a hilar mass may point to adenocarcinoma of the lung as well as indicate that its development is at stage IV (metastatic disease). For this reason, the interventional radiologist must be capable not only of performing percutaneous biopsy but also of performing a thorough pre-biopsy review of a patient's imaging. This ensures that the lesion most suitable for biopsy is targeted not only from a technical standpoint but from the standpoint of overall management. In addition, biopsy may be avoided altogether by additional imaging initiated by an interventional radiologist reviewing the case of a patient referred for possible biopsy. Isolated liver lesions diagnosed by computed tomography (CT) in a patient with colon carcinoma, for example, might be characterized as hemangiomas by magnetic resonance (MR) imaging, making biopsy unnecessary.

Needle types, basic ultrasound (US)-guided techniques, and approaches for biopsy of the liver, adrenal, pancreas, thorax, and bone are reviewed elsewhere in this series of syllabi (*SCVIR Syllabus: Thoracic and*

Visceral Nonvascular Interventions). This chapter reviews some of these topics briefly but focuses on special or modified techniques for lesions not readily accessible by standard percutaneous access.

NEEDLE TYPES

There are two types of needles used to obtain material via percutaneous biopsy. *Aspirating needles* provide material for cytologic analysis. The material is obtained by a rapid to-and-fro motion of the needle through the lesion while gentle suction is applied by a syringe attached to the needle hub. Cutting needles obtain a core of tissue that allows histologic analysis. Cytologic analysis can be performed by performing a "touch prep" by gently touching the tissue core to a slide, thereby creating a single layer of cells smeared onto the slide.[1] *Cutting needles* are available in two basic cutting designs: those that obtain the tissue through the end of the needle (analogous to aspirating needles) and those that obtain tissue in a groove in the side of the needle. Side-cutting needles provide more reliable specimens and are the most common cutting needles in current use (**Fig. 8-1**).

Most cutting needles can be placed through coaxial introducers. The introducer stays in the lesion while the sampling needle is removed for recovery of the sample. This technique allows multiple needle passes to be performed through the introducer with only one puncture through the organ of interest. Likewise, both fine-needle aspirates and cores can be obtained without reentering the lesion. The coaxial introducer is especially useful for deep lesions or lesions that are difficult to access to minimize the risk and effort inherent in obtaining multiple samples.

SPECIMEN ANALYSIS

Routine biopsy specimens in the setting of known or suspected malignancy are sent for routine cytologic and/or histologic evaluation. If the clinical scenario leaves reasonable suspicion for an infectious cause for a mass lesion, then appropriate cultures are also requested. For example, multiple small liver lesions in an immunocompromised patient with lymphoma may represent lymphoma but are more likely to be fungal microabscesses.

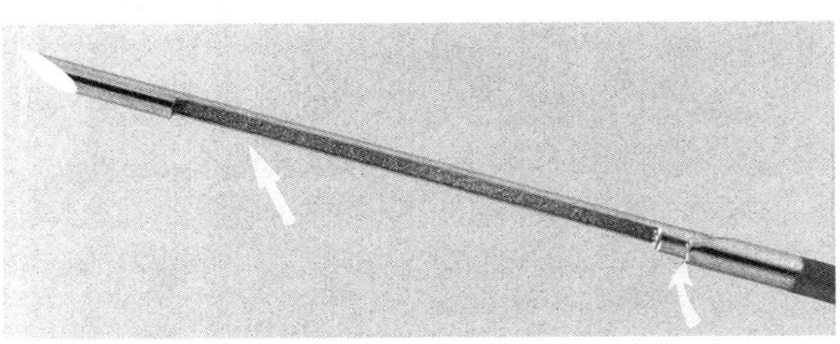

Figure 8-1. Side-cutting core biopsy needle. The specimen is trapped in the side recess (straight arrow) when the outer cutting needle (curved arrow) is fired.

Individual disease processes may require special studies. Biopsy specimens of metastatic lesions in patients with primary breast cancer may require evaluation for estrogen and progesterone receptors. Genetic analysis for the HER-2/neu or the BRCA1 or BRCA2 genes may be required by the patient's treatment protocol. For patients with metastatic breast cancer, the interventional radiologist must consult the oncologist to ensure that all appropriate special laboratory studies are requested. Likewise, flow cytometry has proven useful in patients with lymphoma. Although cell block immunohistochemistry can be performed on core specimens, flow cytometry allows rapid evaluation of a fine-needle aspirate, often confirming the diagnosis of lymphoma faster than the cytologic or histologic analysis. A dedicated needle pass saved entirely in a separate specimen bottle provides optimal material for flow cytometry. Finally, pediatric tumors often require multiple large cores to provide ample material for histologic analysis as well as genetic analysis, such as for aneuploidy and N-*myc* gene amplification in neuroblastoma.

IMAGING MODALITY

CT and US are the imaging modalities used most commonly for percutaneous biopsy. Fluoroscopic guidance can be used for many lung lesions, some bone lesions, and occasional pancreatic lesions, but its use is limited for other soft-tissue biopsies. US provides real-time needle visualization, requires no ionizing radiation, and allows angulation of the needle tract in any plane. Focal lesions can be approached with needle guides or the freehand US techniques described elsewhere in this syllabus series (*SCVIR Syllabus: Thoracic and Visceral Nonvascular Interventions*). For those with the expertise, freehand techniques provide greater flexibility in terms of the approach to the lesion because the needle guide is fixed in position with only one or two possible angles between the needle and US transducer. However, needle guides can be rapidly deployed by those familiar with their use and can facilitate needle placement when a clear window to the target lesion is available.

CT guidance facilitates biopsy of deep lesions or other lesions not well demonstrated by US. The needle path is restricted to the axial plane, although gantry-

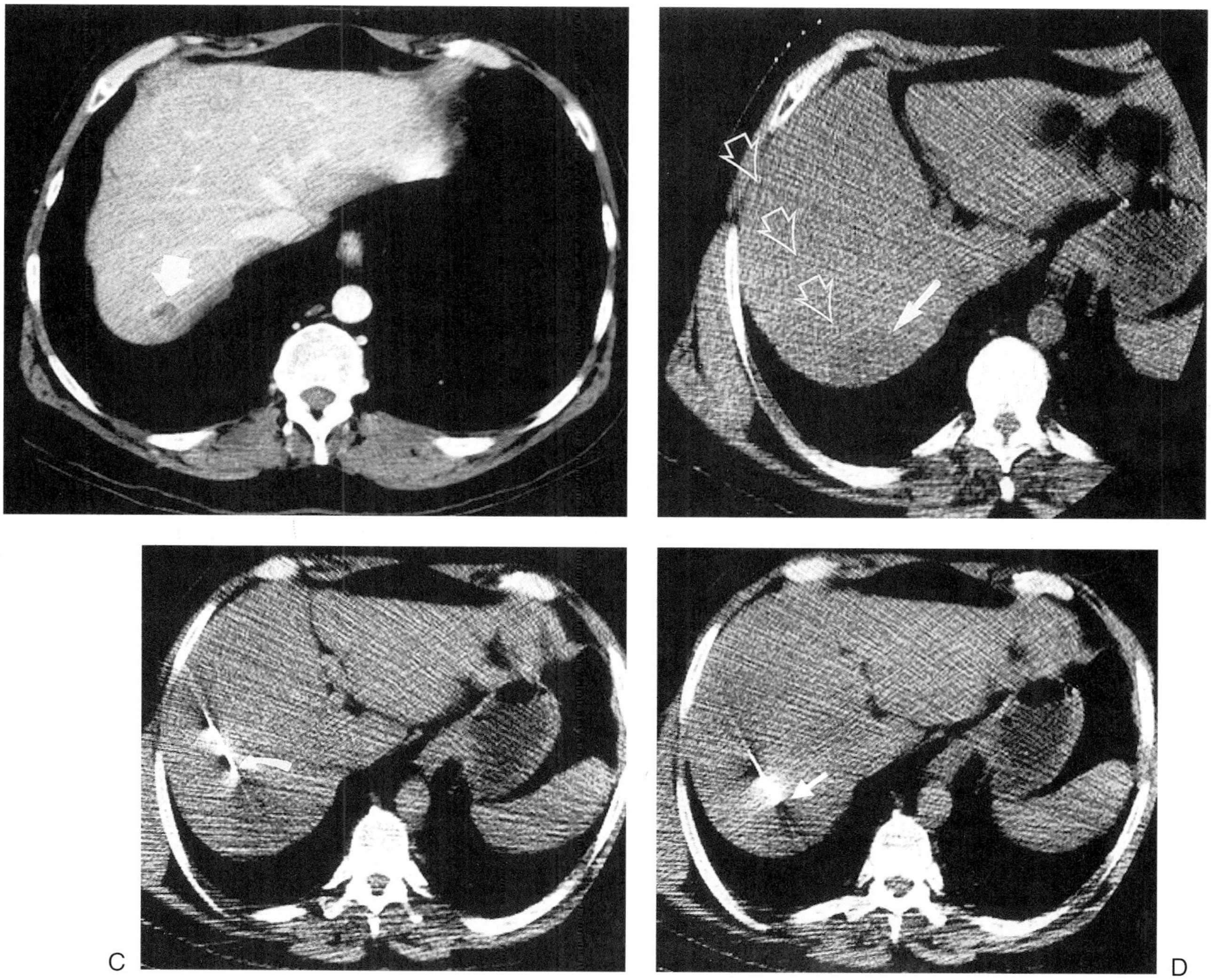

A B C D

Figure 8-2. (A) Computed tomography (CT) scan with intravenous contrast material in a 49-year-old man with colon cancer shows a solitary liver lesion in segment 7 in the dome (arrow). Access to this lesion in the axial plane shown here would involve a transpulmonary approach. However, the lung can be avoided by angling the gantry so that the needle enters more caudal to the lesion. (B) CT scan without contrast material obtained at biopsy with gantry angulation of 22°. The lesion is still visible (arrow), and there is now an anterolateral puncture site that would avoid transgressing the lung (open arrows). (C and D) CT scans during biopsy with gantry angulation show parts of the needle. In this case, the needle is not perfectly in the plane of the CT gantry. In Figure 8-2C, the needle is seen (arrow), but the tip is not identified. In Figure 8-2D, the needle tip artifact is seen confirming tip position (arrow). The biopsy specimen was positive for colon cancer metastasis.

angulation techniques provide cephalocaudal angulation to a degree (**Fig. 8-2**). The recent introduction of CT fluoroscopy allows more rapid imaging of target lesions and the biopsy needle.[2] However, the lower radiation dose used to acquire individual images compromises image quality, in comparison with conventional diagnostic scans. This consideration is of little consequence where the lesion-to-background contrast is high, such as focal lung lesion surrounded by air. However, liver lesions that are difficult to identify on high-quality diagnostic scans may be invisible on CT fluoroscopy images. Recent developments in MR imaging have allowed MR guidance for percutaneous procedures. However, the limited availability of this modality for everyday procedures, as well as the need for special MR-compatible needles, has limited the use of this modality for routine biopsy.

The absolute requirement for the choice of imaging guidance is that the lesion be visible via the modality chosen. If multiple modalities fulfill this requirement, then in practice, the modality chosen often reflects variations in availability of the modality for interventional procedures and the radiologist's skill and degree of confidence with the different modalities.

BIOPSY PREPARATION

Preparation for a percutaneous biopsy involves review of the indications and images at the time of scheduling. Coagulation study results are reviewed if available, and blood is drawn if necessary. Doing coagulation studies for every image-guided percutaneous procedure is controversial and likely not necessary for many superficial biopsies, such as those of the thyroid, superficial lymph nodes, and large superficial chest wall or abdominal masses. However, all patients taking anticoagulants, who have recently undergone chemotherapy that could deplete platelets, or with a personal history or family history of a bleeding disorder should undergo the appropriate laboratory evaluation. In the absence of available recent values, doing coagulation studies (prothrombin time, partial thromboplastin time) and a complete blood cell count is also the practice in our institution prior to doing parenchymal organ biopsies, such as those of the liver, kidney, spleen, and lung.

Patients who are to receive intravenous sedation for the biopsy are told to have nothing to eat after midnight for a morning procedure. For afternoon procedures, patients have nothing by mouth after 6:00 A.M. Oral medications, with the exception of anticoagulants and hypoglycemics, can be taken with very small sips of water in the morning. For outpatients, an adult must accompany the patient home after the patient has been sedated. Intravenous (IV) sedation is administered in keeping with institutional guidelines. In general, these require monitoring of vital signs and oxygen saturation during and after the procedure.[3]

BIOPSIES OF FOCAL LESIONS OF ABDOMINAL PARENCHYMAL ORGANS

Liver Biopsy

Liver biopsy of focal liver lesions can be performed with US or CT guidance. With the US approach, some prefer to choose a subcostal approach even if a longer path to a high lesion results. The theoretic advantage is that the tract can be compressed. Others prefer the most direct route using the intercostal rather than subcostal approach whenever necessary. To optimize the US image for the biopsy, the radiologist must be sure to use an oblique angle of imaging perfectly parallel to the intercostal spaces rather than the usual orthogonal transverse or sagittal images. A purely transverse image will place shadowing ribs in the image, limiting the field of view. An angle parallel to the ribs will avoid interference from the ribs and allow use of the entire transducer field.

If intravenous sedation is used for the liver biopsy, the radiologist may often find that the lesion is no longer optimally seen from a site chosen prior to sedation. This happens as breathing patterns change as a result of the sedation. Often, respirations are not as deep, and the liver is cephalad relative to its position prior to sedation. To avoid having to start again at a different site, the radiologist can choose to sedate first, then choose a site. Alternatively, the site can be chosen prior to sedation, and very light intravenous analgesia with a short-acting narcotic, such as fentanyl citrate, can be administered just prior to advancing the needle. The patient should be awake enough to follow breathing instructions to allow the liver and the focal lesion to remain within the field of view.

Liver biopsy with CT guidance can be performed in the standard axial plane. Difficult-to-reach lesions near the dome can be approached with an angled gantry to avoid lung parenchyma (**Fig. 8-2**). When all else fails, a transpulmonary approach can be used in the absence of emphysema or pulmonary hypertension for lesions high in the dome.[4]

Whether CT or US is used to guide liver biopsy, a mantle of normal liver should be kept in the needle path on the way to the lesion whenever possible. Direct entry to the lesion without including a mantle of liver results in a higher risk of bleeding complications. Liver can almost always be included in the needle tract by angling the needle.

Hemangioma Biopsy

Most cavernous hemangiomas of the liver can be characterized by MR imaging of the liver with dynamic enhancement with gadolinium-based contrast agents. Definitive lesion characterization will allow patients to avoid unnecessary biopsies. However, in rare cases where there remains sufficient doubt or the lesion is absolutely not characteristic of hemangioma, biopsy can be performed safely with both fine needle-aspiration and core biopsies.[5] Again, care should be taken to leave normal liver parenchyma in the needle path to the lesion.

Pancreas Biopsy

Although most lesions are suitable for percutaneous biopsy, biopsy of pancreatic masses is performed most commonly with endoscopic ultrasound (EUS) in institutions where this modality is readily available. In cases of inaccessibility of the lesion to EUS or in cases where the specimen obtained by EUS-guided biopsy is nondiagnostic, the patient is then referred for percutaneous biopsy. Percutaneous access to solid lesions can be achieved through bowel (stomach, colon, small bowel)

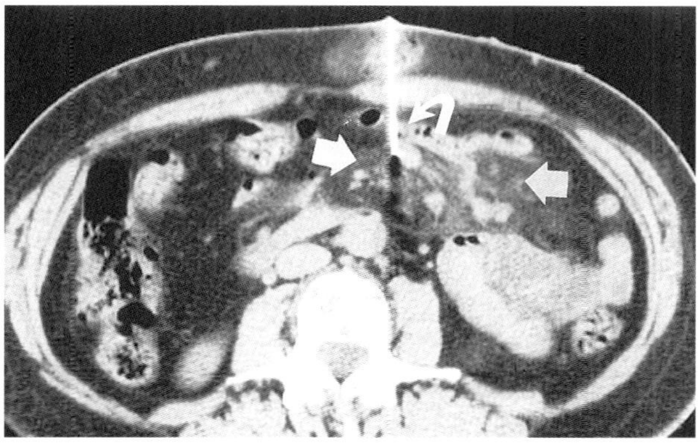

Figure 8-3. Transbowel biopsy. Computed tomography scan during biopsy of mesenteric lymph node shows with enlarged nodes and "misty" mesentery (arrows). The needle crossed a bowel loop (curved arrow) to access the edge of the node. The needle was repositioned slightly, and biopsy revealed lymphoma. Bowel can be crossed to reach target lesions that are solid. If the lesion is fluid, then an approach through the colon risks infecting the collection and should be avoided.

or liver if no direct path exists. However, cystic masses should never be accessed via a percutaneous path that traverses colon, because of the risk of infecting the cystic component with bowel flora. Care should be taken to avoid regions of normal pancreas if possible, because needling areas of normal pancreas places the patient at risk for pancreatitis or pancreatic duct leak. Fluid obtained from cystic pancreatic tumors should be sent for pancreatic fluid analysis of tumor markers such as CA 19-9 and CA 72-4 as well as for cytologic workup to increase the overall diagnostic yield.[6]

Spleen Biopsy

Splenic biopsy is occasionally indicated for diagnosis of infection or differentiation of benign from malignant disease. Keogan et al. achieved a specific diagnosis in 16 of 18 (89%) splenic biopsies including 10 benign and 6 malignant diagnoses.[7] The small series and rarity of reports in the literature are both testament to the rarity of splenic biopsies. In the absence of other target lesions for biopsy elsewhere in the body, splenic biopsy can be performed safely. Keogan et al. reported no complications in 18 biopsies.[7] The main concern with splenic biopsy is hemorrhage, and it has been noted anecdotally that radiologists prefer to include splenic parenchyma in the needle path to the lesion, as is the practice for liver lesions. However, given the sparse data on image-guided splenic biopsy, there is little evidence to either support or refute this practice. In the absence of known malignancy or concern for infection, most splenic lesions are benign, and management can be limited to follow-up imaging to assess stability.

Biopsy of Other Organs

Finally, biopsies of other organs, nodes, and bowel can be performed using the same approaches[8,9] (**Figs. 8-3, 8-4**).

SPECIAL APPROACHES

Deep Pelvic Structures

Transgluteal

Lesions deep in the pelvis often prove difficult to access because of intervening structures. Bowel, bladder, blood vessels, and bones may limit the conventional percutaneous approaches. Whereas passage of the needle through bowel to access a deep lesion is acceptable for solid lesions, the nature of a lesion may be in question prior to biopsy. One would not want to infect a fluid-filled structure or necrotic tumor with bowel flora, for example. In such cases, the CT-guided transgluteal approach is the safest because no transgression of colonized structures is

A

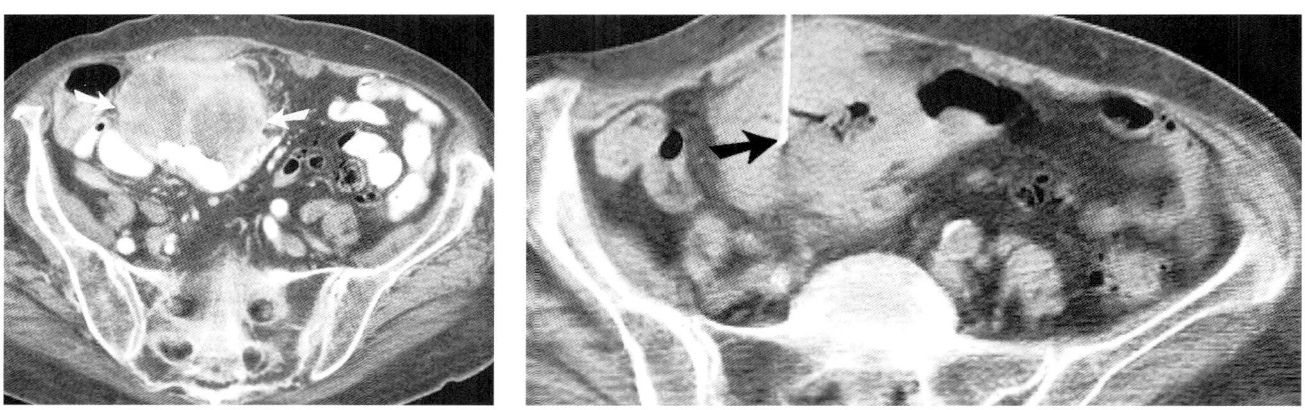

B

Figure 8-4. (A) Computed tomography (CT) in a 62-year-old man with abdominal pain shows a large mass involving the cecum (arrows). (B) CT at needle biopsy shows coaxial introducer needle (arrow) in the mass. The biopsy specimen revealed cecal lymphoma.

involved. The transgluteal approach is also useful when the transrectal approach is precluded, such as after rectal resection and colostomy formation for colon cancer[10] (**Fig. 8-5**). The patient is placed in the lateral decubitus or prone position, and the needle is placed through the greater sciatic foramen. The most medial approach possible is chosen so as to avoid the sciatic nerve, which courses laterally and inferiorly.[11] In the cephalad aspect of the foramen, the needle will traverse the piriformis muscle. In the caudal aspect, the needle may traverse the sacrospinous ligament.

Passage of the needle through several structures may result in pain. Pain at the needle entry site on advancing the introducer needle can be treated with injection of local 1% lidocaine, as for any percutaneous biopsy. Pain radiating down the leg usually indicates irritation of one of the branches of the sacral plexus anterior to the piriformis muscle and ligaments. The pain can be relieved by partially withdrawing the needle and redirecting it at a slightly different angle toward the lesion. Slight reangulation is usually sufficient to avoid the nerve previously irritated. In general, local pain is most commonly related to the muscles traversed to get into the pelvis—the gluteus muscles and, in the cephalad aspect of the greater sciatic foramen, the piriformis muscle. Local pain can be controlled by injection of 1% lidocaine as muscle is crossed with the biopsy introducer. Pain is worse for patients with bulky muscles, usually younger patients. Intravenous narcotics are usually necessary in addition to local analgesia for complete pain control. In addition to patient discomfort, muscular pain often results in contractions of the involved muscles. The contracted muscles in turn deviate the needle from its projected path, further complicating the needle placement. At times, this needle deviation may necessitate pulling the needle back until it is out of the muscle. In this setting, a dose of fentanyl timed 5 to 10 minutes before repositioning the needle, combined with reassurance of the patient, will facilitate accurate needle placement on the next attempt.

Transrectal and Transvaginal Approaches

For solid lesions, transrectal and transvaginal US transducers facilitate biopsy by allowing high-frequency imaging of structures adjacent to the rectum or vagina (**Figs. 8-6, 8-7**). The most common transrectal biopsy performed in clinical practice is likely prostate biopsy, often performed by urologists rather than radiologists. However, many radiologists are familiar with transrectal biopsy because they provide US guidance for the urologist. The simplest approach to transrectal or transvaginal biopsy involves an endoluminal end-firing US transducer with a mounted needle guide (**Fig. 8-8**). Spring-loaded core biopsy needles can be advanced through the guide with accurate placement into the target lesion. Local analgesia is not administered for transvaginal or transrectal biopsy. In both approaches, local discomfort can be minimized by advancing the US probe until resistance is felt. This step stretches the tissues over the transducer and limits the thickness of tissue to be traversed by the needle to the target lesion.

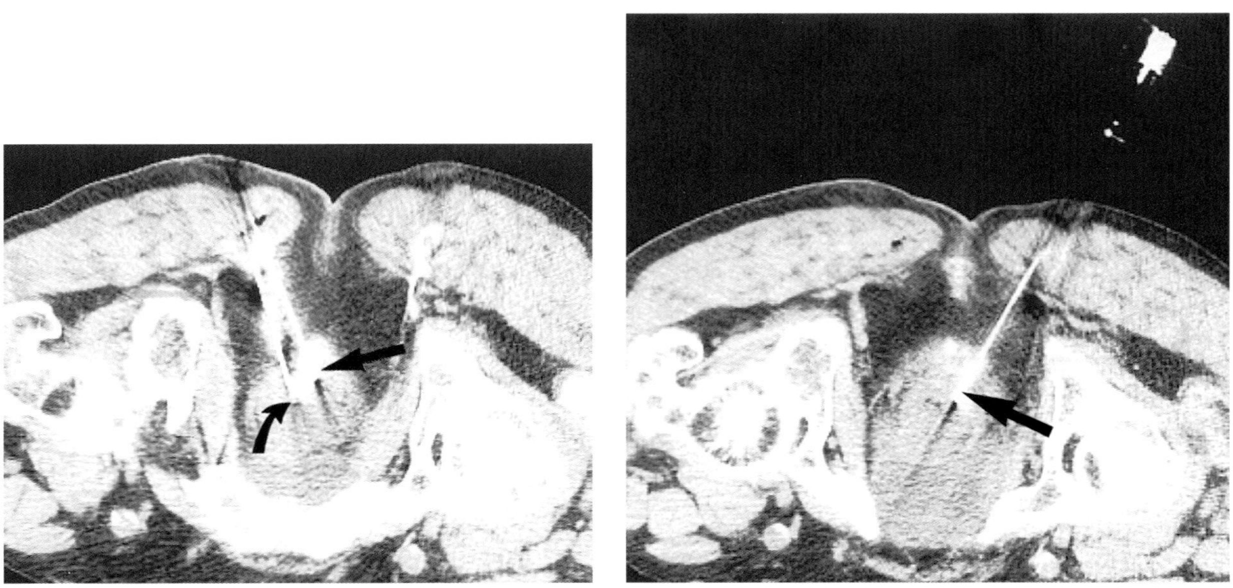

A B

Figure 8-5. Computed tomography–guided transgluteal prostate biopsy in a 56-year-old man with rising levels of prostate-specific antigen. Transrectal biopsy was precluded by prior rectal resection for colorectal carcinoma. Right (A) and left (B) sides are approached separately. A guiding needle is seen here on the right side (curved arrow) next to the biopsy needle (straight arrow). Guiding needles are placed bilaterally. Then, biopsy needles are placed in tandem to the guiding needle, with slight differences in angulation to provide sampling of different areas of the prostate. Most transgluteal biopsies are performed using coaxial introducers, but the prostate must be sampled in many different locations.

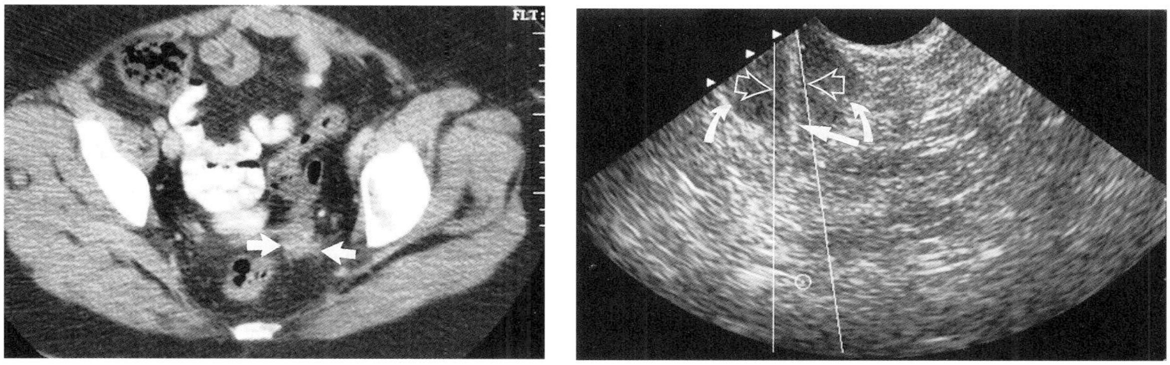

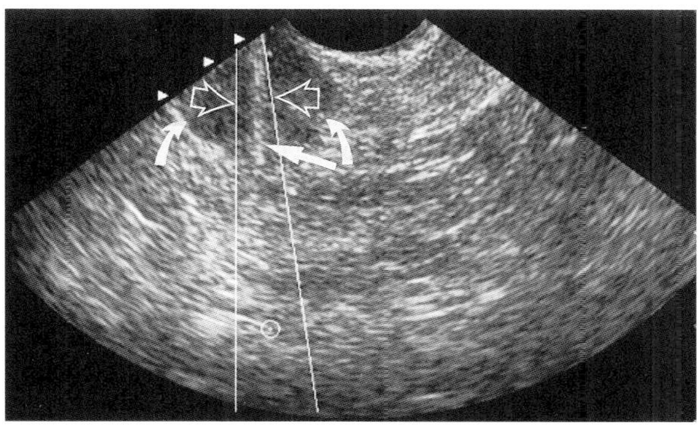

Figure 8-6. (A) Computed tomography of the pelvis in a 55-year-old woman with a remote history of cervical carcinoma. There is a small mass along the left lateral vaginal fornix (arrows). (B) Transvaginal ultrasound (US) allows imaging of the mass (arrows) with high resolution with the US probe in close proximity. (C) Transvaginal US–guided biopsy. Software allows for display of needle guides on the US image (open arrows). The needle, placed on a needle guide, will be within these lines. The US probe is then positioned so that the mass (curved solid arrows) is within the lines, and the needle is fired. US demonstrates the needle (straight solid arrow) within the mass.

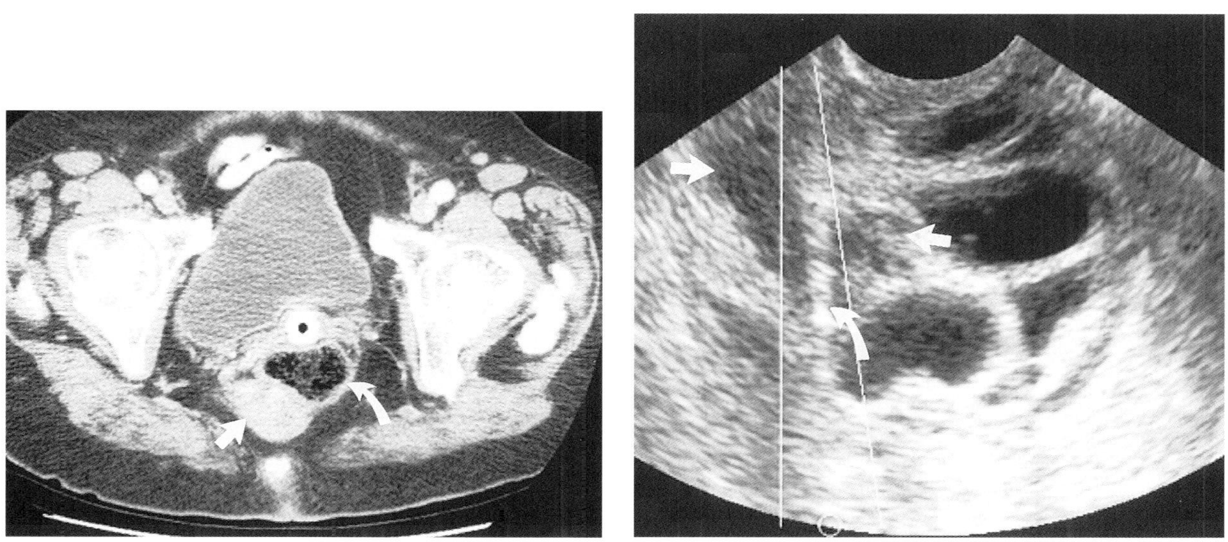

Figure 8-7. (A) Computed tomography of the pelvis in a patient with a history of melanoma and a new isolated soft-tissue mass (arrow) near the rectum (curved arrow). Biopsy was requested. (B) Transrectal ultrasound–guided needle biopsy. The mass (straight arrows) has been imaged so that the needle guide is directly centered, and the needle (curved arrow) is fired directly through the mass.

Patient Preparation for Transrectal or Transvaginal Biopsy

In practice, transrectal biopsy is not a sterile procedure, and transvaginal biopsy is a semi-sterile procedure at best. Prophylactic antibiotic regimens vary among practitioners, but both approaches involve oral and parenteral antibiotics. For routine prostate biopsies at our institution, tobramycin (80 mg, intramuscular [IM]) is administered immediately before the procedure. If the patient has an artificial joint prosthesis or heart valve, administration of this periprocedural dose is IV instead of IM. In addition, ciprofloxacin (500 mg PO BID), is given for 5 to 7 days after the procedure. There is no sterile preparation for transrectal biopsy, although the gel used and US probe covers are sterile at the start of the procedure. Sedation is generally not administered.

Transvaginal biopsies can be performed without sedation, but light sedation with fentanyl and midazolam is often indispensable in reducing the patient's anxiety. After identification of the target lesion with a preliminary limited transvaginal US, the perineum and vagina are prepped with povidone-iodine.[12] Forceps and sponges facilitate the vaginal preparation. IV antibiotics are administered, consisting of gentamicin (80 mg) and clindamycin (1 g). After the procedure, oral clindamycin (300 mg every 6 hours) is prescribed for 5 days. Even with the preparation and IV antibiotic regimen, the transvaginal approach is semi-sterile, and its use is thus limited to solid-lesion biopsies or fluid structures that can be completely drained by needle aspiration.

Modification of a Percutaneous Path by Saline Injection

In some instances with no apparent safe percutaneous approach, sufficient displacement of vital structures can be achieved by adjacent saline installation to allow safe biopsy needle placement (**Fig. 8-9**). This technique has been applied in the anterior mediastinum to

A

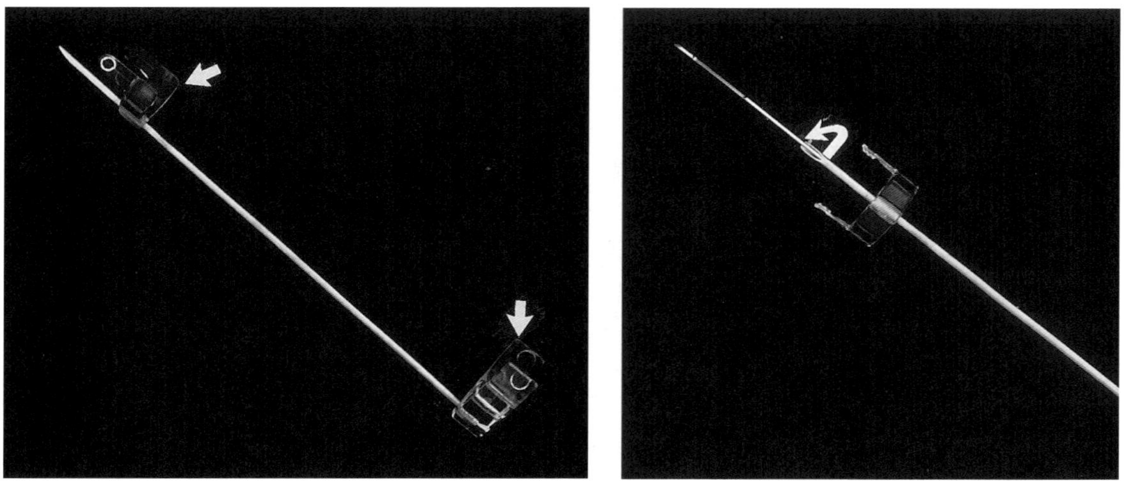

B

C

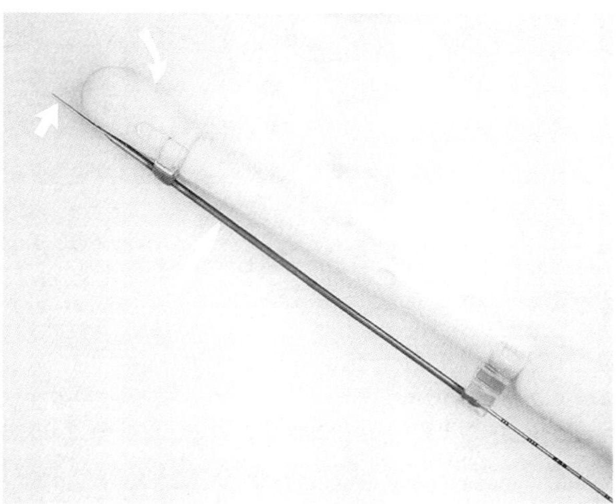

Figure 8-8. (A) Biopsy guide for transvaginal/transrectal ultrasound (US) probe. There are two handles (arrows) that slide onto the US probe and clamp the guide onto the probe. (B) Close-up of the biopsy guide tip with the biopsy needle exiting the guide (curved arrow) (C) Transvaginal/transrectal US probe (curved arrow) with biopsy guide (long straight arrow) mounted and biopsy needle (short straight arrow) exiting the guide tip. This image demonstrates the apparatus at its simplest. In practice, for doing a biopsy, the probe would be covered by a condom/probe cover containing gel at the probe tip. The guide then mounts over the cover, and the needle is advanced through the guide as many times as needed to obtain specimens.

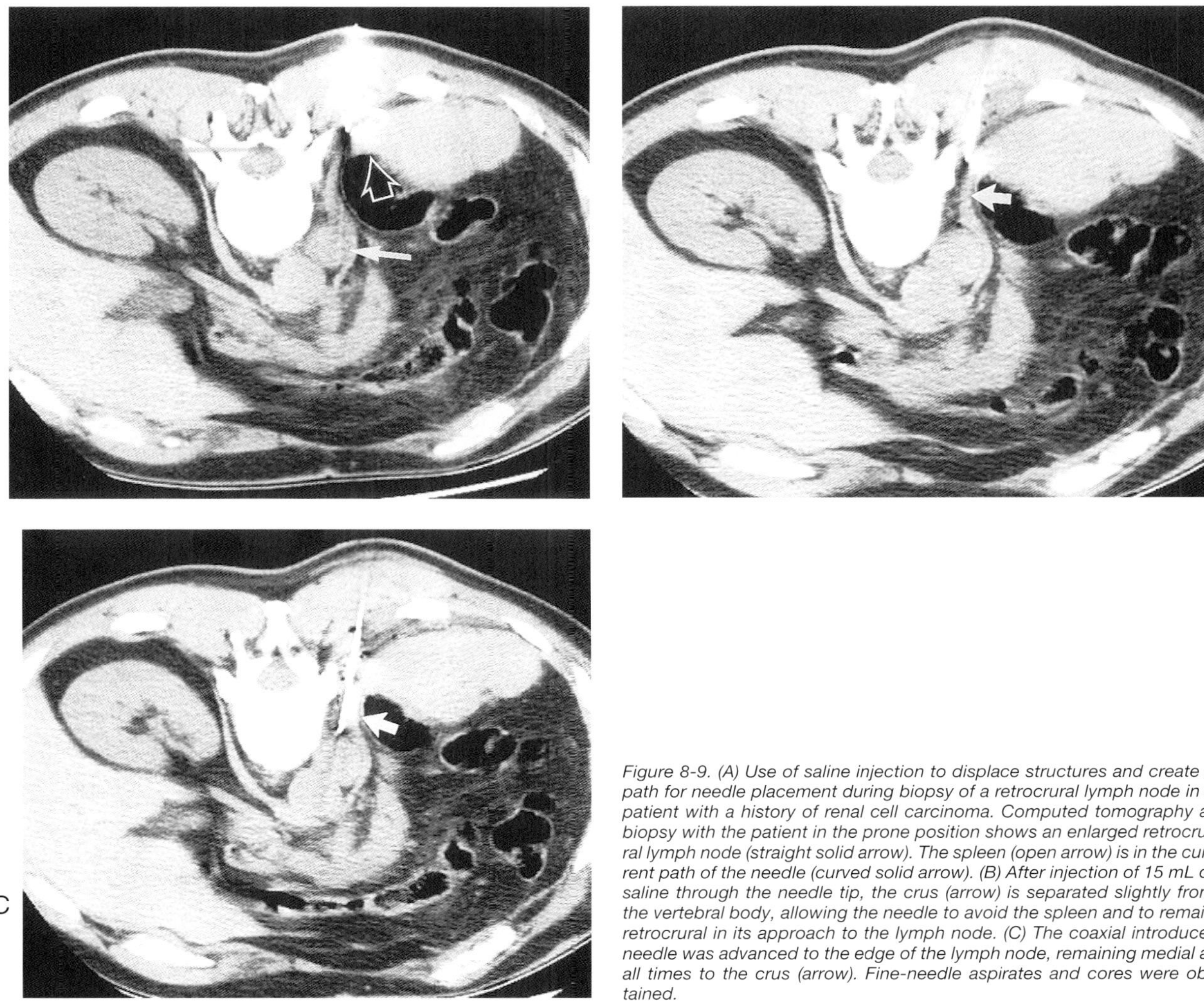

A B C

Figure 8-9. (A) Use of saline injection to displace structures and create a path for needle placement during biopsy of a retrocrural lymph node in a patient with a history of renal cell carcinoma. Computed tomography at biopsy with the patient in the prone position shows an enlarged retrocrural lymph node (straight solid arrow). The spleen (open arrow) is in the current path of the needle (curved solid arrow). (B) After injection of 15 mL of saline through the needle tip, the crus (arrow) is separated slightly from the vertebral body, allowing the needle to avoid the spleen and to remain retrocrural in its approach to the lymph node. (C) The coaxial introducer needle was advanced to the edge of the lymph node, remaining medial at all times to the crus (arrow). Fine-needle aspirates and cores were obtained.

displace internal mammary vessels and in the posterior mediastinum to displace lung.[13–16] In practice, saline displacement can be applied safely elsewhere in the abdomen or pelvis as needed.

Transsternal Approach to the Lung and Mediastinal Structures

An alternative to saline injection for avoiding the internal mammary vessels has been reported. Gupta et al. described a direct transsternal approach to mediastinal and lung tumors.[17] The sternum was traversed with a coaxial introducer system in all cases so that multiple biopsy specimens could be obtained as needed. The sternum was traversed in some cases with needles designed for bone biopsy, and in others with routine biopsy needles to which constant pressure was applied with a rotating motion.[17]

Modified Needles

Modifications of existing needles and development of modified needles have been proposed to approach tumors or nodes difficult to access with a direct approach because of intervening structures. Sze described creating a gentle curve manually on existing biopsy needles to produce an arc that facilitates needle placement into the target lesion while avoiding critical structures such as bowel or large vessels.[18] Sze successfully applied this approach to mediastinal, lung, and abdominal/pelvic biopsies. The investigator cautioned, however, that the arc be created separately in the coaxial outer introducer and in its inner stylet; creation of the arc with the two pieces together results in the inability to remove the inner stylet.[18] Kopecky et al. described a modified coaxial introducer with a sidehole strategically placed adjacent to the structure of interest.[19] The inner stylet is removed, and a curved biopsy needle is advanced out the sidehole and into the target.

EVOLVING ISSUES IN PERCUTANEOUS BIOPSY: RENAL MASSES

Conventional management of focal renal masses is predicated on the assumption that they are almost all renal cell carcinoma and thus are removed surgically. In cases of small masses (< 3 cm) in elderly patients or patients with extensive co-morbidities, follow-up imaging has been advocated because many small renal cell carcinomas grow slowly, and most do not metastasize until they are larger than 3 or 4 cm. In both of these management strategies, percutaneous biopsy has not played a role. Percutaneous aspiration or biopsy has conventionally been limited to cases in which lymphoma is suspected or in cases of focal pyelonephritis if necessary to identify an underlying organism. However, Wood et al. reported a series of 73 patients in which disease management was changed in 41% of patients by the results of the percutaneous biopsy.[20] Patients for whom disease management was changed were usually those with preexisting malignancies in whom metastatic disease rather than renal cell carcinoma was diagnosed. Therefore, in patients with a prior history of malignancy, percutaneous needle biopsy with fine-needle aspiration and core biopsies can be useful and may change disease management from a surgical to a nonsurgical approach.

REFERENCES

1. Hahn PF, Eisenberg PJ, Pitman MB, Gazelle GS, Mueller PR. Cytopathologic touch preparations (imprints) from core needle biopsies: accuracy compared with that of fine-needle aspirates. *Am J Roentgenol* 1995;165:1277–1279.
2. Silverman SG, Tuncali K, Adams DF, et al. CT fluoroscopy-guided abdominal interventions: techniques, results, and radiation exposure. *Radiology* 1999;212:673–681.
3. American Society of Anesthesiologists Task Force on Sedation and Analgesia by Non-Anesthesiologists. Practice guidelines for sedation and analgesia by non-anesthesiologists. *Anesthesiology* 1996;84:459–470.
4. Gervais DA, Gazelle GS, Lu DS, Hahn PF, Mueller PR. Percutaneous transpulmonary CT-guided liver biopsy: a safe and technically easy approach for lesions located near the diaphragm. *Am J Roentgenol* 1996;167:482–483.
5. Cronan JJ, Esparza AR, Dorfman GS, Ridlen MS, Paolella LP. Cavernous hemangioma of the liver: role of percutaneous biopsy. *Radiology* 1988;166:135–138.
6. Sperti C, Pasquali C, Guolo P, et al. Serum tumor markers and cyst fluid analysis are useful for the diagnosis of pancreatic cystic tumors. *Cancer* 1996;78:237–243.
7. Keogan MT, Freed KS, Paulson EK, Nelson RC, Dodd LG. Imaging-guided percutaneous biopsy of focal splenic lesions: update on safety and effectiveness. *Am J Roentgenol* 1999;172:933–937.
8. Fields S, Libson E. CT-guided aspiration core needle biopsy of gastrointestinal wall lesions. *J Comput Assist Tomogr* 2000;24:224–228.
9. Tudor GR, Rodgers PM, West KP. Bowel lesions: percutaneous US-guided 18-gauge needle biopsy—preliminary experience. *Radiology* 1999;212:594–597.
10. Papanicolau N, Eisenberg PJ, Silverman SG, McNicholas MM, Althausen AF. Prostatic biopsy after proctocolectomy: a transgluteal, CT-guided approach. *Am J Roentgenol* 1996;166:1332–1334.
11. Butch RJ, Mueller PR, Ferrucci JT, et al. Drainage of pelvic abscesses through the greater sciatic foramen. *Radiology* 1986;158:487–491.
12. O'Neill MJ, Rafferty EA, Lee SI, et al. Transvaginal interventional procedures: aspiration, biopsy, and catheter drainage. *Radiographics* 2001;21:657–672.
13. Karampekios S, Hatjidakis AA, Drositis J, Gourtsoyiannis N. Artificial paravertebral widening for percutaneous CT-guided adrenal biopsy. *J Comput Assist Tomogr* 1998;22(2):308–310.
14. Grant TH, Stull MA, Kandallu K, Chambliss JF. Percutaneous needle biopsy of mediastinal masses using a computed tomography-guided approach. *J Thorac Imaging* 1998;13:14–19.
15. Langen HJ, Jochims M, Gunther RW. Artificial displacement of kidneys, spleen, and colon by injection of physiologic saline and CO_2 as an aid to percutaneous procedures: experimental results. *J Vasc Interv Radiol* 1995;6:411–416.
16. Moulton JS. Artificial extrapleural window for mediastinal biopsy. *J Vasc Interv Radiol* 1993;4:825–829.
17. Gupta S, Wallace MJ, Morello FA, Ahrar K, Hicks M. CT-guided percutaneous needle biopsy of intrathoracic lesions by using the transsternal approach: experience in 37 patients. *Radiology* 2002;222:57–62.
18. Sze DY. Use of curved needles to perform biopsies and drainages of inaccessible targets. *J Vasc Interv Radiol* 2001;12:1441–1444.
19. Kopecky KK, Broderick LS, Davidson DD, Burney BT. Side-exiting coaxial needle for aspiration biopsy. *Am J Roentgenol* 1996;167:661–662.
20. Wood BJ, Khan MA, McGovern F, et al. Imaging guided biopsy of renal masses: indications, accuracy and impact on clinical management. *J Urol* 1999;161:1470–1474.

CHAPTER 9

ANGIOGRAPHIC DIAGNOSIS OF ABDOMINAL NEOPLASMS

CHRISTOPH BINKERT, MD
ELIAS BROUNTZOS, MD
JOHN KAUFMAN, MD

INTRODUCTION

Before the era of cross-sectional imaging such as ultrasonography, computed tomography, and magnetic resonance imaging, visceral angiography played an important role in the diagnosis of visceral tumors. The noninvasive imaging modalities have now replaced visceral angiography for primary diagnostic workup of abdominal masses.

Why is it still important for an angiographer to know the angiographic appearance of abdominal tumors? On one hand, abdominal aortograms are performed routinely during evaluation of peripheral vascular or aneurysmal disease. Recognition of an incidental tumor is important to enable an early diagnosis and treatment with a potentially more favorable outcome for the patient. On the other hand, visceral angiography can add useful information to the cross-sectional imaging in certain cases. For example, the organ from which a large tumor originates can be difficult to assess with cross-sectional imaging alone. The main arterial supply to a tumor usually derives from its organ of origin, and visceral angiography can be helpful in this setting (**Fig. 9-1**). The presence or absence of involvement of arteries and veins is critical to the planning of surgical tumor resection. Cross-sectional images provide unspecific information, like vessel narrowing or tumor tissue adjacent to an artery or vein; angiography can specifically show tumor encasement and therefore can help define the resectability of a lesion.

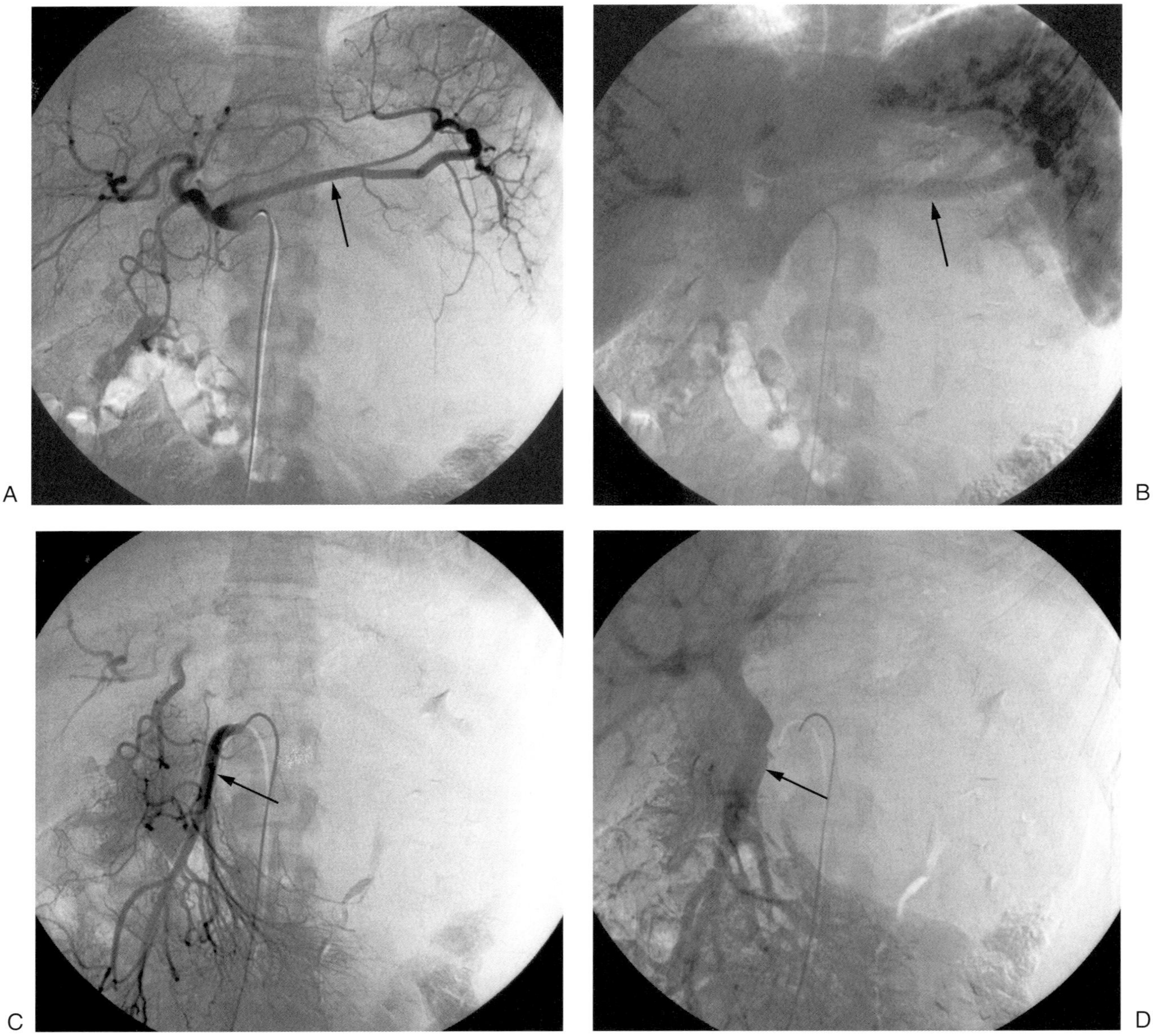

Figure 9-1. (A through E) Angiographic diagnosis of the origin of a large abdominal mass: Selective visceral arteriograms showed displacement of large visceral vessels by a large abdominal mass: (A) splenic artery (arrow) and (B) vein (arrow), (C) superior mesenteric artery (arrow) and (D) vein (arrow). *(Continued on next page.)*

E 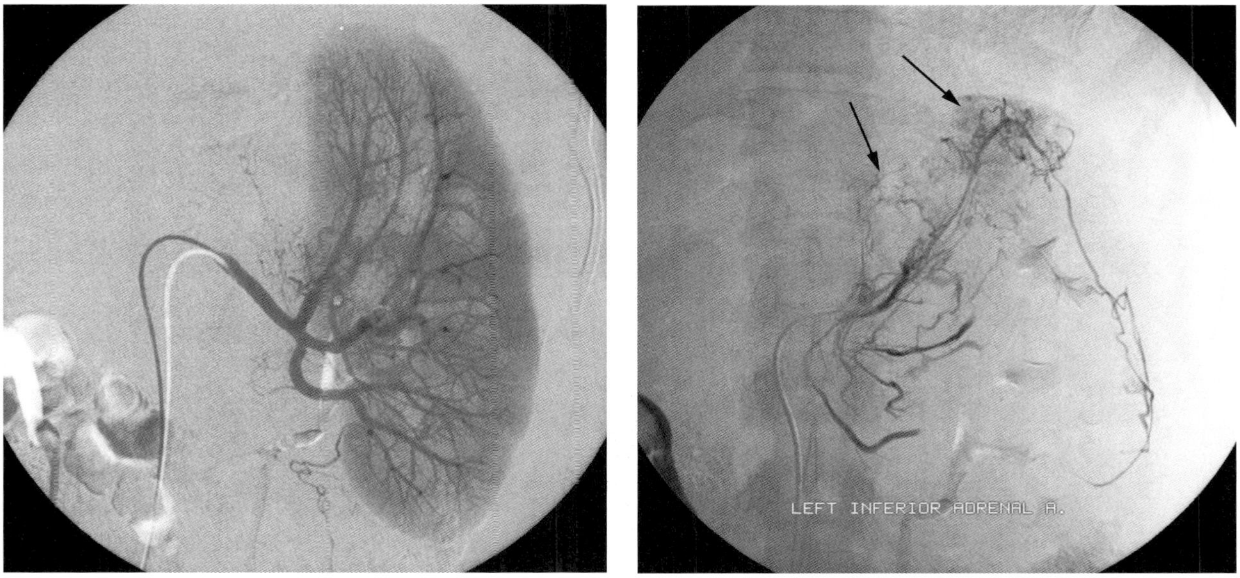 F

Figure 9-1. (Continued). Left renal artery (E). No tumor involvement or tumor vessels were visible. (F) Selective arteriogram of the inferior adrenal artery revealed the organ of origin by showing tumor vessels (arrows) arising from this artery, making the diagnosis of an adrenal carcinoma.

ANGIOGRAPHIC TECHNIQUE

Selective angiography is mandatory for evaluation of abdominal tumors. To avoid arterial spasm, which may lead to the false diagnosis of vessel encasement, the first-order branch of the aorta should be selected by the angiographic catheter alone without a guidewire (**Figs. 9-2, 9-3**). If necessary, more selective catheterization is performed over a guidewire to avoid dissection of the artery.

The rate of injection of contrast material should replace the blood flow of the vessel as usual. The rate is

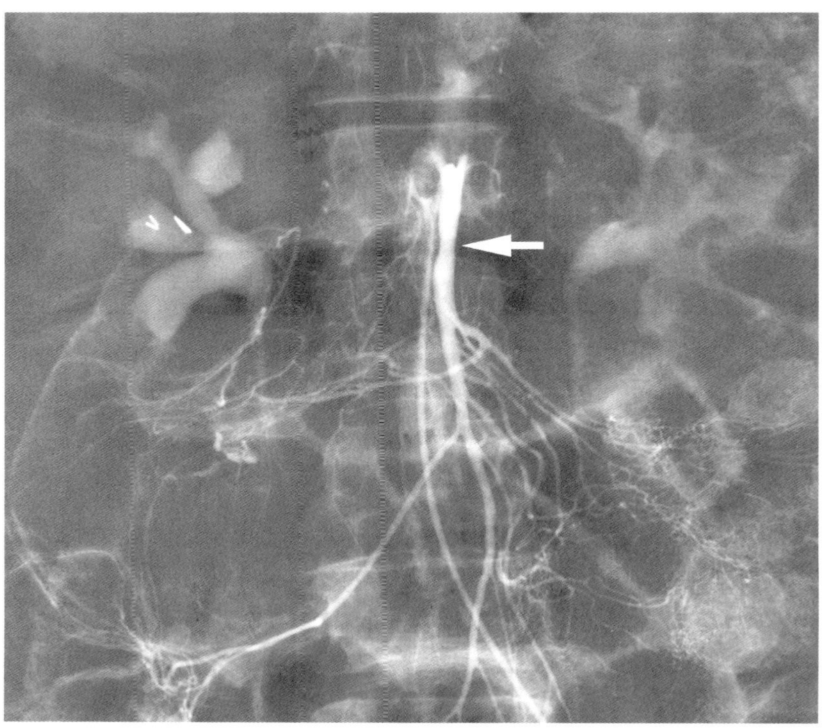

Figure 9-2. Arterial spasm of the superior mesenteric artery (SMA). Smooth segmental narrowing of the this artery (arrow) is caused by infusion of vasopressin.

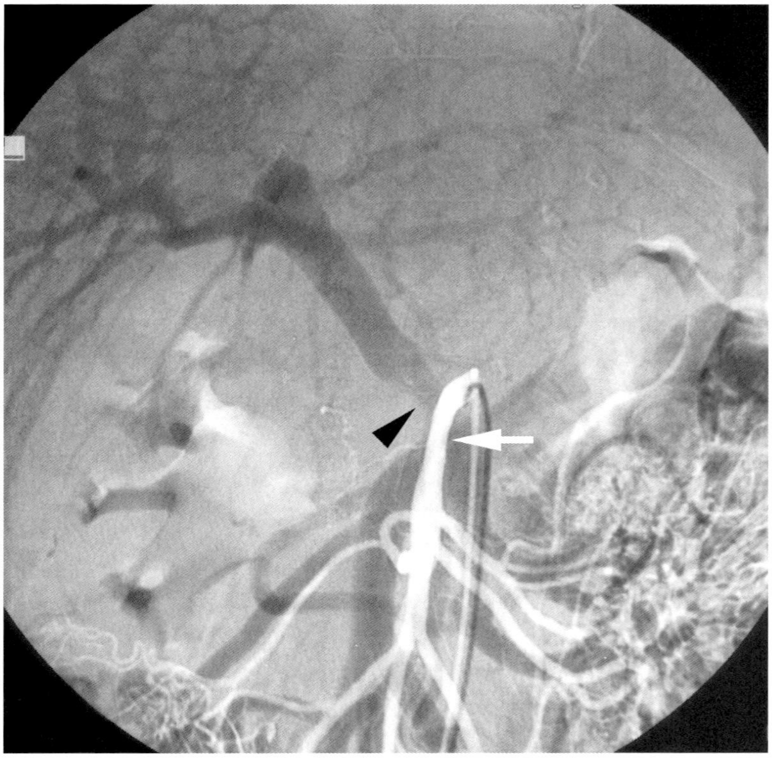

Figure 9-3. Smooth tumor encasement of the proximal superior mesenteric artery (SMA). Smooth narrowing of the proximal SMA (white arrow) is similar to that seen in Figure 9-2. The additional encasement of the adjacent portal vein (black arrowhead) confirmed vascular invasion by a pancreatic head tumor.

6–10 mL/sec for the celiac trunk and superior mesenteric artery (SMA), 6–8 mL/sec for renal arteries, and 3–5 mL/sec for the inferior mesenteric artery (IMA). Larger injections of undiluted contrast material should be used to obtain good filling of the parenchyma and veins, both of which are important for tumor diagnosis. The injection time therefore varies from 3 seconds for renal arteries, to 6–8 seconds for the celiac trunk, to 8–10 seconds for the SMA and IMA. For the same reason, filming should be prolonged, up to 25 seconds for injection of the SMA.[1] If available, cut-film technique is preferred over digital subtraction angiography (DSA) during mesenteric angiography because of the former's (1) higher spatial resolution and (2) absence of artifacts secondary to bowel gas movement. For better visualization, the general angiographic principles, such a second projection and magnification views, apply.

The quality of visceral angiograms can be further improved by administration of pharmacologic agents. If DSA is used, 1 mg of glucagon should be injected intravenously 1 minute before angiography, to decrease bowel movement artifacts. Intra-arterial administration of a vasodilator helps visualization of the portal vein after SMA injection[1]; 25–50 mg of tolazoline (Priscoline), an alpha-adrenergic blocking agent, is slowly injected over a period of 10–15 seconds into the SMA 30 seconds before the angiogram (**Fig. 9-4**). Tolazoline's vasodilatory effect on small arteries can also be used to intensify the parenchymal phase of the liver[2] and pancreas.[3] Alternatively, 100–200 μg of nitroglycerin can be used. The advantage of nitroglycerin is its more transient effect, which facilitates stabilization of potential hypotension.

Another way to enhance tumor vessels is to administer the vasoconstrictor epinephrine.[4] The basis of the epinephrine effect is a preferential vasoconstriction of the normal arteries rather than tumor arteries, which lack a normal musculature layer. After administration of epinephrine, therefore, normal vessels constrict but tumor vessels remain unchanged. Epinephrine-enhanced angiography is used mainly for renal masses in a central location, which are partly obscured by overlapping normal vascularity. The usual dose is 3–5 μg epinephrine, depending on kidney size, injected through the angiographic catheter just before the angiogram.[5] The proper epinephrine effect should be a uniform constriction of the renal arteries with filling of the major and some of the interlobar branches (**Fig. 9-5**).[5]

ANGIOGRAPHIC FINDINGS

Malignant tumors are associated with typical angiographic changes. Tumors with similar histology, such as primary tumors and their corresponding metastases, have similar angiographic findings regardless of their location. **Table 9-1** describes the most typical appearance of each tumor.

Most angiographic findings are nonspecific, however, also appearing with benign tumors or inflammation.[6, 7]

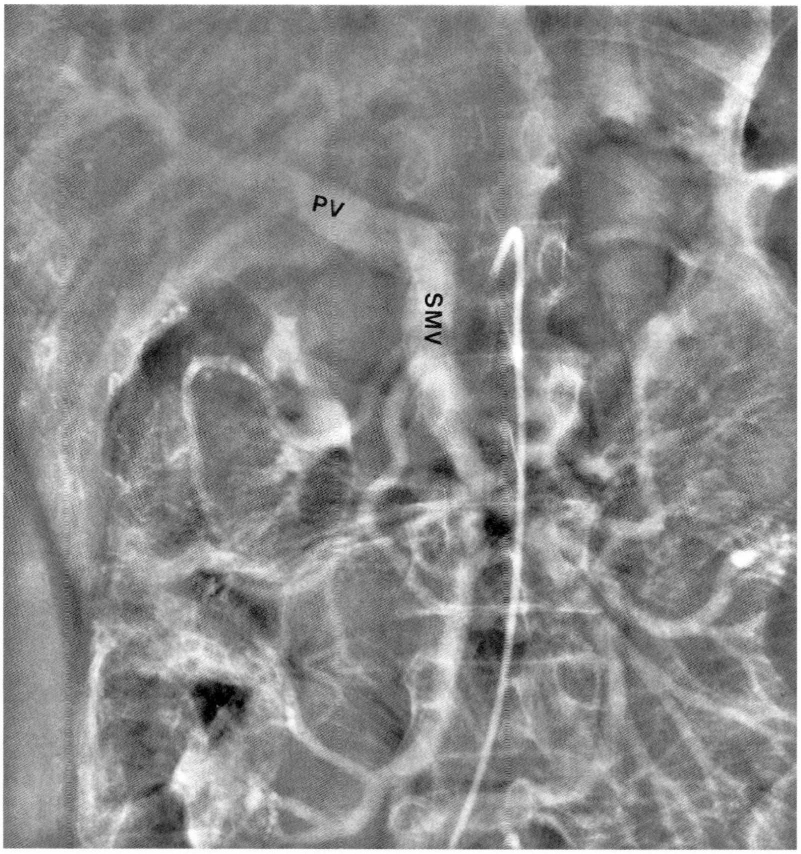

Figure 9-4. Pharmacologically enhanced normal arterial portography. Good visualization is a prerequisite for adequate evaluation of the portal vein (PV). Enhanced contrast filling of the superior mesenteric vein (SMV) and portal vein is achieved by intra-arterial administration of tolazoline (Priscoline) or nitroglycerin prior to the injection of a contrast agent.

A 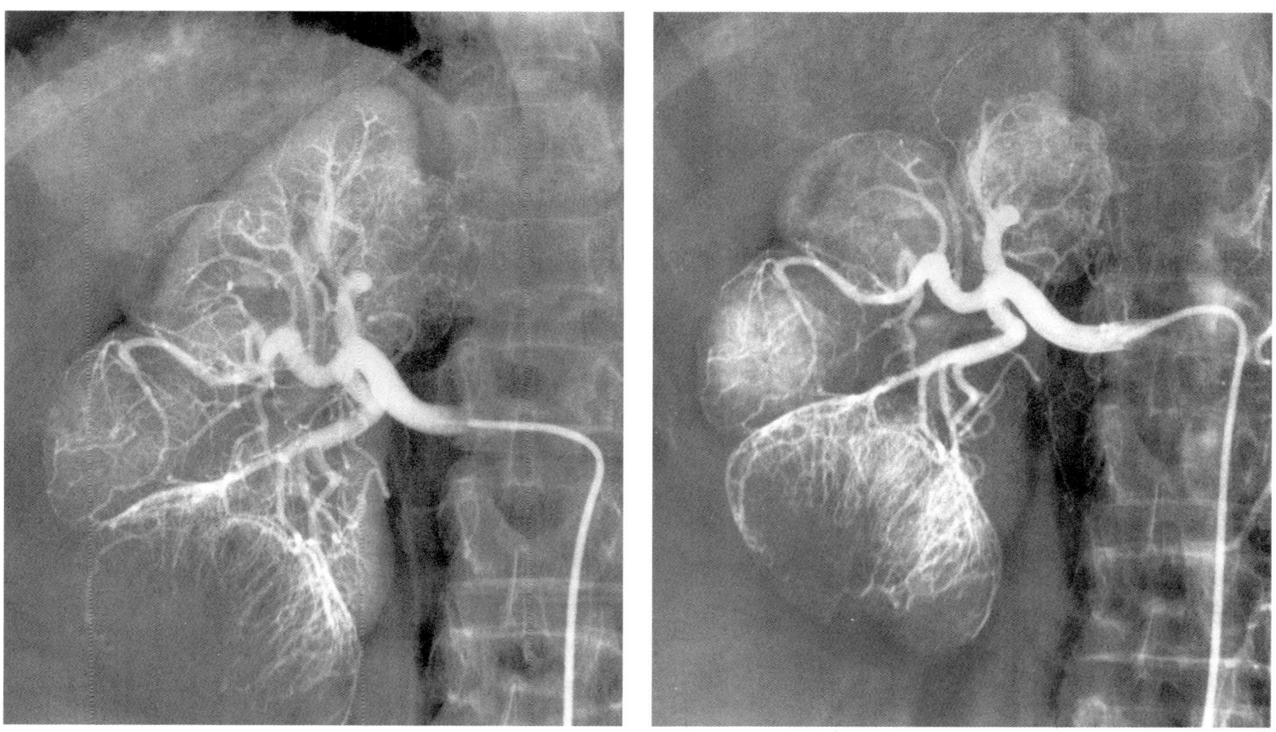 B

Figure 9-5. Epinephrine-enhanced renal angiography in an asymptomatic patient with multiple oncocytomas. (A) Selective right renal angiography suggests four oncocytomas. (B) The tumors are better delineated after injection of epinephrine, which caused spasm of the normal arteries.

TABLE 9-1
Angiographic Features of Abdominal Tumors

Tumor	Arterial phase	Capillary phase	Venous phase	Comment
Liver				
Hepatoma	Enlarged, irregular feeding arteries	Hypervascularity with abnormal tumor vessels and arteriovenous (AV) shunts	Portal vein invasion	Distribution: unifocal-multifocal-diffuse
Cholangiocarcinoma	Encasement of nondilated arteries (may be only abnormality)	Unremarkable, especially if growing through bile ducts	Venous encasement and displacement if large tumor mass	
Adenoma	Bizarre circumferential arterial branches around mass	Rounded homogeneously hypervascular mass	Accummulation of contrast material into venous phase	Associated with oral contraceptives; complication: bleeding
Focal nodular hyperplasia	Peripheral and/or central feeding arteries	Homogeneous granular hypervascularity with central scar	Dilated veins	If no central artery, angiographic features similar to those of adenoma
Hemangioma	Normal arteries displaced around mass	Filling of small peripheral coarse, well-marginated spaces	Contrast material retained in peripheral spaces into venous phase	Tumor may be largely thrombosed
Hemangio-endothelioma	Markedly dilated arteries	Multiple vascular channels with AV shunts to hepatic vein	Early venous filling	Infancy; congestive heart failure if AV shunts are large
Gastrointestinal				
Leiomyomas	Moderately dilated arterial branches; displacement if tumor mass is large	Hypervascular in small bowel, hypovascular in stomach (greater curvature)	Venous displacement if tumor mass is large	
Carcinoid	Kinked, tortuous feeding artery (desmoplastic reaction: starburst)	Primary tumor less hypervascular than metastasis	Tortuous or occluded draining veins	Most common in appendix and terminal ileum
Lymphoma	Unremarkable; displacement if mass is large	Poorly vascularized	Unremarkable; displacement if mass is large	
Pancreas				
Adenocarcinoma	Encasement of nondilated arteries (typical)	Hypovascular to mildly hypervascular	Venous invasion with compression or occlusion of adjacent vein	
Islet cell adenoma	Normal arteries in small lesions; dilated arteries in large lesions	Dense tumor blush	Accummulation of contrast material into venous phase	Usually small: easy to miss if poorly vascularized

(Continues)

TABLE 9-1
Continued

Tumor	Arterial phase	Capillary phase	Venous phase	Comment
Kidney				
Renal cell carcinoma	Encasement of enlarged irregular arteries	Irregular hypervascularity with AV shunts and contrast pooling	Invasion of renal vein and inferior vena cava	
Oncocytoma	Circumferential artery with wheel-spoke pattern	Hypervascular with well-defined borders	Venous displacement if mass is large	Similar on angiography to well-differentiated renal cell carcinoma
Angiomyolipoma	Large tortuous arteries with small aneurysms	Hypervascular with filling of lakes, but no AV shunts	Dilated veins	Associated with tuberous sclerosis; complication: bleeding

Visceral angiography in tumor evaluation must include analysis of arterial, capillary, and venous phases. The assessment of angiographic abnormalities in all three phases is important to categorize a lesion; the higher the number of abnormalities present, the greater the certainty of the diagnosis. The angiographic findings in each phase are discussed separately.

ARTERIAL PHASE

Invasion of normal arteries by tumor leads to narrowing and distortion of the vessel, called *encasement*. Two different types of encasement can be seen[8]:

- *Serrated encasement* (**Fig. 9-6**): The saw-toothed appearance is specific for tumor infiltration and is typically found in larger arteries, such as the hepatic, splenic, left gastric, superior mesenteric, and gastroduodenal arteries.
- *Serpiginous encasement* (**Figs. 9-7, 9-8**): Arteries are abruptly angulated and distorted by tumor; this finding is reasonably specific for carcinoma but is occasionally caused by severe fibrosis (e.g., relapsing pancreatitis) or after extensive radiotherapy.

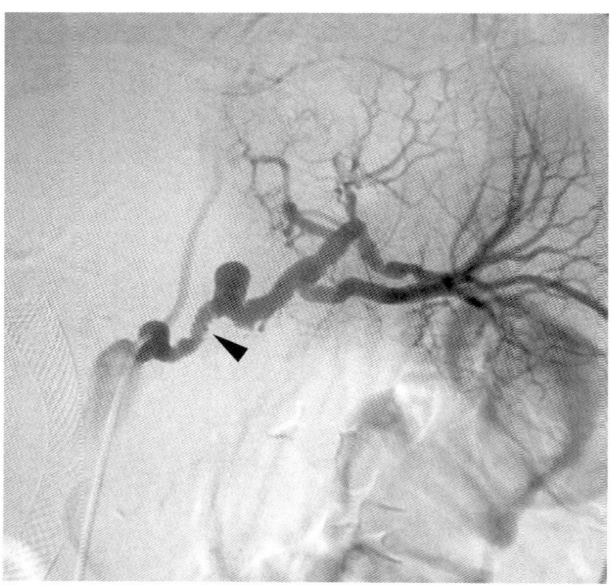

Figure 9-6. Serrated tumor encasement of the splenic artery (arrowhead) in a patient with advanced pancreatic carcinoma.

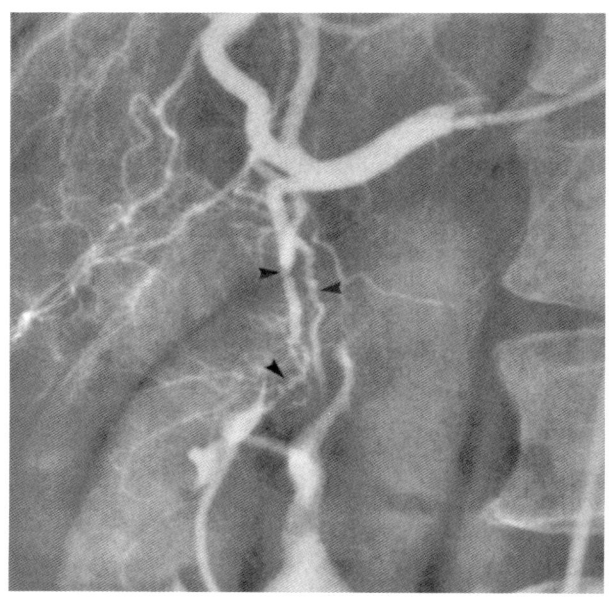

Figure 9-7. Serpiginous type of encasement. Note the distorted course of the gastroduodenal and superior pancreaticoduodenal arteries (arrowheads) in a patient with a pancreatic head carcinoma.

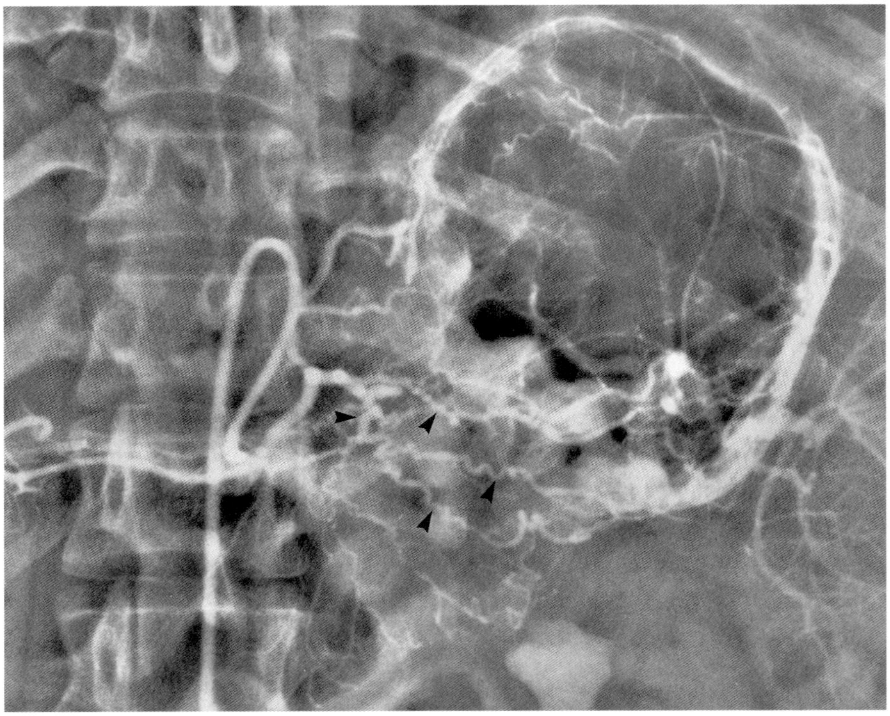

Figure 9-8. In this example of serpiginous encasement, the left gastric artery branches (arrowheads) are involved by an aggressive gastric carcinoma.

Smaller arteries tend to show the pattern of serpiginous encasement with abrupt angulation and frequent variation of caliber. Smooth encasement is nonspecific and is also commonly seen in inflammatory disease (**Fig. 9-9**). Nevertheless, if the artery appears normal on either side of the narrowing and if other signs for a neoplasm are present, tumor encasement can be diagnosed. In addition to being encased, arteries can be occluded by tumors (**Fig. 9-10**). Like smooth narrowing, occlusion is not a specific tumor finding because it is caused by other diseases, such as atherosclerosis.

Malignant neoplasms, like benign tumors, cysts, and abscesses, may displace the surrounding arteries.

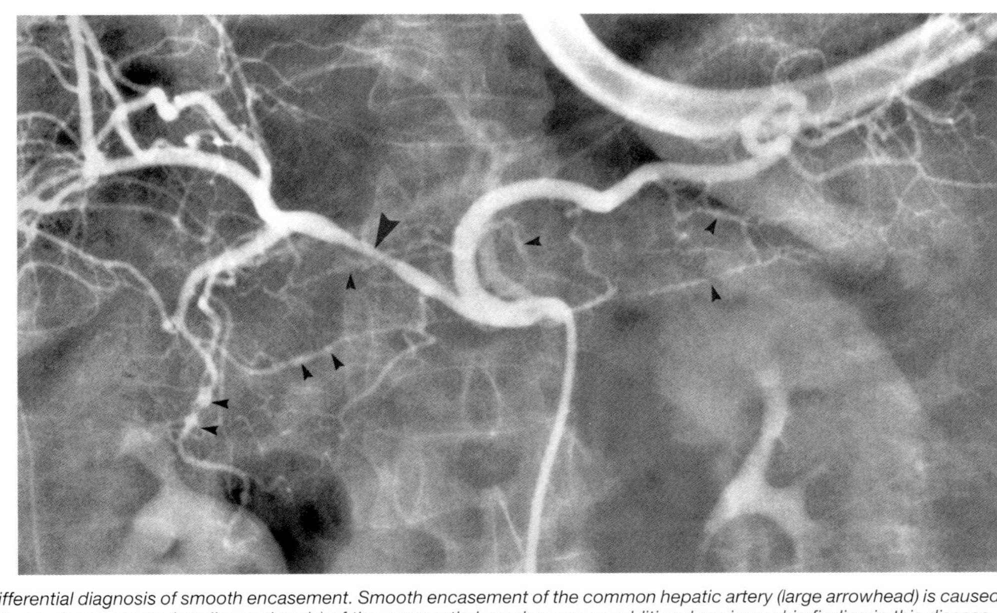

Figure 9-9. Differential diagnosis of smooth encasement. Smooth encasement of the common hepatic artery (large arrowhead) is caused by chronic pancreatitis. Small pseudoaneurysms (small arrowheads) of the pancreatic branches are an additional angiographic finding in this disease.

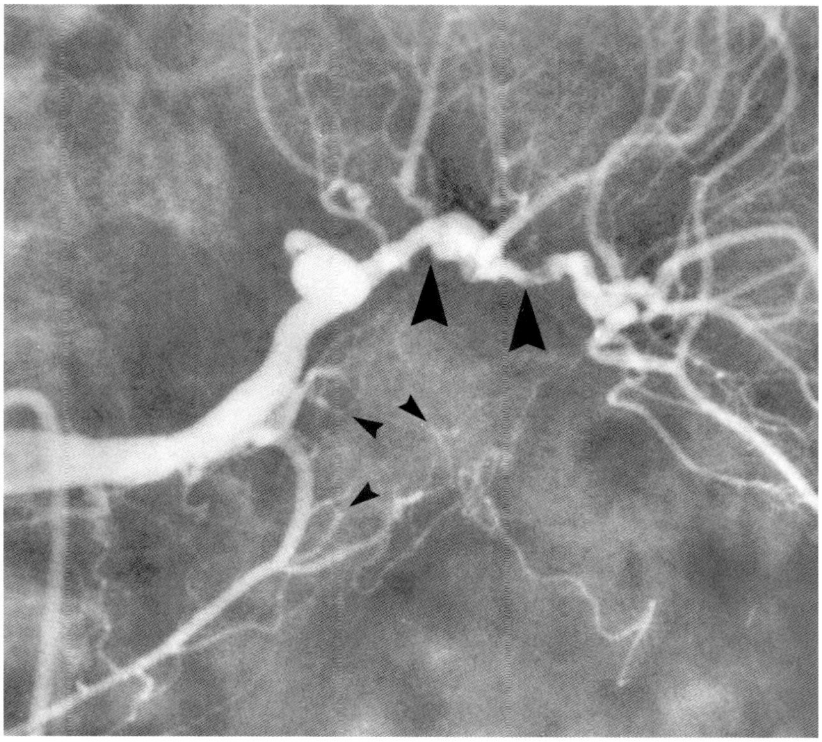

Figure 9-10. Occlusion of multiple intrapancreatic artery branches (small arrowheads) is caused by a pancreatic carcinoma invading the splenic hilum. In addition, serrated encasement of the splenic artery is shown (large arrowheads).

How the artery is pushed away from its original course helps localize the mass (**Fig. 9-11; see Fig. 9-1**). The displaced artery can be normal or dilated; a larger arterial diameter is often seen in malignant tumors as a result of an increase in blood demand.

CAPILLARY PHASE

The growth of solid neoplasms is always accompanied by neovascularization.[9] Neovascularity is characterized by an abundance of small primitive vascular

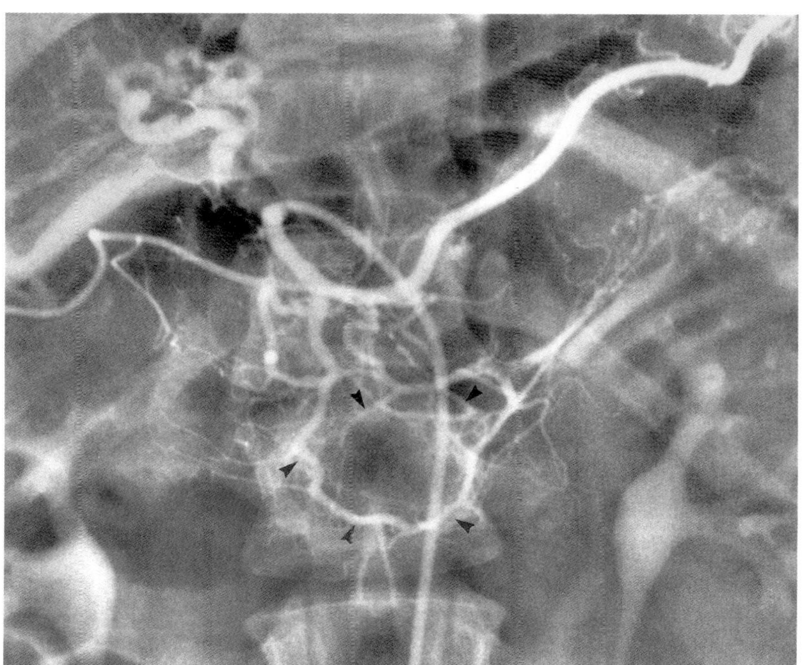

Figure 9-11. Vascular displacement. Pancreatic artery branches (arrowheads) are stretched around a small mass located in the pancreatic head—an unspecific finding. In this case, the mass was a small pseudocyst.

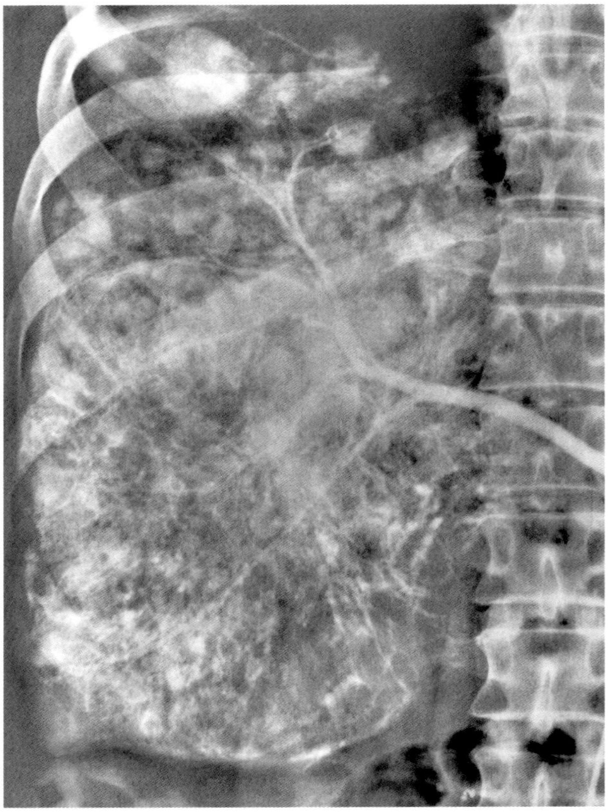

Figure 9-12. The extent of this multifocal hepatocellular carcinoma is depicted by the angiographic blush of the main tumor mass. Satellite lesions around the mass are also visible.

channels without a regular muscular layer. These vessels are often below the limits of angiographic resolution. Instead of appearing as single vessels, a number of these small channels seem to fuse, giving the appearance of increased vascularity that is also called *tumor blush* or *tumor stain* (**Fig. 9-12**). A tumor blush is generally seen in highly vascular tumors and rarely in scirrhous, invasive lesions. If present, the tumor blush is a good indicator of tumor size. If the tumor is hypovascular, its size can often be estimated from the unopacified area within a homogeneously stained organ (**Fig. 9-13**).

Tumor necrosis is usually visualized as an avascular area within the lesion. Occasionally, the area of necrosis communicates with tumor vessels or with blood vessels invaded by the tumor. This invasion leads to filling of the spaces with contrast material ("pooling") (**Fig. 9-14**). The margins of the pools or lakes of contrast material are irregular and poorly defined, in contrast to the well-defined, dilated vascular spaces seen in hemangiomas (**Fig. 9-15**).

Early venous filling can be observed if arteriovenous shunts are present. Arteriovenous shunts occur in some of the more vascular tumors, particularly in well-differentiated hepatomas.[10] The formation of anastomoses between tumor vessels and intrahepatic portal vein branches is considered typical for hepatoma and helps differentiate this tumor angiographically from cholangiocarcinoma (**Fig. 9-16**). The angiographic appearance of arteriovenous shunt consists of (1) opacification of veins in the tumor with visualization of the arteries in the adjacent region or (2) filling of veins in one area several seconds earlier than filling of veins in the surrounding tissue. Arteriovenous shunt is not specific for tumors and can be seen in benign processes, such as inflammation and arteriovenous malformations.

VENOUS PHASE

The presence of a venous abnormality supports the angiographic diagnosis of a neoplasm. Like arteries,

A

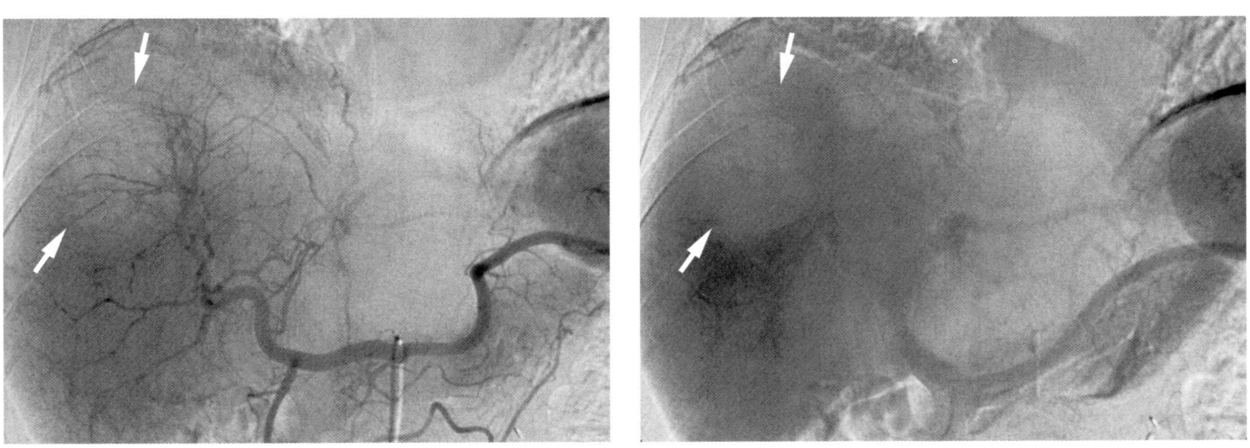

B

Figure 9-13. Hypovascular tumor in a solid organ. (A) Large metastasis of a colorectal carcinoma appeared in the late arterial phase as a hypovascular area (arrows). (B) In the venous phase, the tumor is delineated as a nonopacified area (arrows) within the homogeneously stained liver.

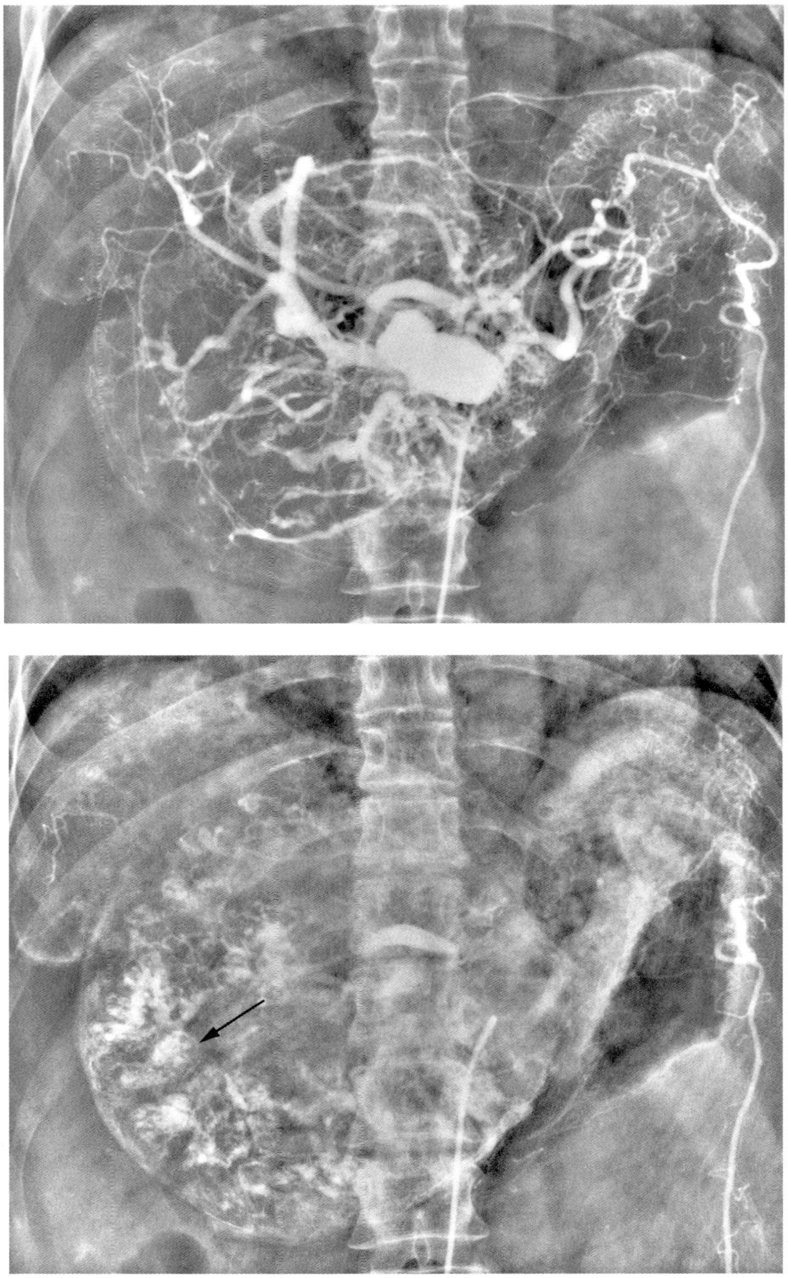

A

B

Figure 9-14. Contrast medium has pooled within necrotic areas (arrow) in a large hepatocellular carcinoma. (A) Arterial phase; (B) capillary phase.

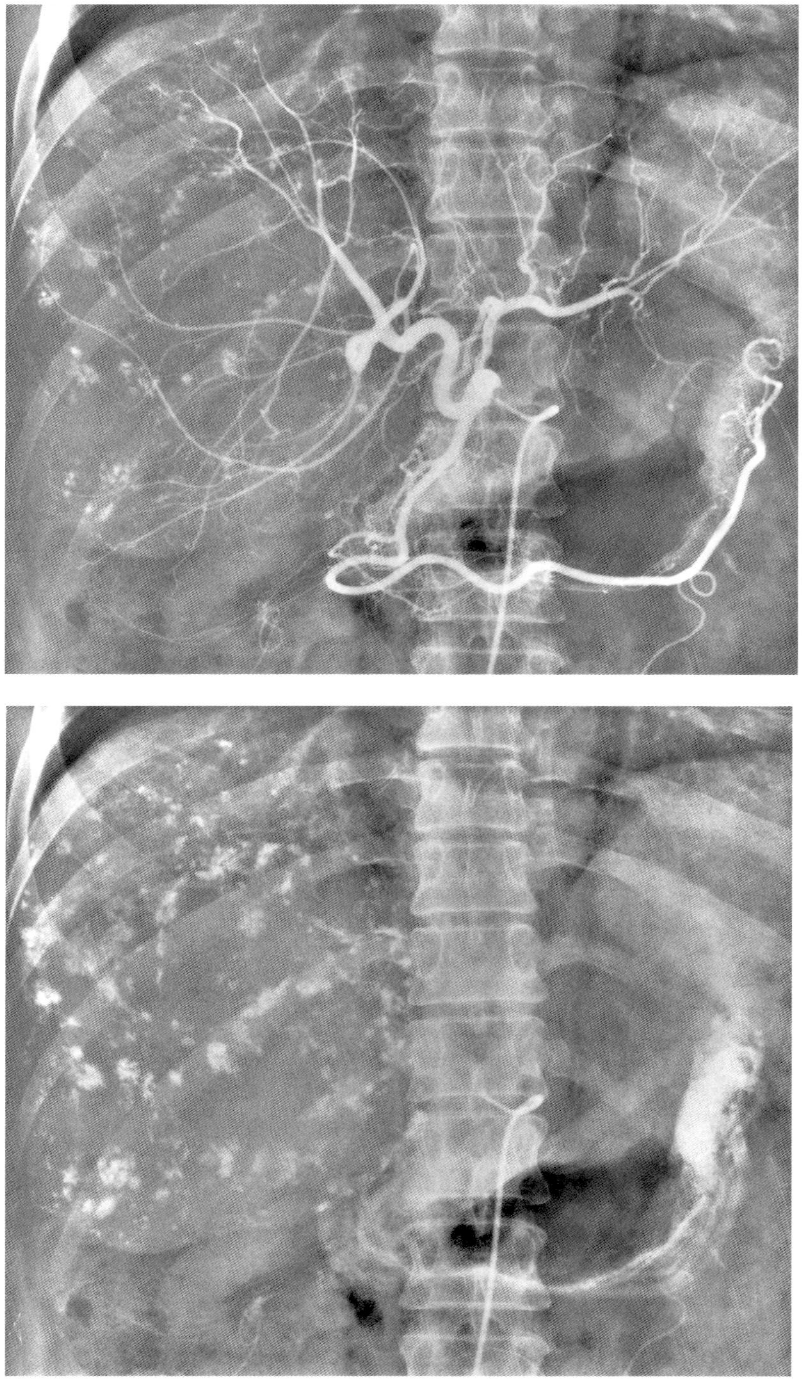

A

B

Figure 9-15. The "cotton-wool" appearance of hemangioma. Dilated vascular spaces of a giant cavernous hemangioma are depicted in the arterial phase (A) and late in the capillary phase (B). Note the well-defined borders (compare with Fig. 9-14).

A

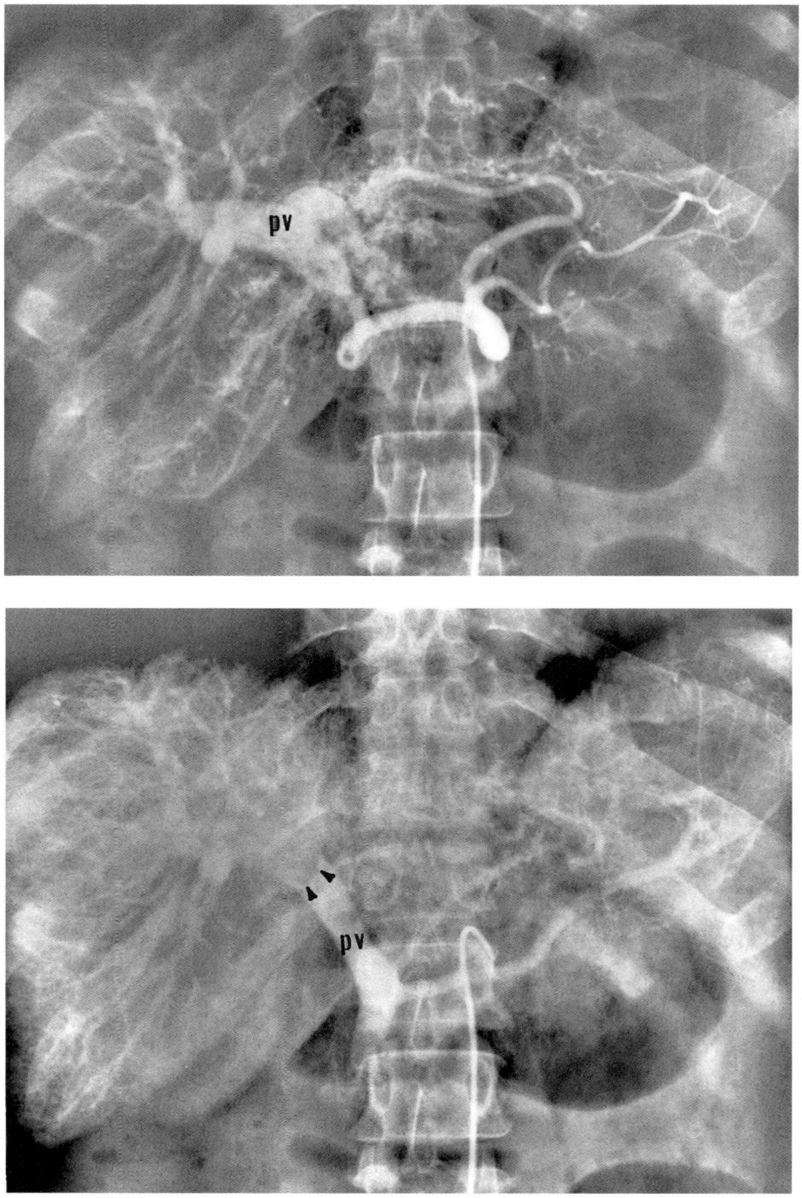

B

Figure 9-16. Arteriovenous shunting and venous invasion, in this case of the portal vein (pv), are typical features of hepatoma. (A) In the arterial phase, shunting is depicted as early filling of the portal vein. (B) During the venous phase, tumor thrombus can be seen within the portal vein (arrowheads).

veins can be displaced or invaded by tumors. Because a vein has a thinner wall than an artery, the angiographic appearances of tumor involvement of veins and arteries are different. A vein is more easily compressed by a tumor mass. If tumor invasion occurs, the vein demonstrates a serrated appearance, like an encased artery (**Fig. 9-17**). The angiographic demonstration of a venous collateral circulation is commonly the only feature other than the absence of the involved vein (**Fig. 9-18**). Certain tumors have a tendency to grow directly into an adjacent vein. Renal cell carcinoma is particularly known for this behavior, invading the renal vein in 13%–23% of cases, with involvement of the inferior vena cava in 5%–13% (**Fig. 9-19**).[11, 12] Portal vein thrombosis associated with hepatocellular carcinoma is found at autopsy in up to 44% of cases.[13] Angiography not only can demonstrate venous thrombosis but can document tumor vessels in the thrombus (**Fig. 9-20**).

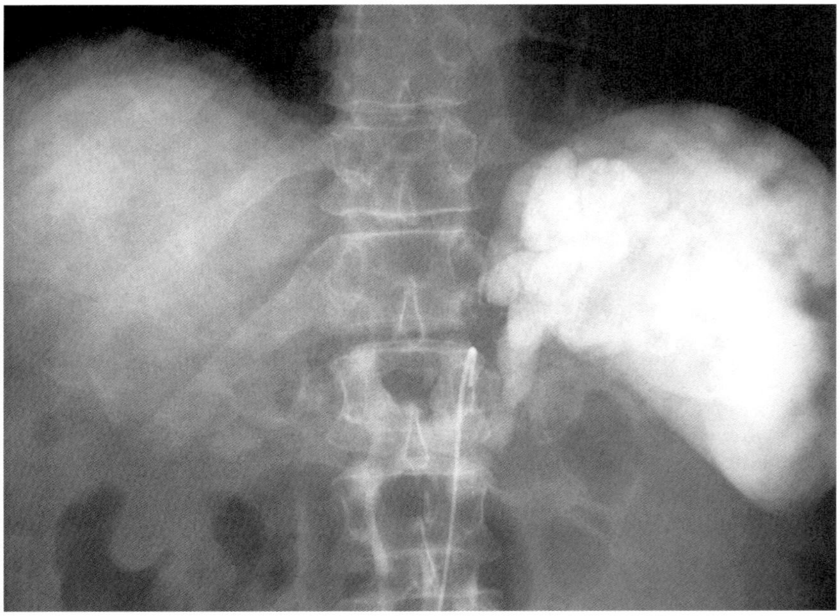

Figure 9-17. Venous occlusion by tumor. Nonappearance of the splenic vein on late-phase images of celiac artery injection indicates that the vein is occluded. Extensive gastric varices function as a collateral pathway.

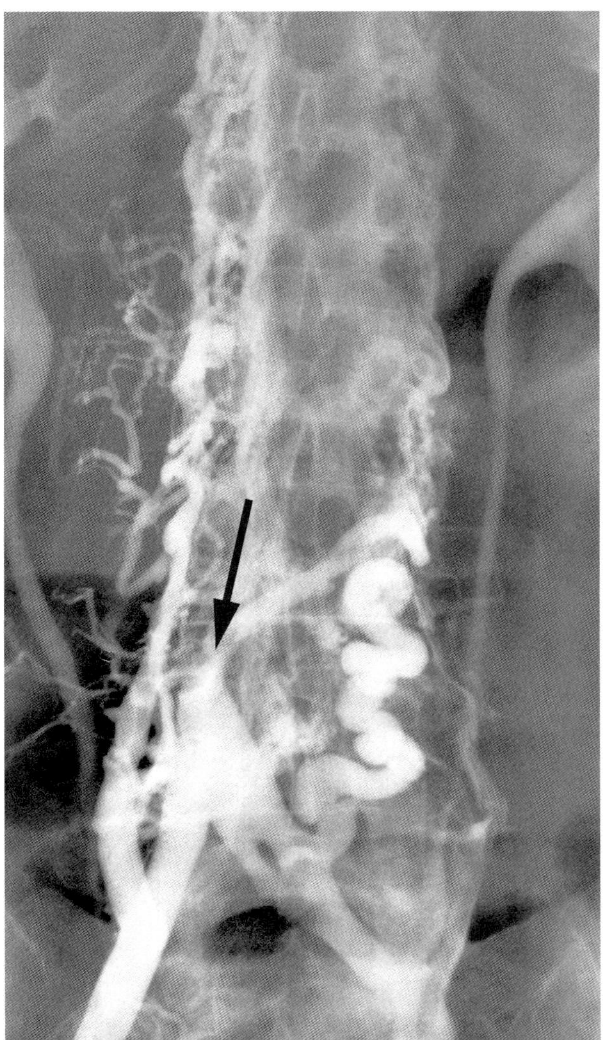

Figure 9-18. Venous occlusion by intrinsic tumor. Occlusion of the inferior vena cava (arrows) is caused by primary leiomyosarcoma, with development of an extensive collateral network.

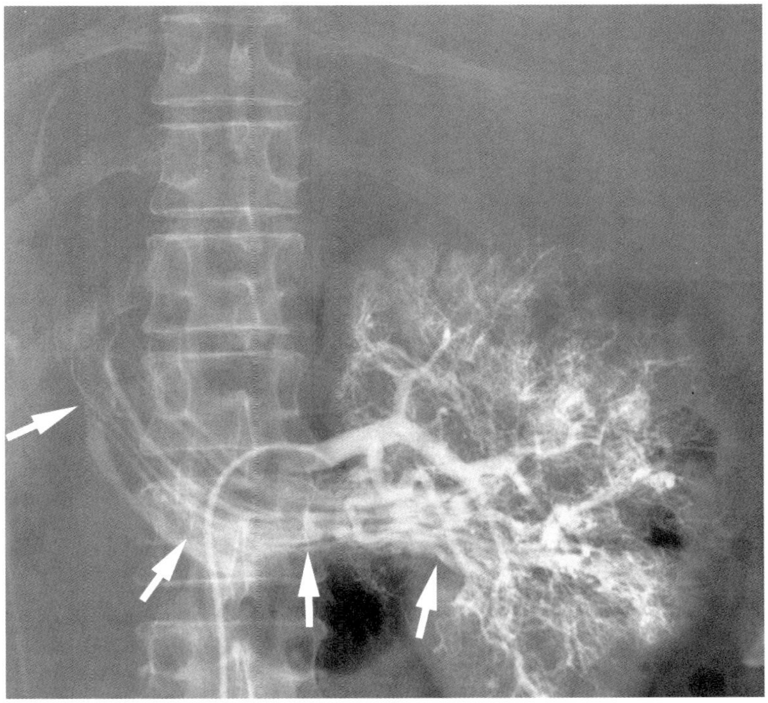

Figure 9-19. Venous invasion by tumor. Renal cell carcinoma has invaded the left renal vein and extended into the inferior vena cava. Multiple arteries are feeding the tumor in the vein (arrows). This finding, typical of tumor thrombus, is known as the "thread-and-streak" sign.

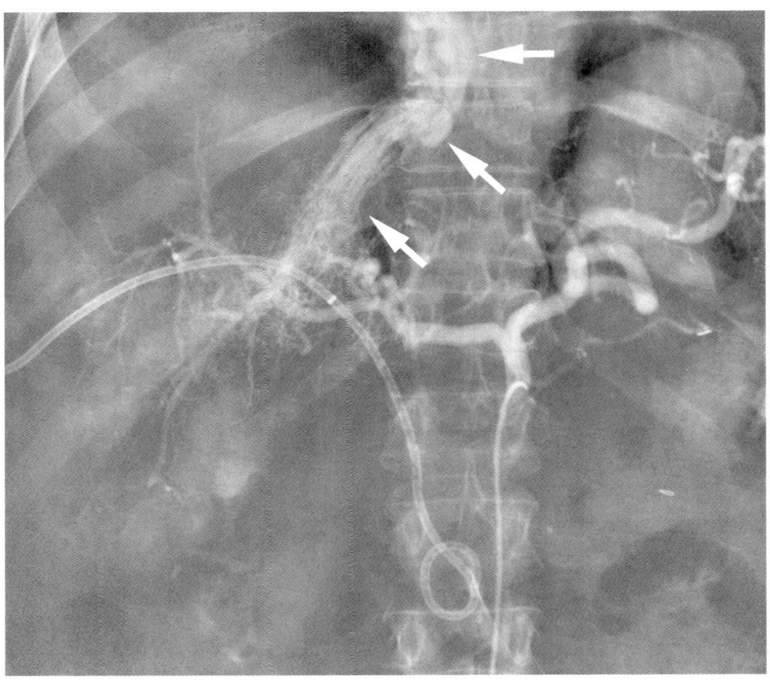

Figure 9-20. Another example of "thread-and-streak" sign. Hepatoma has invaded the right hepatic vein. The tumor thrombus extends into the right atrium (arrows).

REFERENCES

1. Redman HC, Reuter SR, Miller WJ. Improvement of superior mesenteric and portal vein visualization with tolazoline. *Invest Radiol* 1969;4: 24–27.
2. Goldstein HM, Thaggard A, Wallace S, Neiman HL. Priscoline-augmented hepatic angiography. *Radiology* 1976;119:275–279.
3. Goldstein HM, Neiman HL, Bookstein JJ. Angiographic evaluation of pancreatic disease: a further appraisal. *Radiology* 1974;112:275–282.
4. Abrams HL. The response of neoplastic renal vessels to epinephrine in man. *Radiology* 1964;82:217–223.
5. Bosniak MA, Ambos MA, Madayag MA, et al. Epinephrine-enhanced renal angiography in renal mass lesions: is it worth performing? *Am J Roentgenol* 1977;129:647–652.
6. Viamonte M Jr, Roen S, LePage J. Nonspecificity of abnormal vascularity in the angiographic diagnosis of malignant neoplasms. *Radiology* 1973;106:59–63.
7. Levin DC, Wilson R, Abrams HL. The changing role of pancreatic arteriography in the era of computed tomography. *Radiology* 1980;136:245–249.
8. Reuter SR, Redman HC. General angiographic characteristics of gastrointestinal neoplasms. In: *Gastrointestinal Angiography*, 2nd ed. Philadelphia: WB Saunders, 1977:106–117.
9. Folkman J. Tumor angiogenesis: therapeutic implications. *N Engl J Med* 1971;285:1182–1186.
10. Kido C, Sasaki T, Kaneko M. Angiography of primary liver cancer. *Am J Roentgenol Radium Ther Nucl Med* 1971;113:70–81.
11. Vilits P, Colombo T, Hubmer G. [Renal cell carcinoma with venous invasion: therapy–prognosis]. Helv Chir Acta 1990;57:459–461.
12. Ljungberg B, Stenling R, Osterdahl B, et al. Vein invasion in renal cell carcinoma: impact on metastatic behavior and survival. *J Urol* 1995;154:1681–1684.
13. Pirisi M, Avellini C, Fabris C, et al. Portal vein thrombosis in hepatocellular carcinoma: age and sex distribution in an autopsy study. *J Cancer Res Clin Oncol* 1998;124:397–400.

CHAPTER 10

INTERVENTIONAL RADIOLOGY TECHNIQUES FOR LOCALIZATION OF ENDOCRINE TUMORS*†

DONALD L. MILLER, MD

INTRODUCTION

Interventional radiologists are sometimes called upon to assist in the care of patients with endocrine tumors. These patients have hyperfunctioning tumors and clinically evident syndromes of hormone excess. They may have tumors of the pituitary gland, the parathyroid glands, the pancreas, or the adrenal glands.

†The opinions expressed herein are those of the author and do not necessarily reflect the views of the United States Navy, the Department of Defense, or the Department of Health and Human Services.

Arteriography and venous sampling are never used as the initial localization techniques in patients with endocrine disorders, because of the risk and expense. The specific indications for these procedures vary for each organ and disease. Arteriography is generally performed for tumor localization. Venous sampling may be performed for one of two indications: localization of occult tumors, and differentiation between single and multiple gland involvement. Arteriography is now needed less often because of advances in imaging and the introduction of new radiopharmaceutical agents. Conversely, differentiation between single and multiple gland involvement has become an increasingly important indication for venous sampling in patients with hyperaldosteronism.

GENERAL PRINCIPLES OF ENDOCRINE LOCALIZATION

The most basic principle of endocrine localization efforts is *diagnosis first, localization second*. The diagnosis of a disorder of endocrine gland hyperfunction never requires demonstration of a tumor or enlarged gland. Endocrine localization procedures are not intended to establish a diagnosis. Their sole purpose is to identify the location of a source (or sources, in the case of multiple gland hyperplasia) of known hormone overproduction. The results of endocrine arteriographic and venous sampling studies are interpreted with the assumption that a specific endocrine disorder exists. These studies are certain to yield misleading results if the diagnosis is in error.

Venous sampling has definite advantages over other localization techniques. It provides localization by identifying sites of hormone production. Results are derived from measurements of hormone concentration in blood samples obtained from veins draining an endocrine organ. There is no need to visualize the actual lesion responsible for hormone production. Thus, the sensitivity of venous sampling is independent of tumor size. The only requirements for successful detection are that the lesion secrete sufficient hormone to be assayed and that the appropriate vein be sampled.

Venous sampling also has distinct drawbacks. Because the lesion is not visualized during the sampling procedure, it cannot be localized precisely. Venous sampling permits only regionalization—definition of a territory drained by a specific vein or veins, within which the abnormality must lie. In addition, venous sampling techniques are technically demanding, for two reasons. First, venous anatomy is more variable than arterial anatomy. Second, because blood flows from smaller to larger veins, injection of contrast material into main venous trunks does not demonstrate the small tributaries that must be sampled.

Tumor regionalization is based on detection of increased hormone levels in selectively obtained venous blood samples in comparison with the hormone level in peripheral venous blood. Normal glandular tissue is suppressed when an autonomous hormone source, such as an endocrine tumor, is present. In this setting, the normal tissue does not secrete measurable levels of hormone. Hormone levels in veins draining normal tissue approximate those in peripheral venous blood. Elevated hormone concentrations in selectively obtained vein samples are assumed to arise from an autonomous source. *Interpretation of all venous sampling procedures is based on this assumption.* If, however, the diagnosis of an endocrine disorder is wrong, and endocrine function is normal, no glandular suppression is present. In this situation, elevated hormone concentrations in veins draining normal endocrine glands (in comparison with peripheral vein hormone levels) will be misinterpreted as evidence of a nonexistent autonomous source. In short, if venous sampling procedures are performed in normal patients, false-positive results are virtually certain. It is critical that a firm diagnosis of endocrine hyperfunction be established before localization procedures are begun.

Venous sampling is time consuming and requires careful attention to proper labeling and handling (including interim storage) of the samples. All such preparations—documentation of the site from which each sample was obtained, preparation of specimen tubes, and details of specimen handling and transport—should be made and reviewed in advance with the interventional radiology suite technical staff and the hospital chemistry laboratory. This step is particularly important, given the complexity and relative infrequency of the study.

CUSHING SYNDROME

In the normal individual, cortisol production from the adrenal gland exerts negative feedback on the synthesis and release of corticotropin-releasing hormone (CRH) in the hypothalamus and adrenocorticotropic hormone (ACTH) in the pituitary.[1] This mechanism maintains homeostasis of the hypothalamic-pituitary-adrenal axis.

In ACTH-*independent* Cushing syndrome, there is an autonomous source of cortisol. The negative feedback exerted on the pituitary and hypothalamus results in suppression of ACTH production, and ACTH levels are low. ACTH-independent Cushing syndrome is usually caused by an adrenal adenoma or adrenal carcinoma. Rarely, it is due to micronodular hyperplasia (primary pigmented nodular adrenal disease) or massive macronodular hyperplasia. The etiology is established with adrenal CT or MRI.

ACTH-*dependent* Cushing syndrome is characterized by elevations of both cortisol and ACTH. Most patients have a pituitary corticotroph adenoma (Cushing disease), but in 10%–15% of patients the ACTH source is a nonpituitary tumor (ectopic ACTH syndrome). Pseudo-Cushing syndrome, which can be caused by alcoholism, obesity, or major depression, is characterized by excess circulating CRH and can sometimes mimic ACTH-dependent Cushing syndrome.[1]

Differentiation between Cushing disease and the ectopic ACTH syndrome in a patient with ACTH-dependent Cushing syndrome can often be accomplished with endocrine testing. However, stringent criteria are required for evaluation of the test results in order to maximize their specificity and avoid misdiagnosis.[2] A pituitary adenoma can be sought with MRI, but the sensitivity of contrast-enhanced MRI is only 54%–91% in this setting.[3] In addition, pituitary microadenomas are identified in 10% of normal individuals on MRI, so there is a risk of both false-positive and false-negative results.[4]

The obvious method for determining whether the pituitary is secreting ACTH is to perform pituitary venous sampling. Pituitary venous effluent drains into the cavernous sinuses and then via various tributaries into the internal jugular vein. One accessible tributary is the inferior petrosal sinus, which extends from the cavernous sinus to the jugular bulb (**Fig. 10-1**). Inferior petrosal sinus sampling (IPSS) is the standard method for venous sampling in patients with ACTH-dependent Cushing syndrome. IPSS has a higher accuracy rate than endocrine stimulation and suppression testing or MRI.[2, 3, 5] When the procedure has been performed properly, false-negative results are typically due to a type III or type IV anatomic variant of the inferior petrosal sinus (multiple inferior petrosal channels or a hypoplastic inferior petrosal sinus) (**Fig. 10-2**).[6, 7] False-positive results are due to low circulating cortisol levels and incomplete suppression of normal pituitary tissue, or to an incorrect diagnosis of Cushing syndrome.[8]

Pituitary venous sampling may also be performed with microcatheters placed in the cavernous sinus or with standard catheters placed in the internal jugular veins.[9] There does not appear to be any advantage to sampling the cavernous sinuses to offset the increase in cost and complexity of the procedure.[10] Internal jugular vein sampling is less sensitive than IPSS (substantially less so in my own experience).[9] However, it is less demanding technically than IPSS, has a lower complication rate than IPSS, and, if its results are positive, obviates IPSS.

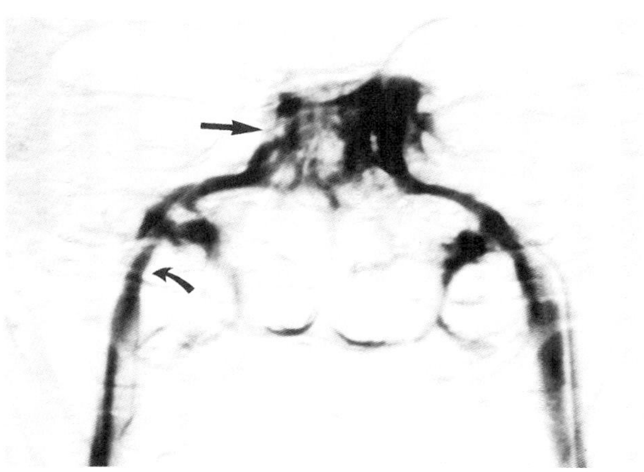

Figure 10-1. Inferior petrosal sinus venogram obtained during inferior petrosal sinus sampling (IPSS). There is a single inferior petrosal sinus on each side, connecting the cavernous sinus (straight arrow) to the internal jugular vein (curved arrow).

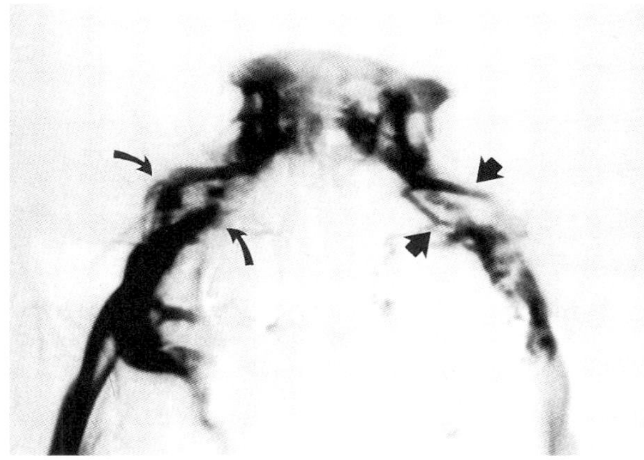

Figure 10-2. Inferior petrosal sinus venogram demonstrating type III inferior petrosal sinus anatomy. There are two inferior petrosal sinuses on the right (curved arrows), and three on the left (broad arrows). A catheter in a small-diameter channel may not accurately sample pituitary venous blood.

IPSS is technically demanding and has a prolonged learning curve. Because it is rarely performed at most institutions, an interventional radiologist working outside a specialized center is unlikely ever to see enough cases to develop expertise. The procedure is not described here, but the technique of IPSS and the anatomy of the inferior petrosal sinus have been reported in detail elsewhere.[6, 11]

Jugular venous sampling is a much less demanding procedure. It may be performed from a femoral vein approach, using standard Seldinger technique, or via direct puncture of the internal jugular veins, using ultrasound guidance and a micropuncture system. In either event, the catheter tips are placed along the medial wall of the internal jugular vein at the level of the mandible. Samples are obtained simultaneously from both jugular vein catheters and a peripheral intravenous catheter (or a femoral vein sheath, if the femoral approach is used). A baseline set of samples is obtained, and then CRH (1 μg/kg) is administered as a slow intravenous injection over a period of 1 minute. Additional sets of samples are obtained from all three sites at 3 minutes, 5 minutes, and 10 minutes after the end of the CRH injection. All samples are carefully labeled and submitted for ACTH assay.

A positive result is defined as a central-to-peripheral ACTH gradient (the ratio of the highest ACTH concentration in either jugular vein sample to the ACTH concentration in the peripheral vein sample) greater than 2 in the baseline sample set and a central-to-peripheral ACTH gradient greater than 3 in any post-CRH stimulation sample set.[9] Lesser gradients are considered negative results. A positive result is considered definitive evidence that the patient has a pituitary source of ACTH. A negative result could be due to ectopic ACTH secretion, but it could also be a false-negative result because internal jugular vein sampling is less sensitive that IPSS. Therefore, patients with negative jugular vein sampling results should undergo IPSS.[10]

HYPERPARATHYROIDISM

In normal individuals, elevated serum calcium concentration inhibits production of parathyroid hormone (PTH) through a negative feedback loop. Patients with primary hyperparathyroidism have excess production of PTH due to loss of the normal feedback inhibition. Primary hyperparathyroidism is one of the most common disorders of hormone excess, with approximately 100,000 cases per year occurring in the United States. Of these, 80% are due to a solitary adenoma, 15% to hyperplasia, 3%–5% to multiple adenomas, and 1% to parathyroid carcinoma.

Evolution in surgical technique, the introduction of sestamibi scintigraphy, and the routine use of preoperative noninvasive imaging techniques (principally sestamibi scanning, ultrasound, and MRI) before the initial neck exploration have reduced surgical failure rates and have permitted less invasive surgery in patients who present with primary hyperparathyroidism.[12–14] Invasive localization studies are very rarely required in these patients.

Patients with persistent or recurrent hypercalcemia after surgery, however, will benefit from the use of all necessary radiologic localization techniques before reoperation, because each additional surgical exploration is more difficult, carries a higher risk of vocal cord paralysis, and is less likely to succeed.[15] Noninvasive studies, being less expensive and less risky, should be performed first. An abnormal parathyroid gland should be demonstrated by at least two of these modalities before localization is considered complete, in order to avoid false-positive localizations. If noninvasive techniques fail to achieve localization, arteriography and venous sampling may be required. The need for these procedures has diminished in recent years as noninvasive techniques have been refined.[16]

Parathyroid Arteriography

Parathyroid arteriography demonstrates an abnormal parathyroid gland in about 60% of patients in whom noninvasive study results are negative or equivocal.[15, 17] Parathyroid venous sampling, the final localization procedure in the evaluation of these patients, permits localization to one side of the neck or to the mediastinum in 80%–90% of the remaining few patients in whom all other studies have failed to image an abnormal gland.

Most individuals have four parathyroid glands, although as few as three and as many as eight have been reported.[18] When the glands are in the normal anatomic position, they are adherent to the posterior surface of the thyroid gland. However, they may also be intrathyroidal (**Fig. 10-3**) or ectopic, and may be located anywhere from the angle of the jaw to the mediastinum. Knowledge of the common locations of normal and ectopic glands is a prerequisite to successful localization. Fortunately, most ectopic glands lie along specific, well-defined pathways of embryologic descent, either in the anterior mediastinum and thymus (**Fig. 10-4**) or in the tracheoesophageal groove and superior mediastinum.[18, 19]

A single artery usually supplies each parathyroid gland.[20, 21] The arterial supply to parathyroid glands located in the normal anatomic position is the same as for the thyroid gland: the paired superior thyroid arteries (from the external carotid artery) and the paired inferior thyroid arteries (from the thyrocervical trunk) (see Fig. 10-3). Branches of the internal mammary artery supply anterior mediastinal and thymic glands (see Fig. 10-4). A branch of the inferior thyroid artery usually supplies

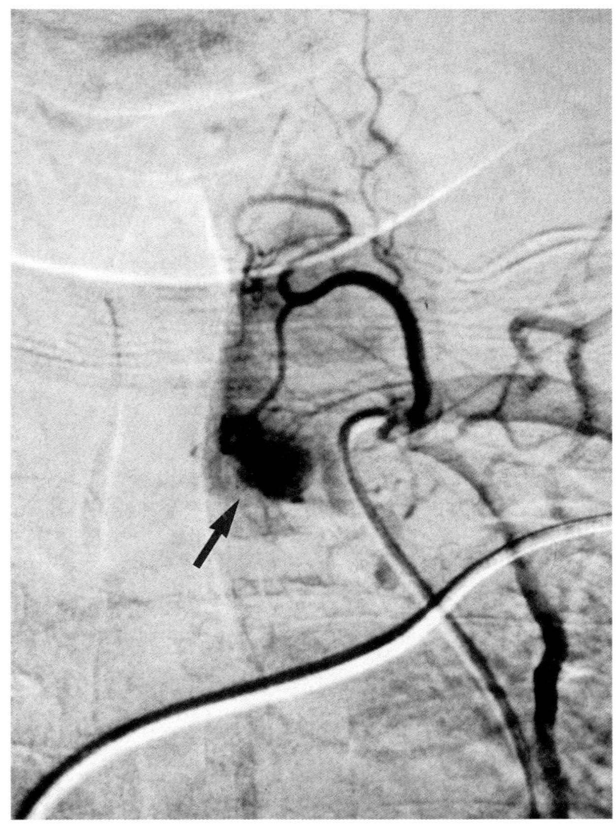

*Figure 10-3. Parathyroid arteriogram with selective injection into the left inferior thyroid artery. Artifact from an electrocardiography lead is present. Note the characteristic inverted **U** loop of the inferior thyroid artery. An intrathyroidal parathyroid adenoma (arrow) is identified as an intensely enhancing, homogeneous, well-marginated lesion. This appearance is not diagnostic of an intrathyroidal lesion, because an adenoma on the normal location on the posterior surface of the thyroid gland would have the same appearance.*

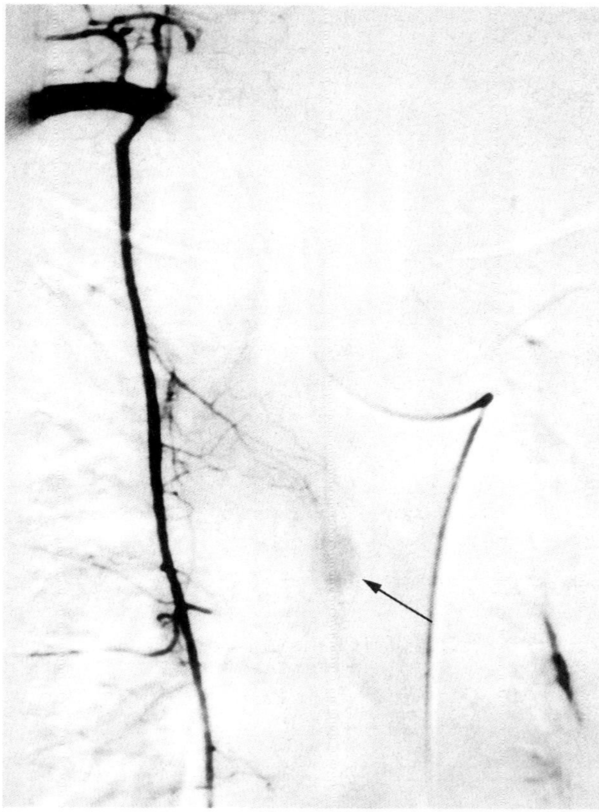

Figure 10-4. A right internal mammary arteriogram demonstrates a mediastinal parathyroid adenoma (arrow). Lesions supplied by the internal mammary artery are located in the thymus or anterior mediastinum.

glands in the superior mediastinum and tracheoesophageal groove.

Parathyroid arteriography is performed with superselective digital subtraction arteriography of both thyrocervical trunks, both internal mammary arteries, and both common carotid arteries.[22] This study also provides "roadmaps" and defines venous drainage patterns that will be useful if venous sampling proves necessary (**Fig. 10-5**). If results of the common carotid artery injections are not clearly negative, bilateral superior thyroid artery injections may be helpful to clarify the arteriographic findings. If all else fails, an arch aortogram may reveal a thyroidea ima artery; present in approximately 6% of individuals, a thyroidea ima artery most commonly arises from the aortic arch, the innominate artery, or the right common carotid artery and supplies variable portions of the thyroid and parathyroid glands.[23,24] This regimen demonstrates an abnormal parathyroid gland in about 60% of patients in whom results of noninvasive imaging are negative or inconclusive, with a very low false-positive rate.[17,25]

The aortic arch, common carotid arteries, and, if necessary, the superior thyroid arteries may be catheterized with standard techniques and catheters. However, these are the least useful vessels for parathyroid localization. Catheterization of the thyrocervical trunk, a critical vessel in parathyroid arteriography, is often more difficult. The most useful catheter is one designed for catheterization of the internal mammary artery. The internal mammary artery should be catheterized first. This vessel arises anteriorly or anteroinferiorly from the subclavian artery, and not directly inferiorly. After internal mammary arteriography is performed, the catheter is slowly withdrawn until it is near the orifice of the internal mammary artery. As gentle puffs of contrast material are injected under fluoroscopic control, the catheter is withdrawn further and rotated anteriorly to engage the orifice of the thyrocervical trunk. The thyrocervical trunk arises from the anterior or anterosuperior aspect of the subclavian artery in close proximity to the internal mammary artery (see Fig. 10-3). One or more thyrocervical trunk branches may share a common origin with the internal mammary artery. In patients with markedly tortuous arch vessels, it can be very difficult to catheterize the right internal mammary artery and right thyrocervical trunk from the groin; in

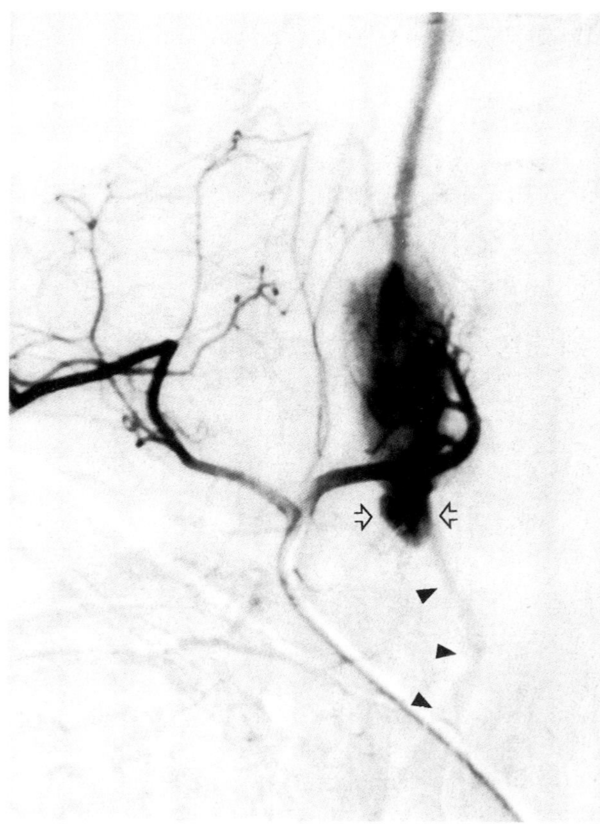

Figure 10-5. A right thyrocervical trunk injection demonstrates a normal thyroid blush and a parathyroid adenoma (open arrows). The inferior thyroid vein is also visible (arrowheads).

these patients, it may be necessary to catheterize these vessels from a right upper extremity approach.

The thyrocervical trunk (see Fig. 10-5) typically gives rise to a medial branch (the inferior thyroid artery), two lateral branches (the suprascapular and transverse cervical arteries) and a superior branch (the ascending cervical artery), although numerous variations exist. It may be recognized from the characteristic looping course of the inferior thyroid artery (see Fig. 10-3). Although the inferior thyroid artery may occasionally have been ligated at the initial operation, failure to identify this vessel usually means that the catheter is in the costocervical trunk, not the thyrocervical trunk. The costocervical trunk arises from the posterosuperior aspect of the subclavian artery, adjacent to the thyrocervical trunk, and is usually much easier to catheterize than the thyrocervical trunk. However, intentional injection of the costocervical trunk should be avoided, because this vessel often supplies a major feeder to the cervical spinal cord.

At arteriography, hyperplastic and adenomatous parathyroid glands appear oval or rounded areas of uniform enhancement, often superimposed on thyroid tissue (see Figs. 10-3 to 10-5). With optimal radiographic technique and collimation, diseased glands as small as 4 to 5 mm may be visible. Normal parathyroid glands are not visualized angiographically in hyperparathyroid patients because their PTH production is suppressed, and the normal glands become quite small (1–2 mm).[26]

Parathyroid Venous Sampling

Parathyroid venous sampling relies on the unilateral elevations in PTH concentrations produced by hyperfunctioning parathyroid glands. Mapping the PTH concentrations in selective samples from draining veins reveals the source of elevated hormone production, because the remaining normal glands are suppressed and their draining veins contain only background levels of PTH. Parathyroid hormone concentrations more than twice the background level are generally considered diagnostic, but gradients are commonly much higher in samples from small veins.[27]

Results of parathyroid venous sampling are positive in 80%–90% of patients in whom results of arteriography are negative.[28] In one series of 86 patients with negative or equivocal results of noninvasive localization studies and arteriograms, parathyroid venous sampling had a sensitivity of 88% and a specificity of 86%.[28]

Venous sampling in patients with hyperparathyroidism due to hyperplasia typically demonstrates bilateral (but unequal) elevations in PTH above background level. For this reason, venous sampling is usually not performed in these patients unless (1) only a single gland remains occult or (2) four glands have been identified and resected at surgery but the patient remains hypercalcemic.

Parathyroid venous sampling is technically far more difficult than parathyroid arteriography. The venous anatomy of the thyroid bed is quite variable, and examples shown in anatomic atlases are invariably oversimplified. Detailed descriptions of the venous anatomy relevant to parathyroid venous sampling should be reviewed before this study is attempted.[29–31]

Venous drainage from the parathyroid glands commonly occurs via ipsilateral superior, middle, and inferior thyroid veins. The superior thyroid vein drains via the facial vein into the internal jugular vein. The middle thyroid vein drains directly into the internal jugular vein. Both inferior thyroid veins commonly drain into the left brachiocephalic vein, either separately or via a combined trunk. Less commonly, the right inferior thyroid vein drains directly into the right brachiocephalic vein. The superior and inferior thyroid veins should be sampled bilaterally, if possible.

In patients who have undergone surgical exploration, ligation of the middle thyroid veins has invariably been performed (failure to perform this ligation is a mark of an inadequate exploration). Often the inferior thyroid veins have been ligated as well. In this situation, venous drainage from the thyroid bed is usually via the vertebral veins, which should always be sampled. Their anatomy has been described in detail elsewhere.[32]

The left thymic vein empties into the left innominate vein. PTH elevations in the thymic vein suggest that the abnormal parathyroid gland is located in the anterior mediastinum. Samples from this vein may be essential to localize an ectopic parathyroid adenoma in the thymus. The anatomy and anastomotic connections of the thymic vein are quite variable, and mediastinal parathyroid glands often drain into the inferior thyroid veins.[33]

Internal jugular vein samples are occasionally helpful. Less selective venous sampling (innominate vein, subclavian vein) generally does not produce gradients sufficiently above background levels to localize the abnormality. Left innominate vein samples are particularly unhelpful because this vein receives drainage from both sides of the neck as well as from the mediastinum.[27, 34]

Venous-phase images from parathyroid arteriography are invaluable, both for clarifying venous anatomy and for guiding interpretation of the results of venous sampling. False-positive rates for parathyroid venous sampling of 6%–18% without arteriography decrease to 0–4% when a preceding arteriogram has been done.[15, 28] Venous sampling should not be performed without a preceding arteriographic study.

Tips and Techniques

Because it is often necessary to use a number of differently shaped catheters to catheterize all of the veins that must be sampled, a sheath should be placed in the femoral vein at the beginning of the procedure. The peripheral vein sample, which defines the baseline PTH concentration, may be drawn through this sheath, at either the beginning or the end of the procedure. A heparin bolus (2000–2500 IU) is given intravenously.

The vertebral, internal jugular, and inferior thyroid veins may all be catheterized with a Berenstein or similarly shaped catheter. Difficulty in advancing the guidewire past the valve at the base of the left internal jugular vein is common. Hyperextension of the neck, combined with repeated advancing and withdrawing of the guidewire while the patient is taking deep breaths, is usually successful.[11]

Catheterization of the superior thyroid and thymic veins is often more difficult. The original literature described the use of a tip-deflecting catheter-guidewire assembly that is no longer manufactured. No really satisfactory substitute is available. If the brachiocephalic and internal jugular veins are large enough, a shepherd's-hook, visceral hook, Mikaelsson, or inferior mesenteric catheter may be used to catheterize the superior thyroid veins. It is often necessary to steam a catheter to an appropriate shape, or modify an existing catheter. A tip-deflecting wire may help. The thymic vein may be approached from the left upper extremity. It is helpful to remember that it originates from the anteroinferior aspect of the left brachiocephalic vein. The thymic vein is usually the most difficult vein to catheterize during parathyroid venous sampling, but it is also one of the most important, so extensive efforts to catheterize it are justified.

After each sample is obtained, and before the catheter is moved, a small amount of contrast material should be injected gently, and a spot film (either conventional or digital) should be obtained to document the position of the catheter tip and the site from which the sample was obtained. In addition, as each sample is obtained, an assistant should record the sample number and the location from which it was obtained. At the conclusion of the procedure, this list should be included as part of the dictated report, a copy of the list should be attached to the patient's chart, and an additional copy should be included in the film jacket with the spot films. It takes several days to a week or longer for the PTH levels to be reported by the laboratory, by which time recollection of the details of the sampling procedure may be hazy. Without the information from the spot films and the sample list, the PTH data are meaningless.

PANCREATIC ENDOCRINE TUMORS

Functioning pancreatic endocrine tumors tend to produce clinical symptoms while still quite small (often less than 1 cm). The two functioning islet cell tumors that most commonly present difficulties in localization are insulinomas and gastrinomas.

Insulinomas, the most common islet cell tumors, tend to be solitary (92%), intrapancreatic (99.5%), benign (90%), and uniformly distributed throughout the pancreas.[35] These tumors are usually easily identified with a combination of intraoperative ultrasound and palpation. Other preoperative localization procedures are far less sensitive.[36–40] A preoperative imaging study is required only to exclude liver metastases.[39]

Unlike insulinomas, 60% of gastrinomas are malignant, 60% are multiple, and more than 30% are extrapancreatic.[35] Seventy-five percent to 90% of gastrinomas are located to the right of the superior mesenteric artery, in the pancreas or duodenum, or in peripancreatic lymph nodes. Gastrinomas are small, with duodenal tumors typically less than 1 cm. No procedure or combination of procedures for localization of gastrinomas approaches the sensitivity of intraoperative ultrasound and palpation for localization of insulinomas.[41, 42] Somatostatin receptor scintigraphy and endoscopic ultrasound are the best available studies, with sensitivities of 55%–65% for localization of primary gastrinomas.[41–44]

In the very uncommon situations of a patient who has multiple endocrine neoplasia type I (MEN I) and insulinoma, a previous attempt at resection of an insulinoma that was unsuccessful, or who has adult nesidioblastosis, investigation with interventional radiologic techniques may be indicated.[39] The procedure, arteriography with arterial stimulation and venous sampling (ASVS), is now rarely required. It is not discussed here, but the technique has been described in detail.[45–48]

HYPERALDOSTERONISM

Primary hyperaldosteronism (Conn syndrome) is the only disorder of the adrenal glands for which venous sampling is required. The adrenal lesions of Cushing syndrome, pheochromocytoma, and virilizing disorders can be characterized or localized by cross-sectional imaging or scintigraphy. Arteriography is not used for characterization or localization in any of these disorders.

Patients with hyperaldosteronism typically present with hypertension and some degree of hypokalemia. It has been estimated that 1%–2% of hypertensive patients have hyperaldosteronism.[49] Demonstration of

A

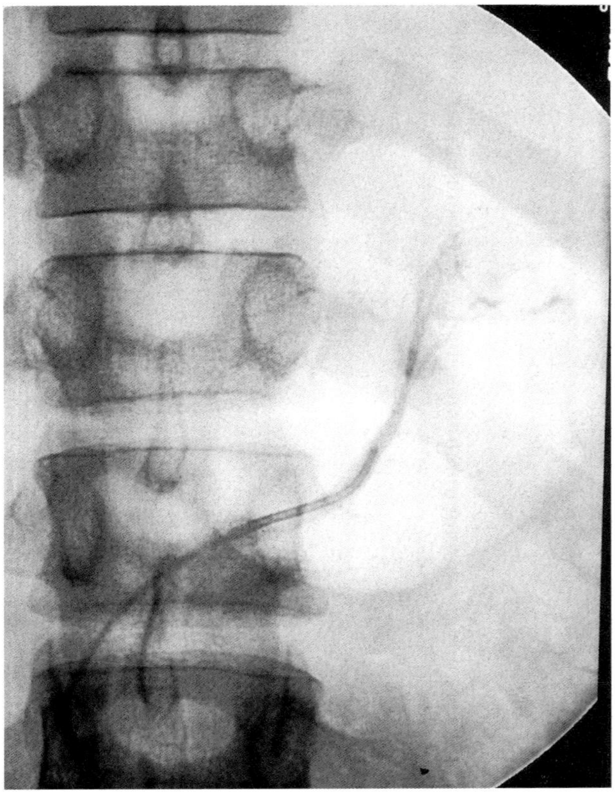

B

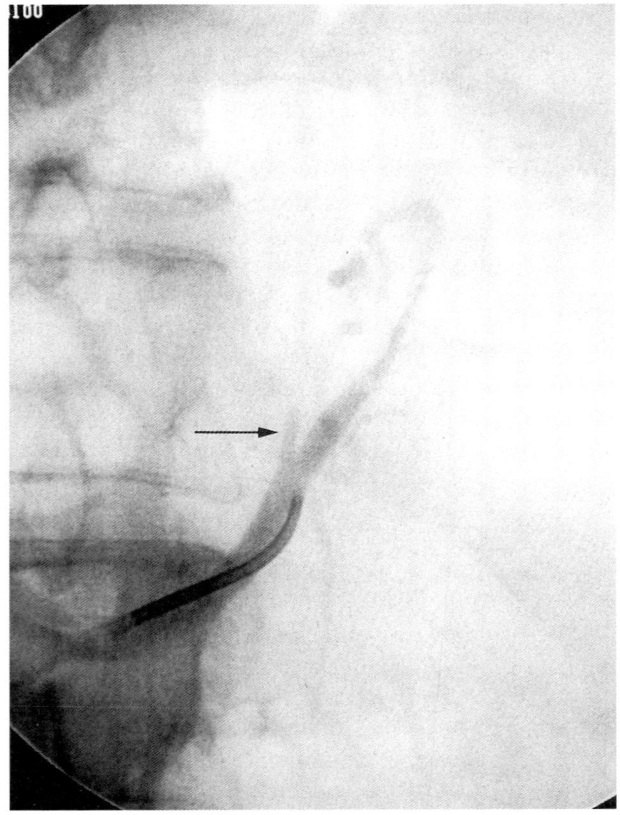

C

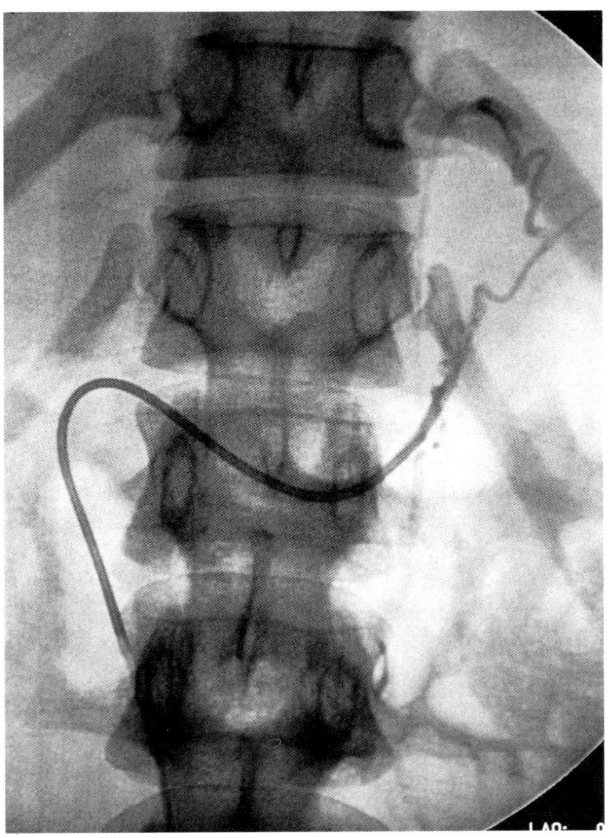

D

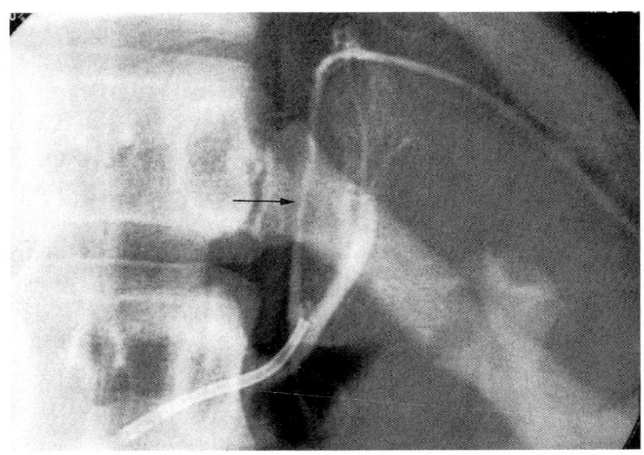

Figure 10-6. (A to D) Left adrenal venograms in four different patients. The left adrenal vein drains into the superior surface of the left renal vein just lateral to the left lateral margin of the spine. A Berenstein or Weinberg catheter is typically used with a tip-deflecting wire, but a Simmons II catheter is occasionally helpful (C). The left inferior phrenic vein (arrow, B and D) drains into the left adrenal vein. The sampling catheter should be placed either more selectively (A) or more centrally (B), but not at the junction of these two veins. In the last venogram (D), the catheter tip is at the junction of the inferior phrenic vein and adrenal vein. With respiratory motion, the tip could slip into the inferior phrenic vein, leading to collection of an inadequate sample. In this patient, the catheter tip was withdrawn slightly before sampling was performed. This view demonstrates the importance of verifying catheter position before sampling.

nonsuppressible aldosterone excretion in conjunction with normal cortisol excretion is diagnostic.

The two most common causes of primary hyperaldosteronism are a unilateral aldosterone-producing adenoma (APA; 54%) and bilateral adrenal hyperplasia (idiopathic hyperaldosteronism; 45%).[49] Rare causes include adrenal carcinoma, primary unilateral adrenal hyperplasia, and glucocorticoid-suppressible hyperaldosteronism (<1% each). The ability to distinguish between bilateral hyperplasia and an APA is a crucial part of the endocrine evaluation, because adenomas are resected but hyperplasia is treated medically.

Incidental adrenal nodules are present with higher frequency in older individuals and in patients with hypertension. As the spatial resolution of cross-sectional imaging studies has improved, these adrenal nodules are detected in more patients. Adrenal nodules detected on imaging studies in patients with hyperaldosteronism may be related to aging or hypertension, may be APAs, may represent nodular adrenal hyperplasia, or may be nonfunctioning adenomas. These entities cannot be distinguished reliably on the basis of imaging.

Noninvasive laboratory and imaging studies together have an accuracy of 70%–80% for distinguishing an APA from bilateral hyperplasia. In the past it has been suggested that a patient in whom endocrine test results are consistent with an APA, and also where CT demonstrates a single adrenal nodule with a normal contralateral adrenal gland may be referred directly for surgery. However, in recent years the accuracy of CT in patients with hyperaldosteronism has been no better than 37%–50%.[50, 51] Iodocholesterol (NP-59) scintigraphy has also fallen out of favor because it is insensitive for APAs smaller than 15 mm.[52]

Most experts now agree that bilateral adrenal vein sampling, which has an accuracy approaching 100%, should be performed in virtually all patients with hyperaldosteronism.[50, 51, 53–56] Adrenal venous sampling is also the best procedure for characterizing unilateral primary adrenal hyperplasia, as this entity's cross-sectional imaging appearance may be confusing.[53, 57]

The anatomy of the left adrenal vein is fairly constant. It virtually always drains into the superior aspect of the left renal vein at the left lateral margin of the vertebral column (**Fig. 10-6**). In the uncommon case of a retroaortic left renal vein, the adrenal vein drains either into the anomalous renal vein or, rarely, directly into the inferior vena cava (IVC). When a circumaortic left renal vein is present, the left adrenal vein drains into the superior portion (**Fig. 10-7**). Very rarely, the left adrenal vein may empty directly in to the IVC when the left renal vein is normal.[58]

The right adrenal vein is usually both small and quite short (5–8 mm) (**Fig. 10-8**). It normally empties directly into the posterior or posterolateral aspect of the IVC, anywhere from the level of the posterior right 10th rib to the level of the posterior right 12th rib, but typically in the vicinity of the posterior right 11th rib. On occasion, the right adrenal vein may drain into a small hepatic vein branch or, rarely, the right renal vein. It is more variable in position than the left adrenal vein and can be very difficult to locate. The right adrenal vein trifurcates almost immediately and often receives one or more renal capsular veins (see Fig. 10-8). These characteristics may help in distinguishing it from intercostal veins and small hepatic veins (**Fig. 10-9**).

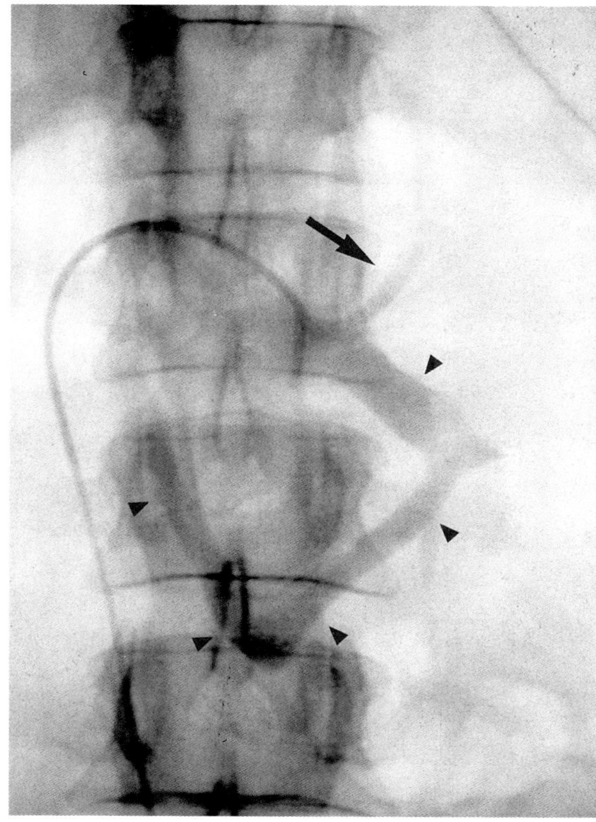

Figure 10-7. Left renal venogram obtained before catheterization of the left adrenal vein. A circumaortic renal vein is present (arrowheads). The left adrenal vein is apparent (straight arrow).

Adrenal Venous Sampling

Bilateral adrenal venous sampling requires simultaneous sampling from a femoral vein sheath and from catheters selectively placed in both adrenal veins via ipsilateral femoral vein punctures. Samples are obtained both before and after the intravenous administration of ACTH. The purpose of sampling is to determine whether one adrenal gland is *not* producing aldosterone.[53] If that is the case, the other adrenal gland is abnormal. Failure

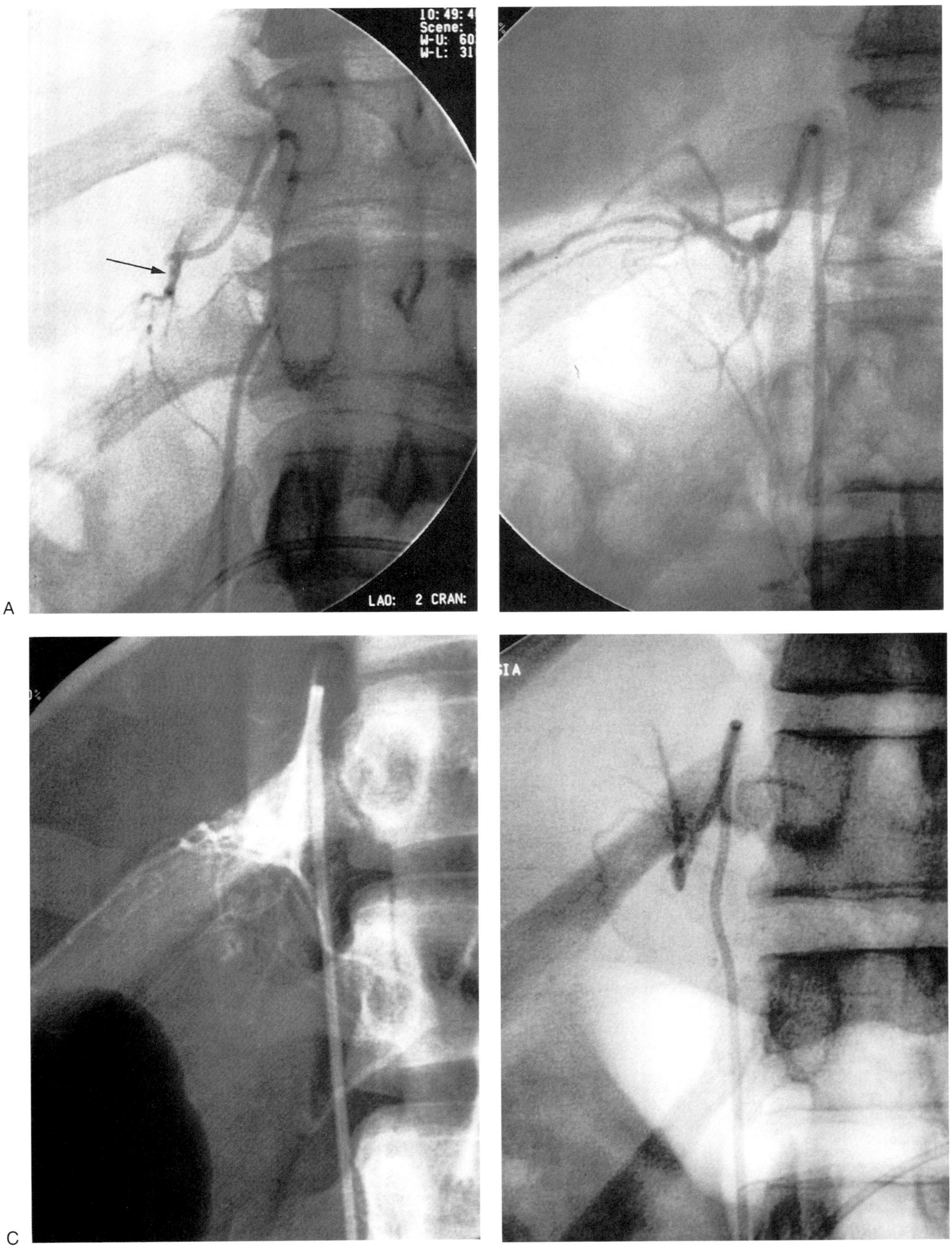

Figure 10-8. (A to D) Right adrenal venograms in four different patients. The right adrenal vein empties into the posterior or right posterolateral surface of the inferior vena cava at the level of the 10th through 12th posterior ribs. It is usually catheterized with a 4F or 5F Simmons I or a Mikaelsson catheter. Typically, only one of these catheters will work. The vein is short (arrow in A). It trifurcates almost immediately into equal-diameter branches and often has capsular branches as well (B and C).

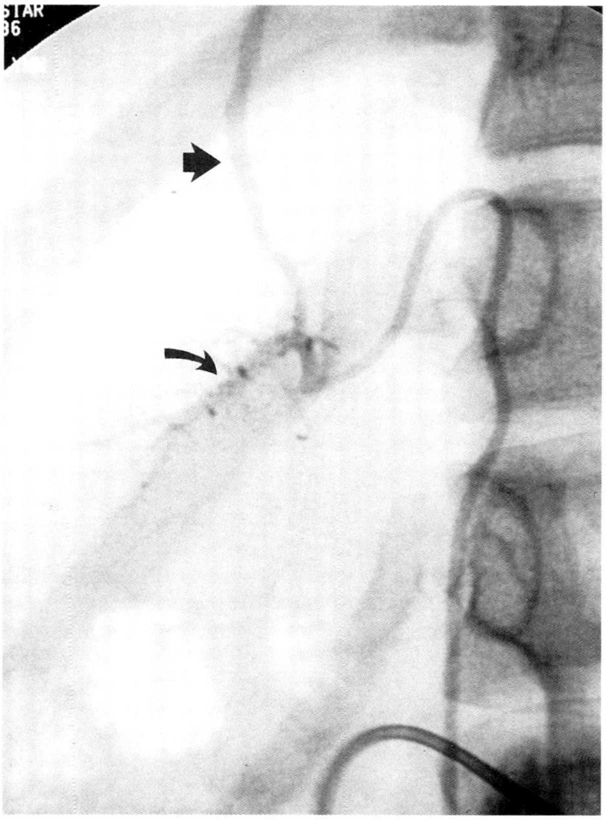

Figure 10-9. Small hepatic vein (curved arrow) encountered during attempted catheterization of the right adrenal vein. The right inferior phrenic vein (broad arrow) appears to drain into this vessel. Note that the hepatic vein does not divide into equal-sized branches. Instead, it has a main trunk with numerous small side branches. This appearance is characteristic.

of an adrenal gland to produce aldosterone after ACTH stimulation confirms that aldosterone production is suppressed and that the gland is therefore normal (ACTH stimulates release of aldosterone as well as cortisol.) If both glands produce aldosterone, the patient has hyperplasia.

A standardized approach to the technical details of the procedure is advisable. A 6F sheath is placed in the right femoral vein using standard techniques and is connected to a heparinized saline drip. A heparin bolus (2000–2500 IU) is given intravenously. The left femoral vein is then catheterized, and an appropriate catheter introduced.

The left adrenal vein is catheterized first. A 4F or 5F Weinberg or Berenstein catheter is guided into the left renal vein with the help of a tip-deflecting wire. Once in the renal vein, the catheter tip usually encounters the orifice of the left adrenal vein at the left lateral margin of the vertebral column. If these catheters do not permit left adrenal vein catheterization, a Simmons II catheter or a 4F straight polyethylene catheter, shaped with the use of steam into an S curve, may be used instead. Alternatively, a 5F Simmons I catheter placed in the left renal vein can be used as a guiding catheter to direct a microcatheter into the left adrenal vein while gentle traction is placed on the guiding catheter to direct its tip superiorly. Note that the left inferior phrenic vein also drains into the left adrenal vein. The catheter tip should not be advanced into the inferior phrenic vein; if it is, samples may not contain blood from the left adrenal gland (see Fig. 10-6D). The catheter is connected to a heparinized saline drip, and attention is then directed to the right side.

With the left adrenal vein catheter in place, the right adrenal vein catheter may be introduced through the right femoral vein sheath. Care is needed to avoid dislodging the tip of the left-sided catheter from the left adrenal vein. A 4F or 5F Mikaelsson or Simmons I catheter is usually effective. Occasionally, a catheter must be steamed to shape. The catheter tip is gently swept in a superior-to-inferior direction along the posterior wall of the inferior vena cava from the level of the 10th posterior rib until either the tip catches on the orifice of a small vein or the level of the 12th posterior rib is reached. A gentle hand injection of contrast material is performed to identify any branch engaged by the tip. If it is not the right adrenal vein, or if no branch is engaged, the catheter tip is rotated very slightly to the right, and the process is repeated. Often, it is not possible to engage the orifice of the right adrenal vein with the first catheter chosen. In this event, the catheter is exchanged over a guidewire for a different shape, and the search process is repeated.

Regardless of the catheter shape used, once the right adrenal vein is catheterized, the catheter tip is often occluded. The end-hole of the catheter may be against the wall of the right adrenal vein or against the adrenal vein trifurcation (see Fig. 10-8A), thus preventing aspiration of right adrenal vein blood. To avoid this phenomenon, a single hole is punched in the superior aspect of the catheter, approximately 3–4 mm from the catheter tip.[53] This maneuver permits collection of venous effluent at the point where the right renal vein joins the IVC. With this technique, sampling of both adrenal veins is consistently possible.

Small, gentle hand injections of contrast material are used to verify catheter position. It is helpful to obtain a spot film or short digital subtraction angiography run when a candidate vein has been catheterized. This practice allows leisurely inspection of the anatomy, helping confirm that the catheter is in the correct vein and that the catheter tip is correctly positioned (see Figs. 10-6D and 10-9). These images also serve as a useful guide during attempts to relocate the vein after the catheter slips out (an almost invariable occurrence with the right adrenal vein).

No attempt should be made to opacify the gland parenchyma or to outline tumors. Diagnostic retrograde venography, performed commonly in the past, is no longer employed because the procedure may cause hemorrhage and/or infarction due to rupture of small adrenal venous radicals.

Catheterization of the right adrenal vein is usually substantially more difficult than catheterization of the left adrenal vein. In a series of 49 attempted adrenal vein sampling procedures reported by Magill et al.,[51] the operator was unable to catheterize and sample both veins in 11 instances (22%). Of these 11 failures, 4 were due to failure to catheterize the left adrenal vein, and 7 to difficulties with right adrenal vein catheterization. In a series of 32 cases, Harper et al.[50] reported successful sampling of the left adrenal vein in 93% of procedures, but of the right adrenal vein in only 61%. If satisfactory samples cannot be obtained, the patient should be referred to an institution where greater expertise is available. There is a prolonged learning curve for this procedure but an experienced operator, using the techniques and catheters described here, can perform bilateral adrenal vein sampling in almost all patients.

After the collection of baseline samples from both adrenal veins and the femoral vein sheath, ACTH is administered intravenously in the form of a 0.25-mg bolus, followed by an infusion of 0.25 mg in 250 mL of normal saline at a rate of 150–200 mL/hr. Both adrenal vein catheters are connected to heparinized saline drips. Fifteen minutes after the start of the infusion, a second set of samples is obtained from both adrenal veins and the femoral vein sheath. The ACTH infusion is then discontinued. All samples are submitted for assay of both aldosterone and cortisol.

Right adrenal vein samples are diluted to an unknown extent by IVC blood. To correct for this dilution, aldosterone/cortisol ratios (A/C ratios) are used. Cortisol production by the two adrenal glands is assumed to be equal. The decrease in right adrenal aldosterone levels due to dilution should be equal in proportion to the decrease in cortisol levels. Use of the A/C ratio corrects for any dilution and allows right and left adrenal vein samples to be compared.

Interpretation of the results is based on the physiologic suppression of aldosterone production in the adrenal gland contralateral to an APA. If an APA is present, the A/C ratio in the contralateral normal gland is typically at or below the background ratio, and the A/C ratio from the ipsilateral gland is much higher than the background ratio. (Background levels are indicated by the sample obtained from the femoral vein sheath.) In patients with bilateral hyperplasia, however, A/C ratios in the two adrenals are comparable. The A/C ratios from both adrenal glands will be greater than that found in the femoral vein sheath sample. When one gland shows suppressed aldosterone production before ACTH stimulation and a reduced aldosterone response (and normal cortisol response) after ACTH stimulation, surgical removal of the contralateral gland produces a high cure rate.[53]

Some investigators have compared the A/C ratios from the two adrenal veins to establish a diagnosis. For distinguishing between APA and hyperplasia, the cutoff value for the ratio between ipsilateral and contralateral adrenal vein A/C ratios has been given as >5, >4, and ≥ 2 in various series.[51, 56, 59]

Adrenal Embolization

Adrenal embolization has been attempted for treatment of adrenal adenomas. Retrograde venous injection is not a reliable method for infarcting the gland. Arterial injection of ethanol produces immediate and severe hypertension and arrhythmias in monkeys, and has the potential to produce the same complications in humans.[60, 61]

CONCLUSION

Endocrine tumors can be some of the smallest lesions but have the direst prognoses in all of medicine. Fortunately, most of these tumors are uncommon. Their localization may require interventional radiology procedures that are complex and technically demanding, and require obsessive attention to detail. However, when performed properly on appropriate patients, they can yield lifesaving information.

REFERENCES

1. Orth DN. Cushing's syndrome. *N Engl J Med* 1995; 332:791–803.
2. Wiggam MI, Heaney AP, McIlrath EM, et al. Bilateral inferior petrosal sinus sampling in the differential diagnosis of adrenocorticotropin-dependent Cushing's syndrome: a comparison with other diagnostic tests. *J Clin Endocrinol Metab* 2000; 85:1525–1532.
3. Booth GL, Redelmeier DA, Grosman H, Kovacs K, Smyth HS, Ezzat S. Improved diagnostic accuracy of inferior petrosal sinus sampling over imaging for localizing pituitary pathology in patients with Cushing's disease. *J Clin Endocrinol Metab* 1998; 83:2291–2295.
4. Hall WA, Luciano MG, Doppman JL, Patronas NJ, Oldfield EH. Pituitary magnetic resonance imaging in normal human volunteers: occult adenomas in the general population. *Ann Intern Med* 1994; 120:817–820.
5. Kaltsas GA, Giannulis MG, Newell-Price JDC, et al. A critical analysis of the value of simultaneous inferior petrosal sinus sampling in Cushing's disease and the occult ectopic adrenocorticotropin syndrome. *J Clin Endocrinol Metab* 1999; 84:487–492.
6. Miller DL, Doppman JL, Chang R. Anatomy of the junction of the inferior petrosal sinus and the internal jugular vein. *Am J Neuroradiol* 1993; 14:1075–1083.
7. Doppman JL, Chang R, Oldfield EH, Chrousos G, Stratakis CA, Nieman

LK. The hypoplastic inferior petrosal sinus: a potential source of false-negative results in petrosal sampling for Cushing's disease. *J Clin Endocrinol Metab* 1999; 84:533–540.

8. Yanovski JA, Cutler GB Jr, Doppman JL, et al. The limited ability of inferior petrosal sinus sampling with corticotropin-releasing hormone to distinguish Cushing's disease from pseudo-Cushing states or normal physiology. *J Clin Endocrinol Metab* 1993; 77:503–509.
9. Doppman JL, Oldfield EH, Nieman LK. Bilateral sampling of the internal jugular vein to distinguish between mechanisms of adrenocorticotropic hormone-dependent Cushing syndrome. *Ann Intern Med* 1998; 128:33–36.
10. Doppman JL, Nieman LK, Chang R, et al. Selective venous sampling from the cavernous sinuses is not a more reliable technique than sampling from the inferior petrosal sinuses in Cushing's syndrome. *J Clin Endocrinol Metab* 1995;80:2485–2489.
11. Miller DL, Doppman JL. Petrosal sinus sampling: technique and rationale. *Radiology* 1991; 178:37–47.
12. Boggs JE, Irvin GL III, Carneiro DM, Molinari AS. The evolution of parathyroidectomy failures. *Surgery* 1999; 126:998–1003.
13. Moka D, Voth E, Dietlein M, Larena-Avellaneda A, Schicha H. Technetium 99m-MIBI-SPECT: a highly sensitive diagnostic tool for localization of parathyroid adenomas. *Surgery* 2000; 128:29–35.
14. Pattou F, Torres G, Mondragon-Sanchez A, et al. Correlation of parathyroid scanning and anatomy in 261 unselected patients with sporadic primary hyperparathyroidism. *Surgery* 1999; 126:1123–1131.
15. Miller DL. Preoperative localization and interventional treatment of parathyroid tumors: when and how? *World J Surg* 1991; 15:706–715.
16. Feingold DL, Alexander HR, Chen CC, et al. Ultrasound and sestamibi scan as the only preoperative imaging tests in reoperation for parathyroid adenomas. *Surgery* 2000; 128:1103–1110.
17. Miller DL, Doppman JL, Krudy AG, et al. Localization of parathyroid adenomas in patients who have undergone surgery: part II: invasive procedures. *Radiology* 1987; 162:138–141.
18. Wang C-A. The anatomic basis of parathyroid surgery. *Ann Surg* 1976; 183:271–275.
19. Kaplan EL, Yashiro T, Salti G. Primary hyperparathyroidism in the 1990s: choice of surgical procedure for this disease. *Ann Surg* 1992; 215:300–317.
20. Jander HP, Diethelm AG, Russinovich NAE. The parathyroid artery. *Am J Roentgenol* 1980; 135:821–828.
21. Nobori M, Saiki S, Tanaka N, Harihara Y, Shindo S, Fujimoto Y. Blood supply of the parathyroid gland from the superior thyroid artery. *Surgery* 1994; 115:417–423.
22. Miller DL, Chang R, Doppman JL, Norton JA. Localization of parathyroid adenomas: superselective arterial DSA versus superselective conventional angiography. *Radiology* 1989; 170:1003–1006.
23. Lippert H, Pabst R. *Arterial Variations in Man: Classification and Frequency*. Munich: J.F. Bergmann Verlag; 1985.
24. Krudy AG, Doppman JL, Brennan MF. The significance of the thyroidea ima artery in arteriographic localization of parathyroid adenomas. *Radiology* 1980; 136:51–55.
25. McIntyre RC Jr, Kumpe DA, Liechty RD. Reexploration and angiographic ablation for hyperparathyroidism. *Arch Surg* 1994; 129:499–504.
26. Doppman JL. Parathyroid localization: arteriography and venous sampling. Radiol Clin North Am 1976; 14:163–188.
27. Monchik JM, Doppman JL, Earll JM, Aurbach GD. Localization of hyperfunctioning parathyroid tissue: radioimmunoassay of parathyroid hormone on samples from the large veins of the neck and thorax and selectively catheterized thyroid veins. *Am J Surg* 1975; 129:413–420.
28. Sugg SL, Fraker DL, Alexander R, et al. Prospective evaluation of selective venous sampling for parathyroid hormone concentration in patients undergoing reoperations for primary hyperparathyroidism. *Surgery* 1993; 114:1004–1011.
29. Doppman JL, Hammond WG. The anatomic basis of parathyroid venous sampling. *Radiology* 1970; 95:603–610.
30. Shimkin PM, Doppman JL, Pearson KD, Powell D. Anatomic considerations in parathyroid venous sampling. *Am J Roentgenol* 1973; 118:654–662.
31. Doppman JL, Melson GL, Evens RG, Hammond WG. Selective superior and inferior thyroid vein catheterization: venographic anatomy and potential applications. *Invest Radiol* 1969; 4:97–99.
32. Ibukuro K, Fukuda H, Mori K, Inoue Y. Topographic anatomy of the vertebral venous system in the thoracic inlet. *Am J Roentgenol* 2001; 176:1059–1065.
33. Doppman JL, Mallette LE, Marx SJ, et al. The localization of abnormal mediastinal parathyroid glands. *Radiology* 1975; 115:31–36.
34. Shimkin PM, Powell D, Doppman JL, et al. Parathyroid venous sampling. *Radiology* 1972; 104:571–574.
35. Miller DL. Islet cell tumors of the pancreas: diagnosis and localization. In: Freeny PC, Stevenson GW, eds. *Margulis and Burhenne's Alimentary Tract Radiology*. 5th ed. Hanover: C.V. Mosby; 1994:1167–1196.
36. Brown CK, Bartlett DL, Doppman JL, et al. Intraarterial calcium stimulation and intraoperative ultrasonography in the localization and resection of insulinomas. *Surgery* 1997; 122:1189–1193.
37. Boukhman MP, Karam JM, Shaver J, Siperstein AE, DeLorimier AA, Clark OH. Localization of insulinomas. *Arch Surg* 1999; 134:818–823.
38. Miller DL, Buetow PC. Imaging procedures for the endocrine pancreas. In: Howard JM, Idezuki Y, Ihse I, Prinz RA, eds. *Surgical Diseases of the Pancreas*. 3 ed. Baltimore: Williams & Wilkins; 1998:703–715.
39. Grant CS. Surgical aspects of hyperinsulinemic hypoglycemia. *Endocrinol Metab Clin North Am* 1999; 28:533–554.
40. Lo CY, Chan FL, Tam SCF, Cheng PW, Fan ST, Lam KSL. Value of intra-arterial calcium stimulated venous sampling for regionalization of pancreatic insulinomas. *Surgery* 2000; 128:903–909.
41. Gibril F, Reynolds JC, Doppman JL, et al. Somatostatin receptor scintigraphy: its sensitivity compared with that of other imaging methods in detecting primary and metastatic gastrinomas: a prospective study. *Ann Intern Med* 1996; 125:26–34.
42. Ruszniewski P, Amouyal P, Amouyal G, et al. Localization of gastrinomas by endoscopic ultrasonography in patients with Zollinger-Ellison syndrome. *Surgery* 1995; 117:629–635.
43. Krausz Y, Bar-Ziv J, de Jong RBJ, et al. Somatostatin-receptor scintigraphy in the management of gastroenteropancreatic tumors. *Am J Gastroenterol* 1998; 93:66–70.
44. Jensen RT, Gibril F. Somatostatin receptor scintigraphy in gastrinomas. *Ital J Gastroenterol Hepatol* 1999; 31(suppl 2):S179-S185.
45. Doppman JL, Chang R, Fraker DL, et al. Localization of insulinomas to regions of the pancreas by intra-arterial stimulation with calcium. *Ann Intern Med* 1995; 123:269–273.
46. Doppman JL, Miller DL, Chang R, Shawker TH, Gorden P, Norton JA. Insulinomas: localization with selective intraarterial injection of calcium. *Radiology* 1991; 178:237–241.
47. Doppman JL, Miller DL, Chang R, Gorden P, Eastman RC, Norton JA. Intraarterial stimulation test for detection of insulinomas. *World J Surg* 1993; 17:439–443.
48. Defreyne L, König K, Lerch MM, et al. Modified intra-arterial calcium stimulation with venous sampling test for preoperative localization of insulinomas. *Abdom Imaging* 1998; 23:322–331.
49. Young WF Jr, Hogan MJ, Klee GG, Grant CS, van Heerden JA. Primary aldosteronism: diagnosis and treatment. *Mayo Clin Proc* 1990; 65:96–110.
50. Harper R, Ferrett CG, McKnight JA, et al. Accuracy of CT scanning and adrenal vein sampling in the pre-operative localization of aldosterone-secreting adrenal adenomas. *Q J Med* 1999; 92:643–650.
51. Magill SB, Raff H, Shaker JL, et al. Comparison of adrenal vein sampling and computed tomography in the differentiation of primary aldosteronism. *J Clin Endocrinol Metab* 2001; 86:1066–1071.
52. Young WF Jr. Pheochromocytoma and primary aldosteronism: diagnostic approaches. *Endocrinol Metab Clin North Am* 1997; 26:801–827.
53. Doppman JL, Gill JR Jr. Hyperaldosteronism: sampling the adrenal veins. *Radiology* 1996; 198:309–312.

54. Gleason PE, Weinberger MH, Pratt JH, et al. Evaluation of diagnostic tests in the differential diagnosis of primary aldosteronism: unilateral adenoma versus bilateral micronodular hyperplasia. *J Urol* 1993; 150:1365–1368.
55. Tokunaga K, Nakamura H, Marukawa T, et al. Adrenal venous sampling analysis of primary aldosteronism: value of ACTH stimulation in the differentiation of adenoma and hyperplasia. *Eur Radiol* 1992; 2:223–229.
56. Rossi GP, Sacchetto A, Chiesura-Corona M, et al. Identification of the etiology of primary aldosteronism with adrenal vein sampling in patients with equivocal computed tomography and magnetic resonance findings: results in 104 consecutive cases. *J Clin Endocrinol Metab* 2001; 86:1083–1090.
57. Morioka M, Kobayashi T, Sone A, Furukawa Y, Tanaka H. Primary aldosteronism due to unilateral adrenal hyperplasia: report of two cases and review of the literature. *Endocr J* 2000;47:443–449.
58. Stack SP, Rösch J, Cook DM, Sheppard BC, Keller FS. Anomalous left adrenal venous drainage directly into the inferior vena cava. *J Vasc Interv Radiol* 2001; 12:385–387.
59. Doppman JL, Gill JR Jr, Miller DL, et al. Distinction between hyperaldosteronism due to bilateral hyperplasia and unilateral aldosteronoma: reliability of CT. *Radiology* 1992; 184:677–682.
60. Fink IJ, Girton M, Doppman JL. Absolute ethanol injection of the adrenal artery: hypertensive reaction. *Radiology* 1985; 154:357–358.
61. Ueno K, Nakajo M, Miyazono N, et al. Transcatheter adrenal arterial embolization of cortisol-producing tumors: two cases of Cushing's syndrome. *Acta Radiol* 1999; 40:100–103.

CHAPTER 11

HEPATIC ARTERIAL INTERVENTIONS

TARA HANJAN, MD

JULIA T. De SANCTIS, MD

Hepatocellular carcinoma (HCC) is one of the most common malignancies worldwide,[1] with an estimated 250,000 to 1 million new cases per year.[2] Surgical resection is the treatment of choice and the only curative option for HCC.[2–5] However, HCCs are considered resectable at initial presentation in only 15%–20% of all patients with such tumors, as determined by extent of intrahepatic tumor involvement, extrahepatic disease, hepatic function, or contraindication for orthotopic liver transplantation.[4,6]

The liver is also the second most frequent site of metastatic disease from extrahepatic primary tumors: colorectal carcinoma, neuroendocrine tumors, gastrointestinal leiomyosarcomas, and ocular melanomas all commonly metastasize to the liver.[7] Ninety-five percent of liver metastases are inoperable[3] and carry a poor prognosis for the patient.[8] Since the 1970s, regional hepatic arterial interventions have been developed for palliation of symptoms and retardation or stabilization of tumor growth.[9] These treatments consist of chemoinfusion therapy,[10] sterile embolization,[11,12] chemoembolization,[5] and injection of radiomicrospheres into the hepatic artery[13,14] (**Table 11-1**).

PHYSIOLOGIC BACKGROUND

The dual blood supply of the liver provides the key physiologic basis for intra-arterial interventions. The hepatic artery supplies approximately 20% of the normal hepatic parenchymal blood flow and the portal vein supplies the remainder.[16,17] Eighty percent of the

TABLE 11-1
Hepatic Intra-arterial Procedures

- Hepatic arterial chemoinfusion
  - Surgically placed infusion pump
  - Percutaneous catheter for prolonged infusion
    - Brachial artery approach
    - Femoral artery approach
- Transcatheter arterial embolization
  - Absorbable substances
    - Gelfoam, Lipiodol, Avitene, blood clot, muscle, dura
  - Nonabsorbable substances[15]
    - Steel coils, sclerosing agents, polyvinyl alcohol, silicone microspheres
- Transcatheter arterial chemoembolization
  - Gelfoam permeated with chemotherapeutic agent such as doxorubicin, mitomycin C, cisplatin, floxuridine (5-fluoro-2′deoxyuridine), 5-fluorouracil
- Transcatheter oily chemoembolization
  - Lipiodol with anticancer agent emulsion plus Gelfoam embolization
  - Lipiodol with anticancer agent emulsion without Gelfoam embolization
- Radiomicrosphere embolization
  - Yttrium-90 microspheres
  - Iodine-131 microspheres

oxygen requirement for normal liver tissue is derived from the portal vein.[18] In contrast, oxygen for hepatic neoplasms is supplied predominantly or exclusively by the hepatic artery.[19] Either circulation can sustain the liver if one system becomes occluded; in the setting of a decrease in blood flow, the liver is able to vary its oxygen extraction from the portal circulation.[20] The percutaneous accessibility and ease of catheterization of the hepatic artery, together with the dominant or exclusive hepatic arterial supply to hepatic neoplasms in the setting of dual but dominantly portal venous supply to normal liver, creates the opportunity for successful hepatic arterial interventions.[21]

PATIENT SELECTION

Hepatic arterial interventions are indicated for patients with selected unresectable tumors confined to the liver, including primary HCC and hypervascular secondary hepatic malignancies, such as metastases from some colorectal carcinomas, neuroendocrine tumors (carcinoid and islet cell tumors), ocular melanoma, and gastrointestinal sarcomas[8,21–26] (**Table 11-2**). Chemoembolization is also performed preoperatively as a neoadjuvant therapy to prevent recurrences of HCC or to facilitate resection of large tumors.[27,28]

TABLE 11-2
Tumors Treated with Hepatic Arterial Interventions

- Unresectable tumor [8]
- Primary hepatic malignancies[24]
- Secondary hepatic malignancies
  - Neuroendocrine metastases
    - Carcinoid tumors[23]
    - Islet cell tumors[22]
  - Colorectal metastases[29]
  - Gastrointestinal leiomyosarcoma metastases[26]
  - Ocular melanoma metastases[21]

Because the majority of hepatic arterial interventions performed are palliative, careful patient selection is vital to maximize outcomes while minimizing morbidity. Absolute and relative contraindications are outlined in **Table 11-3**. The presence of extrahepatic metastases reflects the degree of tumor progression and has been found to have prognostic significance in treatment of unresectable HCC.[30] Replacement of more than 50% of the liver volume by tumor, hepatofugal portal venous

TABLE 11-3
Contraindications for Hepatic Arterial Interventions

- Absolute
  - Uncorrectable bleeding disorder[37]
  - Severe thrombocytopenia; platelet count $<50{,}000$[37]
  - Leukopenia; white blood cell count $<2.5 \times 10^3/\mu L$[8]
  - Hepatic encephalopathy[33]
  - Portal vein obstruction with hepatofugal blood flow[8]
  - Jaundice[8]
  - Biliary obstruction[33]
  - Dilated intrahepatic bile ducts[37]
  - Significant hepatic dysfunction[8]
    1. Lactate dehydrogenase >425 U/L[37]
    2. Aspartate aminotransferase >100 U/L[37]
    3. Total bilirubin >2.0 mg/dL[37]
  - Ascites[33]
  - $>50\%$ of liver volume replaced by tumor[37]
  - Extrahepatic metastases, tumors, or any medical condition resulting in a life expectancy <3 months[8]
  - Cardiac insufficiency[33]
  - Pregnancy[8]
- Relative
  - Anaphylactic reaction to contrast media[33]
  - Main portal vein obstruction[8]
  - Renal insufficiency (serum creatinine >2.0 mg/dL)[8]
  - Immediate contact of large hepatocellular carcinoma to the liver capsule
  - Marked arteriovenous shunting

blood flow, poor liver function with encephalopathy, ascites, and jaundice suggest inadequate hepatic reserve, which limits tolerability of chemoembolization, thereby increasing the likelihood that hepatic failure will occur. Biliary obstruction and dilated intrahepatic bile ducts typically demonstrate concurrent decreased portal venous inflow, which increases susceptibility to hepatic infarction and abscess formation. Adequate decompression of the biliary system should be performed before hepatic artery embolization.[31]

In addition to absolute contraindications, there are several relative contraindications. Portal vein occlusion with hepatopetal flow predisposes the patient to the development of postembolization hepatic failure and infarction and increases the likelihood of liver abscess formation.[31–33] According to Chung et al., transcatheter oily chemoembolization (TOCE) should be performed cautiously in these patients, using a reduced amount of chemoembolic agents with selective administration into tumor-feeding arteries.[31] Song et al. have reported, for patients with portal vein obstruction, an increased incidence of hepatic abscess formation only when gelatin sponge particle embolization is used with TOCE.[34]

Pijl et al. reported a case of fatal liver rupture after transcatheter arterial chemoembolization of a large HCC. They have proposed that immediate juxtaposition of a large HCC and the liver capsule is a relative contraindication for transarterial chemoembolization. This recommendation is based on their experience with capsular necrosis and liver rupture, with subsequent spillage of necrotic tumor into the abdominal cavity and resulting patient mortality. They recommend withholding Gelfoam (Upjohn Co., Kalamazoo, Michigan) embolization whenever a rim of normal liver parenchyma does not encapsulate large HCCs.[35]

Marked arteriovenous shunting to portal or hepatic veins is also a contraindication to embolotherapy, as it may cause embolization of the pulmonary vascular network.[4,31] The use of intra-arterial radiomicrospheres is contraindicated in patients with significant pulmonary shunting (>15%) or shunting of activity to the gastrointestinal region as detected by angioscintigraphic technetium 99m–macroaggregated albumin (^{99m}Tc-MAA) perfusion scans.[13,36]

PREPROCEDURAL EVALUATION

The basic preprocedural evaluation for hepatic arterial chemoinfusion, transcatheter arterial embolization, chemoembolization, and arterial infusion of radiomicrospheres is uniform, with a few notable exceptions. The diagnosis of hepatic malignancy must be documented histologically or based on an elevated serum alpha fetoprotein (AFP value >400 ng/mL) in the presence of a solid hepatic lesion.[7,37–39] Cross-sectional abdominal imaging with computed tomography (CT) or magnetic resonance (MR) imaging is performed to assess tumor location, percentage of liver parenchyma replaced by tumor, and presence or absence of extrahepatic involvement.[7,37] Portal vein patency and direction of flow must be evaluated with duplex ultrasound, CT scanning, MR venography, or angiography.[33,40,41] Chest radiography is performed to exclude pulmonary metastases,[42] and routine laboratory studies, consisting of a complete blood count (CBC), coagulation profile, liver function tests (LFTs), and electrolytes with blood urea nitrogen and creatinine levels, are done.[9,33,37] Tumor markers AFP and carcinoembryonic antigen (CEA) are measured for HCC and metastases from colorectal carcinoma, respectively, and are used in follow-up treatment to assess response to therapy.[30,43] In patients undergoing treatment for carcinoid and neuroendocrine metastases, the biochemical markers 5-hydroxyindoleacetic acid (5-HIAA), chromogranin A (CGA), and neuron-specific enolase (NSE) are obtained to evaluate treatment efficacy.[9]

Hepatic arteriography is performed before the scheduled embolization at some institutions to assess the arterial anatomy, tumor blood flow, and patency of the portal vein.[15] Determination of portal vein patency is an essential preliminary step in verifying an adequate blood supply to the normal liver parenchyma.[32]

Preprocedural evaluation for planned intra-arterial radiomicrosphere therapy includes a number of additional studies. Pulmonary function tests (PFTs), including forced expiratory volume in 1 second, vital capacity, functional residual volume, and diffusion capacity of the lungs for carbon monoxide are performed. Careful patient selection, by excluding those with PFTs values greater than or less than 30% of expected normal parameters, may help reduce the likelihood of developing radiomicrosphere-induced pulmonary toxicity.[36] A diagnostic hepatic arteriogram is usually obtained and, if results are normal, it is immediately followed by a planar hepatic arterial ^{99m}Tc-MAA scan of the abdomen and chest.[13,36] Pretherapeutic diagnostic ^{99m}Tc-MAA angioscintigraphy evaluates the capacity of an individual tumor to retain particles, determines the tumor-to–normal liver tissue uptake ratio, detects reflux and shunting of blood to extrahepatic organs, and allows evaluation of catheter position.[13,36,44] The presence of a significant pulmonary shunt may affect pulmonary function or induce pneumonitis after radioembolization. Furthermore, serious pancreatic and bowel injury can occur as a result of embolization of the therapeutic agent outside the tumor. In the presence of reflux and shunting, reduced doses of the therapeutic agent are

TABLE 11-4
Preprocedural Evaluation

Histologically or clinically proven hepatic malignancy
Cross-sectional abdominal imaging (CT or MR imaging)
Assessment of portal vein patency (duplex ultrasound, CT, MR venography, or angiography)
Hepatic arteriography (may or may not be included)
Chest radiography
Laboratory studies
LFTs
CBC with differential
Platelet count
International normalized ratio (INR)
Partial thromboplastin time
Electrolytes
Blood urea nitrogen and creatinine
Tumor markers (AFP, CEA)[9]
For carcinoid hepatic metastases, biochemical markers[9]
5-HIAA
CGA
NSE
Intra-arterial radiomicrosphere–specific studies
PFTs
Angioscintigraphic ^{99m}Tc-MAA scan of chest and abdomen

5-HIAA = 5-hydroxyindolacetic acid; AFP = alpha fetoprotein; CBC = complete blood count; CEA = carcinoembryonic antigen; CGA = chromogranin A; CT = computed tomography; LFT = liver function test; MR = magnetic resonance; NSE = neuron-specific enolase; PFT = pulmonary function test.

Data from Patel et al.,[7] Drougas et al.,[9] Lau et al.,[13] al-Bassam et al.,[33] Dancey et al.,[36] Ngan et al.,[38] Perry et al.,[40] Soulen,[41] and Walser et al.[44]

used.[44] HCC has been shown to be associated with a greater degree of shunting than colorectal metastases (37% versus 3%, respectively).[44] Although angioscintigraphic imaging with ^{99m}Tc-MAA is routinely used in radioembolization, it may be advantageous to all tumors or embolization techniques[44] (**Table 11-4**).

PATIENT PREPARATION

Hepatic arterial interventions are performed, after an overnight fast, either as a same-day procedure or with hospitalization the night prior to the procedure. Substantial intravenous hydration must be accomplished prior to initiating the procedure and is continued for 24 hours or until the patient resumes full oral intake of fluids.[8] Admission the night prior to the procedure allows slower hydration for those intolerant of rapid hydration.[15,22,32]

Pharmacologic blockade is administered to patients with functioning metastatic neuroendocrine or carcinoid tumors to prevent or reduce the severity of hormonal crisis. These patients receive octreotide (200 μg every 8 hours, subcutaneously), beginning 8–16 hours before the procedure, until they are discharged.[15,32] For patients with Zollinger-Ellison syndrome, omeprazole or an H_2-receptor antagonist is administered.[15] Allopurinol, which decreases uric acid production, is given to prevent urate-induced renal failure, which may occur secondary to tumor lysis. Prophylactic lactulose is administered to curtail postembolization hepatic encephalopathy.[9,22]

Patients are further premedicated with analgesics, such as hydromorphone hydrochloride[8] or acetaminophen/codeine,[24] and are given a sedative and antiemetic such as hydroxyzine orally.[8]

Prophylactic broad-spectrum intravenous antibiotics, commonly ampicillin/sulbactam, or cefazolin and metronidazole, are typically administered immediately before the procedure[8,22,24,37,40,45] and continued for 4–7 days after the procedure. However, the efficacy of prophylaxis remains open to debate. Chung et al. and Tarazov et al. do not recommend the routine use of prophylactic antibiotics, except for those patients with risk factors for development of infectious complications.[31,46] Such factors include nonselective placement of the catheter during TOCE, high doses of cytostatics and iodized oil, use of small-diameter embolic agents, liver function disorders, previous surgery on the liver and bile ducts, and obstruction of the bile ducts and/or portal vein branches.[46]

Throughout the procedure, conscious sedation is provided with a combination of intravenous midazolam hydrochloride and fentanyl citrate.[8,37] A Foley catheter is placed to monitor urine output and provide patient comfort.[33]

HEPATIC ARTERIAL EMBOLIZATION

Hepatic arterial particulate embolization was primarily used in the 1970s and 1980s.[11,23,47,48] A randomized controlled trial by Lin et al. showed that hepatic arterial embolization was superior to systemic chemotherapy.[48] Percutaneous particulate embolization was advantageous relative to surgical hepatic arterial ligation because it eliminated the need for general anesthesia and provided improved obliteration of tumor circulation.[47] Agents used included polyvinyl alcohol (PVA), Gelfoam (gelatin surgical sponge), collagen, degradable starch microspheres, and stainless-steel coils.[21]

CHEMOEMBOLIZATION

During the same time period that hepatic arterial embolization was being investigated, transarterial chemoembolization using gelatin sponge particles permeated with anticancer agents was also being performed.[27,49–51] Chemoembolization for HCC is an interventional procedure combining hepatic arterial administration of chemotherapeutic agents with selective vascular occlusion, using various embolic particles.[21,52] This procedure aims to induce ischemia; an additional effect of the decreased arterial flow is to increase the contact time between the cytotoxic agents and the neoplasm.[53] Furthermore, the increased local drug concentration within the tumor bed is enhanced by the increased tissue permeability caused by anoxia.[54] These factors ultimately result in increased tumor cell destruction.[53]

During the 1970s, transarterial embolization of HCC was carried out with occlusive materials alone (transcatheter arterial embolization [TAE]) or with embolic substances combined with anticancer drugs (transcatheter arterial chemoembolization [TACE]).[15,49,55] Subsequently, in the early 1980s, Lipiodol (Savage Laboratories, Melville, New York), an oily contrast medium, was introduced in combination with TOCE.[56] Lipiodol, or ethiodized oil, is an ethyl ester of the fatty acid of poppy seed oil containing 38% iodine.[4,17,57] It distributes diffusely within the liver parenchyma, with localized greater depositions in hepatic tumors.[30,57] It is delivered via the bloodstream into the main tumor, areas of capsular invasion, tiny intrahepatic metastatic nodules, and tumor thrombi.[58] This property enables Lipiodol to act both as a carrier for the anticancer drug and as an embolic material.[30,56,59]

There are two major advantages of TOCE over hepatic arterial chemotherapy and conventional hepatic arterial embolization. First, Lipiodol injected in the hepatic artery reaches the sinusoids via arterioportal communications (**Fig. 11-1**). As a result, nonencapsulated infiltrative lesions and proliferative daughter nodules, fed by sinusoids as well as by the hepatic artery, demonstrate greater tumor necrosis and a better clinical response; arterial embolization without Lipiodol produces low survival rates when performed in patients with nonencapsulated and infiltrative tumors or those with intrahepatic daughter metastatic nodules. Second, Lipiodol is selectively retained in the tumor and can be detected easily on CT scans[43] (**Fig. 11-2**). Evaluation of Lipiodol accumulation on CT scans is useful for assessing the therapeutic effect of the treatment.[55]

Use of both TOCE, with a mixture of Lipiodol and an anticancer agent, and Gelfoam embolization has been reported to result in a better cumulative survival rate than that achieved with systemic chemotherapy and nonoily chemoembolization.[28,55,56]

PROCEDURAL TECHNIQUE

The steps involved in TAE, TACE, and TOCE are essentially the same until the time of actual embolization. Although multiple embolization and chemoembolic regimens exist, there is no consensus on the best protocol.

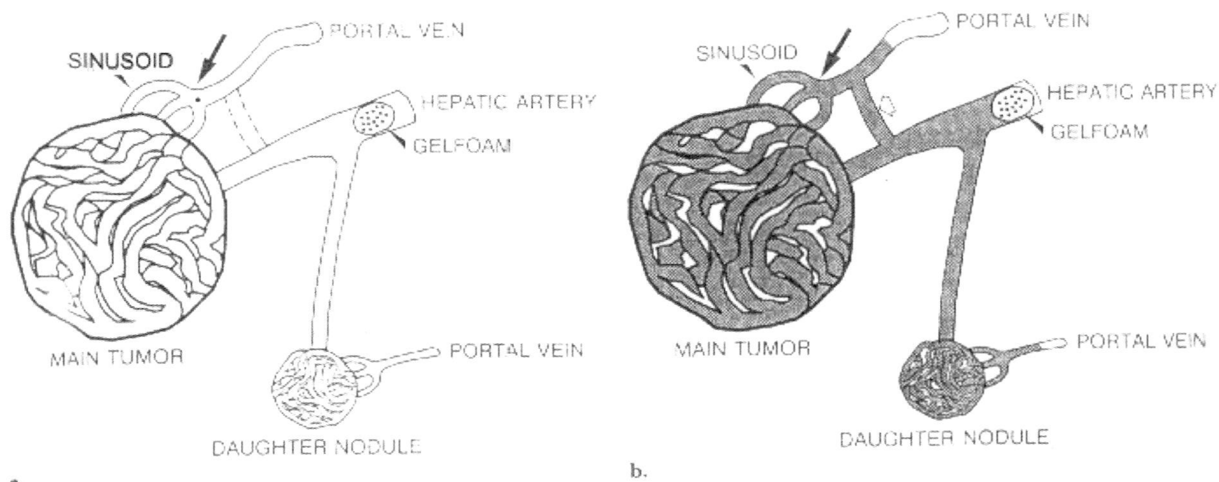

Figure 11-1. (A) Diagram of Gelfoam embolization. Peripheral infiltrative portions of the tumor and daughter nodules are fed not only by hepatic arteries but also by the sinusoids that communicate directly with the portal vein (arrow). Dotted lines represent the potential arterioportal communications (transvasal and transplexal). Gelfoam embolizes only tumor-feeding arteries. (B) Diagram of transcatheter oily chemoembolization. Lipiodol with an anticancer agent (gray) remains in the fine tumor vessels, sinusoids, and portal vein, as well as in the feeding arteries distal to the Gelfoam. Lipiodol can enter the potential arterioportal communications (solid arrow, transsinusoidal; open arrow, transvasal and transplexal communications). An intrahepatic daughter nodule is also filled with Lipiodol. (From Nakagawa et al.,[43] with permission.)

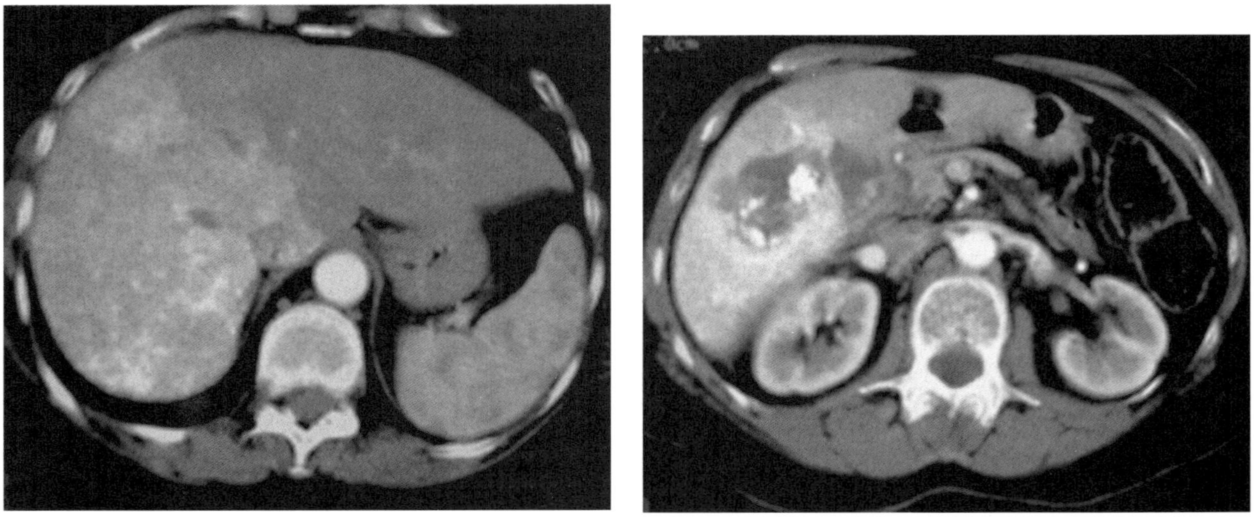

A B

Figure 11-2. A large right hepatic-lobe hepatoma in a 61-year-old woman who underwent staged chemoembolization procedures in an attempt to decrease the tumor size before surgery. Selective oily chemoembolization was performed via the right hepatic artery. (A) Axial computed tomography (CT) scan performed 1 day after the initial oily chemoembolization demonstrates the presence of residual Lipiodol in the right hepatic artery distribution, as noted by the increased density of the entire right hepatic lobe. (B) Axial CT scan performed 2 months after an oily chemoembolization demonstrates accumulation of Lipiodol within the necrotic tumor.

A department nurse is present throughout the procedure for noninvasive hemodynamic and respiratory monitoring while the patient is receiving intraprocedural anesthesia. Local anesthesia is provided with infiltration of 1% Xylocaine, and arterial access is obtained using the Seldinger technique. Although access via the common femoral artery is the most commonly used approach, Watanabe et al. demonstrated that the left brachial approach is a safe and effective alternative to the transfemoral approach for catheterization and embolization.[60] Patients with occlusive diseases of the aortic bifurcation or iliac arteries, aneurysms of the abdominal aorta, severe lumbago, kyphosis, or with difficulty maintaining the supine position required for angiography from the femoral route are good candidates for the brachial approach.[60]

Angiographic catheters used range in size from 4 F to 6 F.[28,40,60,61] Initial diagnostic mesenteric and hepatic arteriograms are performed for anatomic mapping and assessment of tumor location, size, and vascularity.[40] A superior mesenteric artery injection is performed to exclude aberrant hepatic arterial supply and to outline the portal venous circulation and confirm portal vein patency[28,37,40,51,62,63] (**Fig. 11-3**). Celiac axis catheteri-

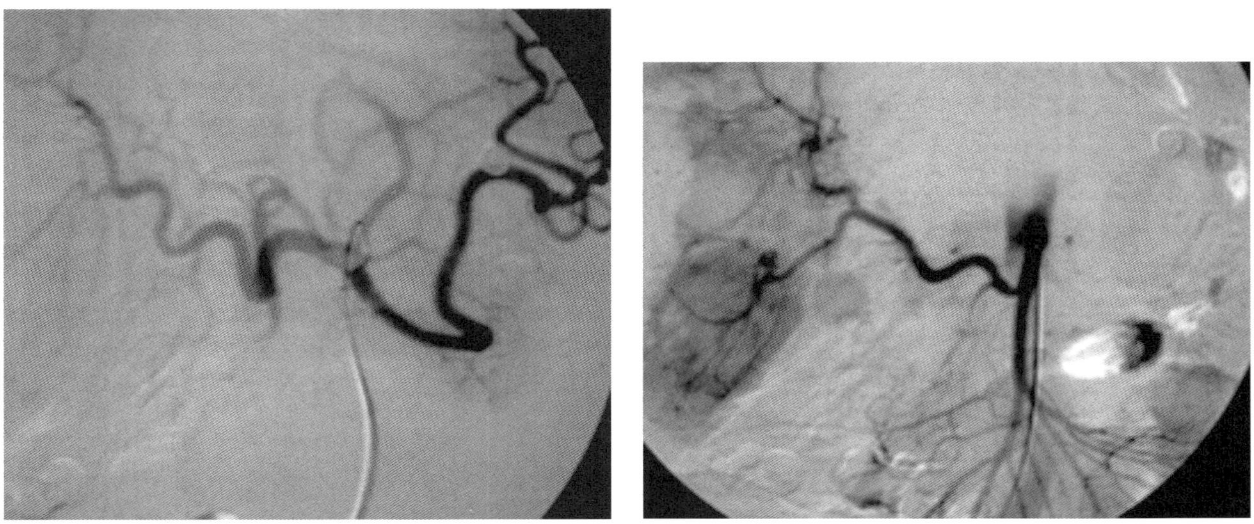

A B

Figure 11-3. 40-year old female with metastatic neuroendocrine tumor. Diagnostic angiography was performed prior to chemoembolization to determine vascular anatomy. A. Digital subtraction angiography obtained during a celiac artery injection demonstrates apparently normal hepatic arterial anatomy. B. Digital subtraction angiography obtained during a superior mesenteric artery injection demonstrates an accessory right hepatic artery supplying multiple hypervascular metastases.

zation and arteriography are performed, and the common hepatic artery is evaluated. The hepatic lobe with the largest tumor burden, as determined by preprocedural imaging, is selected for chemoembolization,[37] leaving the other lobe unaffected to support the normal metabolic functions of the liver.[15] The entire vascular supply of tumor in both lobes of the liver is not occluded at one setting, because it may result in fatal liver insufficiency. In patients with hepatic neuroendocrine metastases being treated for pain control, the side containing the pain-inducing lesions is treated. If the disease is symmetric and localized and pain is not the issue, then the side technically easiest to access is embolized first.[64] Sequential embolizations are performed at varying intervals[15,23] and repeated only when deemed necessary on the basis of findings on follow-up CT or MRI or of clinical symptomatology.[65]

To prevent inadvertent embolization of the bowel and pancreas, protective coil embolization of the gastroduodenal artery or gastric branches of a left gastrohepatic trunk or a right hepatic artery may be necessary[22,33,66,67] (**Fig. 11-4**).

The efficacy and tolerability of TACE increase when it is used selectively and repeated only when necessary—that is, only when the results of follow-up CT and MR imaging indicate that it is necessary.[65] After diagnostic angiography, a 4- to 6-F catheter is introduced into the celiac trunk and advanced beyond the gastroduodenal artery. Depending on the size, location, and arterial supply of the tumor and its satellites, superselective catheterization of the segmental arteries is performed using a coaxial technique with a 3-F microcatheter (e.g., Tracker catheter, Boston Scientific/Target Therapeutics, Fremont, California).[28,60,68,69] The microcatheter is inserted into the feeding vessel up to the third-order branch of the hepatic artery.[68] A superselective arteriogram should be obtained to confirm the safety of the final catheter position before injection of chemotherapeutic drugs.[70] Intra-arterial 1% Xylocaine may be administered during chemoembolization to reduce the severity and duration of pain, resulting in faster recovery and a shorter hospital stay.[37,71] After satisfactory catheter positioning, 20–30 mg of intra-arterial Xylocaine is injected before chemoembolization, with 10- to 30-mg bolus injections between each aliquot of chemoembolic emulsion.[24,71] In addition, 20–50 mg of Xylocaine may be added to a gelatin sponge slurry.[71] The total dose of Xylocaine should not exceed 200–300 mg.[37,71]

Various chemoembolic mixtures exist (**Table 11-5**) and can be tailored for each individual by the oncologist.

The cytotoxic agent and Lipiodol emulsion is created by manual mixing of the agents with a pumping method, using two syringes connected by a three-way stopcock. This mixing continues until a homogeneous "water-in-oil" emulsion is formed.[43] The optimum dose (volume in mL) of Lipiodol for TAE was determined, by a retrospective multivariate analysis by Nakao et al., to be up to 1.5 times the absolute value of the tumor diameter in centimeters.[72] In an experimental study, Kan

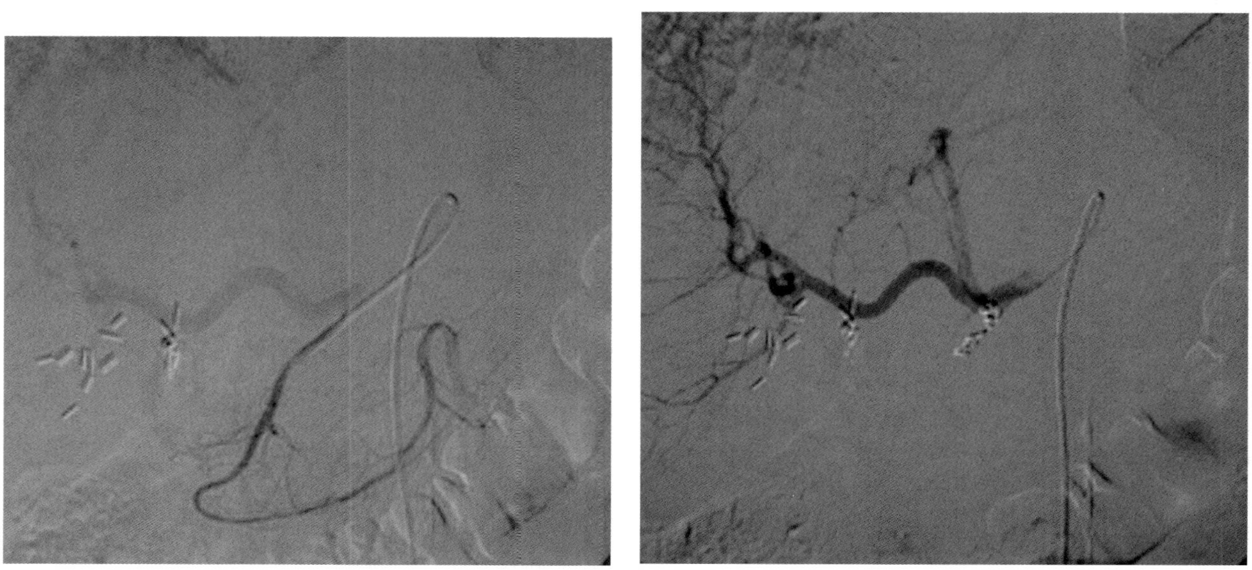

A B

Figure 11-4. A multifocal hepatoma in a 51-year-old man. A diagnostic angiogram was performed prior to surgical placement of a hepatic arterial infusion pump. To protect the gastroduodenal artery (GDA) distribution from chemotherapy given via the hepatic artery catheter, coils were placed into the GDA. (A) Digital subtraction angiogram of the GDA demonstrates a normal appearance of the GDA and its branches. Reflux into the proper hepatic artery is noted. (B) Digital subtraction angiogram of the common hepatic artery demonstrates complete occlusion of the GDA at its origin. The coil pack can be seen at the origin of the GDA.

TABLE 11-5
Various Chemoembolic Regimens

Author	Year	Tumor	Embolic mixture/regimen: Lipiodol (mL)	Isovue (mL)	Chemotherapeutic agents (mg)	Particulate embolization
Rajan et al.[67]	2001	Leiomyosarcoma metastases	10	10	MMC 10 mg ADR, 50 mg Cisp, 100 mg	PVA
Leung et al.[24]	2001	HCC	10	10	MMC, 10 mg ADR, 50 mg Cisp, 100 mg	PVA (150–250 μm)
Okusaka et al.[55]	2000	HCC	10	NR	ADR, 20–30 mg Epirub, 30–50 mg *or* Pirarub, 30–50 mg	Gelatin sponge
Vogl et al.[69]	2000	HCC	10	NR	ADR, 50 mg Cisp, 50 mg	Amilomer microspheres
Savastano et al.[39]	1999	HCC	~10	10	Epirub, ~ 46.5 mg	Gelatin sponge
Ernst et al.[65]	1999	HCC	10–15	NR	ADR, 50–70 mg	With or without Gelfoam
Brown et al.[64]	1999	NE metastases	0	0	0	PVA
Arora et al.[95]	1999	NE metastases Colorectal metastases Gastrointestinal sarcoma metastases	10	10	MMC, 10 mg ADR, 50 mg Cisp, 100 mg	PVA
al-Bassam et al.[33]	1999	HCC NE metastases Leiomyosarcoma metastases	20	20	ADR, 30–60 mg	Gelfoam powder
		Colorectal metastases	20	10	5-FU, 1 g MMC, 10 mg	Gelfoam powder
Drougas et al.[9]	1998	Carcinoid metastases	NR	NR	MMC, 30 mg ADR, 60 mg Cisp, 100 mg	PVA
Gates et al.[8]	1999	HCC NE metastases	20	10	ADR, 60 mg	Gelatin sponge
		Colorectal metastases	20	10	5-FU, 1 g MMC, 10 mg	Gelatin sponge
Clouse et al.[22]	1994	NE metastases	20	10	ADR, 40–80 mg	Gelfoam powder
Lang and Brown[122]	1993	Colorectal metastases	7–20	NR	ADR, 50–100 mg	None
Llado et al.[6]	2000	HCC	5–22	NR	ADR, 13–65 mg	Gelatin sponge

5-FU = 5-fluorouracil; ADR = doxorubicin; cisp = cisplatin; epirub = epirubicin; HCC = hepatocellular carcinoma; MMC = mitomycin C; NE = neuroendocrine; NR = not reported; pirarub = pirarubicin; PVA = polyvinyl alcohol.

et al. determined the optimal dose of Lipiodol to be in the range of 0.1–0.3 mL/kg based on the distribution of the iodized oil and observation of systemic embolism or significant hepatic infarction with higher doses.[73] Chung et al. consider the maximum safe dose of iodized oil injected into the hepatic artery to be between 15 and 20 mL, because pulmonary embolisms were observed in patients undergoing TOCE with greater than 20 mL of iodized oil.[74] The total volume of Lipiodol–chemotherapeutic agent emulsion administered depends on the size of the tumor,[38,55] the patient's underlying liver function, and, if such information is available, the response of the tumor to previous chemoembolization.[38]

At some institutions, oily chemoembolization is not followed by particulate embolization,[30,38,63,75] or it is applied only to large (>9 cm) tumors.[30] The more common approach is to follow administration of Lipiodol–chemotherapeutic emulsion with particulate embolization using absorbable gelatin powder or pledgets mixed with 2 mL of absolute ethanol and 30–50 mL of water-soluble iodinated contrast.[40,56,76,77] PVA particles are used for the particulate embolization by some institutions.[7,24,37,38,67] Infusion of the emulsion is stopped when blood flow in the artery supplying the tumor slows down but before occlusion occurs, with or without the appearance of iodized oil in portal vein branches.[4,31,34,38,66] After embolization, devascularization is confirmed with an additional angiographic study of the hepatic artery.[69]

Proponents of particulate embolization following oily chemoembolization believe that inhibition of hepatic arterial blood flow with the gelatin sponge enhances the effect of the iodized oil by increasing the retention of the anticancer agent in tumor tissues.[43,56] Furthermore, light Gelfoam embolization does not produce permanent occlusion of the hepatic artery, allowing repeated performance of TACE at intervals of 6–12 weeks.[4] Those in favor of TOCE without the use of Gelfoam believe that preserving the hepatic arterial flow for a long time makes repeated chemoembolization for recurrent tumors possible. If particulate embolization is performed, it should be ensured that some antegrade flow through the hepatic artery is noted at the end of the procedure (**Fig. 11-5**). If no antegrade flow is noted, the entire hepatic artery may occlude because of the lack of outflow. Obstruction of the hepatic artery by particulate embolization may lead to the development of complicated collateral circulation, making repeated use of TACE difficult.[30]

HEPATIC ARTERIAL CHEMOINFUSION

Regional intra-arterial infusion chemotherapy of primary and secondary hepatic tumors through percutaneous or surgically placed catheters is another method directed at improving the efficiency of chemotherapy by delivering high doses selectively to the tumors.[10,18,54,78–82] The chemotherapeutic agent may be administered directly through a subcutaneously placed port or via a continuous infusion pump (e.g., the Infusaid model 400, Infusaid Corp., Norwood, Massachusetts).

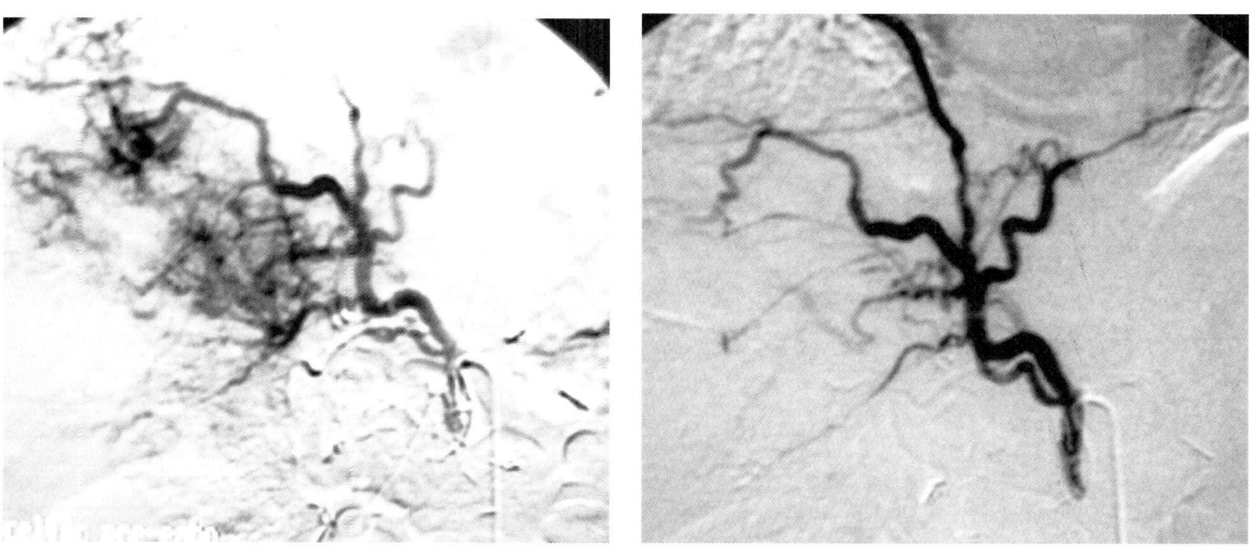

A B

Figure 11-5. A metastatic neuroendocrine tumor that has persisted for 7 years in a 58-year-old man despite cryotherapy, use of a hepatic arterial infusion pump, and systemic chemotherapy. (A) Digital subtraction angiogram obtained during celiac injection demonstrates multiple hypervascular metastases arising from the hepatic artery distribution. (B) Digital subtraction angiogram obtained after hepatic arterial chemoembolization demonstrates some persistent antegrade flow through the hepatic artery. This persistent outflow is essential in keeping the hepatic artery patent for repeat embolization procedures.

Hepatic arterial infusion, as compared with systemic infusion, produces increased concentrations in the liver on the order of 100-fold for 5-fluorouracil (5-FU) and 400-fold for floxuridine (5-fluoro-2′deoxyuridine, or FUDR).[18] With both techniques, it is important to occlude aberrant hepatic vessels and to temporarily or permanently embolize branch vessels supplying other organs by using steel coils or Gelfoam pledgets.[10,54,82] Embolization of multiple hepatic arteries redistributes flow, thereby allowing infusion of the entire liver through a single catheter in the dominant artery.[10,54] Branch vessels that may require protective coil embolization or ligation are the gastroduodenal, right gastric, and accessory left gastric arteries. Their occlusion maximizes tumor infusion and minimizes exposure of normal tissues to chemotherapeutic agents, thereby decreasing gastric, duodenal, and pancreatic complications.[54,82]

For the surgical method, a catheter is placed into the gastroduodenal artery by laparotomy and is positioned at its junction with the hepatic artery.[10,79,80] The catheter is then connected either to an implantable port[83] or to an Infusaid pump; the port or pump is implanted in the right or left lower quadrant in a subcutaneous pouch.[80] After surgery, catheter positioning is verified with a ^{99m}Tc-MAA perfusion scan via the pump to confirm hepatic distribution of the pump effluent.[79]

The chemotherapeutic agent is administered either via bolus infusion or continuous infusion through a pump. Continuous infusion may have an advantage over bolus infusion.[79] The Infusaid pump allows continuous infusion of FUDR, which is continued for 14 days at a dose of 0.3 mg/kg/day, followed by 14 days of continuous saline infusion.[79,80] Heparin (10,000 U) is placed in the 50-mL pump reservoir with each refill of drug.[79,84]

Percutaneous hepatic arterial infusion catheters have been placed percutaneously via the left femoral, brachial, and left axillary arterial approaches.[82,85] The advantage of percutaneous implantation of the chemoinfusion device is that laparotomy and general anesthesia are avoided.[85] For the left brachial artery approach, mid- to high brachial artery access is obtained with use of a 21-gauge micropuncture introducer system. Catheters used with the brachial approach include the 4- or 5-F Cobra, H-1-H, and Simmons 2 catheters (Cook, Inc., Bloomington, Indiana). For the femoral artery approach, access is obtained with a single-wall-puncture technique with an 18-gauge needle, and the catheters used are 5-F Cobra and 5- or 6-F Simmons 2. Diagnostic angiography of the celiac axis and superior mesenteric artery is performed to determine hepatic arterial supply and portal vein patency. The catheter is advanced into the hepatic arterial system, with the goal of providing flow to the lobe with the majority of tumor burden, and is connected to a port or infusion pump.[18,85] Presence or absence of gastrointestinal tract perfusion and adequate hepatic perfusion are assessed with the aid of a ^{99m}Tc-MAA scan. After satisfactory catheter positioning, a course of chemoinfusion is started. A solution of normal saline with 10 U of heparin per milliliter is infused at 40mL/h prior to beginning the chemoinfusion.[82]

A variety of different chemoinfusion regimens exist. The most commonly used anticancer agents are FUDR, 5-FU, and mitomycin C.[18,26,54,82,85,86] The left brachial artery and left axillary approaches are generally preferred over the femoral approach because they allow patients to remain ambulatory during chemoinfusion.[82] However, Habbe et al. noted an increased incidence of complications related to the brachial approach and recommend its use only when femoral artery access is not possible.[82]

INTRAHEPATIC ARTERIAL RADIOMICROSPHERES

HCC is responsive to a large dose of conventional radiotherapy; however, delivery of a tumoricidal dose of radiation is limited by the low tolerance of hepatocytes. External-beam radiotherapy therefore has a very limited role in the treatment of HCC because of the adverse effects of irradiation, which lead to hepatic fibrosis of normal liver tissue.[4,87] Intrahepatic arterial injection of radioactive isotopes allows selective deposition within the tumor vasculature and spares the normal tissue, producing a local tumoricidal effect. With hepatic arterial administration of radiomicrospheres, significantly higher doses of radiation are delivered to the liver, with an approximate threefold or greater radiation dose in the tumor nodules relative to normal liver.[36] The optimal tumoricidal dose suggested for HCC is greater than 120 Gy.[87,88]

Radiomicrospheres used include iodine 131–Lipiodol (^{131}I-Lipiodol), yttrium 90, phosphorus 32, and rhenium glass microshperes.[36,88–91] The most commonly used are ^{131}I-Lipiodol and yttrium 90. The latter has a shorter half-life (64 hours) and lacks gamma-ray emissions, which eliminates the need for patient isolation. Yttrium 90, however, is not amenable to dosimetry measurements. It has a long beta energy range, with a cytotoxic range of 11 mm, few shielding problems, and little radiation dose to surrounding normal tissues.[14,92] Conversely, iodine 131 has a half-life of approximately 8 days and is actively excreted in body fluids, which may cause radiation protection problems. Both beta and gamma radiation are produced by its decay. The beta energy is low, giving it a cytotoxic range of only 2 mm. The presence of gamma radiation allows accurate dosimetry measurements to be made using external scintigraphy.[14]

The radioisotopes can be administered through a percutaneously placed angiocatheter via the femoral artery[36,87,91] or through an implantable port system placed via laparotomy.[93] Treatment with radiomicrospheres causes less toxicity than systemic or hepatic arterial chemotherapy or hepatic arterial chemoembolization.[36]

POST-PROCEDURAL CARE AND FOLLOW-UP TREATMENT

Patients are admitted immediately after the procedure for continued intravenous hydration and pain control. The antiemetic prochlorperazine is administered as needed.[24] Antibiotics are continued for 5–7 days.[9,38] Daily blood work, consisting of a CBC, creatinine, LFTs, prothrombin time (PT), and partial thromboplastin time (PTT), are done to monitor hepatic, renal, and bone marrow function. With chemoembolization, liver enzymes peak at 12–24 hours and typically return to baseline levels within 1 week; with particulate embolization, liver enzymes peak at 5–6 days and return to baseline within 9–10 days.[22] Only patients with elevated tumor marker levels prior to treatment are monitored with serial blood work. Patients are discharged home when their hepatic and renal functions return to baseline, they no longer require parenteral analgesics, and they are tolerating an oral diet.[9,24]

Follow-up CT scans and CBC, PT, PTT, LFTs, and creatinine levels are obtained 1 month after the procedure and at 3-month intervals thereafter.[8,22,24,67,87] CT scans are used to assess changes in tumor morphology, changes in tumor size, the pattern of ethiodized oil uptake and changes in the pattern of ethiodized oil distribution, resorption of ethiodized oil, overall liver size, and the development of new lesions or metastases.[8] A morphologic response to treatment is defined as cessation of growth of tumor with evidence of tumor necrosis, or decrease in the size of lesions in the treated territory.[64] Levels of tumor markers (AFP for HCC; CEA for metastases from colorectal carcinoma; 5-HIAA, NSE, and CGA for neuroendocrine tumors) are measured routinely at the same intervals as follow-up CT is done. A fall in tumor marker levels indicates a response to chemoembolization; a subsequent rise indicates tumor recurrence.[8]

FACTORS AFFECTING PROGNOSIS

Ueno et al. performed chemoembolization without particulate embolization and found the presence of extrahepatic metastases, elevation of serum tumor markers, and progress of portal vein involvement to be associated with a poor prognosis.[30] Savastano et al. reported the presence of ascites, elevated bilirubin levels, elevated AFP values, a tumor diameter greater than 5 cm, and the absence of a tumor capsulelike rim to be associated with significantly worse survival rates.[39] A decrease of AFP after TOCE is a useful post-procedural predictor of a good tumor response.[39]

COMPLICATIONS

Complications of hepatic arterial interventions may be related either to the method of vascular access or to the specific therapeutic modality employed (**Table 11-6**).

According to Tarazov et al., certain variables lead to the development of complications after TACE. These include nonselective placement of the catheter, high

TABLE 11-6
Complications of Hepatic Arterial Interventions

Complications
Common
Post-embolization syndrome
Elevation of liver enzymes
Ascites
Ischemic cholecystitis
Less common
Vascular access complications
Gastric and duodenal ulcers
Gastrointestinal hemorrhage
Duodenal perforation
Pancreatitis
Ischemic cholangitis
Acute hepatic failure
Liver infarction
Liver abscess
Liver rupture
Jaundice
Splenic infarction and abscess
Encephalopathy
Pulmonary edema
Pulmonary Lipiodol embolism
Cutaneous complications (supraumbilical rash, ulceration, necrosis, painful erythema)
Acute renal failure
Septicemia
Hypertensive crisis (in patient with carcinoid metastases)
Dysuria
Hiccups
Inguinal hematoma

(Data from from Leung et al.,[24] Jeng and Ching,[27] Chung et al.,[31] Song et al.,[34] Ngan et al.,[38] Tarazov et al.,[46] and Cohen et al.[94–102])

doses of cytostatics and iodized oil, use of small-diameter embolic agents, preexisting functional liver disorders, previous surgery on the liver and bile ducts, and obstruction of the bile ducts and/or portal vein branches.[46]

The most common complication related to arterial access is development of a local hematoma. Other associated complications are arterial thrombosis, development of a pseudoaneurysm or arteriovenous fistula, and arterial dissection. Iatrogenic dissection of the celiac and proximal hepatic arteries has been reported, at an incidence of 1.3%–3.2%.[60,101] Subsequent hepatic arterial interventions may be performed successfully within 1–2 months after iatrogenic dissection of the celiac artery in most patients, because spontaneous recanalization occurs in over 70%.[101] Celiac artery dissection has not been observed with the left brachial artery approach.[60] However, cerebral infarctions, acute brachial artery thromboses, and transient loss of the radial pulse have occurred with the left brachial approach.[18,60,82]

Major complications occur with approximately 2%–7% of hepatic arterial embolization procedures.[24] Post-embolization syndrome (PES), the most common complication, is seen in 15%–90% of patients[24,31,99] and is characterized by abdominal pain, fever, nausea, and vomiting.[7,24,31,37] It is a self-limited process that requires supportive management with intravenous hydration and parenteral narcotics. The cause of PES is not known; however, it is thought to be related to tissue ischemia and an inflammatory response to the embolization. Severe PES is more common when patients have tumors larger than 6 cm in diameter.[35] Gallbladder embolization and the chemoembolic dose administered have been found to be associated with an increased risk of PES.[24]

Transient elevation of LFTs and serum bilirubin occur in most patients.[38] The deterioration of hepatic function is transient in most patients, with liver enzymes and serum bilirubin reaching peak levels 2–3 days after the procedure and returning to preembolization values within 5 days to 4 weeks after the procedure.[31,94] In some patients, the deterioration of liver function becomes irreversible and progresses to acute hepatic failure, with ascites, encephalopathy, and eventual death.[31,94]

Serious ischemic complications such as cholecystitis, pancreatitis, bile duct necrosis, and liver and splenic abscesses occur in about 5% of patients undergoing chemoembolization. These complications do not worsen survival rates.[46] Development of a liver abscess is a rare complication, with a reported incidence ranging between 0% and 3.3%.[31,34,97] The abscess develops when necrotic tumor tissue is contaminated with bacteria introduced either exogenously during the procedure or from the bowel.[28,31,34,94,97,99]

Other serious but less common complications are gastric and duodenal mucosal erosions; duodenal perforation and gastrointestinal hemorrhage; gallbladder, liver, and splenic infarction; liver rupture; pulmonary edema; pulmonary embolism; acute tumor lysis syndrome; and septicemia.[27,28,31,34,35,46,94,97,99,100,103]

Complications seen more specifically with hepatic artery chemoinfusion consist of port-pocket infection, catheter thrombosis, catheter dislodgement, catheter malposition with misperfusion, and obstructive jaundice secondary to chemotherapy-induced biliary sclerosis.[42,82,104]

Complications restricted to hepatic intra-arterial radiomicrosphere embolization are radiation pneumonitis, hepatitis, and cholecystitis. Pulmonary fibrosis, reversible gastritis or duodenitis, and development of a chronic atrophic and contracted stomach have also been reported.[13,14,36,88,105,106]

OUTCOMES AND SURVIVAL

Although the controlled randomized trial by Groupe d'Etude et de Traitment du Carcinome Hepatocellulaire failed to demonstrate a significant efficacy of transarterial chemoembolization,[107] multiple studies have demonstrated that chemoembolization is an effective palliative therapeutic option for patients with unresectable HCC. Reported survival rates for patients who have undergone chemoembolization range from 34% to 88% at 1 year, 33% to 64% at 2 years, and 18% to 51% at 3 years.[4,6,9,10,30,37,39,52,65,77,86,108,109] Survival rates after TOCE for hepatomas are likely dependent on the degree of the patient's underlying liver disease. Bismuth et al. demonstrated 2-year survival rates for patients with class A cirrhosis (modified Pugh's classification) to far exceed the survival of patients with class C cirrhosis (49% and 9%, respectively).[28]

Although there have been very few studies comparing one treatment methodology with another, two groups of investigators have demonstrated improved survival—one by adding Lipiodol to the chemoembolic mixture[56] and the other by adding Gelfoam particles to the mixture.[110]

In addition to improved survival rates, investigators have demonstrated the benefit of using TOCE in hepatomas by monitoring the post-procedural appearance of embolized tumors using either CT[111,112] or contrast-enhanced MR imaging.[113] In addition, Schilling et al. described the immediate post-TOCE appearance of hepatomas using phosphorus 32 MR spectroscopy.[114] In this report, it was noted that the effects of successful chemoembolization procedures became apparent during the first few hours after the procedure. The prognostic benefits of this type of study have yet to be fully elicited.

Unlike the treatment of hepatomas, the goal of chemoembolization for neuroendocrine tumor metastases is not increased survival but rather the control of symptoms related to hormone production, arrest of tumor growth, and control of pain. Because individuals with metastatic neuroendocrine tumors can have very long survivals without any therapy at all, the goal of chemoembolic therapy is purely palliative. In this regard, the results of chemoembolization are excellent. In up to 90% of patients, hormonal symptoms respond to embolotherapy or chemoembolization, and nearly 100% of patients treated have palliation of tumor-related pain and/or cessation of tumor growth.[9,15,22,23,32,40,64,66] In separate studies, Clouse et al. and Perry et al., using TOCE, found that hormone secretion decreased by a mean of 90%, with relief of symptoms in all patients with hormonally active tumors.[22,40] For all patients, there was a demonstrated reduction in the size of metastases by 84% at 1 week to 3 months after TOCE.

Unlike its cutaneous counterpart, primary ocular melanoma presents with metastatic disease in up to 50% of all patients; metastases may occur many months or years after resection of the primary tumor. Survival rates are poor—with median survival times reported as being less than 6 months—after the development of metastatic disease.[25,115] Typically, metastatic disease is limited to the liver, making local therapy a viable option. Results with TCE are promising; however, because of the relative rarity of the disease, firm results are lacking. In what is likely the largest study to date, Mavligit et al. treated 30 patients with metastatic ocular melanoma using a combination of cisplatin and PVA particles.[25] The median survival time in this study was 11 months, and although there was no control group, the results compared favorably with those for historical controls. Similar results have been found by other investigators.[116–118]

The results for chemoembolization of the liver with colorectal metastases are marginal. Owing to the high incidence of colorectal disease metastasizing to the liver, hopes were high that TCE would demonstrate some benefit against the disease. Hepatic arterial infusion of chemotherapy, without embolization, preceded chemoembolization as a treatment modality. Early results were promising[79,119,120]; however, toxicity of infused chemotherapeutic agents proved limiting.[121] Because most metastases from colorectal primaries are hypovascular, the benefit from adding embolization therapy to chemoinfusion was anticipated to be minor. Two studies, however, have described a benefit to patients receiving such therapy.

Lang and Brown performed TOCE in 46 patients with colorectal metastases to the liver.[122] Their results were exceptional, demonstrating complete cure, as assessed by radiology and by tumor marker levels, in 8 patients (17%). Additionally, 72% of patients who survived 3 years or more demonstrated no tumor progression after TOCE. In a separate study, Civalleri et al. infused chemotherapy and biodegradable starch microspheres into both the hepatic arterial and portal venous systems in an attempt to expose the tumor to TCE via both vascular systems.[123] Early promising results were limited by technical difficulties. An intriguing study was recently performed that assessed the cost-effectiveness of chemoembolization for colorectal metastases to the liver.[124] Its authors determined that a survival of close to 5 months must be proved to make the procedure cost-effective.

REFERENCES

1. Bruix J. Treatment of hepatocellular carcinoma. *Hepatology* 1997;25(2):259–261.
2. Caturelli E, Siena DA, Gusilli S, et al. Transcatheter arterial chemoembolization for hepatocellular carcinoma in patients with cirrhosis: evaluation of damage to nontumorous liver tissue—long-term prospective study. *Radiology* 2000;215(1):123–128.
3. Cho KJ, Andrews JC, Williams DM, Doenz F, Guy GE. Hepatic arterial chemotherapy: role of angiography. *Radiology* 1989;173(3):783–791.
4. Liu C-L, Fan S-t. Nonresectional therapies for hepatocellular carcinoma. *Am J Surg* 1997;173:358–365.
5. Palma LD. Diagnostic imaging and interventional therapy of hepatocellular carcinoma. *Br J Radiol* 1998;71:808–818.
6. Llado L, Virgili J, Figueras J, et al. A prognostic index of the survival of patients with unresectable hepatocellular carcinoma after transcatheter arterial chemoembolization. *Cancer* 2000;88(1):50–57.
7. Patel NH, Hahn D, Rapp S, Bergan K, Coldwell DM. Hepatic artery embolization: factors predisposing to postembolization pain and nausea. *J Vasc Interv Radiol* 2000;11(4):453–460.
8. Gates J, Hartnell GG, Stuart KE, Clouse ME. Chemoembolization of hepatic neoplasms: safety, complications and when to worry. *Radiographics* 1999;19(2):399–414.
9. Drougas JG, Anthony LB, Blair TK. Hepatic artery chemoembolization for management of patients with advanced metastatic carcinoid tumors. *Am J Surg* 1998;175:408–412.
10. Sterchi JM, Richards F, White DR, et al. Chemoinfusion of the hepatic artery for metastases to the liver. *Surg Gynecol Obstet* 1989;168(4):291–295.
11. Chuang VP, Wallace S. Hepatic artery embolization in the treatment of hepatic neoplasms. *Radiology* 1981;140:51–58.
12. Brown KT, Nevins AB, Getrajdman GI, et al. Particle embolization for hepatocellular carcinoma. *J Vasc Interv Radiol* 1998;9(5):822–828.
13. Lau WY, Leung TWT, Ho S, et al. Diagnostic pharmaco-scintigraphy with hepatic intra-arterial technetium-99m macroaggregated albumin in the determination of tumour to non-tumour uptake ratio in hepatocellular carcinoma. *Br J Radiol* 1994;67:136–139.
14. Novell JR, Hilson A, Hobbs KE. Therapeutic aspects of radio-isotopes in hepatobiliary malignancy. *Br J Surg* 1991;78(8):901–906.
15. Ajani JA, Carrasco HC, Wallace S. Neuroendocrine tumors metastatic to the liver—vascular occlusion therapy. *Ann N Y Acad Sci* 1994;733:479–487.
16. Farmer DG, Seu P, Swenson K, Economou J, Busuttil RW. Current and future treatment modalities for hepatocellular carcinoma. *Clin Liv Dis* 1997;1(2):361–396.

17. Rose DM, Chapman WC, Brockenbrough AT, et al. Transcatheter arterial chemoembolization as primary treatment for hepatocellular carcinoma. *Am J Surg* 1999;177:405–410.
18. Clouse ME, Ahmed R, Ryan RB, et al. Complications of long term transbrachial hepatic infusion chemotherapy. *Am J Roentgenol* 1977;129:799–803.
19. Breedis C, Young G. The blood supply of neoplasms in the liver. *Am J Pathol* 1954:969–977.
20. Lautt W, Greenway D. Conceptual review of the hepatic vascular bed. *Hepatology* 1987;7:952–963.
21. Pentecost MJ. Transcatheter treatment of hepatic metastases. *Am J Roentgenol* 1993;160:1171–1175.
22. Clouse M, Perry L, Stuart K, Stokes KR. Hepatic arterial chemoembolization for metastatic neuroendocrine tumors. *Digestion* 1994;55(suppl 3):92–97.
23. Carrasco CH, Charnsangavej C, Ajani J, et al. The carcinoid syndrome: palliation by hepatic artery embolization. *Am J Roentgenol* 1986;147:149–154.
24. Leung DA, Goin JE, Sickles C, et al. Determinants of postembolization syndrome after hepatic chemoembolization. *J Vasc Interv Radiol* 2001;12:321–326.
25. Mavligit GM, Charnsangavej C, Carrasco CH, et al. Regression of ocular melanoma metastatic to the liver after hepatic arterial chemoembolization with cisplatin and polyvinyl sponge. *JAMA* 1988;260(7):974–976.
26. Paquet KJ, Kalk JF, Cuan-Orozco F, et al. Hepatic chemoinfusion of 5-FU in metastasis of gastrointestinal cancer and advanced primary hepatocellular carcinoma. *Eur J Surg Oncol* 1992;18:156–161.
27. Jeng K-S, Ching H-J. The role of surgery in the management of unusual complications of transcatheter arterial embolization for hepatocellular carcinoma. *World J Surg* 1988;12(3):362–368.
28. Bismuth H, Morino M, Sherlock D, et al. Primary treatment of hepatocellular carcinoma by arterial chemoembolization. *Am J Surg* 1992;163:387–394.
29. Ramming KP, O'Toole K. The use of the implantable chemoinfusion pump in the treatment of hepatic metastases of colorectal cancer. *Arch Surg* 1986;121:1440–1444.
30. Ueno K, Miyazono N, Inoue H, et al. Transcatheter arterial chemoembolization therapy using iodized oil for patients with unresectable hepatocellular carcinoma. *Cancer* 2000;88(7):1574–1581.
31. Chung JW, Park JH, Han JK, et al. Hepatic tumors: predisposing factors for complications of transcatheter oily chemoembolization. *Radiology* 1996;198(1):33–40.
32. Diamandidou E, Ajani JA, Yang DJ, et al. Two-phase study of hepatic artery vascular occlusion with microencapsulated cisplatin in patients with liver metastases from neuroendocrine tumors. *Am J Roentgenol* 1998;170:339–344.
33. al-Bassam SH, Munk PL, Sallomi DF, et al. Chemo-embolization of hepatic tumours. *Diagn Radiol* 1999;43:165–174.
34. Song S-Y, Chung JW, Han JK, et al. Liver abscess after transcatheter oily chemoembolization for hepatic tumors: incidence, predisposing factors, and clinical outcome. *J Vasc Interv Radiol* 2001;12(3):313–320.
35. Pijl MEJ, Pattynama PMT, Hoek BV. Liver rupture after transcatheter arterial chemoembolization of a giant hepatocellular carcinoma. *J Vasc Interv Radiol* 1999;10:895–897.
36. Dancey JE, Shepherd FA, Paul K, et al. Treatment of nonresectable hepatocellular carcinoma with intrahepatic ^{90}Y-microspheres. *J Nucl Med* 2000;41(10):1673–1681.
37. Solomon B, Soulen MC, Baum RA, et al. Chemoembolization of hepatocellular carcinoma with cisplatin, doxorubicin, mitomycin-C, ethiodol, and polyvinyl alcohol: prospective evaluation of response and survival in a U.S. population. *J Vasc Interv Radiol* 1999;10(6):793–798.
38. Ngan H, Lai C-L, Fan S-T, et al. Transcatheter arterial chemoembolization in inoperable hepatocellular carcinoma: four-year follow-up. *J Vasc Interv Radiol* 1996;7(3):419–425.
39. Savastano S, Miotto D, Casarrubea G, et al. Transcatheter arterial chemoembolization for hepatocellular carcinoma in patients with Child's grade A or B cirrhosis. *J Clin Gastroenterol* 1999;28(4):334–340.
40. Perry LJ, Stuart K, Stokes KR. Hepatic arterial chemoembolization for metastatic neuroendocrine tumors. *Surgery* 1994;116:1111–1117.
41. Soulen MC. Chemoembolization of hepatic malignancies. *Oncology* 1994;8(4):77–84.
42. Pozniak MA, Babel SG, Trump DL. Complications of hepatic arterial infusion chemotherapy. *Radiographics* 1991;11:67–79.
43. Nakagawa N, Cornelius AS, Kao SCS, Nakajima Y, Nakada K. Transcatheter oily chemoembolization for unresectable malignant liver tumors in children. *J Vasc Interv Radiol* 1993;4(3):353–358.
44. Walser RH, Haldemann AR, Rosler H, et al. Diagnostic angioscintigraphic evaluation of malignant hepatic tumors before catheter embolization: determination of shunt, flow distribution, and reflux. *Cardiovasc Intervent Radiol* 1996;19:77–81.
45. McDermott VG, Schuster MG, Smith JP. Antibiotic prophylaxis in vascular and interventional radiology. *Am J Roentgenol* 1997;169(1):31–38.
46. Tarazov PG, Polysalov VN, Prozorovskij KV, et al. Ischemic complications of transcatheter arterial chemoembolization in liver malignancies. *Acta Radiologica* 2000;41:156–160.
47. Allison DJ, Booth A. Arterial embolization in the management of liver metastases. *Cardiovasc Intervent Radiol* 1990;13:161–168.
48. Lin D-Y, Liaw Y-F, Lee T-Y, Lai C-M. Hepatic arterial embolization in patients with unresectable hepatocellular carcinoma—a randomized controlled trial. *Gastroenterology* 1988;94(2):453–456.
49. Yamada R, Sato M, Kawabata M, et al. Hepatic artery embolization in 120 patients with unresectable hepatoma. *Radiology* 1983;148:397–401.
50. Yoshioka H, Sato M, Sonomura T, et al. Factors associated with survival exceeding 5 years after transcatheter arterial embolization for hepatocellular carcinoma. *Semin Oncol* 1997;24(suppl 6):S6-29–S6-37.
51. Yamada R, Kishi K, Sonomura T, et al. Transcatheter arterial embolization in unresectable hepatocellular carcinoma. *Cardiovasc Intervent Radiol* 1990;13:135–139.
52. Harada T, Matsuo K, Inoue T, et al. Is preoperative hepatic arterial chemoembolization safe and effective for hepatocellular carcinoma? *Ann Surg* 1996;224(1)4–9.
53. Wallace S, Kan Z, Li C. Hepatic chemoembolization: clinical and experimental correlation. *Acta Gastroenterol Belg* 2000;63(2):169–173.
54. Wallace S, Carrasco CH, Charnsangavej C, et al. Hepatic artery infusion and chemoembolization in the management of liver metastases. *Cardiovasc Intervent Radiol* 1990;13:153–160.
55. Okusaka T, Okada S, Ueno H, et al. Evaluation of the therapeutic effect of transcatheter arterial embolization for hepatocellular carcinoma. *Oncology* 2000;58:293–299.
56. Nakamura H, Hashimoto T, Oi H, Sawada S. Transcatheter oily chemoembolization of hepatocellular carcinoma. *Radiology* 1989;170(3):783–786.
57. Yumoto Y, Jinno K, Tokuyama K, Ishimitsu T, et al. Hepatocellular carcinoma detected by iodized oil. *Radiology* 1985;154(1):19–24.
58. Jin-no K, Hyodo I, Tanimizu M. Total necrosis of hepatocellular carcinoma with a combination therapy of arterial infusion of chemotherapeutic Lipiodol and transcatheter arterial embolization: report of 14 cases. *Semin Oncol* 1997;24(2, suppl 6):S6-71–S6-80.
59. Ravoet C, Bleiberg H, Gerard B. Non-surgical treatment of hepatocarcinoma. *J Surg Oncol* 1993;3(suppl):104–111.
60. Watanabe S, Minami A, Nishioka M, Ohjawa M, Koui F. Left brachial approach for transcatheter arterial embolization therapy in patients with hepatocellular carcinoma. *Dig Dis Sci* 1997;42(1):47–58.
61. Terayama N, Miyayama S, Tatsu H, et al. Subsegmental transcatheter arterial embolization for hepatocellular carcinoma in the caudate lobe. *J Vasc Interv Radiol* 1998;9(3):501.

62. Venook A, Stagg RJ, Lewis BJ, et al. Chemoembolization for hepatocellular carcinoma. *J Clin Oncol* 1990;8(6):1108–1114.
63. Lang E, Brown C. Colorectal metastases to the liver: selective chemoembolization. *Radiology* 1993;189(2):417–422.
64. Brown KT, Koh BY, Brody LA, et al. Particle embolization of hepatic neuroendocrine metastases for control of pain and hormonal symptoms. *J Vasc Interv Radiol* 1999;10(4):397–403.
65. Ernst O, Sergent G, Mizrahi D, et al. Treatment of hepatocellular carcinoma by transcatheter arterial chemoembolization: comparison of planned periodic chemoembolization and chemoembolization based on tumor response. *Am J Roentgenol* 1999;172:59–64.
66. Stokes KR, Keith S, Clouse M. Hepatic arterial chemoembolization for metastatic endocrine tumors. *J Vasc Interv Radiol* 1993;4(3):341–345.
67. Rajan DK, Soulen MC, Clark TWI, et al. Sarcomas metastatic to the liver: response and survival after cisplatin, doxorubicin, mitomycin-C, ethiodol, and polyvinyl alcohol chemoembolization. *J Vasc Interv Radiol* 2001;12(2):187–193.
68. Park JH, Han JK, Chung JW, et al. Superselective transcatheter arterial embolization with ethanol and iodized oil for hepatocellular carcinoma. *J Vasc Interv Radiol* 1993;4(3):333–339.
69. Vogl TJ, Trapp M, Schroeder H, et al. Transarterial chemoembolization for hepatocellular carcinoma: volumetric and morphologic CT criteria for assessment of prognosis and therapeutic success—results from a liver transplantation center. *Radiology* 2000;214(2):349–357.
70. Kim JH, Chung JW, Han JK, et al. Transcatheter arterial embolization of the internal mammary artery in hepatocellular carcinoma. *J Vasc Interv Radiol* 1995;6(1):71–77.
71. Hartnell GG, Gates J, Stuart K, et al. Hepatic chemoembolization: effect of intraarterial lidocaine on pain and postprocedure recovery. *Cardiovasc Intervent Radiol* 1999;22:293–297.
72. Nakao N, Uchida H, Kamino K, et al. Determination of the optimum dose level of Lipiodol in transcatheter arterial embolization of primary hepatocellular carcinoma based on retrospective multivariate analysis. *Cardiovasc Intervent Radiol* 1994;17:76–80.
73. Kan Z, Sato M, Ivancev K, Uchida B, et al. Distribution and effect of iodized poppyseed oil in the liver after hepatic artery embolization: experimental study in several animal species. *Radiology* 1993;186(3):861–866.
74. Chung JW, Park JH, Im J-G, et al. Pulmonary oil embolism after transcatheter oily chemoembolization of hepatocellular carcinoma. *Radiology* 1993;187(3):689–693.
75. Madden MV, Krige JEJ, Bailey S, et al. Randomised trial of targeted chemotherapy with Lipiodol and 5-epidoxorubicin compared with symptomatic treatment for hepatoma. *Gut* 1993;34:1598–1600.
76. Shirato K, Numata K, Mitsui K, et al. Color Doppler sonography for evaluating response to transcatheter arterial embolization and percutaneous ethanol injection therapy and for detecting recurrence of hepatocellular carcinoma. *J Ultrasound Med* 2000;19:807–814.
77. Takayasu K, Suzuki M, Uesaka K, et al. Hepatic artery embolization for inoperable hepatocellular carcinoma; prognosis and risk factors. *Cancer Chemother Pharmacol* 1989;23(suppl):23–25.
78. Cady B, Oberfield RA. Arterial infusion chemotherapy of hepatoma. *Surg Gynecol Obstet* 1974;138:381–384.
79. Kemeny N, Daly J, Reichman B, et al. Intrahepatic or systemic infusion of fluorodeoxyuridine in patients with liver metastases from colorectal carcinoma. *Ann Intern Med* 1987;107(4):459–465.
80. Rougier P, Laplanche A, Huguier M, et al. Hepatic arterial infusion of floxuridine in patients with liver metastases from colorectal carcinoma: long-term results of a prospective randomized trial. *J Clinl Oncol* 1992;10(7):1112–1118.
81. Martin JK, O'Connell MJ, Wieand HS, et al. Intra-arterial floxuridine vs systemic fluorouracil for hepatic metastases from colorectal cancer. *Arch Surg* 1990;125:1022–1027.
82. Habbe TG, McCowan TC, Goertzen TC, et al. Complications and technical limitations of hepatic arterial infusion catheter placement for chemotherapy. *J Vasc Interv Radiol* 1998;9(2):233–239.
83. Goey SH, Eggermont AMM, Oskam R, et al. Prolonged continuous hepatic artery infusion with interleukin-2 in unresectable liver metastases of colorectal cancer: a phase IA-B study. *Ann Oncol* 1996:317–319.
84. Daly J, Kemeny N, Oderman P, Botet J. Long-term hepatic arterial infusion chemotherapy. *Arch Surg* 1984;119:936–941.
85. Yoshikawa M, Ebara M, Nakano T, et al. Percutaneous transaxillary catheter insertion for hepatic artery infusion chemotherapy. *Am J Roentgenol* 1992;158:885–886.
86. Kusano S, Katayama M, Uematsu M, et al. Intraarterial infusion of dibutyryl cyclic adenosine monophosphate plus mitomycin C for unresectable hepatocellular carcinoma: long-term survival and response to tumor growth inhibition. *Acad Radiol* 1995;2(4):286–292.
87. Lau WY, Leung WT, Ho S, et al. Treatment of inoperable hepatocellular carcinoma with intrahepatic arterial yttrium-90 microspheres: a phase I and II study. *Br J Cancer* 1994;70:994–999.
88. Ho S, Lau WY, Leung TWT, Johnson PJ. Internal radiation therapy for patients with primary or metastatic hepatic cancer. *Cancer* 1998;83(9):1894–1907.
89. Conzone SD, Hafeli UO, Day DE, Ehrhardt GJ. Preparation and properties of radioactive rhenium glass microspheres intended for in vivo radioembolization therapy. *J Biomed Mater Res* 1998;42:617–625.
90. Meade VM, Burton MA, Gray BN, Self GW. Distribution of different sized microspheres in experimental hepatic tumours. *Eur J Cancer Clin Oncol* 1987;23(1):37–41.
91. Mantravadi RVP, Spigos DG, Tan WS, Felix EL. Intraarterial yttrium-90 in the treatment of hepatic malignancy. *Radiology* 1982;142(3):783–786.
92. Wang S-J, Lin W-Y, Lui W-Y, et al. Hepatic artery injection of yttrium-90-Lipiodol: biodistribution in rats with hepatoma. *J Nucl Med* 1996;37(2):332–335.
93. Lin W-Y, Tsai S-C, Hsieh J-F, Wang S-J. Effects of ^{90}Y-microspheres on liver tumors: comparison of intratumoral injection method and intra-arterial injection method. *J Nucl Med* 2000;41(11):1892–1897.
94. Cohen SE, Safadi R, Verstandig A, et al. Liver–spleen infarcts following transcatheter chemoembolization. *Dig Dis Sci* 1997;24(5):938–943.
95. Arora R, Soulen MC, Haskal ZJ. Cutaneous complications of hepatic chemoembolization via extrahepatic collaterals. *J Vasc Interv Radiol* 1999;10(10):1351–1356.
96. Balestrero LM, Beaver CR, Rigas JR. Hypertensive crisis following meperidine administration and chemoembolization of a carcinoid tumor. *Arch Intern Med* 2000;160:2394–2395.
97. Chen C, Chen P-J, Yang P-M, et al. Clinical and microbiological features of liver abscess after transarterial embolization for hepatocellular carcinoma. *Am J Gastroenterol* 1997;92(12):2257–2259.
98. Kim M-J, Lee SW, Kim GA, Song JH. Acute renal failure after transarterial chemoembolization progressing to chronic renal failure in hepatocellular carcinoma. *Nephrol Dial Transplant* 2000;15:741–742.
99. Wong E, Khardori N, Carrasco CH, et al. Infectious complications of hepatic artery catheterization procedures in patients with cancer. *Rev Infect Dis* 1991;13:583–586.
100. Yamaura K, Higashi M, Akiyoshi K, et al. Pulmonary Lipiodol embolism during transcatheter arterial chemoembolization for hepatoblastoma under general anaesthesia. *Eur J Anaesthesiol* 2000;17(11):704–708.
101. Yoon DY, Park JH, Chung JW, et al. Iatrogenic dissection of the celiac artery and its branches during transcatheter arterial embolization for hepatocellular carcinoma: outcome in 40 patients. *Cardiovasc Intervent Radiol* 1995;18:16–19.
102. Hasegawa K, Kubota K, Aoki T, et al. Ischemic cholangitis caused by transcatheter hepatic arterial chemoembolization 10 months after resection of the extrahepatic bile duct. *Cardiovasc Intervent Radiol* 2000;23(4):304–306.
103. Burney IA. Acute tumor lysis syndrome after transcatheter chemoembolization of hepatocellular carcinoma. *South Med J* 1998;91(5):467–470.
104. Brown KT, Kemeny N, Berger MF, et al. Obstructive jaundice in

patients receiving hepatic artery infusional chemotherapy: etiology, treatment implications, and complications after transhepatic biliary drainage. *J Vasc Interv Radiol* 1997;8(2):229–234.

105. Lin M. Radiation pneumonitis caused by yttrium-90 microspheres: radiologic findings. *Am J Roentgenol* 1994;162:1300–1302.
106. Andrews JC, Walker SC, Ackermann RJ, et al. Hepatic radioembolization with yttrium-90 containing glass microspheres: preliminary results and clinical follow-up. *J Nucl Med* 1994;35(10):1637–1644.
107. Goupe d'Etude et de Traitment du Carcinome Hepatocellulaire. A comparison of Lipiodol chemoembolization and conservative treatment for unresectable hepatocellular carcinoma. *N Engl J Med* 1995;332:1256–1261.
108. Arii S, Yamaoka Y, Futagawa S, et al. Results of surgical and nonsurgical treatment for small-sized hepatocellular carcinomas: a retrospective and nationwide survey in Japan. *Hepatology* 2000;32(6):1224–1229.
109. Yamamoto K, Shimizu T, Narabayashi I. Intraarterial infusion chemotherapy with Lipiodol-CDDP suspension for hepatocellular carcinoma. *Cardiovasc Intervent Radiol* 2000;23:26–39.
110. Ngan H, Lai CL, Fan ST, et al. Treatment of inoperable hepatocellular carcinoma by transcatheter arterial chemoembolization using an emulsion of cisplatinum in iodized oil and Gelfoam. *Clin Radiol* 1993;47:315–320.
111. Choi BI, Kim HC, Han JK, et al. Therapeutic effect of transcatheter oily chemoembolization therapy for encapsulated nodular hepatocellular carcinoma: CT and pathologic findings. *Radiology* 1992;182:709–713.
112. Imaeda T, Yamawaki Y, Seki M, et al. Lipiodol retention and massive necrosis after Lipiodol-chemoembolization of hepatocellular carcinoma: correlation between computed tomography and histopathology. *Cardiovasc Intervent Radiol* 1993;16:209–213.
113. Murakami T, Nakamura H, Hori S, et al. Detection of viable tumor cells in hepatocellular carcinoma following transcatheter arterial chemoembolization with iodized oil: pathologic correlation with dynamic turbo-flash MR imaging with Gd-DTPA. *Acta Radiol* 1993;34:399–403.
114. Schilling A, Gewiese B, Gerger G, et al. Liver tumors: follow-up with P-31 MR spectroscopy after local chemotherapy and chemoembolization. *Radiology* 1992;182:887–890.
115. Lorigan JG, Wallace S, et al. The prevalence and location of metastases from ocular melanoma: imaging study in 110 patients. *Am J Roentgenol* 1991;157:1279–1281.
116. Morassut S, Fiorentini G, Balestreri L, et al. Chemoembolization of liver metastases from ocular melanoma: preliminary results. *Reg Cancer Treat* 1995;8:173–176.
117. Carrasco CH, Wallace S, Sharnsangavej C, et al. Treatment of hepatic metastases in ocular melanoma. Embolization of the hepatic artery with polyvinyl sponge and cisplatin. *JAMA* 1986;255:3152–3154.
118. Feun LG, Reddy KR, Scagnelli T, et al. A phase I study of chemoembolization with cisplatin, thiotepa, and Lipiodol for primary and metastatic liver cancer. *Am J Clin Oncol* 1999;22:375–380.
119. Pettavel J, Leyvraz S, Douglas P. Arterial chemotherapy of colorectal liver metastases. An update. *Reg Cancer Treat* 1993;2:62–66.
120. Niederhuber JE, Ensminger W, Gyves J, et al. Regional chemotherapy of colorectal cancer metastatic to the liver. *Cancer* 1984;53:1336–1343.
121. Chang AE, Schneider PD, Sugarbaker PH, et al. A prospective randomized trial of regional versus systemic continuous 5-fluorodeoxyuridine chemotherapy in the treatment of colorectal liver metastases. *Ann Surg* 1897;206:685–693.
122. Lang EK, Brown CL Jr. Colorectal metastases to the liver: selective chemoembolization. *Radiology* 1993;189:417–422.
123. Civalleri D, Pector JC, Hakansson L, et al. Treatment of patients with irresectable liver metastases from colorectal cancer by chemo-occlusion with degradable starch microspheres. *Br J Surg* 1994;81:1338–1341.
124. Abramson RG, Rosen MP, Perry LJ, et al. Cost-effectiveness of hepatic arterial chemoembolization for colorectal liver metastases refractory to systemic chemotherapy. *Radiology* 2000;216:485–491.

CHAPTER 12

PREOPERATIVE PORTAL VEIN EMBOLIZATION TO INCREASE SAFETY OF MAJOR HEPATECTOMIES FOR HEPATOBILIARY MALIGNANCIES

DAVID C. MADOFF, M.D.
JEAN-NICOLAS VAUTHEY, M.D.
MARSHALL E. HICKS, M.D.

INTRODUCTION

At present, major advances in hepatobiliary surgical techniques have led to improved perioperative outcomes in patients selected for hepatic resection. Although fatal liver failure after resection is now exceedingly rare, complications associated with cholestasis, fluid retention, and impaired synthetic function still contribute to prolonged recovery time and extended hospital stay.[1] Because patients in whom more than 70% of the functional liver mass is resected are generally considered at higher risk for these complications, portal vein embolization (PVE) has been advocated in an attempt to reduce these complications by increasing the functional liver mass after resection. PVE induces selective hypertrophy of the non-diseased portion of the liver so that patients with primary or secondary hepatobiliary malignancies with small estimated future liver remnants (FLRs) may have fewer complications and shorter hospital stays after resection.[2,3] In addition, PVE performed in patients in whom hepatobiliary tumors were initially considered unresectable for lack of sufficient remaining normal parenchyma may add to the pool of candidates for surgical treatment.

Before performing PVE, interventional radiologists should be able to recognize both normal and variant portal venous anatomy, should understand the mechanisms and pathophysiology of liver regeneration, and should be aware of the different approaches and embolic agents that can be used. This chapter discusses those issues, deals with the indications for and limitations of

PVE, and provides an up-to-date review of the results (for PVE and hepatic resection).

ANATOMIC CONSIDERATIONS

Couinaud and Anglo-Saxon Classification Systems of Liver Segments

A comprehensive knowledge of functional liver anatomy is imperative for anyone performing PVE. The most widely used classification system was described by Couinaud[4] and is shown in **Figure 12-1**. The liver is divided into two hemilivers (left and right, separated by the main portal fissure) and eight segments. Hepatic segmentation is based on the distribution of the portal pedicles and the location of the hepatic veins. The Couinaud classification with the corresponding Anglo-Saxon classification is shown in **Table 12-1** and Figure 12-1.

Portal Venous Anatomy

The portal vein (PV) is formed in the retroperitoneum by the confluence of the superior mesenteric vein (SMV) and the splenic vein (SV) behind the neck of the pancreas, and it courses behind the duodenal bulb. The portal bifurcation may be extrahepatic (48%), intrahepatic (26%), or located right at the liver entrance (26%).[5,6] Figure 12-1 illustrates the most commonly observed portal venous anatomy. On the right, there are usually two sectoral branches (the anterior and posterior); on the left, there are two parts of the left PV (the main left PV)—the extrahepatic portion (pars horizontalis, i.e., the horizontal part) and the intrahepatic portion (pars umbilicalis, i.e., the umbilical [vertical] part).

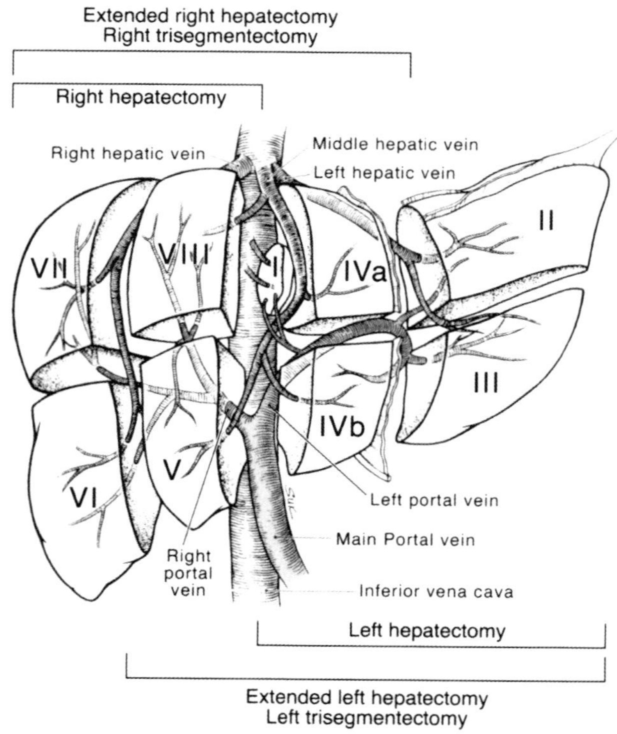

Figure 12-1. Schematic of segmental liver anatomy shows normal portal venous structures. The possible hepatic resection procedures are also shown.

In general, the sectoral branches divide into a number of segmental portal branches, which in turn supply segments. One segmental branch is typically found for segments II, VI, and VII, and more rarely for segment III.

TABLE 12-1
Classifications of Hepatic Lobar and Segmental Anatomy

Couinaud classification	Anglo-Saxon classification
Dorsal Sector (segment 1)	Caudate lobe
Left liver	Left lobe
Left paramedian sector	Anterior medial segment (quadrate lobe)
Segment 4	Anterior inferior subsegment (lateral segment)
Segment 3	Posterior superior subsegment (lateral segment)
Left lateral sector	Right lobe
Segment 2	Anterior segment
Right liver	Anterior inferior subsegment
Right paramedian sector	Anterior superior subsegment
Segment 5	Posterior segment
Segment 8	Posterior inferior subsegment
Right lateral sector	Posterior superior subsegment
Segment 6	
Segment 7	

Frequently, segments IV, V, and VIII are supplied by more than one segmental branch. Segmental veins are then divided into subsegmental branches and further into small veins leading to the portal venule of the liver acinus.

Portal Vein Variants

Anatomic variations of the PV are uncommon, occurring in 10%–15% of patients (**Fig. 12-2**).[7] However, when present, they are important to recognize because they may have profound implications on whether or not PVE and/or subsequent resection can be performed successfully. In a small proportion of the population (11%), the PV divides into one left and two right portal branches. This variant, known as portal trifurcation, is present if three branches stem from the main portal trunk—posterior branch, anterior branch, and the left main branch. In addition, the right anterior segment PV may branch from the left main PV (4%), or the left main PV may branch from the right anterior PV. In another variant, the right posterior branch stems from the main portal trunk, and the anterior branch forms a bifurcation with the left PV (5%). Quadrifurcation of the PV can also occur: there would be a branch for segment VII, a branch for segment VI, an anterior branch, and a left main portal branch (left PV). In extraordinary cases, a branch for subsegment IVb or an additional branch for segment VI, VII, or even VIII may stem from the portal bifurcation. Rarely (1%), the bifurcation of the PV is completely absent (i.e., no right PV)[8, 9]; the solitary portal vein in the hilum passes through the entire liver either from left to right or from right to left. Failure to identify this variation in the setting of hilar portal ligation leads to hepatic failure and/or death. Resection or liver transplantation may require PV resection and reconstruction, significantly increasing the complexity of the procedure.[8, 9]

Further variations can occur in both the right and left portal systems. Maintaining an awareness of portal anomalies is exceedingly important, as failure to do so can lead to non-target embolization with possible risk to the FLR.

PHYSIOLOGY OF PORTAL VEIN EMBOLIZATION

Mechanism of Liver Regeneration

PVE has been developed because the liver has the ability to regenerate and hypertrophy. Rous and Larimore[10] first reported this phenomenon in 1920, when they ligated portal vein branches in rabbits and noticed that the ligated (ipsilateral) lobe atrophied and the non-ligated (contralateral) lobe hypertrophied. Later, other researchers reported that PV occlusion secondary to tumor invasion or ligation leads to atrophy of the ipsilateral lobe and hypertrophy of the contralateral lobe for patients.[11–13] To this end, major hepatic resections (that constitute up to 75% of the liver) can be performed, provided that the future liver remnant is not functionally compromised (e.g., by cirrhosis).[14–16]

The liver regenerates after extended right or left hepatectomies or other major atypical resections provided that two or three contiguous segments remain.[17, 18] Liver regeneration is a crucial parameter of the liver's response to injury. There are two underlying mechanisms for liver regeneration. First, the hepatocytes' ability to dedifferentiate and clonally expand leads to increases in hepatocyte cell mass and number.[3] Second, intrahepatic factors (e.g., hepatocyte growth factor [HGF]) and extrahepatic factors contribute to induction and control of hepatocyte growth and are released in response to hepatocellular injury. Mitogenic factors (e.g., epidermal growth factor [EGF], transforming growth factor-α) and cytokines (e.g., tumor necrosis factor-α, interleukin-6) also lead to prompt gene induction and regeneration. Notably, insulin is co-mitogenic with HGF, contributing to the slower hypertrophy rates seen for patients with diabetes.[19, 20] Extrahepatic factors are transported primarily by the portal vein and not by the hepatic artery.[3, 21–23]

Rate of Liver Regeneration

Hepatocyte regeneration occurs early after PVE or resection. Regeneration is determined by the DNA index, which may rise 14 hours after resection and, in some studies, may climax by 24 hours.[24] Important to the discussion of liver regeneration is the observation that cirrhotic (i.e., injured) liver has less capacity to regenerate than normal (i.e., non-injured) liver.[25] This difference may be the result of the diminished capacity of hepatocytes to respond to hepatotrophic factors and/or because parenchymal damage (fibrosis) leads to slower portal flow rates. Regeneration rates are directly related to portal venous flow.[26]

In swine, Duncan et al.[27] found that hepatocyte changes mirrored PVE clinically. Replication peaked at 7 days, occurring in approximately 14% of hepatocytes. Replication decreased to baseline levels by day 12. The peak replication after PVE, compared with that after resection, is delayed approximately 3 to 4 days, suggesting that the stimulus of hepatocyte removal is superior to apoptosis seen with PVE.[25]

Regeneration rates are greater in normal liver than in cirrhotic liver. Lee et al.,[25] evaluating rats with normal and chemically-induced cirrhosis, found that the weight of the liver increased after 24 hours, tripled after

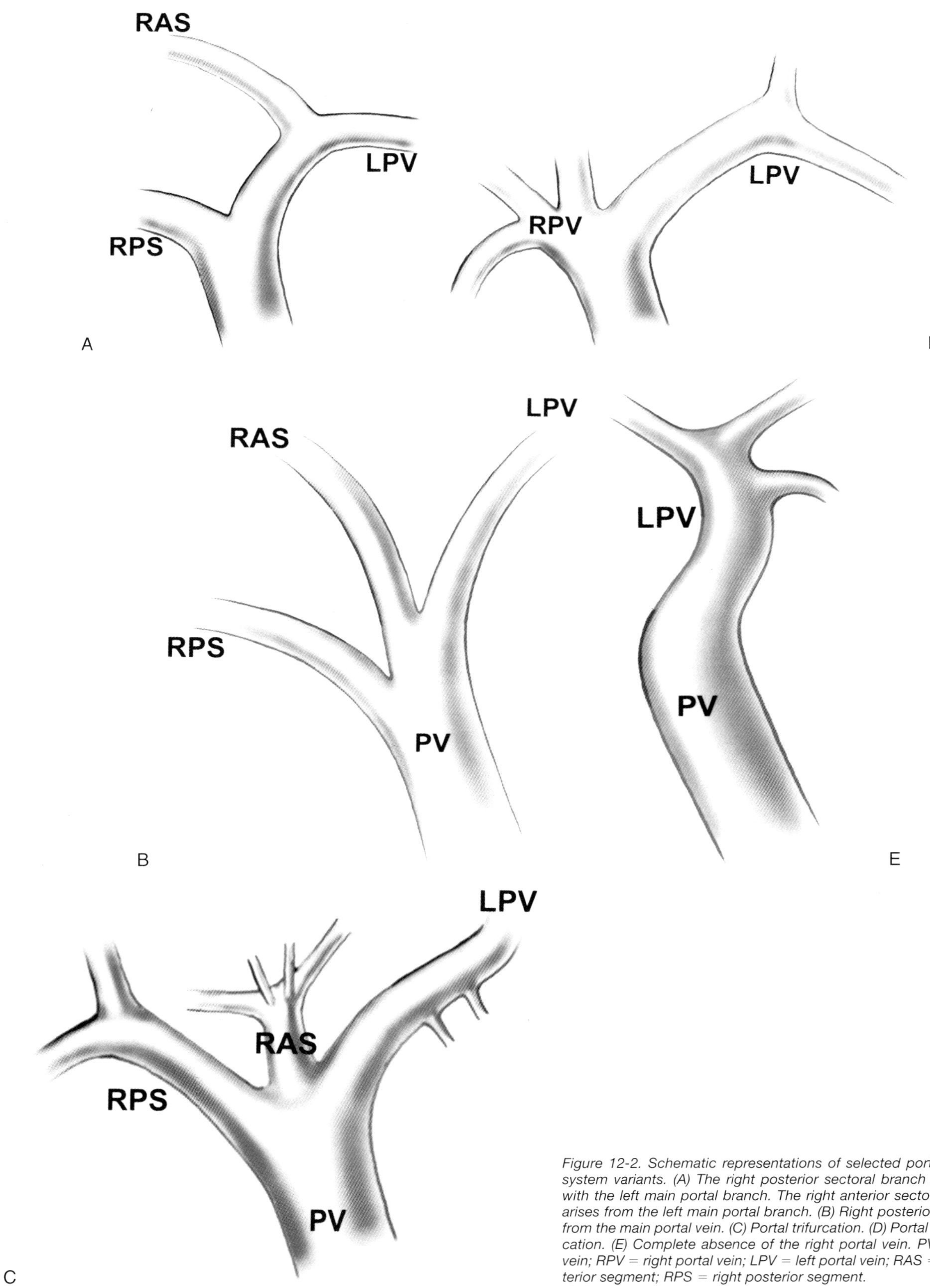

Figure 12-2. Schematic representations of selected portal venous system variants. (A) The right posterior sectoral branch bifurcates with the left main portal branch. The right anterior sectoral branch arises from the left main portal branch. (B) Right posterior segment from the main portal vein. (C) Portal trifurcation. (D) Portal quadrifurcation. (E) Complete absence of the right portal vein. PV = portal vein; RPV = right portal vein; LPV = left portal vein; RAS = right anterior segment; RPS = right posterior segment.

7 days, and reached a plateau between 7 and 14 days. The rate of regeneration in the cirrhotic animals was delayed and of a lesser magnitude.[25] In patient studies the findings are similar. Non-cirrhotic livers regenerate fastest (12 to 21 cm^3, 11 cm^3, and 6 cm^3 at 2 weeks, 4 weeks, and 32 days post-PVE, respectively).[20, 28] The rates of hypertrophy are slower (9 cm^3 at 2 weeks) in cirrhotic livers. Nagino et al.[20] found comparable rates in diabetic patients.

Pathophysiology of Portal Vein Embolization Prior to Major Liver Resection

Transcatheter PVE was first reported in 1986 by Kinoshita et al.,[29] who combined intra-arterial chemoembolization with PVE in an attempt to decrease portal tumor thrombi from hepatocellular carcinoma before hepatic resection. Makuuchi et al.[14] later reported the initial use of preoperative PVE performed solely for inducing left lobe hypertrophy before major hepatic resection. The rationale for using PVE in this setting is that PVE minimizes the abrupt rise in portal pressure at resection that can lead to hepatocellular damage in the liver remnant. The effect of operative manipulation may combine with the alteration in portal pressure to cause hepatic congestion and post-resection dysfunction.[30–32] Metabolic changes are also diminished after resection performed following PVE; a lesser relative decrease in hepatocyte cell mass may improve overall tolerance to major resection. Finally, portal blood flow to the non-embolized hepatic segments measured by Doppler ultrasound increased significantly, then decreased towards (without reaching) the baseline value after 11 days. The resultant hypertrophy rate correlated with the flow rate measurements.[3, 26]

After PVE, changes in liver function test values are usually minor and transient; 50% of patients have no appreciable change. When transaminase levels increase, they usually peak at less than three times baseline 1–3 days after embolization and return to baseline within 7–10 days, regardless of the embolic agent used. A slight change in total bilirubin value and white blood cell count may be seen. Synthetic functions (e.g., prothrombin time) are almost never affected.

PVE is much less toxic than arterial embolization, and side effects are typically minimal.[3] Symptoms of post-embolization syndrome, such as nausea and vomiting, are unusual, and pain and fever are infrequent. This is because PVE produces no distortion of anatomy, only nominal inflammation except immediately around the embolized vein, and not much, if any, parenchymal or tumor necrosis.[14, 33] Research performed on animals has shown that hepatocytes undergo apoptosis but not necrosis after portal venous occlusion.[27, 34]

TECHNIQUES OF PORTAL VEIN EMBOLIZATION

Approaches

PVE is performed to redirect portal flow to the hepatic segments that will remain after surgery (i.e., the FLR). To ensure adequate hypertrophy, embolization of portal branches must be as complete as possible so that the occluded portal system does not recanalize. Occlusion of the entire portal tree to be resected is necessary to avoid development of intrahepatic porto-portal collaterals that may limit regeneration.[35]

PVE can be performed by three approaches: contralateral approach, ipsilateral approach, and transileocolic vein approach. The contralateral approach, developed by Kinoshita et al.,[29] is most often used in Japan and Europe (**Fig. 12-3**). Using this approach, Kinoshita et al.[29] accessed a branch of the left portal system and advanced a 6-F double-lumen catheter through an introducer into branches of the right portal tree for embolization. Modifications of this technique have been made since their initial report.[36] The major advantage of the contralateral approach is that catheterization of the desired right portal branches is more direct via the left system than a puncture from the right system, making the former procedure technically easier. However, the disadvantage of the contralateral approach is the potential injury to the FLR. A large multi-center European study reported on procedure-related FLR injuries, including hematoma, portal vein wall dissection, and portal vein thrombosis.[37] These injuries may compromise the integrity of the future liver remnant and may make the planned resection more difficult.

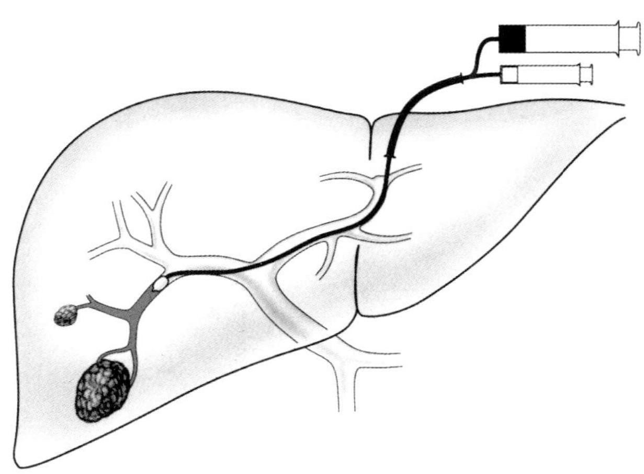

Figure 12-3. Schematic representation of the contralateral approach for PVE as described by Kinoshita et al.[29] An occlusion balloon catheter is placed into the right portal branch with delivery of embolic agent in antegrade direction.

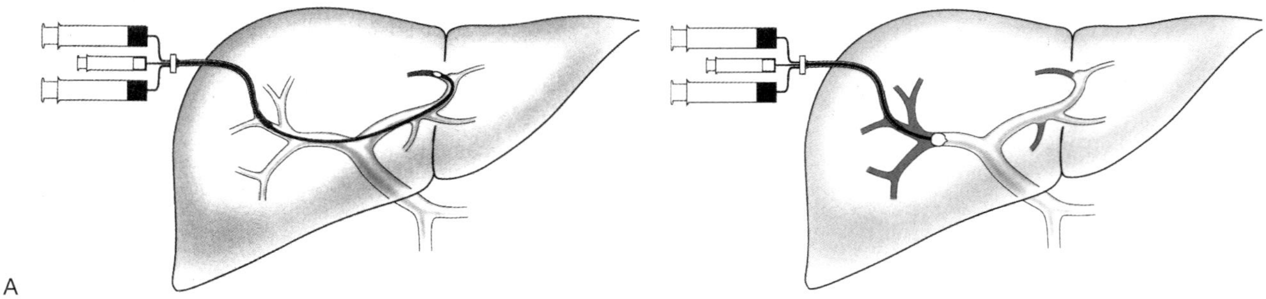

Figure 12-4. Schematic representation of the ipsilateral approach for right PVE as described by Nagino et al.[38] (A) Type 1 catheter used for antegrade embolization of segment 4 veins. (B) Type 2 catheter used for retrograde delivery of embolic agent into right portal system.

The ipsilateral approach has been advocated by Nagino et al.[38] (**Fig. 12-4**). For this approach, a peripheral right portal branch is accessed, through which a 6-F sheath is advanced. An occlusion balloon is then advanced over a guidewire into the right portal branches. Nagino et al.[38] designed two types of balloon catheters, type 1 and type 2. Both catheters are 5.5-F and have three lumens; one is a lumen to the balloon, the other two have holes that are either at the catheter tip (type 1) or with holes just proximal to the balloon (type 2). These catheters serve distinct functions of targeting embolization with adhesive agents proximal or distal to balloon placement. Once in the right portal system, embolization can be done in the right and left (segment 4 if trisectoral embolization) portal branches. Left-sided PVE can also be performed through this ipsilateral approach (**Fig. 12-5**). Nagino et al.[38] strongly recommend leaving a "proximal" segment of approximately 1 cm long unembolized within the right portal trunk. They believe this segment is important because it facilitates the division and closure of the right portal vein during surgery and prevents post-resection stenoses of the portal bifurcation.

A modification of the ipsilateral technique has been advocated at M. D. Anderson Cancer Center for particulate embolization (**Fig. 12-6**).[39] PVE is performed after a 6-F sheath is placed into the right portal venous system. If trisectoral PVE is necessary, embolization of segments IVa and IVb is performed first. A microcatheter is advanced coaxially into segment IVa and IVb branches. Once segment IV embolization is completed, a 5-F reverse-curved catheter is used for right PVE. Embolization of the access tract is performed with coils to promote hemostasis.

One benefit of the ipsilateral approach is that the anticipated liver remnant is not injured. However, catheterization of the right portal branches may be more difficult because of severe angulations between right portal branches. A disadvantage of this approach is that some embolic material could be displaced upon removal of the catheter, leading to non-target embolization.

The last technique, the transileocolic vein approach, is performed by direct cannulation of the ileocolic vein at laparotomy, followed by advancement of a balloon catheter into the portal vein for subsequent embolization.[40] Although preferred by many surgeons in Asia, this approach is often performed when interventional radiology suites are not available, if the percutaneous approach is not feasible, or if additional treatment is needed during the same surgical exploration.[41] A disadvantage of the transileocolic vein approach is the need for general anesthesia with its inherent risks.

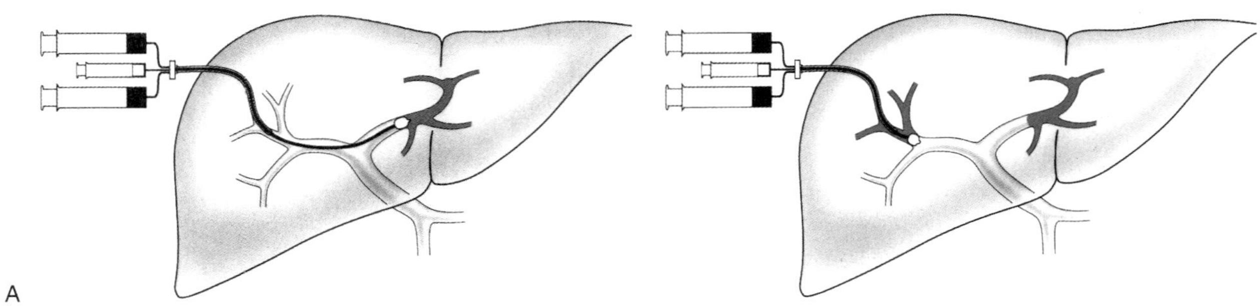

Figure 12-5. (A) Schematic representation of the ipsilateral approach for left trisectoral PVE as described by Nagino et al.[38] (B) Type 2 catheter used for retrograde delivery of embolic agent into the right anterior portal system.

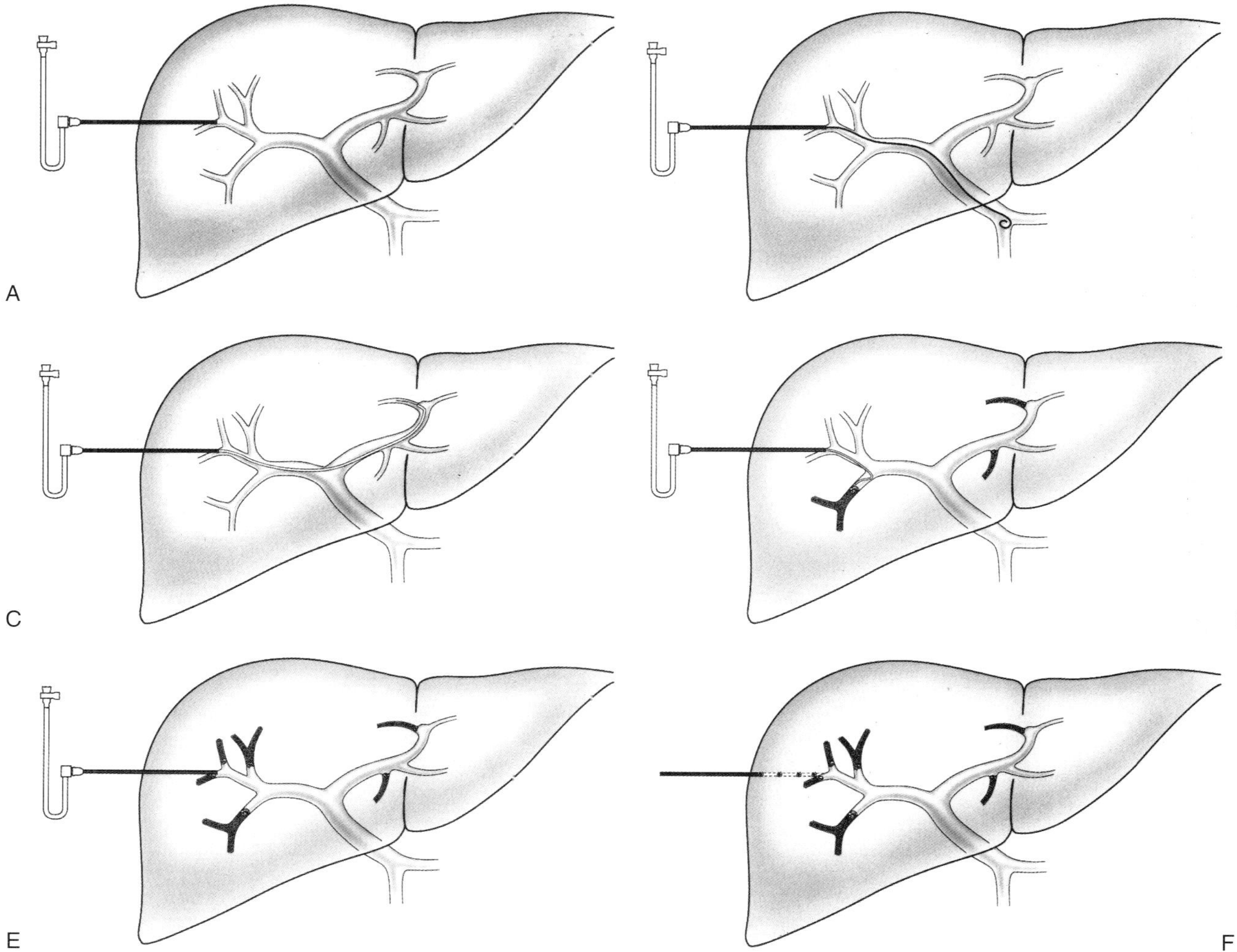

Figure 12-6. Schematic diagrams showing modification of the ipsilateral technique for right trisectoral PVE performed at M. D. Anderson Cancer Center. (A) Placement of a 6-F vascular sheath into the right portal branch. (B) Flush catheter is then placed into the main portal vein for planning portography. (C) An angled guide catheter is placed into the left portal system with subsequent placement of microcatheter into the segment 4 branch. Particulate embolization is performed, followed by placement of coils. (D) After complete PVE of segment 4, the angled guide catheter and microcatheter are exchanged for a 5-F reverse-curve catheter for right PVE. Particulate embolization is performed, followed by coil placement. (E) Complete right trisectoral PVE. (F, Coil embolization of access tract with placement of coils via vascular sheath.

Embolic Materials for Portal Vein Embolization

Many embolic materials have been used for PVE without significant differences in degrees or rates of hypertrophy.[3] These agents include, but are not limited to, fibrin glue, cyanoacrylate-ethiodized oil, absorbable gelatin sponge (Gelfoam) and thrombin, coils, microparticles (i.e., polyvinyl alcohol particles, *tris*-acryl microspheres), and absolute alcohol. Newer agents are currently being developed to provide more complete and more nearly permanent occlusions, so as to reduce recanalization and ultimately provide better and faster hypertrophy.

Gelfoam (mixed with diatrizoate sodium meglumine and gentamicin) was used in the initial procedures reported by Makuuchi et al.[14, 42] However, frequent portal recanalization was observed within 2 weeks after PVE.[14, 16] In comparison with other embolic agents, Gelfoam seems less efficient at 4 weeks in term of hypertrophy. Kaneko et al.[43] have proposed a combination of gelatin sponge with a sclerosing agent (polidocanol). This emulsion, used in a canine model, allowed prolonged embolization of the desired portal branches for up to 8 weeks after PVE.

Some investigators prefer cyanoacrylate mixed with ethoidized oil, as its use leads to fast, reliable hypertrophy and minimizes the delay to definitive resection.[16] This material ensures portal vein occlusion, which persists after 4 weeks, whereas the combination of absorbable gelatin sponge and thrombin tends to permit recanalization.[44] de Baere et al.[15] reported that cyanoacrylate embolization led to a 90% increase in liver volume after 30 days, and that the gelatin sponge–thrombin combination resulted in only a 53% volume increase after 43 days. Two potential drawbacks of cyanoacrylate embolization have been noted. First, there is induction of an inflammatory process (peribiliary fibrosis, casting of the portal vein), which may increase the difficulty of the subsequent surgical procedure.[16, 45] Second, the agent is difficult to use in clinical practice, especially in patients with reduced portal flow (e.g., from chronic liver disease), possibly leading to non-target embolization in other segments.[16]

PVE using absolute alcohol has been found to be particularly useful in the treatment of hepatocellular carcinoma because of the agent's strong coagulation effect. Shimamura et al.[46] reported that volumes of 20mL injected via the contralateral approach are adequate to produce complete portal occlusion; this group reported a 27% increase (n = 7) in FLR size (pre-PVE 32%; post-PVE 59%).[46] Ogasawara et al.[47] demonstrated near doubling of the left lobe volume within 4 weeks in patients with chronic liver disease and hepatocellular carcinoma. Unfortunately, the greatest changes in liver function test values, leading to poor patient tolerance, are also found with absolute alcohol.[48] Although this agent causes considerable periportal fibrosis, endothelial destruction, and necrosis, recanalization is rare. Clinical reports show higher rates of hypertrophy, but the numbers of patients in these reports is too small for the result to be conclusive.[46, 47]

Another commonly used agent is a combination of fibrin glue mixed with ethiodized oil. PVE with this material usually induces less than 75% portal obstruction at 2 weeks and less than 25% portal obstruction at 4 weeks.[44] Preferred by Nagino et al.,[18, 20, 49] PVE with this agent has led to FLR volume increases ranging from 10% to 20% after a mean of 18 days.

Recently, microparticles such as polyvinyl alcohol (PVA) particles have been proposed.[27, 39, 50] They are relatively inexpensive and are easy to administer.[3] PVA is safe, causes little periportal reaction, and generates durable portal vein occlusion when used in combination with coils.[27] Theoretically, PVA achieves occlusion to small "outflow" vessels (third-order branches and smaller), and the coils provide "inflow" occlusion of large vessels (second-order branches). In a single patient described in one report, no recanalization of the right portal vein was observed 5 weeks after embolization with PVA alone.[50] Results from use of PVA and coils at the M. D. Anderson Cancer Center (n = 26) revealed an increase in the ratio of FLR to total estimated liver volume (FLR/TELV ratio) of 7.8% (pre-PVE FLR/TELV, 17.6%; post-PVE FLR/ TELV, 25.4%) and a mean absolute increase in FLR of 47% after PVE.[39] Examples of right PVE and right trisectoral PVE using this technique are shown in **Figures 12-7** and **12-8**.

Methods of Follow-up

Computed tomography (CT) with volumetric assessment is fundamental for planning surgical resection of the liver.[3] Because there are different methods of calculating liver volumes, comparison between results achieved at various institutions is difficult. Two methods are described here. With either technique, measurements are obtained by outlining the contours of the hepatic segments and calculating the liver volume from these surface measurements on each slice. CT must be performed after intravenous administration of a contrast agent to demarcate the vascular landmarks of the hepatic segments. With this technique, the total liver volume and the future remnant liver can be calculated within 15 minutes of scanning.[14, 51]

The first method measures the resected and total liver volumes and estimates the "normal liver" by sub-

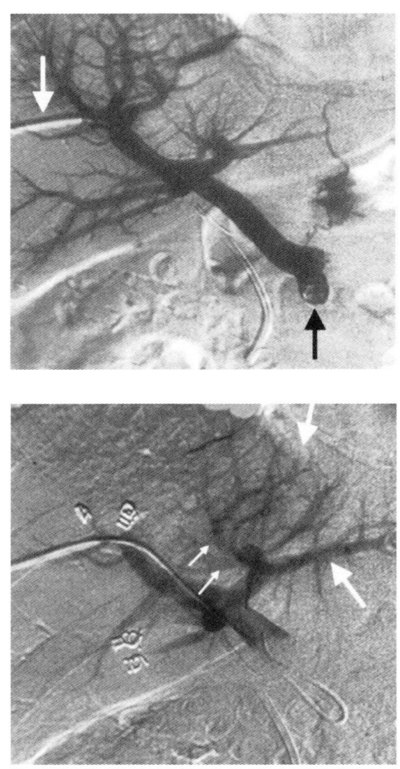

A

B

Figure 12-7. Right portal vein embolization procedure. (A) Anterior-posterior portal venography performed using a 5-F pigtail flush catheter (black arrow) placed through a 6-F vascular sheath (white arrows). (B) Post-PVE portogram demonstrates complete occlusion of right portal system. The left lateral segment (FLR) portal branches continue to have blood flow (arrows). The portal veins supplying segment 4 are shown by the small white arrows. Courtesy of D.C. Madoff, M.D., adapted from reference 39)

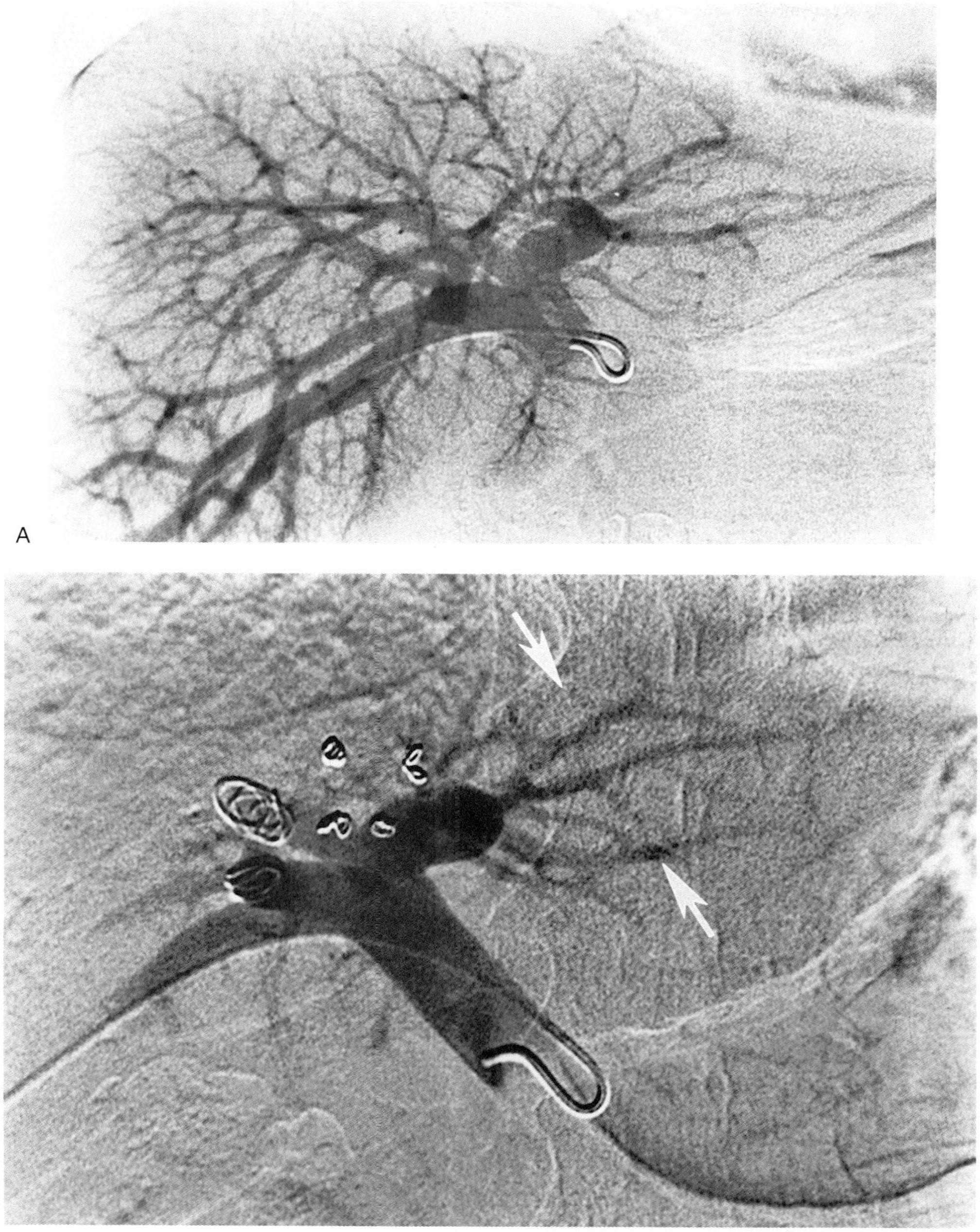

A

B

Figure 12-8. (A) Pre-PVE portogram demonstrating normal portal anatomy. (B) Post-PVE portogram demonstrating successful trisectoral embolization. Portal flow to the left lateral segment is maintained (arrows).

tracting tumor volume: (resected volume − tumor volume)/(total liver volume − tumor volume).[51, 52] This method can be very challenging with multiple tumors and does not account for the actual functional liver volume when there is vascular obstruction, chronic liver disease, or biliary dilatation.[2, 52, 53]

At our institution, we measure directly the FLR and estimate the TELV with a formula (based on the patient's body weight and body surface area) previously described so that the FLR/TELV ratio can be calculated. This method allows for uniform comparison of FLR volume before extended resection with or without preoperative PVE.[2, 3, 54] From this method of calculation, a correlation between FLR and operative outcome was established.[2] CT scans are performed immediately before PVE and approximately 2–4 weeks after PVE to assess the degree of FLR hypertrophy. Two examples of significant FLR hypertrophy after PVE are shown in **Figures 12-9** and **12-10**.

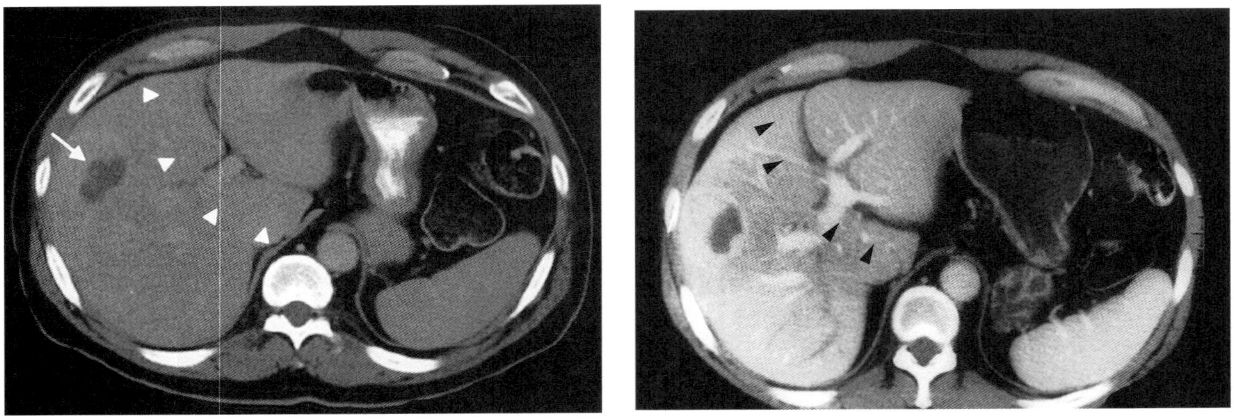

A B

Figure 12-9. A 63-year-old man with hepatocellular carcinoma and a pancreatic mass. (A) Non-contrast axial CT scan shows a 5-cm necrotic mass (arrow) in segments VI and VII. The future liver remnant (FLR) (segments I–IV) is shown by arrowheads. The FLR/TELV ratio was 22.3%. (B) After PVE, the FLR (arrowheads) changed, and the ratio of FLR to total estimated liver volume (TELV) (FLR/TELV ratio) was 37.9%, an increase of 15.6%. The patient subsequently underwent successful right hepatic hepatectomy and pancreaticoduodenectomy. (Courtesy of D.C. Madoff, M.D., adapted from reference 39)

Developments in nuclear imaging technology are currently being evaluated. In an attempt to measure differences in liver volume, both anatomically and functionally, a new radiolabeled compound, technetium-99m diethylenetriamine-penta-acetic acid galactosamyl human serum albumin, has been advocated. This agent binds specifically to asialoglycoprotein receptors (ASGP-Rs) on hepatocyte cell membranes. Distribution of this agent can be closely monitored using single photon emission computed tomography (SPECT) for the evaluation of functional hepatic reserve. This method has been shown to correlate precisely with indocyanine

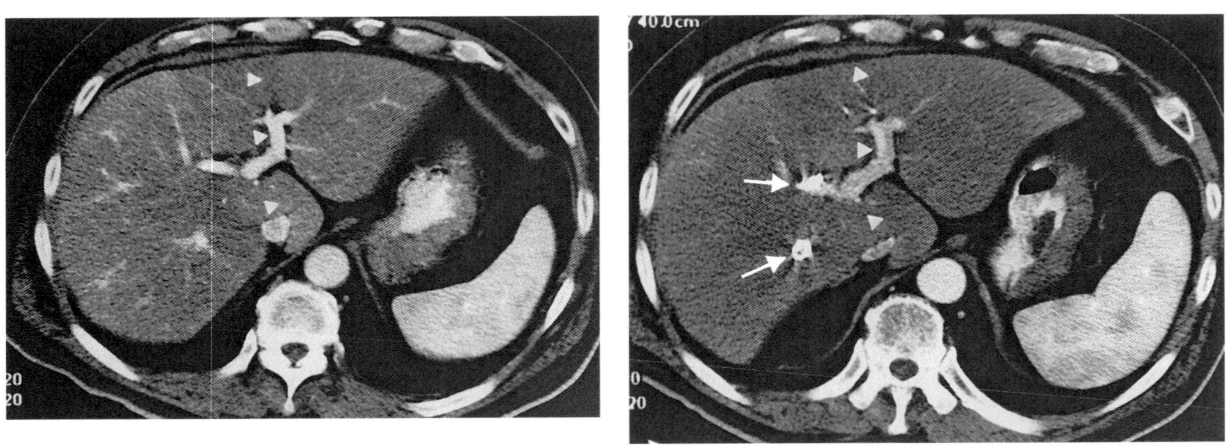

A B

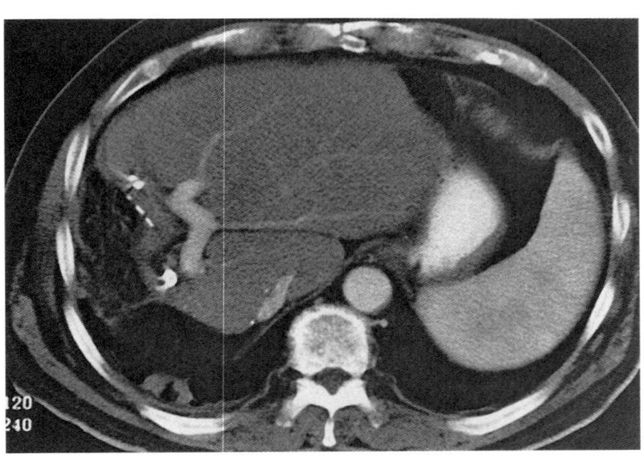

C

Figure 12-10. (A) A 63-year-old man with hepatocellular carcinoma and a small future liver segment FLR (segments I–III) is shown (arrowheads). Axial CT scan demonstrates a small left lateral lobe with a FLR/TELV ratio of 17.0%. (B) After PVE, the ratio of FLR to total estimated liver volume (TELV) (FLR/TELV ratio) was 25.2%, an increase of 8.2%. Coils are seen in the right hepatic lobe portal veins (arrows). (C) After resection, a massive liver remnant is seen.

green (ICG) clearance measurements.[55] With axial image reconstruction, the differential functions of right and left lobes can be determined. This technique shows potential, because close correlation with CT could accurately predict changes in liver volume and function between the right and left lobes after PVE.

INDICATIONS FOR PORTAL VEIN EMBOLIZATION

General Indications

Five factors must be considered in the decision whether to perform PVE. First, the future liver remnant FLR/TELV ratio should be calculated. Second, whether or not the patient has underlying liver disease determines how much FLR is needed, so as to reduce postoperative morbidity and mortality. A FLR/TELV ratio of less than 25% is recommended in patients with otherwise normal livers and a ratio of less than 40% in patients in whom the liver is considered compromised (i.e., chronic liver disease, high-dose chemotherapy).[2, 3, 25, 46] Third, overall liver function may be evaluated. This is especially important for patients with chronic liver disease. In some later series, patients underwent PVE only if surgery was considered to pose a high risk and they were expected to have an FLR/TELV of less than 40% and/or they had a IGC retention rate greater than 10% at 15 minutes.[51, 52] Fourth, the presence or absence of systemic disease such as diabetes mellitus may limit hypertrophy. As mentioned previously, insulin is co-mitogenic with HGF, leading to lower rates of regeneration.[19, 20] Fifth, planning for the type and extent of the anticipated surgical procedure (i.e., hepatectomy and pancreaticoduodenectomy) is crucial, because more functional hepatic reserve may be required to reduce post-operative morbidity.

General Contraindications

Currently, we have found no absolute contraindications for PVE. Relative contraindications are (1) tumor extension to the FLR or extrahepatic metastatic disease (including periportal lymphadenopathy), (2) uncorrectable coagulopathy, (3) tumor invasion of the portal vein, (4) tumor precluding safe transhepatic access, (5) biliary dilation (if biliary tree is obstructed, drainage is recommended), (6) portal hypertension, and (7) renal failure. PVE in cases of tumor invasion of the portal vein may not be justified because the procedure may be of no significant benefit. Tumor precluding safe transhepatic access can occur if the tumor burden is great but is also unlikely, as there is no realistic concern for aiding tumor spread or injuring the diseased segments. If concern does exist, the contralateral approach (access through the FLR) can be chosen.

SPECIFIC INDICATIONS AND RESULTS

Hepatocellular Carcinoma

Hepatocellular carcinoma (HCC) is the one of the most common neoplasms worldwide, with an estimated incidence of 1 million new cases each year.[56] Although advances have been made in percutaneous therapies, curative resection and liver transplantation remain the only chances for long-term disease-free survival.[51, 57, 58] Because of the high incidence of cirrhosis or fibrosis and the nature of the tumor, as characterized by intrahepatic spread and/or vascular invasion, resectability rates have remained low (approximately 10% in Western countries).[59] Although postoperative mortality from liver failure has decreased with surgical experience, death rates after major hepatic resection for HCC remain high (up to 32%), being directly attributed to the remaining functional liver mass.[59–63] For patients in whom resection of HCC may be technically feasible, resection may be contraindicated by the lack of adequate FLR volume and function with the attendant higher risks of lethal liver failure. For this group, PVE has been advocated in an attempt to increase HCC resectability and survival.

PVE prior to hepatic resection for HCC was first described by Kinoshita et al.[29] in 1986. At that time, they had performed only transarterial embolization (TAE), which was effective against liver cancer. Unfortunately, TAE had almost no effect on portal tumor thrombi, which continued to contribute to overall poor prognoses. In an effort to reduce the risk of portal tumor thrombi, these investigators performed a combination PVE and TAE prior to hepatic resection. They observed hypertrophy of the unembolized liver in 21 patients with HCC. No major PVE complications were reported, and 100% of the patients had successful resection.[29]

The indications for utilizing PVE for HCC are highly variable because the selection criteria for resection differ considerably among institutions. Some investigators support the use of PVE in every patient considered a candidate for right hepatectomy[25, 64] or only in patients with poor surgical prognoses.[46, 51, 65, 66] In other series, the only patients who underwent PVE were those for whom surgery was considered to pose a high risk for and for whom estimated FLR volume was less than 40% and/or a ICG retention rate greater than 10% at 15 minutes.[52]

Later studies have demonstrated the clinical efficacy of preoperative PVE performed for patients with HCC (injured liver) in whom surgery was considered untenable for lack of sufficient future liver volume. Azoulay et al.[51] reported on the long-term outcome of liver resection for HCC with and without PVE. They performed preoperative PVE in 10 of 19 patients before resection of three or more liver segments in whom the estimated FLR volume was less than 40%. After PVE, there were significant increases in the FLR volume compared with the pre-PVE value. Liver resection was performed after PVE in 9 of 10 patients without any postoperative liver failure or death within 60 days. The overall actuarial survival rates in patients undergoing hepatectomy with PVE were 89% at 1 year, 67% at 3 years, and 44% at 5 years, compared with 80%, 53%, and 53%, respectively, in patients undergoing hepatectomy without PVE. The disease-free actuarial survival rates were 86%, 64%, and 21% with PVE and 55%, 17%, and 17% without PVE, at 1, 3, and 5 years, respectively. Because the results were comparable for the PVE and non-PVE groups, Azoulay et al.[51] concluded that PVE enabled more patients with previously unresectable HCC in injured liver to benefit from resection.

Tanaka et al.[67] also reported the effect of PVE on long-term outcomes in a large series of patients (n = 71) with impaired hepatic function undergoing right hepatectomy for HCC. Preoperative PVE was used for group 1 (n = 33) but not for group 2 (n = 38), and outcomes after resection were compared. The patients were further divided according to the median tumor diameter (cut-off 6 cm) and ICG retention rate at 15 minutes ($ICGR_{15}$) (cut-off 13%). Although tumor-free survival rates were similar, cumulative survival rates were significantly higher for group 1 than for patients in group 2 with an $ICGR_{15}$ of 13% or higher. The survival rate after tumor recurrence was better for patients with sufficient residual hepatic function to tolerate further treatment (i.e., second hepatic resection). More patients who underwent PVE were able to tolerate treatment for recurrent tumor, despite worse hepatic function before the original operation. To this end, preoperative PVE may preserve hepatic function and allow for further treatment after tumor recurrence.[67]

Although PVE before major hepatic resection for HCC has been shown to reduce rates of postoperative liver failure and death after extended resection, some researchers suggest that overall survival rate is not affected by PVE. Wakabayashi et al.[65] reported on a retrospective analysis of patients with advanced HCC (stages 3 and 4) who underwent resection with or without preoperative PVE. They noted a higher incidence of distant metastases in the PVE group, but the overall survivals were similar for two groups. The belief that distant metastases are more common after PVE may reflect the more advanced stage of disease of the patients undergoing preoperative PVE who would not have been candidates for resection without preoperative PVE.

Embolization techniques are variable for HCC. The increases in non-embolized liver volumes are variable (range: 28% to 46%) 4 weeks after PVE. These rates of hypertrophy are less than those observed for patients with non-injured liver bearing liver metastases. The two key factors affecting hypertrophy rates are the pre-PVE volumes of non-embolized liver and the prior use of transarterial chemoembolization (TACE).[64] The degree of parenchymal fibrosis is also alleged to participate in limiting regeneration, but this theory has never been statistically proven.[51] The complication rates appear higher in these patients than in those with normal liver, because there is the possibility of secondary portal vein thrombosis after PVE, presumably from slow flow in the portal vein trunk after PVE.[37]

Liver Metastases

Hepatic resection is the only chance for long-term survival for patients with colorectal liver metastases, in whom 5-year survival rates are 25% to 40%.[68, 69] Unfortunately, only a small number of patients (5% to 10%) are considered surgical candidates because most have bilobar involvement.[69] As the overall survival of patients with inoperable liver metastases is dismal, various techniques have been utilized to increase the number of surgical candidates.[70] Intravenous chemotherapy and/or TACE may be beneficial in those patients whose tumor characteristics (e.g., location, multifocality, volume) are the reason for unresectability.[71] However, if patients are not surgical candidates because of insufficient FLR volume, PVE may be performed to induce selective hypertrophy and decrease the risk of post-resection hepatic failure.[72] Although no consensus among institutions regarding the FLR volume necessary to avoid post-resection liver failure for this indication has been reached, most reports use between 20% and 40%.

Many investigators have performed PVE for patients with colorectal liver metastases in an attempt to increase the pool of surgical candidates. Kawasaki et al.[73] performed PVE in 5 patients with numerous bilobar colorectal liver metastases before they underwent extensive liver resection. After right PVE, extended right hepatectomy was carried out in 4 patients, 2 of whom underwent additional wedge resection of nodules located in the left lateral segment. The other patient underwent right hepatectomy associated with local resection of the tumor in the left lobe. All 5 patients had an uneventful postoperative course with no serious complications or liver dysfunction. Although 1 patient had tumor recurrence after 28 months, the remaining 4 patients were alive and free of cancer between 36 and 74 months after resection. Therefore, in a selected patient population, PVE was effective for improving the safety of hepatectomy for patients with small metastases who needed major right-sided resection combined with wedge resection of the left lobe.[70]

Elias et al.[74] later demonstrated that PVE performed for patients (n = 41) in whom malignant hepatic disease was deemed unresectable at presentation (for insufficient FLR volume) underwent successful hepatectomy. Of particular interest was a subset of patients (n = 27) with metastatic hepatic colorectal cancer. The 5-year survival rates (including 2 postoperative deaths) for all patients and for patients with colorectal hepatic metastases were similar at 31% and 29%, respectively, showing the significant benefit of preoperative PVE. Azoulay et al.[72] then compared patients with colorectal hepatic metastases who had small FLRs requiring PVE with patients who had similar disease but had sufficient future hepatic parenchyma. These investigators found that the actuarial survival rates after hepatectomy with and without PVE were comparable (40% versus 38% at 5 years, respectively).

When PVE is being considered in the preoperative management of liver metastases, two fascinating issues arise. First, an idea exists that PVE may help proliferate intrahepatic colorectal metastases by reducing the tumor doubling time. This hypothesis was first proposed in 1999 by Elias et al.,[75] who observed during hepatic regeneration or hypertrophy that in non-injured liver (n = 5), the growth rate of metastases was more rapid than that of the normal parenchyma. Kokudo et al.[76] tested this hypothesis in a larger series of patients who underwent PVE before extended hepatectomy. These researchers found no significant change in long-term survival between the PVE and non-PVE groups. However, the rate of recurrence for the PVE group was considerably worse. Kokudo et al.[76] concluded that PVE increases tumor growth and is probably associated with enhanced recurrence of disease. However, there were flaws in this study that may account for misleading conclusions. First, there were significant differences in maximal tumor lesion diameter between the PVE group (6.80 ± 1.00 cm) and the non-PVE group (4.86 ± 0.66 cm). Second, different proportions of patients received adjuvant chemotherapy after hepatic resection; only 6 of 18 (33%) patients of the PVE group received such treatment, compared with 16 of 29 (55%) patients in the non-PVE group. Third, only 3 of 18 (17%) patients in the PVE group had tumors within the non-embolized lobe. Therefore, tumor growth was being assessed in the embolized segments with an increased hepatic arterial flow to the tumors, possibly accounting for the tumor growth. For these reasons, definite conclusions regarding tumor growth and increased rates of metastases cannot be made.

The second issue is the potential benefit of combining PVE with radiofrequency ablation (RFA) for patients with bilobar metastatic disease. Because most patients with colorectal liver metastases have good hepatic reserve, hepatic resection may be appropriate for the majority of patients without distant spread. However, for patients considered poor surgical candidates, resection could be performed in one segment or lobe and multiple small metastatic foci in the remaining lobe could be treated with RFA. The first report of this technique was made by Jiao et al.,[77] who demonstrated success in 13 of 35 patients (27 with metastatic disease and 8 with HCC), increasing the resectability of tumors in those patients. Operation was originally considered untenable in 27 patients with liver metastases, who received PVE and later underwent resection and RFA to treat the remaining lesions in the remnant liver. Although not reported, right PVE combined with RFA of small lesions in the left lobe during the same session may be used to reduce the risk of rapid progression of tumors in the left lobe and to improve the resectability rate in patients with bilobar metastases. Further study of this particular use of PVE is necessary before this approach can become common practice.[78]

Cholangiocarcinoma

Cholangiocarcinoma is rare, accounting for less than 4000 deaths in the United States annually.[79–81] Although technologic advances in imaging have significantly contributed to the diagnosis of hepatobiliary disease, cholangiocarcinoma continues to be encountered at advanced stages.[82, 83] Surgical resection offers the only significant 5-year survival rates, but only a minority of patients with cholangiocarcinoma are candidates for surgery.[84] Patients with unresectable disease usually die within 6 months to 1 year of diagnosis, generally from liver failure or cholangitis secondary to biliary obstruction.[85, 86] Palliation of sequelae of biliary obstruction is vital to improve the quality of life and is often the primary goal in caring for these patients.[87] Nevertheless, aggressive surgical approaches have been tried with varying degrees of success.[83, 88, 89] Nimura et al.[83] reported 26% 5-year survival rates for surgical resection of cholangiocarcinoma.

Extended liver resections are performed with the goal of achieving cure by complete tumor resection with tumor-free margins. Although good long-term results can be achieved, postoperative complications remain considerable.[88, 89] For this reason, preoperative PVE has been advocated to induce FLR hypertrophy in selected patients undergoing extended hepatic resections. A key factor in this population is that they often have bilateral biliary obstruction that is causing hepatic atrophy. PVE performed in this situation is of little benefit and is associated with a high risk of peritoneal biliary fistula if performed percutaneously.[78] Many investigators insist that, to avoid this complication, internal biliary decompression with internal biliary drainage must be performed prior to PVE.[14, 18, 78] If drainage is not performed, hypertrophy does not occur. If and when bilirubin levels return to normal, PVE should be performed.

Portal vein embolization for cholangiocarcinoma was first described by Makuuchi et al.,[14] who reported their experience with PVE performed before extended hepatectomy in patients (n = 14) with hilar bile duct carcinoma in whom more than 70% of the liver mass was removed. Eleven patients with jaundice were treated with biliary drainage prior to PVE, and no complications were reported after PVE. Hepatectomies with bile duct resection and lymphadenectomy were performed at a range of 6 to 41 days after PVE, at which time the ipsilateral (embolized) lobe was atrophied (n = 12). One patient died in the perioperative period from suppurative cholangitis, and 1 patient died 3 months after surgery from aggravated hepatitis. From their initial results, Makuuchi et al.[14] made the following conclusions: (1) PVE is safe, (2) PVE does not complicate subsequent surgical resection, and (3) liver failure may be less common if PVE is performed before resection.

Interpretation of the results of preoperative PVE for patients with cholangiocarcinoma is often problematic because of four important factors. First, only a small number of patients have the disease. Second, only a small number of surgeons perform these aggressive resections. Third, the results of PVE for cholangiocarcinoma are often pooled with results for other hepatobiliary malignancies, making true surgical outcomes for this patient population difficult to interpret. Fourth, because volumetric changes of the liver are a combination of the positive effect (volume increase) of PVE and of the negative effect (volume decrease) of the liver after biliary decompression, an accurate measurement of regeneration may be difficult.[78]

Few researchers have reported experiences with only cholangiocarcinoma. Kawasaki et al.[90] reported the clinical outcomes of 12 patients with cholangiocarcinoma who underwent right PVE followed by right extended hepatectomy. PVE induced a substantial increase in FLR volume: pre-PVE volume was 437 ± 88 cm^3 (FLR/TL: 34%) and post-PVE volume was 544 ± 97 cm^3 (FLR/TLV: 42%). No complications were noted after PVE. The mean time from embolization to resection was 17 days, with no perioperative mortality.[90]

An important issue is that many patients require trisegmentectomy for cure. Nagino et al.[18] first described the use of trisectoral PVE in four patients with advanced hilar cholangiocarcinoma (right trisectoral PVE [n = 1] and left trisectoral [n = 3]) before right or left hepatic trisegmentectomy. PVE was performed via the ipsilateral approach with a fibrin glue–Lipiodol mixture. No patients experienced complications after PVE, and the perioperative mortality was 0. The mean time from PVE to resection was 18 days. The FLR volume was 31% before PVE and 41% after PVE and (an increase of 10%) of the total liver volume. Three patients eventually underwent trisegmentectomy. Two patients had uneventful hospital courses, and the third suffered from transient postoperative liver failure. These investigators concluded that trisectoral PVE is effective in the preoperative management for trisegmentectomy, improving the safety of the operation.[18]

This same group of investigators then compared left lateral segment hypertrophy after right trisectoral PVE in 16 patients who had biliary tract disease (bile duct carcinoma in 15, primary sclerosing cholangitis in 1) with 16 patients who underwent only right PVE for cholangiocarcinoma.[17] The right lobe significantly atrophied (pre-PVE volume 650 ± 161 cm^3; post-PVE volume 585 ± 143 cm^3); the left lateral segment significantly hypertrophied (from 240 ± 58 cm^3 to 361 ± 66 cm^3). The volume gain of the left lateral segment was larger for patients undergoing right trisectoral PVE than for patients undergoing only right PVE (122 ± 39 cm^3 versus 66 ± 35 cm^3, respectively). Fourteen of 16 patients underwent right hepatic trisegmentectomy with caudate lobectomy. One patient died of liver failure 87 days after surgery, a mortality rate of 7.1%. From these results, Nagino et al.[17] concluded that right trisectoral PVE is more useful than standard right PVE in preparation for right hepatic trisegmentectomy and has the potential to increase the safety of this high-risk surgery for patients with biliary tract carcinoma.

FUTURE PROSPECTS

Many novel ideas have been proposed for PVE in the setting of hepatobiliary malignancy. A 2000 report showed benefit from combining PVE with TAE to promote hepatic hypertrophy in patients with poor hepatic reserve.[91] In this circumstance, adequate hypertrophy did not occur after PVE in 2 patients with bile duct cancer after adequate biliary drainage. One patient required a left trisegmentectomy but the FLR (right posterior segment) did not change at 51 days after PVE (pre-PVE FLR 485 cm^3; post-PVE FLR 470 cm^3). After TAE, the FLR volume increased to 685 cm^3 (increase of 215 cm^3). The second patient required a right lobectomy for cure after right PVE. After PVE, no significant volume change was noted (pre-PVE FLR 643 cm^3; post-PVE FLR 649 cm^3). After TAE, the left lobe volume was 789 cm^3 (increase of 140 cm^3). Both patients underwent successful hepatic resection after staged PVE/TAE procedure. However, because both arterial and portal systems are blood-deprived, there is a possibility of massive hepatic necrosis with this approach. For this reason, only half of the target segments were embolized by means of superselective embolization.

Another idea is to perform preoperative TAE using various embolic agents to occlude both hepatic arteries and the portal veins for unresectable HCC. Cheng et al.[92] reported that embolization with an Ethiodol-ethanol mixture in 20 patients resulted in a better survival rate because it increased the resectability for inoperable HCC. TAE was performed by slow infusion of the mixture into the artery supplying the tumor until dual hepatic artery and portal vein embolization was achieved. Decreased tumor size (n = 15), improved liver function as shown by ICG-15 (n = 8), and increased volume of the unembolized lobe (n = 10) were noted. The operations performed were right hepatectomy (n = 11), extended right hepatectomy (n = 3), left hepatectomy (n = 2), extended left hepatectomy (n = 2), and wedge resection (n = 2), which was performed in patients who did not want to undergo major hepatectomy. Complete tumor necrosis was found in seven cases, and all patients survived (1-year survival rate: 95%). with no associated complications. The investigators concluded that use of the mixture was a safe, efficacious method for treating HCC because it effectively decreased tumor size, caused compensatory hepatic hypertrophy, and improved liver function, allowing a wider range of patients to undergo liver surgery and achieve better survival.[92]

CONCLUSION

Portal vein embolization is a safe, effective method for inducing selective hepatic hypertrophy in the appropriate clinical setting. As presented here, a thorough knowledge of hepatic segmentation and portal venous anatomy is essential. The indications, contraindications, methods for evaluating for hepatic lobar hypertrophy, when to operate, and possible complications that can occur also need to be understood fully by anyone contemplating performing these procedures. Although technique may vary according to the operator, further research is necessary to identify the best embolic agents available, to determine the expected rates of liver regeneration for PVE, and to better elucidate the indications for PVE in patients with hepatobiliary malignancy.

REFERENCES

1. Tsao JI, Loftus JP, Nagorney DM, Adson MA, Ilstrup DM. Trends in morbidity and mortality of hepatic resection for malignancy: a matched comparative analysis. *Ann Surg* 1994; 220:199–205.
2. Vauthey JN, Chaoui A, Do KA, et al. Standardized measurement of the future liver remnant prior to extended liver resection: methodology and clinical associations. *Surgery* 2000; 127:512–519.
3. Abdalla EK, Hicks ME, Vauthey JN. Portal vein embolization: rationale, technique and future prospects. *Br J Surg* 2001; 88:165–175.
4. Couinaud C. Le foie. *Etudes anatomiques et chirurgicales*. Paris: Masson Edit., 1957:75.
5. Schultz SR, LaBerge JM, Gordon RL, et al. Anatomy of the portal vein bifurcation: intra- versus extrahepatic location: implications for transjugular intrahepatic portosystemic shunts. *J Vasc Intervent Radiol* 1994; 5:457–459.
6. Yamane T, Mori K, Sakamoto K, et al. Intrahepatic ramification of the portal vein in the right and caudate lobes of the liver. *Acta Anat* 1988; 133:162–172.
7. Atri M, Bret PM, Fraser-Hill MA. Intrahepatic portal venous variations: prevalence with ultrasound. *Radiology* 1992; 184:523–526.
8. Couinaud C. Absence de la bifurcation porté. *J Chir (Paris)* 1993; 130:111–115.
9. Hardy KJ, Jones RM. Failure of the portal vein to bifurcate. *Surgery* 1997; 121:226–228.
10. Rous P, Larimore LD. Relation of the portal blood flow to liver maintenance: a demonstration of liver atrophy conditional on compensation. *J Exp Med* 1920; 31:609–632.
11. Schalm L, Bax HR, Mansens BJ. Atrophy of the liver after occlusion of the bile ducts or portal vein and compensatory hypertrophy of the unoccluded portion and its clinical importance. *Gastroenterology* 1956; 31:131–155.
12. Honjo I, Suzuki T, Ozawa K, Takasan H, Kitamura O, Ishikawa T. Ligation of a branch of the portal vein for carcinoma of the liver. *Am J Surg* 1975; 130:296–302.
13. Takayasu K, Matsumura Y, Shima Y, Moriyama N, Yamada T, Makuuchi M. Hepatic lobar hypertrophy following obstruction of the ipsilateral portal vein from cholangiocarcinoma. *Radiology* 1986; 160:389–393.
14. Makuuchi M, Thai BL, Takayasu K, et al. Preoperative portal vein embolization to increase safety of major hepatectomy for hilar bile duct carcinoma: a preliminary report. *Surgery* 1990; 107:521–527.
15. de Baere T, Roche A, Vavasseur D, et al. Portal vein embolization: utility for inducing left hepatic lobe hypertrophy before surgery. *Radiology* 1993; 188:73–77.
16. de Baere T, Roche A, Elias D, Lasser P, Lagrange C, Bousson V. Preoperative portal vein embolization for extension of hepatectomy indications. *Hepatology* 1996; 24:1386–1391.
17. Nagino M, Kamiya J, Kanai M, et al. Right trisegment portal vein embolization for biliary tract carcinoma: technique and clinical utility. *Surgery* 2000; 127:155–160.
18. Nagino M, Nimura Y, Kamiya J, et al. Right or left trisegment portal vein embolization before hepatic trisegmentectomy for hilar bile duct carcinoma: utility. *Surgery* 1995; 117:677–681.
19. Starzl TE, Francavilla A, Porter KA, Benichou J, Jones AF. The effect of splanchnic viscera removal upon canine liver regeneration. *Surg Gynecol Obstet* 1978; 147:193–207.
20. Nagino M, Nimura Y, Kamiya J, et al. Changes in hepatic lobe volume in biliary tract cancer patients after right portal vein embolization. *Hepatology* 1995; 21:434–439.
21. Kock NG, Hahnloser P, Roding B, Schenk WG Jr. Interaction between portal venous and hepatic arterial blood flow: an experimental study in the dog. *Surgery* 1972; 72:414–419.
22. Michalopoulos GK, DeFrances MC. Liver regeneration. *Science* 1997; 276:60–66.
23. Michalopoulos GK, Zarnegar R. Hepatocyte growth factor. *Hepatology* 1992; 15:149–155.
24. Bucher NLR, Swaffield MN. Regulation of hepatic regeneration in rats by synergistic action of insulin and glucagon. *Proc Natl Acad Sci U S A* 1975; 72:1157–1160.
25. Lee KC, Kinoshita H, Hirohashi K, Kubo S, Iwasa R. Extension of surgi-

cal indication for hepatocellular carcinoma by portal vein embolization. *World J Surg* 1993; 17:109–115.
26. Goto Y, Nagino M, Nimura Y. Doppler estimation of portal blood flow after percutaneous transhepatic portal vein embolization. *Ann Surg* 1998; 228:209–213.
27. Duncan JR, Hicks ME, Cai SR, Brunt EM, Ponder KP. Embolization of portal vein branches induces hepatocyte hypertrophy in swine: a potential step in hepatic gene therapy. *Radiology* 1999; 210:467–477.
28. Yamanaka N, Okamoto E, Kawamura E, et al. Dynamics of normal and injured liver regeneration after hepatectomy as assessed on the basis of computed tomography and liver function. *Hepatology* 1993; 18:79–85.
29. Kinoshita H, Sakai K, Hirohashi K, Igawa S, Yamasaki O, Kubo S. Preoperative portal vein embolization for hepatocellular carcinoma. *World J Surg* 1986;10:803–808.
30. Makuuchi M, Takayasu K, Takuma T, et al. Preoperative transcatheter embolization of the portal venous branch for patients receiving extended lobectomy due to the bile duct carcinoma. *Nihon Rinshogeka Gakkai Zasshi* 1984; 45:1558–1564.
31. Lin TY, Lee CS, Chen CC, Liau KY, Lin WSJ. Regeneration of human liver after hepatic lobectomy studied by repeated by liver scanning and repeated needle biopsy. *Ann Surg* 1979; 190:48–53.
32. Chen M, Hwang T, Hung C. Human liver regeneration after major hepatectomy: a study of liver volume by computed tomography. *Ann Surg* 1991; 213:227–229.
33. Shibayama Y, Hashimoto K, Nakata K. Recovery from hepatic necrosis following acute portal vein embolism with special reference to reconstruction of occluded vessels. *J Pathol* 1991; 165:255–261.
34. Ikeda K, Kinoshita H, Hirohashi K, Kubo S, Kaneda K. The ultrastructure, kinetics and intralobular distribution of apoptotic hepatocytes after portal branch ligation with special reference to their relationship to necrotic hepatocytes. *Arch Histol Cytol* 1995; 58:171–184.
35. Denys AL, Abehsera M, Sauvanet A, Sibert A, Belghiti J, Menu Y. Failure of right portal vein ligation to induce left lobe hypertrophy due to intrahepatic portoportal collaterals: successful treatment with portal vein embolization. *Am J Roentgenol* 1999;173:633–635.
36. De Baere T, Roche A, Elias D, Lasser P, Lagrange C, Bousson V. Preoperative portal vein embolization for extension of hepatectomy indications. *Hepatology* 1996;24:1386–1391.
37. Di Stefano D, Bartoli J, De Baere T, Denys AL, Gorin G, Lecrivain F. Incidents et complications des embolisations portales percutanées. *J Radiol* 2000; 81:1488–1489.
38. Nagino M, Nimura Y, Kamiya J, Kondo S, Kanai M. Selective percutaneous transhepatic embolization of the portal vein in preparation for extensive liver resection: the ipsilateral approach. *Radiology* 1996; 200:559–563.
39. Madoff DC, Hicks ME, Abdalla EK, Morris JS, Vauthey JN. Portal vein embolization using polyvinyl alcohol particles and coils in preparation for major liver resection for hepatobiliary malignancy: safety and effectiveness—study in 26 patients. Radiology 2003;227:251–260.
40. Miyagawa S, Makuucki M, Kawasaki S. Preoperative portal embolization to increase safety of major hepatectomies for liver tumors. In: Dionigi R, Madariaga JR, eds. Karger Landes Systems Basel (Switzerland) *New Technologies for Liver Resections* 1997:113–118.
41. Azoulay D, Raccuia JS, Castaing D, Bismuth H. Right portal vein embolization in preparation for major hepatic resection. *J Am Coll Surg* 1995; 181:266–269.
42. Makuuchi M, Kosuge T, Lygidakis NJ. New possibilities for major liver surgery in patients with Klatskin tumors or primary hepatocellular carcinoma—an old problem revisited. *Hepatogastroenterology* 1991; 38:329–336.
43. Kaneko T, Nakao A, Takagi H. Experimental study of new embolizing material for portal vein embolization. *Hepatogastroenterology* 2000; 47:790–794.
44. Matsuoka T. Experimental studies of intrahepatic portal vein embolization and embolic materials. *Nippon Igaku Hoshasen Gakkai Zasshi* 1989; 49:593–606.
45. Imamura H, Shimada R, Kubota M, et al. Preoperative portal vein embolization: an audit of 84 patients. *Hepatology* 1999; 29:1099–1105.
46. Shimamura T, Nakajima Y, Une Y, et al. Efficacy and safety of preoperative percutaneous transhepatic portal embolization with absolute ethanol: a clinical study. *Surgery* 1997; 121:135–141.
47. Ogasawara K, Uchino J, Une Y, Fujioka Y. Selective portal vein embolization with absolute ethanol induces hepatic hypertrophy and makes more extensive hepatectomy possible. *Hepatology* 1996; 23:338–345.
48. Yamakado K, Takeda K, Nishide Y, et al. Portal vein embolization with steel coils and absolute ethanol: a comparative study with canine liver. *Hepatology* 1995; 22:1812–1818.
49. Nagino M, Nimura Y, Hayakawa N. Percutaneous transhepatic portal embolization using newly devised catheters: preliminary report. *World J Surg* 1993; 17:520–524.
50. Brown K, Brody L, Decorato D, Getrajdman G. Portal vein embolization with use of polyvinyl alcohol. *J Vasc Interv Radiol* 2001; 12:882–886.
51. Azoulay D, Castaing D, Krissat J, et al. Percutaneous portal vein embolization increases the feasibility and safety of major liver resection for hepatocellular carcinoma in injured liver. *Ann Surg* 2000; 232:665–672.
52. Kubota K, Makuuchi M, Kusaka K, et al. Measurement of liver volume and hepatic functional reserve as a guide to decision-making in resectional surgery for hepatic tumors. *Hepatology* 1997; 26:1176–1181.
53. Ogasawara K, Une Y, Nakajima Y, Uchino J. The significance of measuring liver volume using computed tomographic images before and after hepatectomy. *Surg Today* 1995; 25:43–48.
54. Vauthey JN, Abdalla EK, Doherty DA, et al. Body surface area and body weight predict total liver volume in western adults. *Liver Transpl* 2002 8:233–240.
55. Mitsumori A, Nagaya I, Kimoto S, et al. Preoperative evaluation of hepatic functional reserve following hepatectomy by technetium-99m galactosyl human serum albumin liver scintigraphy and computed tomography. *Eur J Nucl Med* 1998; 25:1377–1382.
56. Marsh JW, Dvorchik I, Subotin M, et al. The prediction of risk of recurrence and time to recurrence of hepatocellular carcinoma after orthotopic liver transplantation: a pilot study. *Hepatology* 1997; 26:444–450.
57. Livraghi T. Guidelines for treatment of liver cancer. *Eur J Ultrasound* 2001; 13:167–176.
58. Sugarawa Y, Yamamoto J, Higashi H, et al. Preoperative portal vein embolization in patients with hepatocellular carcinoma. *World J Surg* 2002; 26:105–110.
59. Mor E, Kaspa RT, Sheiner P, Schwartz M. Treatment of hepatocellular carcinoma associated with cirrhosis in the era of liver transplantation. Ann Intern Med 1998; 129:643–653.
60. Fan ST, Lo CM, Liu CL, et al. Hepatectomy for hepatocellular carcinoma: towards zero mortality. *Ann Surg* 1999; 229:322–330.
61. Farges O, Malassagne B, Flejou JF, et al. Risk of major liver resection in patients with underlying chronic liver disease. *Ann Surg* 1999; 229:210–215.
62. Fong, Y, Sun, RL, Jarnagin W, Blumgart LH. An Analysis of 412 cases of hepatocellular carcinoma at a western center. *Ann Surg* 1999; 229:790–800.
63. Shirabe K, Shimada M, Gion T, et al. Postoperative liver failure after major hepatic resection for hepatocellular carcinoma in the modern era with special reference to remnant liver volume. *J Am Coll Surg* 1999; 188:304–307.
64. Yamakado K, Takeda K, Matsumura K, et al. Regeneration of the unembolized liver parenchyma following portal vein embolization. *J Hepatol* 1997; 27:871–880.
65. Wakabayashi H, Ishimura K, Okana K, et al. Is preoperative portal vein embolization effective in improving prognosis after major hepatic resection in patients with advanced-stage hepatocellular carcinoma? *Cancer* 2001; 92:2384–2390.

66. Wakabayashi H, Yachida S, Maeba T, Maeta H. Indications for portal vein embolization combined with major hepatic resection for advanced-stage hepatocellular carcinomas: a preliminary clinical study. *Dig Surg* 2000; 17:587–594.
67. Tanaka H, Hirohashi K, Shuto T, et al. Preoperative portal vein embolization improves prognosis after right hepatectomy for hepatocellular carcinoma in patients with impaired hepatic function. *Br J Surg* 2000; 87:879–882.
68. August DA, Ottow RT, Sugarbaker PH. Clinical perspective of human colorectal cancer metastasis. *Cancer Metastasis Rev* 1984; 3:303–324.
69. Fortner JG, Silva JS, Cox EB, Golbey RB, Gallowitz H, Maclean BJ. Multivariate analysis of a personal series of 247 patients with liver metastases from colorectal cancer. II: treatment by intrahepatic chemotherapy. *Ann Surg* 1984; 199:317–324.
70. Jaeck D, Bachellier P, Guiguet M, et al. Long-term survival following resection of colorectal hepatic metastases: Association Francaise de Chirurgie. *Br J Surg* 1997; 84:977–980.
71. Bismuth H, Adam R, Levi F, et al. Resection of nonresectable liver metastases from colorectal cancer after neoadjuvant chemotherapy. *Ann Surg* 1996; 224:509–520; discussion 520–522.
72. Azoulay D, Castaing D, Smail A, et al. Resection of nonresectable liver metastases from colorectal cancer after percutaneous portal vein embolization. *Ann Surg* 2000; 231:480–486.
73. Kawasaki S, Makuuchi M, Kakazu T, et al. Resection for multiple metastatic liver tumors after portal embolization. *Surgery* 1994; 115:674–677.
74. Elias D, Cavalcanti A, de Baere T, Roche A, Lasser P. [Long-term oncological results of hepatectomy performed after selective portal embolization]. *Ann Chir* 1999; 53:559–564.
75. Elias D, De Baere T, Roche A, Mducreux, Leclere J, Lasser P. During liver regeneration following right portal embolization the growth rate of liver metastases is more rapid than that of the liver parenchyma. *Br J Surg* 1999; 86:784–788.
76. Kokudo N, Tada K, Seki M, et al. Proliferative activity of intrahepatic colorectal metastases after preoperative hemihepatic portal vein embolization. *Hepatology* 2001; 34:267–272.
77. Jiao LR, Hansen PD, Havlik R, Mitry RR, Pignatelli M, Habib N. Clinical short-term results of radiofrequency ablation in primary and secondary liver tumors. *Am J Surg* 1999; 177:303–306.
78. Denys A, Madoff DC, Doenz F, et al. Indications for and limitations of portal vein embolization prior to major hepatic resection for hepatobiliary malignancy. *Surg Oncol Clin North Am* 2002;11: 955–968.
79. Marcos-Alvarez A, Jenkins RL. Cholangiocarcinoma. *Surg Oncol Clin North Am* 1996; 5:301–316.
80. Ottow RT, August DA, Sugarbaker PH. Treatment of proximal biliary tract cancer: an overview of techniques and results. *Surgery* 1985; 97:251–262.
81. Kuvshinoff BW, Fong Y, Blumgart LH. Proximal bile duct tumors. *Surg Oncol Clin North Am* 1996; 5: 317–335.
82. Saldinger PF, Blumgart LH. Resection of hilar cholangiocarcinoma—a European and United States experience. *J Hepatobiliary Pancreat Surg* 2000; 7:111–114.
83. Nimura Y, Kamiya J, Kondo S, et al. Aggressive preoperative management and extended surgery for hilar cholangiocarcinoma: Nagoya experience. *J Hepatobil Pancreat Surg* 2000; 7:155–162.
84. Janargin WR. Cholangiocarcinoma of the extrahepatic bile ducts. *Semin Surg Oncol* 2000; 19:156–176.
85. Nordack IH, Pitt HA, Coleman J, et al: Unresectable hilar cholangiocarcinoma. Surgery 1993; 115:597–603.
86. Pitt HA, Nakeeb A, Abrams RA, et al: Perihilar cholangiocarcinoma: postoperative radiotherapy does not improve survival. *Ann Surg* 1995; 221:788–798.
87. Cameron JL, Pitt HA, Zinner MJ, Kaufman SL, Coleman J. Management of proximal cholangiocarcinomas by surgical resection and radiotherapy. *Am J Surg* 1990; 159:91–97; discussion 97–98.
88. Blumgart LH, Hadjis NS, Benjamin IS, Beazley R. Surgical approaches to cholangiocarcinoma at confluence of hepatic ducts. *Lancet* 1984; 1(8368):66–70.
89. Bengmark S, Ekberg H, Evander A, Klofver-Stahl B, Tranberg KG. Major liver resection for hilar cholangiocarcinoma. *Ann Surg* 1988; 207:120–125.
90. Kawasaki S, Makuuchi M, Miyagawa S, Kakazu T. Radical operation after portal embolization for tumor of hilar bile duct. *J Am Coll Surg* 1994; 178:480–486.
91. Nagino M, Kanai M, Morioka A, et al. Portal and arterial embolization before extensive liver resection in patients with markedly poor functional reserve. *J Vasc Interv Radiol* 2000; 11:1063–1068.
92. Cheng Y, Kan Z, Chen C, et al. Efficacy and safety of preoperative lobar and segmental ablation via transarterial administration of ethiodol and ethanol mixture for treatment of hepatocellular carcinoma: clinical study. *World J Surg* 2000; 24:844–850.

CHAPTER 13

MULTIMODALITY THERAPY FOR HEPATIC MALIGNANCIES

LILY Y. KERNAGIS, MD

MICHAEL C. SOULEN, MD

INTRODUCTION

Hepatic malignancies are one of the most difficult therapeutic challenges in oncologic care. Cure is usually not possible because of the predilection for intrahepatic recurrence despite complete resection or ablation of the initial tumor. Nonetheless, durable local control can be achieved through vigilant monitoring and aggressive multimodality therapy coordinated by a multidisciplinary team of specialists in medical, surgical, and interventional oncology. For tumors that tend not to metastasize aggressively beyond the liver, durable regional control may provide benefit in preservation of quality of life and in overall survival.

Individual procedures are reviewed in detail in other chapters. This chapter focuses on the results of various combinations of liver-directed and systemic therapies for treatment of primary and secondary hepatic malignancies.

COMBINATION THERAPIES FOR HEPATOCELLULAR CARCINOMA

Adjuvant Therapy

Surgical resection is considered the only potentially curative therapeutic option for hepatocellular carcinoma (HCC). The 5-year survival after hepatectomy for HCC is 20%–30%, with late morbidity resulting from recurrence of cancer, followed by liver failure, gastrointestinal bleeding, and infection.[1–3] Regional therapy may play a role in improving outcome after resection.

Retrospective studies of postoperative hepatic arterial therapy have yielded favorable results, with decreased recurrence, improvement in disease-free survival (DFS), or improvement in overall survival (OS) compared with patients who undergo resection alone[4–7] (**Table 13-1**). Tanaka et al.[6] evaluated the efficacy of transcatheter arterial infusion of mitomycin C, doxorubicin, and Lipiodol after hepatic resection in 24 patients with tumor capsular invasion, intraportal spread, or intrahepatic metastasis. Hepatic arterial infusion (HAI) appeared to be effective, with significant improvement in cumulative survival and decreased residual liver recurrence. Asahara et al.[7] demonstrated similar findings using doxorubicin and Lipiodol in 68 patients after radical hepatectomy. In patients with adjuvant HAI, survival was improved but not statistically significant at 3, 5, and 7 years (79.1%, 54.5%, 39.9%, respectively), compared with patients who received hepatectomy alone (69.2%, 38.1%, 26.8%, respectively). There was significant improvement in DFS in the adjuvant HAI group at 3, 5, and 7 years (50.8%, 31.7%, 25.6%, respectively), compared with the group without adjuvant therapy (25.7%, 20.6%, 6.4%, respectively; $P = 0.006$).

Randomized control trials, however, have demonstrated contradictory results.[8–11] Ueno et al.[9] found better DFS in patients who received adjuvant HAI, whereas Ono et al.[10] failed to show an improvement in recurrence rate, DFS, or OS. Lai et al.[11] found no improvement and even demonstrated statistically significant adverse effects of adjuvant HAI on 3-year DFS (18% in the adjuvant group versus 48% in the control group). It has been suggested that this difference in outcomes may be due to an adverse effect of the addition of systemic chemotherapy to the adjuvant therapy regimen.[12] Further randomized clinical trials would be needed to evaluate the effectiveness of adjuvant regional therapy.

Neoadjuvant Therapy

Resection and transplantation are effective methods of improving survival in patients with primary liver tumors. Orthotopic liver transplantation (OLT) has been shown to be the best treatment for early-stage HCC.[13–15] Neoadjuvant therapies have been explored in attempts to control tumor growth, prevent growth of latent hepatic foci, induce necrosis, and convert unresectable tumors to resectable tumors to improve DSF and long-term OS (**Table 13-2**).

Preoperative transarterial chemoembolization (TACE) has been shown to be capable of developing partial necrosis in HCC.[16] Complete necrosis occurs less commonly but has also been demonstrated.[16–18] Oldhafer et al.[17] found that 29% of 21 pretransplant patients who received TACE developed complete necrosis, whereas 67% developed partial necrosis; no survival benefit was noted, however. The addition of percutaneous ethanol injection (PEI) to TACE for neoadjuvant therapy was attempted to improve induction of necrosis. Veltri et al.[18] demonstrated that 100% of patients who received preoperative TACE and PEI had complete necrosis, whereas neoadjuvant TACE alone led to complete necrosis in 24% of patients and PEI alone led to complete necrosis in 80% of patients. Tumors recurred in patients

TABLE 13-1
Adjuvant Arterial Chemotherapy for Hepatocellular Carcinoma

	No. of patients	Recurrence rate (versus control)	3-year disease-free survival (versus control)	3-year overall survival (versus control)	Effective?
Takenaka et al.[4] (1995)	17	18% (74%*)	86% (15%*)	—	Y
Nakashima et al.[5] (1996)	26	—	27% (12%*)	71% (32%*)	Y
Asahara et al.[7] (1999)	68	66% (85%*)	51% (26%*)	79% (69%)	Y
Tanaka et al.[6] (1999)	24	50% (81%*)	67% (30%*)	90% (63%*)	Y
Kohno et al.[8] (1996)—RCT	48	—	37% (32%)	49% (50%)	N
Ono et al.[10] (1997)—RCT	24	66% (70%)	32% (42%)	72% (82%)	N
Lai et al.[11] (1998)—RCT	30	77% (47%*)	18% (48%*)	66% (65%)	N (adverse effects)
Ueno et al.[9] (1999)—RCT	10	—	72% (28%*)	—	Y

RCT = randomized control trial.
**Statistically significant. $p \leq 0.05$*

TABLE 13-2
Neoadjuvant Treatment for Hepatocellular Carcinoma

	No. of patients	Recurrence rate (versus control)	3-year disease-free survival (versus control)	3-year overall survival (versus control)	Effective?
Adachi et al.[30] (1993)	46	—	52% (49%)	—	N
Uchida et al.[31] (1996)	60	43% (52%)	—	61% (71%)	N
Harada et al.[27] (1996)	105	—	38% (34%)	78% (68%)	N
Majno et al.[26] (1997)	49	57% (81%*)	29% (26%)	57% (47%)	Y (if downstaged or complete necrosis)
Paye et al.[23] (1998)	24	58% (53%)	33% (32%)	62% (66%)	N
Oldhafer et al.[17] (1998)	21	—	—	48% (54%)	N
Veltri et al.[18] (1998)	38	12% (15%)	—	—	N
Di Carlo et al.[21] (1998)	55	—	40% (20%*)	70% (38%*)	Y (in cirrhosis)
Lu et al.[20] (1999)	20	—	55% (22%)	53% (33%*)	Y (in tumor > 8 cm)
Wu et al.[24] (1995) RCT	24	78% (53%)	—	—	N

RCT = randomized control trial.
**Statistically significant, p ≤ 0.05*

who had TACE only and in patients in whom there was no demonstrable tumor necrosis; however, patients selected to receive TACE alone had more advanced disease. Despite the 100% rate of complete necrosis, neoadjuvant therapy with PEI and TACE did not significantly alter the recurrence rate or patients' prognoses. Pre-OLT administration of TACE was shown not to increase the risk of hepatic artery complications such as hepatic artery thrombosis after patients underwent OLT.[19]

Although pre-OLT TACE trials did not appear to significantly alter patient outcomes, several additional studies for evaluation of preoperative TACE for HCC prior to liver resection were examined with conflicting results. Lu et al.[20] performed a retrospective analysis of 120 cases involving patients with TNM classification stage II or III HCC who underwent hepatectomy. Forty-four patients underwent TACE preoperatively (20 of whom had a tumor > 8 cm). In patients with tumors large than 8 cm, the relative risk of preoperative TACE for OS was 0.38 ($P = 0.017$), demonstrating that there may be some benefit to preoperative TACE in patients with stage II/III tumors larger than 8 cm undergoing hepatectomy. In another study,[21] patients with tumors larger than 8 cm were shown to benefit from preoperative TACE. Di Carlo et al. found that there was a significant improvement in 3-year OS (70% versus 38%; $P < 0.02$) and 3-year DFS (40% versus 20%; $P < 0.05$) in patients who had not yet undergone liver resection who had tumors 5 cm or smaller in diameter and who received TACE for HCC. A retrospective analysis performed by Zhang et al.[22] showed that in 120 patients who had received preoperative TACE, of 1725 patients in total who underwent hepatectomy for HCC, there was a greater DFS in patients who had received more than two TACE treatments. In contrast, a comparative study by Paye et al.[23] demonstrated that neoadjuvant TACE induced no significant decrease in tumor size or increase in DFS. Additionally, Wu et al.[24] demonstrated, in a randomized controlled trial, an increased risk of extrahepatic recurrence and worse actuarial survival in patients who received TACE prior to liver resection.

Preoperative TACE has led to variable effects on preresection tumor size. In a study by Wu et al.,[24] patients with a large HCC (maximum diameter of ≥ 10 cm) were demonstrated to be resectable by the amount of functional liver reserve and anatomic extent of the tumor. Tumor volume was decreased by a mean of 42.8% in 16 patients receiving TACE. TACE did not lead to complete necrosis, and there was no change in DFS. Additional studies regarding the effect of neoadjuvant therapy on tumor size and conversion of unresectable tumors to resectable have led to more favorable conclusions.[25–28] In a study by Majno et al.,[26] improvement in DFS was demonstrated in patients whose tumors were downstaged or had complete necrosis, compared with patients with no response or patients who did not receive preoperative TACE. Additionally, tumors became resectable in 10% of patients after downstaging, which occurred more frequently with tumors larger than 5 cm. An additional study[27] demonstrated no significant improvement in OS and DFS; however, nearly 50% of patients undergoing neoadjuvant TACE demonstrated at least a 25% decrease in maximum tumor diameter (69.6% of patients with tumors < 5 cm). Although the data on TACE conversion of unresectable to resectable HCC have been variable, a study by Sitzmann[28] using chemoradiation as neoadjuvant therapy showed that patients with tumors that were converted to resectable after chemoradiation survived as long as patients whose tumors were initially resectable.

Majno et al.[26] showed that patients who received preoperative TACE had an increased rate of resection of adjacent organs (58% versus 25%; $p = 0.003$) compared with patients in the control group. Other complications included adhesion of the tumor to the diaphragm, thickening of the gallbladder wall, and thickening of the hepatoduodenal ligament.[29] It appears as if preoperative TACE may be effective in inducing at least partial necrosis, and more complete necrosis when PEI is added to the neoadjuvant regimen, but impact on survival is unclear.[30–31] It has been suggested that preoperative neoadjuvant therapy should be reserved for patients with unresectable or locally advanced tumors because preoperative TACE may delay surgery and can complicate further TACE.[12]

Treatment Combinations Without Surgical Resection

Various nonsurgical treatment combinations have been attempted for patients with HCC to improve prognosis. These include liver-directed therapies such as radiofrequency ablation (RFA), microwave ablation, laser ablation, cryoablation, chemical ablation, chemoembolization, and radioembolization, as well as traditional systemic and radiation treatments.

Prospective randomized trials have demonstrated a significant improvement in response in patients who received TACE and ethanol injection compared with patients who received TACE alone.[32–36] Yamakado et al.[34] demonstrated that 26 patients with unresectable HCC who received TACE and transportal ethanol had 1-, 3-, and 5-year survival rates of 87%, 72%, and 51%, respectively (18 patients received a second round of chemoembolization). Similarly, Bartolozzi et al.[35] found significantly greater therapeutic response, lower tumor recurrence rates, and a better rate of survival without recurrence in patients treated with TACE followed by PEI, compared with patients who received repeated TACE treatment for large HCCs (3.1–8.0 cm in diameter). Although patients undergoing both TACE and PEI had better survival rates (100%, 87%, and 72% versus 93%, 70%, and 43% at 1, 2, and 3 years, respectively) than those who underwent only repeated TACE, the differences were not statistically significant. Additionally, patients who received TACE and transportal ethanol injections were shown to develop more complete tumor necrosis.[36]

Although there are fewer studies demonstrating other treatment combinations as a primary treatment, preliminary results have been encouraging. Percutaneous microwave coagulation therapy was given within 1 to 2 days of TACE to 18 patients with HCCs (2–3 cm in diameter) and cirrhosis.[37] Seventeen of 18 (94%) patients demonstrated complete tumor necrosis. Although 1 patient developed a pleural effusion, no fatal complications occurred, and all patients were alive at follow-up evaluation at between 12 and 31 months.

Laser thermal ablation (LTA) uses low-power laser light energy delivered from implanted optical fibers; its use was investigated in combination with TACE in patients with large HCCs (3.5–9.6 cm in diameter).[38] LTA preceded TACE in an attempt to make the tumor more amenable to TACE. Complete tumor necrosis was present in 90% of treated patients, with a cumulative survival rate of 92%, 68%, and 40% at 1, 2, and 3 years, respectively. DFS rates were 74% and 34% at 1 and 2 years, respectively, and no major complications resulted from LTA.

Radiotherapy has also been shown to be effective in patients with HCC. In a study by Seong et al.,[39] a mean tumor dose of 44 Gy with daily 1.8-Gy fractions was delivered to 30 patients 7–10 days after TACE; a 63.3% response rate was noted. Survival rates were 67%, 33.3%, and 22.2% at 1, 2, and 3 years, respectively (median survival, 17 months). Furthermore, combined treatment with radiotherapy and TACE was shown to provide better control of HCC than radiotherapy alone.[40]

RFA is another regional therapy that can be used to create local tumor destruction and can be used as an adjunct to other therapies for tumor control. Rossi et al.[41] delivered percutaneous RFA in 56 patients with nonresectable HCCs after tumor arterial occlusion. One-year survival was 87%, with 2 patients subsequently undergoing surgical resection.

Other treatment combinations using systemic interferon have been attempted. Chung et al.[42] evaluated the use of intra-arterial cisplatin along with systemic interferon-α in patients with major portal vein thrombosis or distal metastases and found that the partial response and survival rate was higher for the patients who received dual therapy compared with those who received intra-arterial chemotherapy alone. Further studies to evaluate effectiveness of regional treatment combinations for HCC need to be developed to assess improvement in DFS and OS.

TREATMENT FOR LIVER METASTASES

The liver is the most common site for colorectal cancer metastases. Patients with colorectal cancer metastases to the liver have a poor prognosis. Liver resection is the only potentially curative option, with a 30% 5-year survival rate.[43] Conversely, patients with unresectable colorectal liver metastases have a median survival of 6–9 months without treatment.[44] Multimodality treatment options with and without resection have been sought to improve outcomes in patients with liver metastases.

Thus far, chemoembolization in combination with systemic treatment has not demonstrated promising results. In a study by Leichman et al.,[45] chemoembolization (doxorubicin/mitomycin C/cisplatin) and systemic 5-fluorouracil (5-FU) with leucovorin was administered to 31 patients, resulting in no improvement in survival compared with systemic treatment alone, with an overall response of 29%, 1-year survival of 58%, and median time to progression of 8 months. An additional study using cisplatin and systemic 5-FU[46] yielded a median survival of 14.3 months and an OS of 57% at 1 year and 19% at 2 years in 27 patients.

Several combination therapies have been tested as an adjunct to resection of liver metastases with more favorable results. Tono et al.[47] demonstrated a beneficial effect of prophylactic hepatic arterial infusion of 5-FU after resection of colorectal metastases in 9 patients (10 controls). Median DFS was 78%, 78%, and 67% at 1, 2, 3 years, respectively, for the treated group, versus 50%, 30%, and 20%, respectively, for the control group.

Additionally, Kemeny et al.[48] studied adjuvant hepatic arterial infusion of chemotherapy (floxuridine/dexamethasone) through an implantable pump after resection of hepatic metastases from colorectal cancer in 74 patients. There was significant improvement in OS (86% versus 72%) and hepatic progression-free survival (90% versus 60%) at 2 years. The morbidity risk ratio was 2.34 (95% confidence interval; range, 1.10–4.98), indicating that postoperative hepatic arterial infusion of chemotherapeutic agents improved 2-year outcome.

A randomized control trial by Lorenz et al.[49] demonstrated minor but not significant improvement in 226 patients with colorectal cancer metastases to the liver who underwent TACE after curative resection. Patients had a median survival of 34.5 months versus 46.8 months in the control group and time to progression of 14.2 months versus 13.7 months.

Rose et al.[50] evaluated RFA in patients with hepatic metastases as a primary treatment or as an adjunct to resection, cryosurgical ablation, or hepatic artery infusion and demonstrated no RFA-associated deaths and only minimal local and systemic complications. This was confirmed in a study by Elias et al.[51] in patients who received RFA for a central metastasis or as an adjunct to hepatectomy in patients with multiple bilateral metastases, where RFA increased the rate of curative resection without complications related to RFA. Further studies are needed to evaluate effect on survival and recurrence.

SUMMARY

The role of neoadjuvant and adjuvant liver-directed therapies in patients undergoing resection of liver tumors remains controversial, though recent trials of postoperative HAI for metastatic colorectal cancer are encouraging. The majority of patients have unresectable disease; in these patients, an impressive armamentarium of techniques is available for image-guided treatment. Combinations of these therapies may improve the efficiency of tumor cell kill and result in better immediate local control. Whether this improvement in local response alters the natural history of the disease remains to be evaluated in carefully designed and controlled trials.

REFERENCES

1. Franco D, Capussotti L, Smadja C, et al. Resection of hepatocellular carcinomas: results in 72 European patients with cirrhosis. *Gastroenterology* 1990;98(3):733–738.
2. Nagao T, Inoue S, Goto S, et al. Hepatic resection for hepatocellular carcinoma: clinical features and long-term prognosis. *Ann Surg* 1987;205:33–40.
3. Iwatsuki S, Starzl TE, Sheahan DG, et al. Hepatic resection versus transplantation for hepatocellular carcinoma. *Ann Surg* 1991;214:221–229.
4. Takenaka K, Yoshida K, Nishizaki T, et al. Postoperative prophylactic lipiodolization reduces the intrahepatic recurrence of hepatocellular carcinoma. *Am J Surg* 1995;169:400–404.
5. Nakashima K, Kitano S, Kim YI, Aramaki M, Kawano K. Postoperative adjuvant arterial infusion chemotherapy for patients with hepatocellular carcinoma. *Hepatogastroenterology* 1996;43:1410–1414.
6. Tanaka K, Shimada H, Togo S, et al. Use of transcatheter arterial infusion of anti-cancer agents with Lipiodol to prevent recurrence of hepatocellular carcinoma after hepatic resection. *Hepatogastroenterology* 1999;46:1083–1088.
7. Asahara H, Itamoto T, Katayama K, et al. Adjuvant arterial infusion chemotherapy after radical hepatectomy for hepatocellular carcinoma—results of long-term follow-up. *Hepatogastroenterology* 1999;46:1042–1048.
8. Kohno H, Nagasue N, Hayashi T, et al. Postoperative adjuvant chemotherapy after radical hepatic resection for hepatocellular carcinoma (HCC). *Hepatogastroenterology* 1996;43:1405–1409.
9. Ueno S, Tanabe G, Yoshida A, et al. Postoperative prediction of and strategy for metastatic recurrent hepatocellular carcinoma according to histologic activity of hepatitis. *Cancer* 1999;86:248–254.
10. Ono T, Nagasue N, Kohno H, et al. Adjuvant chemotherapy with epirubicin and carmofur after radical resection of hepatocellular carcinoma: a prospective randomized study. *Semin Oncol* 1997;24(suppl 6):S6–S25.
11. Lai E, Lo C-M, Fan S-T, Liu C-L, Wong J. Postoperative adjuvant chemotherapy after curative resection of hepatocellular carcinoma. *Arch Surg* 1998;133:183–188.
12. Poon R, Fan S-T, Wong J. Risk factors, prevention, and management of postoperative recurrence after resection of hepatocellular carcinoma. *Ann Surg* 2000;232(1):10–24.

13. Mazzaferro V, Regalia E, Doci R, et al. Liver transplantation for the treatment of small hepatocellular carcinomas in patients with cirrhosis. *N Eng J Med* 1996;334(11):693–699.
14. Pichlmayr R, Weimann A, Oldhafer KJ, et al. Role of liver transplantation for the treatment of unresectable liver cancer. *World J Surg* 1995;19(6):807–813.
15. Selby R, Kadry Z, Carr B, et al. Liver transplantation for hepatocellular carcinoma. *World J Surg* 1995;19(1):53–58.
16. Spreafico C, Marchiano A, Regalia E, et al. Chemoembolization of hepatocellular carcinoma in patients who undergo liver transplantation. *Radiology* 1994;192:687–690.
17. Oldhafer KJ, Chavan A, Fruhauf NR, et al. Arterial chemoembolization before liver transplantation in patients with hepatocellular carcinoma: marked tumor necrosis, but no survival benefit? *J Hepatology* 1998;29:953–959.
18. Veltri A, Grosso M, Martina MC, et al. Effect of preoperative radiological treatment of hepatocellular carcinoma before liver transplantation: a retrospective study. *Cardiovasc Intervent Radiol* 1998;21:393–398.
19. Richard III HM, Silberzweig JE, Mitty HA, et al. Hepatic arterial complications in liver transplant recipients treated with pretransplantation chemoembolization for hepatocellular carcinoma. *Radiology* 2000;214:775–779.
20. Lu C-D, Peng S-Y, Jiang X-C, Chiba Y, Tanigawa N. Pre-operative transcatheter arterial chemoembolization and prognosis of patients with hepatocellular carcinomas: retrospective analysis of 120 cases. *World J Surg* 1999;23:293–300.
21. Di Carlo V, Ferrari G, Castoldi R, et al. Preoperative chemoembolization of hepatocellular carcinoma in cirrhotic patients. *Hepatogastroenterology* 1998;45:1950–1954.
22. Zhang Z, Liu Q, He J, et al. The effect of preoperative transcatheter hepatic arterial chemoembolization on disease-free survival after hepatectomy for hepatocellular carcinoma. *Cancer* 2000;89:2606–2612.
23. Paye F, Jagot P, Vilgrain V, et al. Preoperative chemoembolization of hepatocellular carcinoma. *Arch Surg* 1998;133:767–772.
24. Wu C-C, Ho Y-Z, Ho WL, et al. Preoperative transcatheter arterial chemoembolization for resectable large hepatocellular carcinoma: a reappraisal. *Br J Surg* 1995;85:122–126.
25. Tang Z-Y, Yu Y-Q, Zhou X-D, et al. Cytoreduction and sequential resection for surgically verified unresectable hepatocellular carcinoma: evaluation with analysis of 72 patients. *World J Surg* 1995;19:784–789.
26. Majno PE, Adam R, Bismuth H, et al. Influence of preoperative transarterial Lipiodol chemoembolization on resection and transplantation for hepatocellular carcinoma in patients with cirrhosis. *Ann Surg* 1997;226(6):688–703.
27. Harada T, Matsuo K, Inoue T, et al. Is preoperative hepatic arterial chemoembolization safe and effective for hepatocellular carcinoma? *Ann Surg* 1996;224(1):4–9.
28. Sitzmann J. Conversion of unresectable liver cancer: an approach and follow-up study. *World J Surg* 1995;19:790–794.
29. Yu Y-Q, Xu D-B, Zhou X-D, et al. Experience with liver resection after hepatic arterial chemoembolization for hepatocellular carcinoma. *Cancer* 1993;71:62–65.
30. Adachi E, Matsumata T, Nishizaki T, et al. Effects of preoperative transcatheter arterial chemoembolization for hepatocellular carcinoma: the relationship between postoperative course and tumor necrosis. *Cancer* 1993;72:3593–3598.
31. Uchida M, Kohno H, Kubota H, et al. Role of preoperative transcatheter arterial oily chemoembolization for resectable hepatocellular carcinoma. *World J Surg* 1996;20:326–331.
32. Tanaka K, Nakamura S, Numata K, et al. Hepatocellular carcinoma: treatment with percutaneous ethanol injection and transcatheter arterial embolization. *Radiology* 1992;185:457–460.
33. Matsui O, Kadoya M, Yoshikawa J, et al. Small hepatocellular carcinoma: treatment with subsegmental transcatheter arterial embolization. *Radiology* 1993;188:79–83.
34. Yamakado K, Nakatsuka A, Tanaka N, et al. Long-term follow-up arterial chemoembolization combined with transportal ethanol injection used to treat hepatocellular carcinoma. *J Vasc Interv Radiol* 1999;10: 641–647.
35. Bartolozzi C, Lencioni R, Caramella D, et al. Treatment of large HCC: transcatheter arterial chemoembolization combined with percutaneous ethanol injection versus repeated transcatheter arterial chemoembolization. *Radiology* 1995;197:812–818.
36. Yamakado K, Hirano T, Kato N, et al. Hepatocellular carcinoma: treatment with a combination of transcatheter arterial chemoembolization and transportal ethanol injection. *Radiology* 1994;193:75–80.
37. Seki T, Tamai T, Nakagawa T, et al. Combination therapy with transcatheter arterial chemoembolization and percutaneous microwave coagulation therapy for hepatocellular carcinoma. *Cancer* 2000;89(6):1245–1251.
38. Pacella C, Bizzarri G, Cecconi P, et al. Hepatocellular carcinoma: long-term results of combined treatment with laser thermal ablation and transcatheter arterial chemoembolization. *Radiology* 2001;219:669–678.
39. Seong J, Keum KC, Han KH, et al. Combined transcatheter arterial chemoembolization and local radiotherapy of unresectable hepatocellular carcinoma. *Int J Radiat Oncol Biol Phys* 1999;43(2):393–397.
40. Cheng J, Chuang VP, Cheng SH, et al. Local radiotherapy with or without transcatheter arterial chemoembolization for patients with unresectable hepatocellular carcinoma. *Int J Radiat Oncol Biol Phys* 2000;47(2):435–442.
41. Rossi S, Garbagnati F, Lencioni R, et al. Percutaneous radio-frequency thermal ablation of nonresectable hepatocellular carcinoma after occlusion of tumor blood supply. *Radiology* 2000;217:119–126.
42. Chung Y-H, Song IH, Song B-C, et al. Combined therapy consisting of intraarterial cisplatin infusion and systemic interferon-α for hepatocellular carcinoma patients with major portal vein thrombosis or distant metastasis. *Cancer* 2000;88:1986–1991.
43. Registry of Hepatic Metastases. Resection of the liver for colorectal carcinoma metastases: a multi-institutional study of indications for resection. *Surgery* 1988;103(3):278–288.
44. Wagner JS, Adson MA, Van Heerden JA, Adson MH, Ilstrup DM. The natural history of hepatic metastases from colorectal cancer: a comparison with resective treatment. *Ann Surg* 1984;199(5):502–508.
45. Leichman CG, Jacobson JR, Modiano M, et al. Hepatic chemoembolization combined with systemic infusion of 5-fluorouracil and bolus leucovorin for patients with metastatic colorectal carcinoma. *Cancer* 1999;86(5):775–781.
46. Bavisotto LM, Patel NH, Althaus SJ, et al. Hepatic transcatheter arterial chemoembolization alternating with systemic protracted continuous infusion 5-fluorouracil for gastrointestinal malignancies metastatic to liver: a phase II trial of the Puget Sound Consortium (PSOC 1104). *Clin Cancer Res* 1999;5(1):95–109.
47. Tono T, Hasuike Y, Ohzato H, Takatsuka Y, Kikkawa N. Limited but definite efficacy of prophylactic hepatic arterial infusion chemotherapy after curative resection of colorectal liver metastases. *Cancer* 2000;88(7):1549–1556.
48. Kemeny N, Huang Y, Cohen AM, et al. Hepatic arterial infusion of chemotherapy after resection of hepatic metastases from colorectal cancer. *N Engl J Med* 1999;341(27):2039–2048.
49. Lorenz M, Muller H-H, Schramm H, et al. Randomized trial of surgery versus surgery followed by adjuvant hepatic arterial infusion with 5-fluorouracil and folinic acid for liver metastases of colorectal cancer. *Ann Surg* 1998;228(6):756–762.
50. Rose DM, Allegra DP, Bostick PJ, Foshag LJ, Bilchik AJ. Radiofrequency ablation: a novel primary and adjunctive ablative technique for hepatic malignancies. *Am Surg* 1999;65:1009–1014.
51. Elias D, Debaere T, Muttillo I, et al. Intraoperative use of radiofrequency treatment allows an increase in the rate of curative resection. *J Surg Oncol* 1998;67:190–191.

CHAPTER 14

VASCULAR INTERVENTIONS IN NONHEPATIC MALIGNANCIES

SANJAY GUPTA, MD

INTRODUCTION

Vascular interventional techniques used for management of malignant tumors include (1) embolization of the arterial supply of the tumor to induce ischemia and tumor necrosis, (2) regional intra-arterial infusion of cytotoxic or immunotherapeutic agents to enhance the tumoricidal effect, and (3) chemoembolization, a combination of the two aforementioned techniques. This chapter discusses some of the vascular interventional procedures commonly used in the management of various nonhepatic malignancies.

ARTERIAL EMBOLIZATION FOR RENAL CELL CARCINOMA

Indications

Since its introduction in the early 1970s, renal artery embolization has been widely used for preoperative and palliative ablation of renal cell carcinoma, but the use of this technique remains controversial.[1–7] Preoperative embolization is performed with the goal of facilitating surgical excision by reducing intraoperative blood loss and the duration of surgery. Palliative

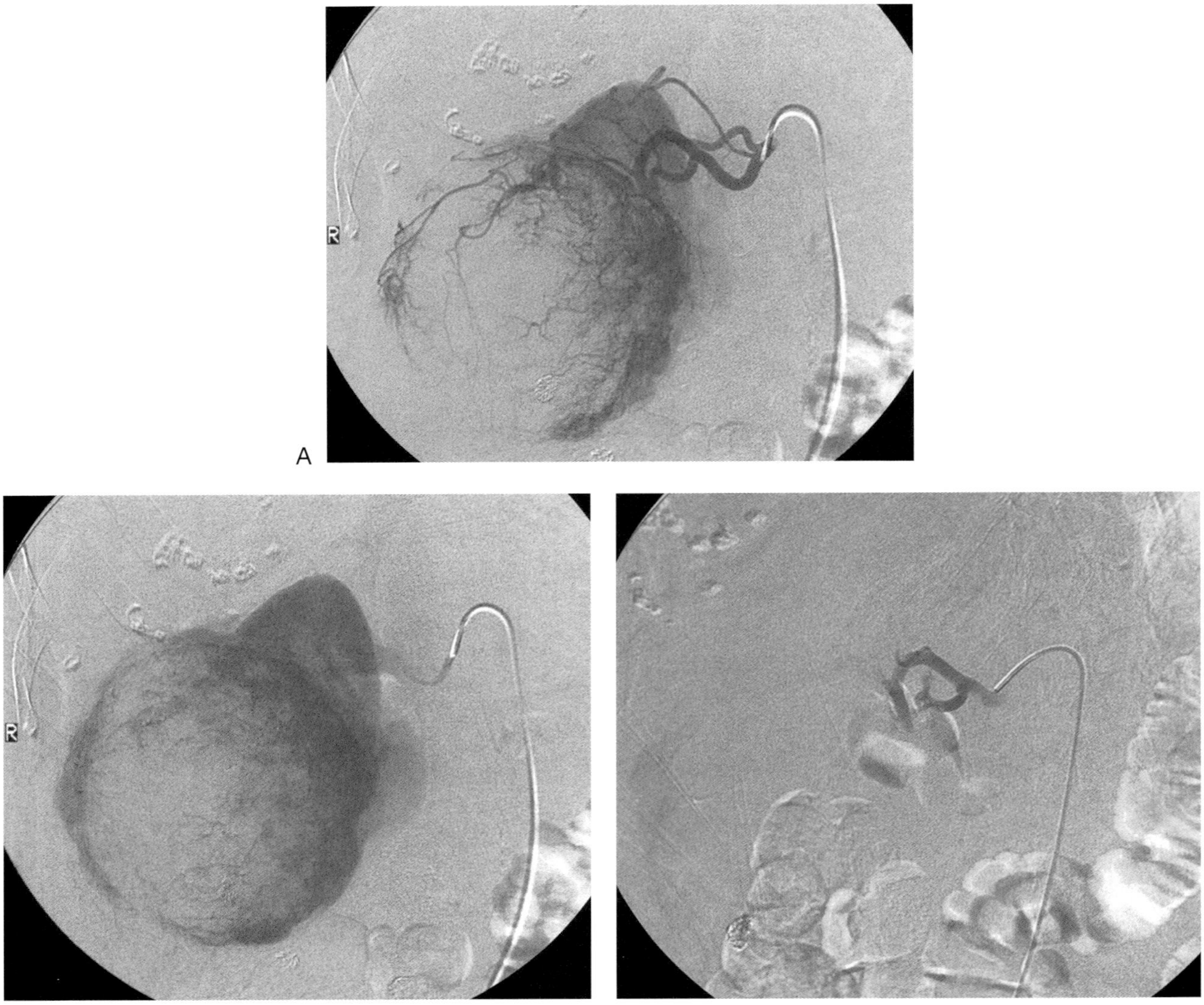

Figure 14-1. Preoperative embolization for renal cell carcinoma. (A and B) Selective renal arteriogram shows hypervascular tumor involving most of the right kidney. (C) Angiogram after embolization with polyvinyl alcohol (PVA) particles shows complete occlusion of the renal arteries.

embolization is performed in patients with nonresectable tumors in an attempt to control tumor-related signs and symptoms, such as hemorrhage, pain related to tumor bulk, polycythemia, hypercalcemia, congestive heart failure from large arteriovenous shunts, and hypertension.

Technical Considerations

Before arterial embolization is performed in a patient with renal cell carcinoma, non-selective abdominal aortography and selective renal arteriography are performed to evaluate the vascular anatomy and to identify all potential collateral blood supply to the tumor. Experimental studies have shown that central embolization of the renal artery alone results in incomplete tumor necrosis, which can be associated with recurrent hematuria and tumor progression. Embolization of the entire vascular bed of the tumor to the level of the capillaries is necessary to achieve good results. Usually the entire kidney is embolized (**Fig. 14-1**); however, selective embolization of branches supplying the tumor in an attempt to spare the normal renal parenchyma is preferable for palliation in patients with impaired renal function or neoplasm in a solitary kidney (**Fig. 14-2**).

Various embolic agents have been used for arterial embolization of renal cell carcinoma.[1–11] The choice of embolic agent depends on the interventional radiologist's experience with the agent, tumor vascularity, and the extent of arteriovenous shunting. In the presence of large arteriovenous shunting, embolization should be performed with sclerosing agents or larger particles. In rare cases, a balloon-occlusion catheter may be placed in the draining vein to prevent pulmonary embolization in patients with large arteriovenous shunts.

The most commonly used technique is embolization with particulate material—for example, absorbable gelatin sponge (Gelfoam), polyvinyl alcohol (PVA) particles, or, more recently, Endosphere® Microspheres (Biospheres Medical, Rockland, MA)—occasionally followed by coil embolization of the proximal renal artery. Coils are placed in the distal main renal artery or its branches to allow easy clamping and transection during surgery. Coils are occasionally used alone for renal artery occlusion in the presence of extensive arteriovenous shunting.

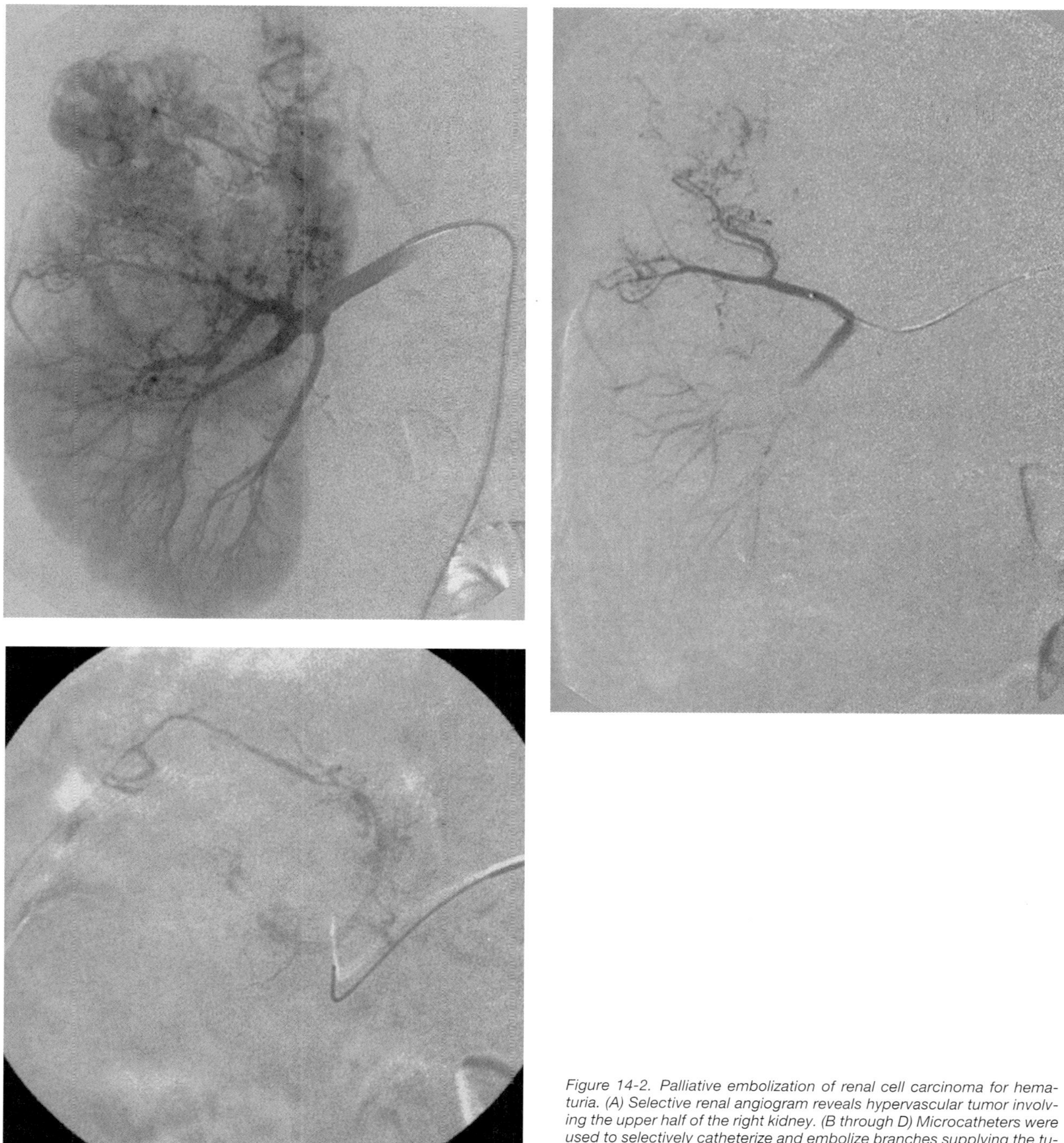

A B C

Figure 14-2. Palliative embolization of renal cell carcinoma for hematuria. (A) Selective renal angiogram reveals hypervascular tumor involving the upper half of the right kidney. (B through D) Microcatheters were used to selectively catheterize and embolize branches supplying the tumor. *(continued on next page)*

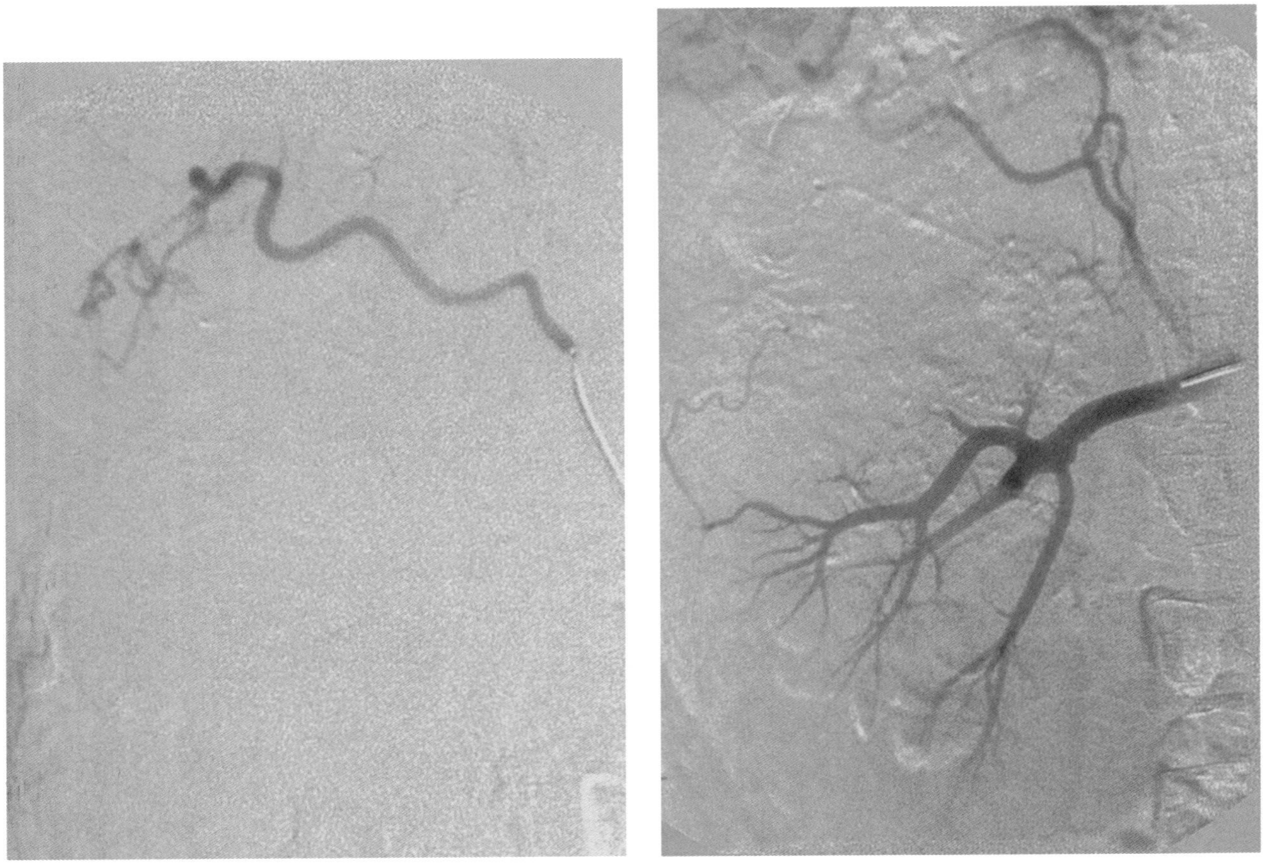

D E

Figure 14-2. (continued) (E) Postembolization angiogram shows occlusion of embolized vessels, absence of tumor blush, and preservation of arterial supply to the lower, uninvolved portion of the kidney.

Liquid agents such as ethanol, Ethibloc, (Ethicon Norderstedt, Germany) and n-butyl-2-cyanoacrylate (Histoacryl, B. Braun, Melsunger, Germany) can also be used for renal tumor embolization.[8–11] Ethanol is cheap, easily available in a sterile form, and easy to infuse through a small catheter. Ethanol is an excellent agent for ablation because it reaches the capillary level and causes necrosis of endothelium and perivascular tissue, sludging of erythrocytes, sloughing of endothelium, and microvascular occlusion, resulting in ischemic necrosis. Complications that can result from reflux of ethanol include mesenteric artery embolism, spinal cord ischemia, and thrombosis of the inferior vena cava, all of which can be avoided with the use of a balloon occlusion catheter.[7, 12, 13] The occlusion balloon should be placed in the midportion of the renal artery distal to the origin of the adrenal and gonadal arteries. Intra-arterial administration of lidocaine can be used to decrease the pain during embolization. A test injection of contrast material through the balloon-occlusion catheter is used to estimate the volume of ethanol needed for embolization. The balloon-occlusion catheter should be kept inflated for about 5 minutes after ethanol infusion. Ethibloc is a saturated alcoholic solution of corn protein mixed with radiopaque iodized oil.[11] After intravascular injection, its ethanol component diffuses, and the Ethibloc precipitates. Ethibloc should also be administered via a balloon-occlusion catheter.

In general, nephrectomy is performed within 24 to 48 hours of embolization to take maximum advantage of the infarction-induced edematous rim around the kidney and also to reduce the distress from postembolization syndrome. Delay of more than 3 days can make surgery difficult because of an increase in collateral circulation.

Complications

Postembolization syndrome, consisting of fever, flank pain, nausea, vomiting, and leukocytosis, is the most common side effect of arterial embolization for renal cell carcinoma and typically occurs 1 to 3 days after the procedure. Symptoms are managed with supportive care and usually resolve after several days. Although some researchers have reported that ethanol embolization may be associated with a milder syndrome compared with other agents, other investigators have not had a similar experience.[8] Gas in the embolized tumor is not uncommonly seen on follow-up imaging; it is the result of either tissue necrosis or air introduced during the embolization procedure and does not necessarily indicate infection.[14]

Major complications are relatively uncommon. Renal failure, renal abscess formation, and transient hypertension during or immediately after the procedure have been reported.[7] Unintentional embolization of nontarget organs, such as the bowel, spinal cord, contralateral kidney, and testes, as a result of either reflux of embolic agent into the aorta or passage of embolic agent through the collateral circulation, is a potential complication. However, this complication is uncommon and can be avoided by scrupulous attention to technique on the part of the interventional radiologist.

Results

Preoperative Embolization

Large, hypervascular renal cell carcinomas usually have dilated tortuous veins covering the surface of the tumor and the renal hilum. Access to the renal artery during surgery may be impeded by these large collateral veins or by tumor thrombus in the renal vein or inferior vena cava. Preoperative arterial embolization with resultant collapse of the veins may facilitate surgery. Although some surgeons believe that embolization produces a plane of edema around the infarcted kidney, facilitating nephrectomy and reducing the operating time, this concept is not universally accepted. Klimberg et al.[10] reported a shorter operating time for nephrectomy after embolization compared with previous studies reporting nephrectomy in non-embolized tumors. However, Mebust et al.[4] found no operating time advantage for preoperative embolization.

The role of preoperative embolization in reducing blood loss during surgery is also controversial. Although some studies have shown reduced intraoperative blood loss after embolization, other studies did not find any significant difference in blood loss between embolization and non-embolization groups. In a study comparing 24 patients who underwent arterial embolization before surgery with 69 patients who did not, Bakal et al.[1] concluded that embolization significantly reduced the volume of blood transfused during nephrectomy for large hypervascular renal cell carcinomas. However, Lanigan et al.[3], in a survey of 210 urologists in Britain and Ireland, found that only 7% of urologists supported the use of preoperative embolization for renal cell carcinomas. In the same study, these investigators also evaluated 70 patients who underwent nephrectomy for renal cell carcinoma (35 with and 40 without embolization) and found that embolization did not reduce operative blood loss and actually prolonged the hospital stay.

At The University of Texas M. D. Anderson Cancer Center, preoperative arterial embolization is only occasionally performed for patients with renal cell carcinoma, usually those with a large vena caval thrombus.[7] In patients with extension of tumor thrombus into the renal vein or inferior vena cava, preoperative arterial embolization may decrease the size and extent of the thrombus, facilitating surgery.

Palliative Embolization

Transcatheter arterial embolization may be performed for palliation of tumor-related signs and symptoms in patients with renal cell carcinoma who are not candidates for surgery because of their general medical condition or the extent of metastatic disease. Palliative embolization has been used with varying degrees of success for control of hemorrhage, flank pain, polycythemia, hypertension, hypercalcemia, and congestive heart failure resulting from arteriovenous shunting.[1–7] Kalman and Varenhorst,[2] reviewing all the available literature on arterial embolization for renal cell carcinoma published between 1973 and 1997, concluded that although a small group of patients with massive hematuria, flank pain, or paraneoplastic syndrome may benefit from palliative embolization, the effectiveness of this procedure in symptom palliation awaits validation.

Other Uses of Embolization

A report from M. D. Anderson Cancer Center suggested that embolization-induced tumor necrosis might stimulate the immune system and that a 4- to 7-day delay between embolization and nephrectomy might allow the body to produce tumor antibodies, which might cause regression of metastases.[5] This idea, although attractive, remains to be proven. In another study by Sella et al.[15], embolization was found to be as effective as nephrectomy in reducing the tumor bulk; also, the reduction in tumor bulk enhanced the efficacy of chemoimmunotherapy for metastases.

ARTERIAL EMBOLIZATION FOR BONE METASTASES

Indications and Results

Transcatheter arterial embolization for hypervascular bone metastases is generally performed preoperatively to reduce blood loss during surgery. Embolization is also used for inhibition of tumor growth and for palliation of pain or bleeding in patients with unresectable tumors.[16–22]

Preoperative arterial embolization has been reported for bone metastases from renal cell, thyroid, breast, melanoma, and lung malignancies. Hypervascular bone metastases are seen in 30% to 45% of patients with renal cell and thyroid carcinoma,[16] which are by far the most commonly embolized bone metastases. Surgical treatment is indicated in patients with pathologic fracture or impending fracture, in patients with spinal cord compression, in patients in whom radiation therapy has failed to control symptoms, and in patients with intractable pain unresponsive to other therapies. However, owing to the hypervascular nature of these lesions, surgical intervention can be complicated by excessive, uncontrollable bleeding. Arterial embolization before surgery has been shown to significantly reduce intraoperative blood loss.

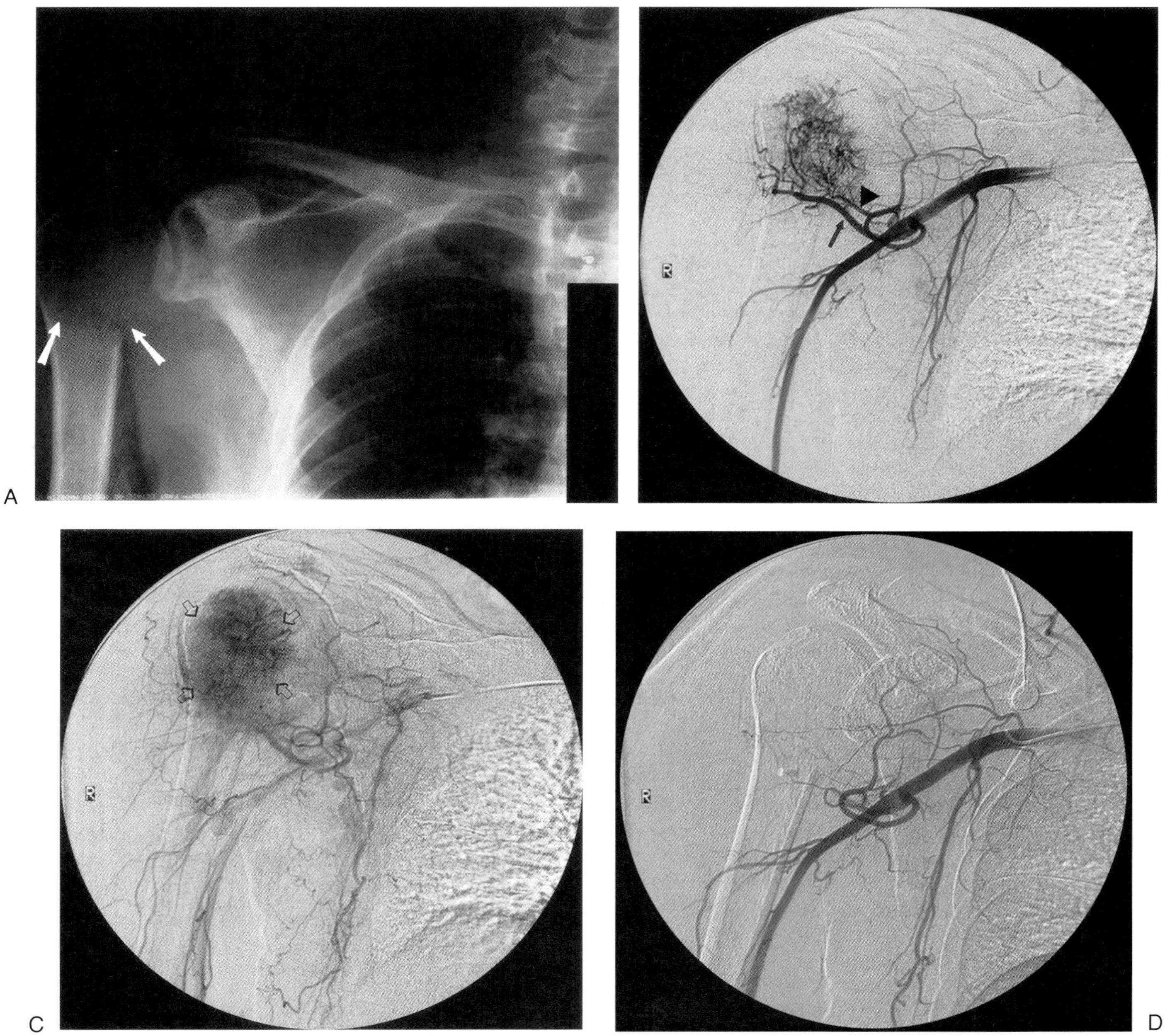

Figure 14-3. Embolization of bone metastases from renal cell carcinoma. (A) Plain radiograph shows large osteolytic lesion (arrows) involving the right humerus. (B and C) Early and late arterial phases of a right subclavian angiogram shows a hypervascular tumor with dense tumor stain (open arrows) supplied by anterior (arrow) and posterior (arrowhead) circumflex humeral branches of the axillary artery.

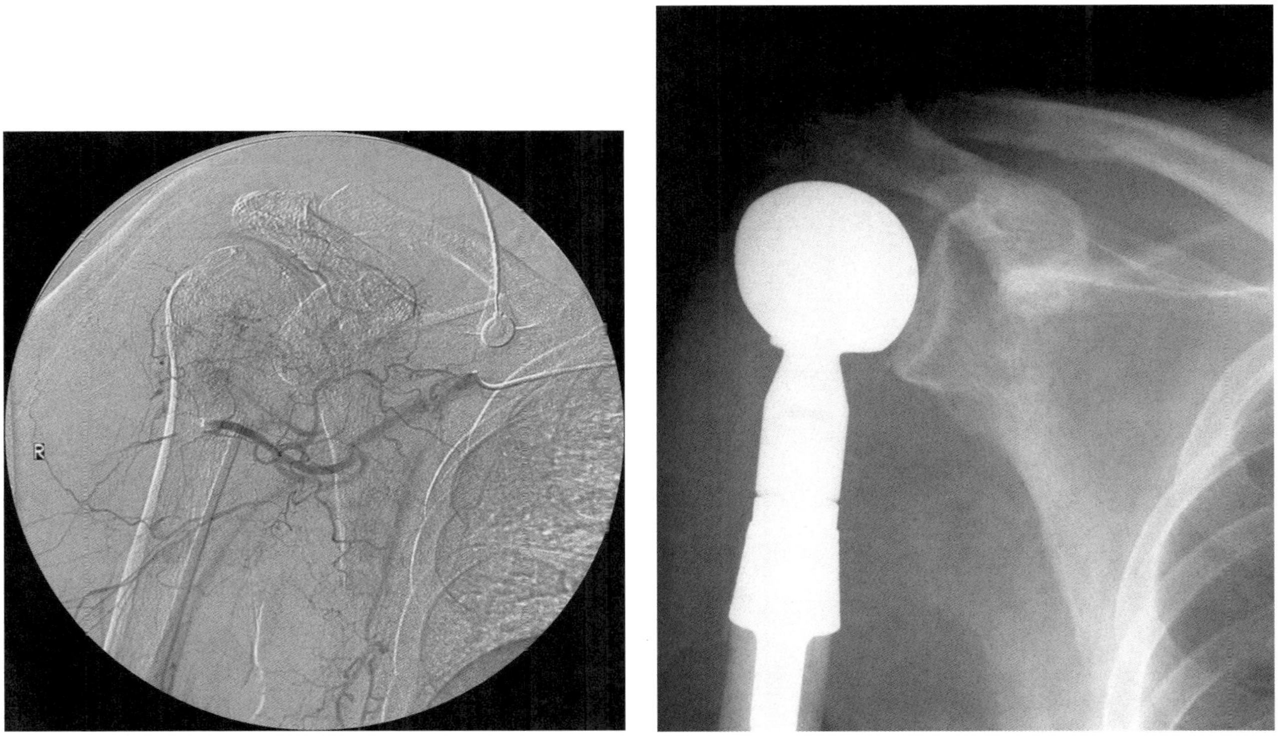

E F

Figure 14-3. (continued) (D and E) Early and late arterial phases of angiogram obtained after superselective embolization of circumflex humeral arteries with polyvinyl alcohol (PVA) particles shows occlusion of the embolized vessels and significant reduction in tumor stain. (F) Patient underwent surgical resection followed within 24 hours by prosthetic reconstruction, with minimal blood loss.

Technical Considerations

A pre-embolization angiogram should be obtained to assess the vascularity of the tumor and to identify all the major vessels supplying it. Many studies have shown that metastases that are less than completely embolized are associated with significantly greater operative blood loss than those that are completely devascularized.[16, 17, 19] Hence, attempts should be made to embolize all arterial feeders to the metastasis (**Figs. 14-3 and 14-4**). A postembolization angiogram that includes all possible collateral pathways should be obtained because small nonembolized feeders may become more prominent after occlusion of the major vessels supplying the metastases.

The choice of embolic agent depends on the tumor location, the anatomic relationship between the tumor and the adjacent organs, the preference of the interventional radiologist, the presence and size of arteriovenous fistula, and the purpose of the occlusion. Almost all available embolic agents—including particulate material, liquid agents, and metal coils—have been used for embolization of bone metastases, with similar results.[16–22] Although coils have been used as the only embolic agent, most investigators believe that only proximal embolization of feeding vessels without embolization of tumor capillary bed is ineffective. Hence, coils are typically used for proximal vessel occlusion after distal embolization with particulate or liquid material.

Ideally, surgery should be performed within 24 hours after embolization to prevent revascularization of the tumor from collateral vessels. This timing is especially important when temporary embolic agents such as absorbable gelatin sponge (Gelfoam) is used for embolization, because resorption of such agents and subsequent recanalization can occur after this time. Even with a permanent or semipermanent agent like polyvinyl alcohol (PVA) or Embospheres® Microspheres, surgery should not be delayed for more than 3 days, because hypervascular tumors can recruit collateral vessels.

Complications

Postembolization syndrome, the most common side effect of arterial embolization for treatment of bone metastases, generally subsides completely within 3 to 5 days after therapy.[16–18, 20] Reported complications include nontarget embolization, skin necrosis, and ischemic ulcers.[20] Although complications can be greatly reduced by adherence to proper technique,

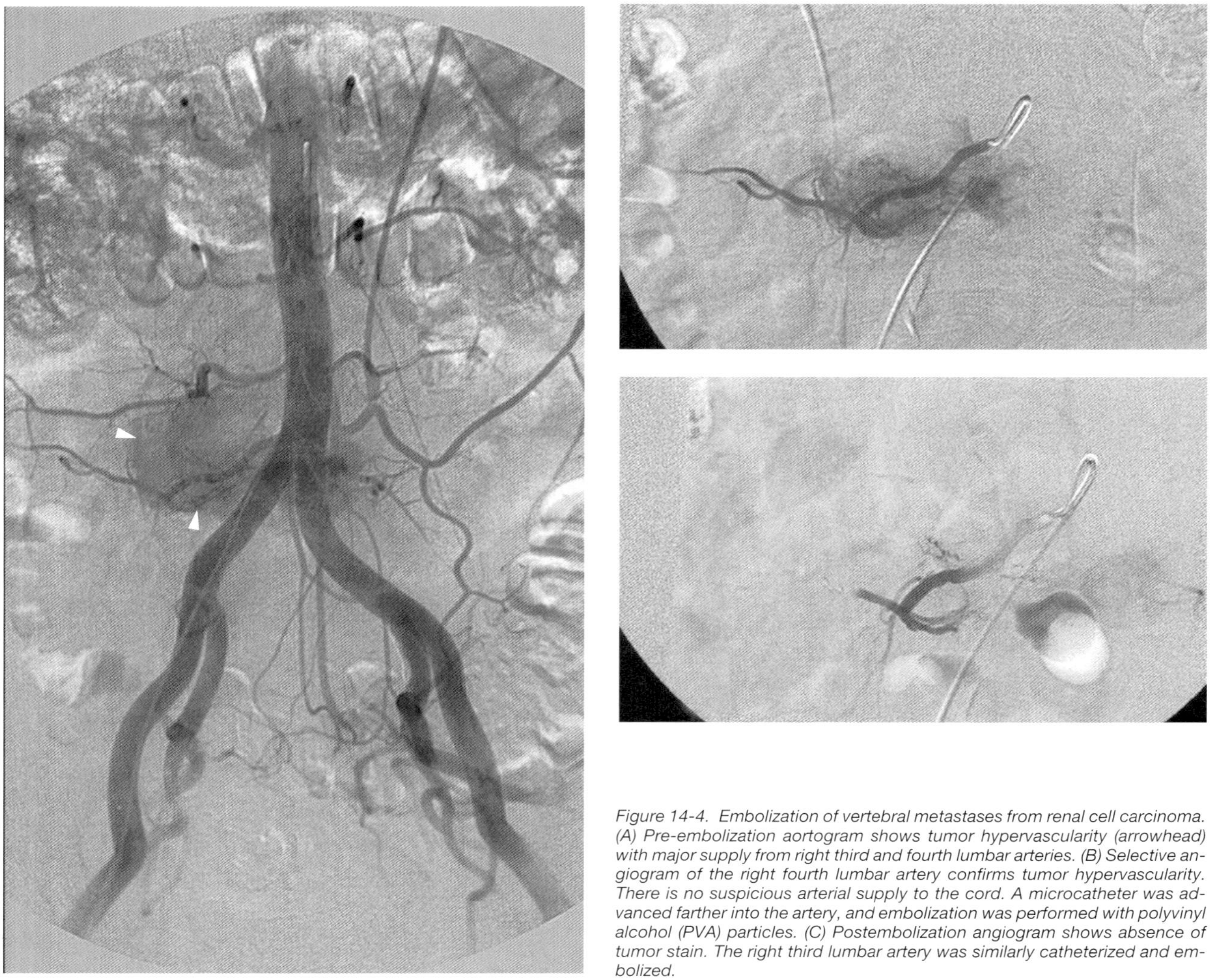

A B C

Figure 14-4. Embolization of vertebral metastases from renal cell carcinoma. (A) Pre-embolization aortogram shows tumor hypervascularity (arrowhead) with major supply from right third and fourth lumbar arteries. (B) Selective angiogram of the right fourth lumbar artery confirms tumor hypervascularity. There is no suspicious arterial supply to the cord. A microcatheter was advanced farther into the artery, and embolization was performed with polyvinyl alcohol (PVA) particles. (C) Postembolization angiogram shows absence of tumor stain. The right third lumbar artery was similarly catheterized and embolized.

risks are higher in certain anatomic locations. Vertebral tumor embolization can result in spinal cord ischemia due to reflux of embolic agent or embolization of unrecognized arterial supply to the cord.[16, 19, 21] During pelvic embolization, occlusion of neural vessels supplying the sciatic nerve can cause ischemic neuropathy; this complication can be prevented by sparing of the inferior gluteal artery during embolization.[16, 23] Also, muscle branches of the superior gluteal artery should be avoided to prevent buttock claudication or necrosis. Coil embolization can be done before particle embolization of the feeders to avoid inadvertent embolization of peripheral normal tissue. Occasionally, a large anastomosis between the inferior gluteal or the obturator arteries and the femoral artery may allow particles to escape into the femoral artery and its branches. To prevent ischemic complications, the size of the embolic particles should be adjusted to the size of these collateral vessels.

REGIONAL INTRA-ARTERIAL INFUSION OF CHEMOTHERAPY

Regional intra-arterial infusion of chemotherapy has the advantage of delivering a high concentration of chemotherapeutic agents directly into the tumor bed with minimal systemic toxicity. This advantage is mainly secondary to intratumoral first-pass extraction. Intra-arterial chemotherapy has been most commonly used for hepatic and musculoskeletal malignancies. Regional chemotherapy has also been used for other malignancies, including breast, stomach, lung, pancreas, pelvic, and head and neck tumors; however, experience with regional intra-arterial chemotherapy for such tumors is limited and the effectiveness of the therapy has not yet been proven.

Osseous and Soft Tissue Sarcomas

Over the past two decades, the surgical treatment of high-grade osseous and soft tissue sarcomas of the extremity has changed considerably, amputation largely being supplanted by limb-sparing surgery. This change in therapeutic practice has been brought about by the use of a multimodality approach that combines surgery with preoperative chemotherapy and radiation therapy. Preoperative chemotherapy is intended to eradicate distant micrometastases, which are already present at the time of initial diagnosis in the majority of patients, and also to control the local tumor. Unfortunately, with preoperative systemic chemotherapy, primary tumor response rates are disappointing, with no significant improvement in limb salvage rates. Radiation therapy has been shown to achieve local tumor control in 70% to 100% of patients.[24] However, wound complications and limb dysfunction secondary to radiation-induced necrosis and fibrosis can be major problems with potentially therapeutic doses, and attempts to reduce the dose to avoid local toxicity have had a negative impact on local tumor control. In this context, intra-arterial infusion of chemotherapy has been advocated to achieve more effective local tumor control.

Intra-arterial infusion results in higher local drug concentrations than standard intravenous infusion, leading to greater tumor necrosis. At the same time, the drug escaping the local area can potentially provide systemic tumoricidal effects. In a study from M. D. Anderson Cancer Center, Stewart et al.[25] found that systemic blood levels after intra-arterial infusion of cisplatin were equivalent to those after intravenous administration, but local levels were 1.5 to 4 times higher. Generally, however, intra-arterial chemotherapy is combined with intravenous chemotherapy to achieve adequate local and systemic effects.

Intra-Arterial Chemotheraphy in Osteosarcomas

Intra-arterial chemotherapy has been most commonly used for the treatment of osteosarcomas. Results of various studies suggest that regional intra-arterial chemotherapy is effective in inducing local tumor regression in patients with osteosarcoma, permitting limb-sparing surgery in the majority of these patients without adversely affecting either the local recurrence rate or long-term survival.[26, 27]

Of the various agents with proven activity against osteosarcomas, cisplatin is the drug most commonly used for intra-arterial infusion. Doxorubicin is associated with a high risk of local complications; hence, it can be infused only in large vessels. Ifosfamide requires hepatic activation before becoming effective. Intra-arterial administration of methotrexate has no added advantage, because large doses can be safely given systemically [28]

In a study from the M. D. Anderson Cancer Center, comprising 96 patients with extremity osteosarcomas treated with intravenous doxorubicin and intra-arterial cisplatin, the limb salvage rate increased from 8% to 80% as a direct result of the response to chemotherapy.[26] A ≥90% tumor necrosis was seen in 68% of the tumors. The local recurrence rate was only 6%, which is less than that seen after amputation. The 5-year disease-free survival rate was around 60%, similar to that seen after amputation and adjuvant chemotherapy. Similar results were reported by Picci et al.[27] from Istituto Rizzoli in Italy, who treated 144 patients with systemic methotrexate and doxorubicin along with intra-arterial cisplatin before resection. The limb salvage rate increased to 91% (from a rate of only 4% seen without preoperative therapy), and the local recurrence rate was only 1.5%.

The controlled, prospective COSS 86 study conducted by Winkler et al.[29] did not demonstrate any increase in local tumor response to intra-arterial cisplatin compared with systemic cisplatin; the percentage of tumors showing more than 90% necrosis was similar in the two groups (68% in the intra-arterial group and 69% in the intravenous group). This study, however, used only two courses of preoperative intra-arterial cisplatin; Jeff et al.[30] found that more than three cycles are needed to achieve good results.

Although the value of regional chemotherapy is still disputed by some investigators, most institutions use preoperative regional intra-arterial chemotherapy as part of the multimodality treatment regimen for patients with osteosarcomas.

Intra-arterial Chemotherapy in Soft Tissue Sarcomas

Experience with the use of regional chemotherapy for nonosseous soft tissue sarcomas is limited. Azzarelli et al.[31] treated 101 patients with large soft tissue sarcomas with two cycles of preoperative intra-arterial doxorubicin. Limb salvage was achieved in 80% of patients, and the 5-year survival rate was 54%. However, the local recurrence rate was high, at 29%. In the series reported by Soulen et al.[32], in which 15 patients with very large high-grade sarcomas were treated with intra-arterial chemotherapy using a combination of multiple chemotherapeutic agents, limb-sparing resection was possible in 87% of patients. Eighty percent to 100%

necrosis was seen in 11 of the 15 tumors. These limited studies suggest that intra-arterial chemotherapy has a potential role in the treatment of soft tissue sarcomas, but its effectiveness is yet to be determined.

Technique and Complications of Intra-arterial Chemotherapy in the Extremities

When intra-arterial chemotherapy is administered for tumors in the extremities, a site remote from the involved extremity—the femoral artery for upper extremity tumors and the contralateral femoral artery for lower extremity tumors—is selected for arterial access. Initially, diagnostic arteriography is performed to delineate the vascular supply to the tumor. Most extremity sarcomas are supplied by multiple feeders; for infusion of chemotherapy, a 4F or 5F straight endhole catheter can be used with the tip positioned proximal to the multiple branches supplying the tumor. If the tumor is supplied by a single vessel, that vessel can be catheterized for infusion.

Curved or angled catheter tip configurations should be avoided to decrease the chances for the tip of the catheter migrating into a side branch.[33] Also, the tip of a curved catheter may abut the vessel wall, possibly leading to chemotherapy-induced endothelial injury. A microcatheter placed coaxially through the 5F catheter may be used for tumors in the distal extremity. Another potential problem with the use of endhole catheters for infusion is inhomogeneous distribution of the infused chemotherapeutic agent because of laminar flow and streaming. This may result in the flow of a large portion of the drug into a side branch supplying normal tissue, leading to necrosis of this tissue. A pulsatile pump, which infuses in short bursts, creating turbulence and disrupting laminar flow, can be used to allow better mixing and a more homogenous distribution of chemotherapeutic agents.[33]

At M. D. Anderson Cancer Center, we use multi–sidehole infusion catheters or infusion wires placed coaxially through 4F or 5F guide catheters, with the sideholes aligned to include the multiple branches feeding the tumor (**Fig. 14-5**). Exit of the chemotherapeutic agent from the multiple sideholes allows for better mixing with the flowing blood. Also, because these catheters do not have any endhole, migration of the catheter tip into a side branch would not have serious side effects.

After catheter placement, a nuclear flow study may be performed to ensure adequate distribution of the drug to the tumor.[33] This is especially important when end-hole catheters are used, to make sure that the tip is not lodged in a side branch. Studies conducted at M. D. Anderson Cancer Center have shown that angiographic demonstration of a decrease in tumor vascularity correlates reasonably well with the histologic response; angiography can therefore be used to monitor response to treatment (see Fig. 14-5).[33, 34]

Localized drug deposition in the muscles can lead to muscle spasm or necrosis. Deposition of chemotherapeutic agents in the skin and subcutaneous tissues can lead to necrosis, manifesting as pain, erythema, induration, and ulceration. These manifestations are uncommon and, if mild, can be managed with aspirin and localized application of heat. However, painful myositis or dermatitis should prompt cessation of chemotherapy and removal or repositioning of the catheter to prevent further damage.[33, 35] Myocutaneous inflammatory changes are more common with intra-arterial administration of doxorubicin than of cisplatin.

The rate of catheter-related complications rises with the duration of infusion. Arterial thrombosis requiring termination of therapy, thrombectomy, bypass, or even amputation has been reported, mostly after prolonged infusion of multiple agents.[33, 35] Other reported complications are venous thrombosis, catheter dislodgment, catheter occlusion, and fever requiring catheter removal.

Pancreatic Cancer

The majority of pancreatic cancers are unresectable at the time of diagnosis. Treatment of unresectable tumors with systemic chemotherapy and/or radiation therapy has been unsatisfactory. One of the reasons for the ineffectiveness of systemic chemotherapy is the inadequate delivery of the anticancer drug to the tumor because of the hypovascularity of pancreatic tumors. Regional intra-arterial chemotherapy has been attempted as a means of increasing the local drug concentration.

Different delivery techniques have been evaluated for arterial infusion for pancreatic cancer: celiac axis infusion, abdominal aortic infusion, gastroduodenal or splenic artery infusion, and arterial infusion combined with vena caval hemofiltration. Because the pancreas is supplied by multiple branches from the celiac, superior mesenteric, and splenic arteries, infusion into the celiac artery or aorta results in inadequate delivery of drug to the tumor. Homma et al.[36] described a novel intra-arterial infusion technique involving superselective coil embolization of all pancreatic blood vessels except those arising from the splenic artery, followed by placement of an infusion catheter into the splenic artery. These investigators believe that hemodynamic changes resulting from vascular redistribution after embolization lead to better delivery of drug to the local tumor. Splenic artery infusion also allows the chemotherapeutic agent to flow into the portal vein via the splenic vein, serving as intraportal chemotherapy for liver metastases.

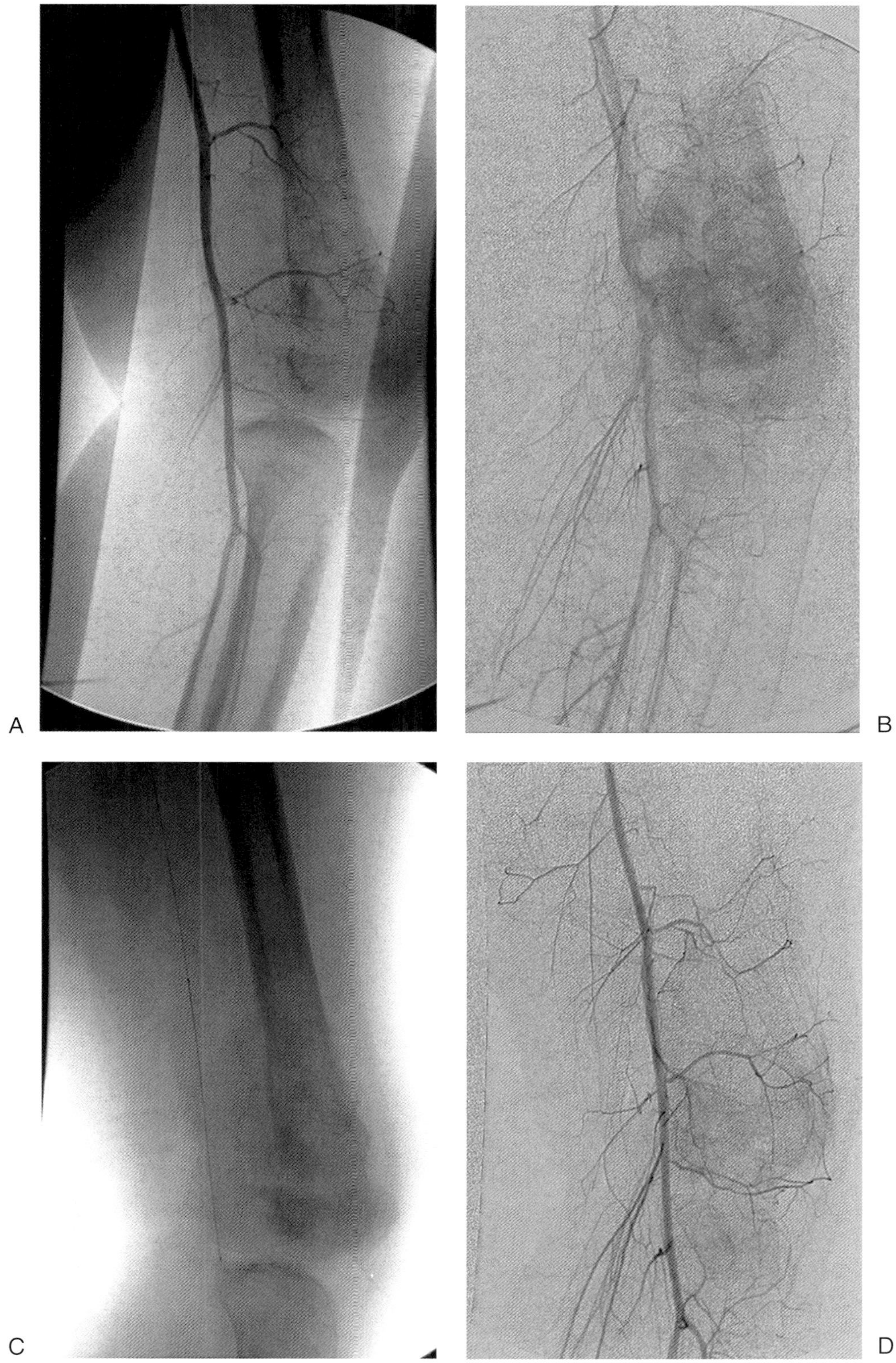

Figure 14-5. Intra-arterial chemotherapy for osteosarcoma of the femur. (A and B) Angiogram reveals hypervascular tumor in the distal femur with multiple feeders from the popliteal artery. (C) Multi–sidehole infusion wire advanced coaxially through the 5F catheter was placed in the popliteal artery with the infusion segment positioned to include the major vessels supplying the tumor. (D) Angiogram after two courses of chemotherapy shows significant reduction in tumor vascularity.

Although the data on intra-arterial chemotherapy in pancreatic cancer are limited, results from small, non-randomized studies suggest that pancreatic cancer is sensitive to regional chemotherapy.[36–38] Muchmore et al.[37] treated 12 patients with unresectable, locally advanced pancreatic tumors using celiac artery infusion of mitomycin C and fluorouracil, along with hemofiltration in the inferior vena cava. A partial response was seen in five patients, stable disease in six patients, and progression of disease in one patient. Curative resection was possible in one of the four patients who underwent a surgical reexploration. Homma et al.[36] reported a response rate of 73.9% and a mean survival of 18 months in their series of 23 patients treated with splenic artery infusion of fluorouracil and cisplatin.

Bronchogenic Cancer

Limited data are available describing bronchial artery infusion for lung cancer.[39–41] Bronchial artery infusion has been used primarily for centrally located, early stage lung cancer in patients who are not candidates for surgery. In 1990, Watanabe et al[41] reported a study in which 106 patients with stage IIIA and IIIB lung cancer were treated with bronchial artery infusion; response rates of 40% and 84% with single-agent and multi-agent infusions, respectively, were achieved. The only complication encountered was transient hemiplegia in one patient. In the study reported by Neyazaki et al.[39], 27 patients (stage of cancer not mentioned) were treated with up to four separate infusions of mitomycin C, and a decrease in tumor size was observed in 14 patients. Chemical pneumonitis was seen in two patients, and erythema was seen in one patient.

In a later study, Osaki et al.[40] treated seven patients with centrally located, early stage squamous cell lung carcinoma using a bronchial artery infusion of cisplatin. All lesions showed complete remission within 1 to 6 weeks, and six patients had no disease relapse at a median follow-up time of 19.8 months. Three patients experienced bronchial ulcers, and one patient died of pulmonary hemorrhage 3 months after bronchial artery infusion. From the available data, it appears that bronchial artery infusion of chemotherapeutic agents is technically feasible, is relatively safe, and can produce radiologic and clinical responses. However, more studies are needed to assess the clinical usefulness of this therapy.

Pelvic Malignancies

Regional intra-arterial chemotherapy has been used for the treatment of various pelvic malignancies, including uterine cervical cancer, bladder tumors, prostate cancer, vaginal cancer, and recurrent rectal cancer. The use of intra-arterial chemotherapy in the management of patients with uterine cervical and bladder carcinoma is discussed later, because this treatment has been used most often for these two malignancies.

Uterine Cervical Carcinoma

Uterine cervical carcinoma is one of the most common malignancies in women. Neoadjuvant chemotherapy is highly effective for patients with locally advanced cervical carcinoma and has been shown to improve the response rate and also the survival rate in such patients. Pelvic intra-arterial infusion therapy has been advocated to maximize the efficacy of the chemotherapeutic drugs. Cisplatin, either alone or in combination with other agents, is the drug most commonly used for intra-arterial infusion. Several studies have reported that intra-arterial infusion chemotherapy, especially in combination with radical surgery, is useful in the management of advanced uterine cervical carcinoma. Kigawa et al.[42], who treated 25 patients with stage IIB to IIIB uterine cervical carcinoma using intra-arterial cisplatin and bleomycin followed by surgery or radiation therapy, achieved a clinical response rate of 80% and an operability rate of 72%. The 3-year survival rate for the patients who underwent surgery was 85.7%.

Nagata et al.[43] treated 97 patients with cervical cancer with two to three sessions of bilateral internal arterial infusion therapy using cisplatin, doxorubicin, mitomycin, and fluorouracil followed by radical hysterectomy in 75 patients, radiation therapy in 12 patients, and no further treatment in the other 10 patients, who had distant metastases at surgery. The overall 5-year survival rates for the patients with stages I, II, and III disease were 93.3%, 58.7%, and 69.7%, respectively. The 5-year survival rates for the patients with stages I, II, and III disease who underwent surgery were 100%, 60.5%, and 63.6%, respectively. Also, histologic evaluation of the resected specimens indicated that arterial infusion therapy might have caused "downstaging" of tumors.

In patients with advanced cervical cancer and distant metastases, intra-arterial chemotherapy may be combined with systemic chemotherapy to achieve adequate control of distant disease. Also, some investigators advocate the use of uterine artery embolization after chemotherapy infusion to enhance the local therapeutic effect. Adachi et al.[44] achieved an overall response rate of 100% in their series of 15 patients with advanced cervical cancer (stages I to IV) who were treated with intravenous nedaplatin and intra-arterial cisplatin infusion followed by uterine artery embolization. Motoyama et al.[45] reported the use of super-high-dose intra-arterial cisplatin infusion (140 to 240 mg/m^2) with extracorporeal chemofiltration to increase the antitumor effect and reduce systemic toxicity. Outcomes were as follows: overall radiologic tumor response rate, 95%; tumor "downstaging" rate, 85%; histologic response rate, 95%; and percentage of patients undergoing radical surgery after two courses of the treatment, 70%. There were no serious side effects.

Urinary Bladder Cancer

Intra-arterial chemotherapy has been used in patients with locally invasive bladder cancer in an attempt to improve both local control and survival rates while maintaining normal bladder function. Results of several studies suggest that a high tumor response rate with bladder preservation can be achieved by intra-arterial chemotherapy plus radiation therapy in patients with muscle-invasive bladder cancer.[46–50] In their series of 104 patients with muscle-invasive bladder cancer treated with intra-arterial cisplatin in combination with radiation therapy, Eapen et al.[46] reported a complete response rate of 90% and a bladder preservation rate of 74%. Mokarim et al.[47] treated 35 patients with muscle-invasive (clinical stage, T2–T4N0M0) bladder carcinoma with intra-arterial cisplatin and doxorubicin followed by radiation therapy. These researchers observed complete response in 26 patients (74%), in all of whom the bladder was preserved.

Intra-arterial cisplatin is readily taken up by the tumor, thereby minimizing the systemic toxicity. Hence, it can also be used as an alternative treatment modality for patients with bladder cancer who are not candidates for systemic chemotherapy. Ganaha et al.[49] used intra-arterial cisplatin and radiotherapy to treat 13 patients with residual invasive bladder cancer after transurethral resection; all of the patients were considered unsuitable candidates for systemic chemotherapy because of age, performance status, poor renal function, or preexisting other malignancy. Complete response was achieved in seven patients (54%). Cause-specific and disease-free survival rates at 4 years were 85% and 28%, respectively. The regimen was well tolerated, with no dose-limiting toxic events. Intra-arterial chemotherapy has also been successfully used as a preoperative adjuvant chemotherapy with the aim of "downstaging" tumor in patients diagnosed as having stage T2 and T3a tumor or stage T1, multiple, large tumors that would be difficult to treat with transurethral resection.[50]

Technique and Complications of Intra-Arterial Chemotherapy for Pelvic Malignancies

For intra-arterial chemotherapy for pelvic malignancies, iliac artery infusion is generally preferred over superselective (e.g., uterine or vesical arteries) infusion because of the presence of collateral supply to the tumor from other branches of the internal iliac artery in a significant number of patients and also because internal iliac artery infusion allows the chemotherapeutic agent to reach the regional lymph nodes. Unilateral or bilateral arterial infusion is performed, depending on the location and vascular supply of the tumor. The infusion catheter is introduced via an ipsilateral or contralateral common femoral arteral access and its tip is positioned in either the internal iliac (hypogastric) artery or the anterior division of the internal iliac artery (**Fig. 14-6**). The tip of the catheter should be distal to the lateral sacral artery to avoid infusion to the sacral plexus. The proximal portion of the superior and inferior gluteal arteries can be embolized with coils to maximize the drug dose to the tumor and also to reduce the risk of muscle or skin necrosis and neurotoxic side effects that may result from infusion of chemotherapeutic agents into the territories of these vessels. Radionuclide angiography with technetium 99m–macroaggregated albumin may be performed after catheter placement to confirm the selective drug distribution to the tumor.

Some investigators advocate the use of balloon-occlusion catheters to infuse the chemotherapeutic agent into both internal iliac arteries to achieve higher local drug concentration as well as reduced systemic toxicity.[50] For bilateral infusion, the dose allocation of the chemotherapeutic agent is based on the laterality and vascularity of the tumor as judged from diagnostic angiography. Ganaha et al.[49] described the use of an

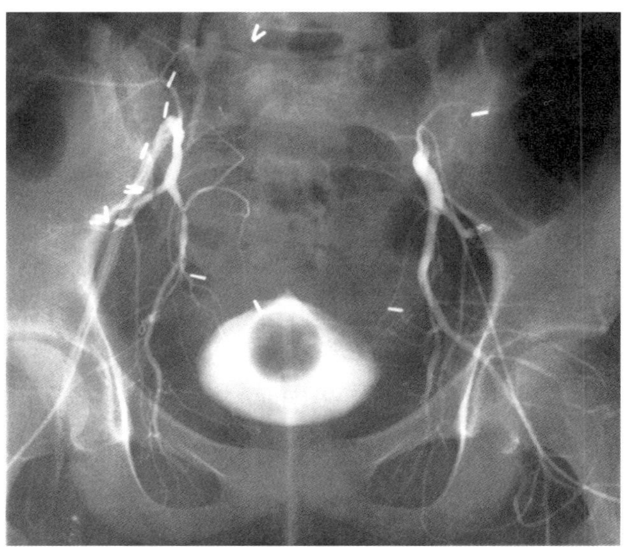

Figure 14-6. Intra-arterial chemotherapy in a patient with cervical carcinoma. This frontal angiogram shows bilateral internal iliac catheters placed via ipsilateral common femoral arterial access. Bilateral superior gluteal arteries (arrows) and right inferior gluteal artery (arrowhead) were embolized with coils before infusion.

indwelling catheter connected to a subcutaneously implantable port to achieve prolonged chemoinfusion in patients with bladder cancer.

Pelvic intra-arterial chemotherapy can be associated with local side effects. Transient rash, buttock pain and ulceration, transient neuropathies involving the sacral or femoral nerves and resulting in numbness and paresthesia, and, rarely, paralysis and muscle atrophy of the lower extremities and hip have been described.[50, 51] Sugimoto et al.[51] reported that balloon-occlusion catheter infusion of both internal iliac arteries can cause cystitis and, rarely, bladder wall necrosis because of the high anticancer drug concentration in the bladder wall. In their series of 22 patients treated with 34 courses of balloon-occlusion catheter infusion, 11 patients (50%) suffered from complications, seven (31.8%) from neurologic complications, and four (18.2%) from cystitis-like symptoms. These researchers concluded that a smaller dose of the chemotherapeutic agent should be used to avoid complications.

Head and Neck Cancer

Intra-arterial infusion of chemotherapy is used as neoadjuvant therapy in head and neck cancer before surgery or radiation therapy or for palliation in patients with advanced cancer. Several studies have shown that intra-arterial infusion of chemotherapeutic agents combined with definitive local treatment (surgery and/or radiation therapy) may improve organ preservation rates and overall survival in patients with advanced squamous cell carcinoma of the head and neck.

In most of the earlier studies of this technique, investigators performed selective infusions into the external carotid artery.[52, 53] The results of these trials demonstrated only a marginal improvement over the therapeutic effectiveness of systemic chemotherapy. Superselective catheterization techniques and high-dose chemotherapy have been advocated to improve the effectiveness of regional intra-arterial chemotherapy.

Cisplatin has been the chemotherapeutic agent most commonly used for intra-arterial infusion in head and neck cancers because sodium thiosulfate can be used as a systemic antagonist. In experimental and clinical studies involving high-dose intra-arterial cisplatin therapy, Robbins et al.[54] found that tumor response rates depended on dose intensity, with higher-intensity regimens producing substantially greater response rates in patients with head and neck cancer. In another study, Robbins et al.[55] treated 213 patients with stage III or IV squamous cell carcinoma of the head and neck at the University of Tennessee, Memphis, with (a) rapid intra-arterial infusion of high doses of cisplatin (150 mg/m^2 weekly $\times$ 4) through a microcatheter selectively placed in the vessel supplying the bulk of the tumor, (b) simultaneous intravenous thiosulfate for systemic drug neutralization, and (c) conventional external-beam radiation therapy. Complete response in the primary and regional sites was obtained in 80% and 61% of patients, respectively.[55] The Kaplan-Meier plot projections for overall and cancer-related 5-year survival rates were 38.8% and 53.6%, respectively.

Other investigators have reported similar response rates with superselective infusion therapies using relatively small doses of chemotherapeutic agents.[56, 57] In a series of 13 patients with squamous cell carcinoma of the mouth who were treated with 30 to 40 mg/m^2 of cisplatin once a week, Korogi et al.[56] observed complete response in 38% of patients and partial response in 54%. In patients with multiple feeding arteries, all feeding arteries were individually catheterized with a coaxial microcatheter system and infused in one session. The dose of cisplatin for each feeding artery was determined by the percentage of tumor stained with indigocarmine dye on each vascular injection.

Catheterization is generally performed using a common femoral arterial access obtained by the Seldinger technique. Preliminary diagnostic angiographic studies are performed to study the vascular anatomy on both sides, to identify the vessels feeding the tumor, and to rule out any abnormal communication between the vessels supplying the tumor and the branches of the internal carotid artery. A 5F catheter or, more commonly, a coaxially introduced microcatheter is placed in the appropriate feeding artery. The catheter tip should be advanced as far distally as possible as to avoid infusion into the mucosal and muscular branches **(Fig. 14-7)**.

Some investigators have described a technique that involves placement of a temporary indwelling catheter via superficial temporal arterial access to perform repeated superselective infusions.[58] After a preliminary diagnostic angiographic study performed via the common femoral arterial approach, the superficial temporal artery is accessed via a preauricular skin incision, and the feeding artery is catheterized with a coaxial microcatheter system under fluoroscopic control. Attempts to catheterize small vessels may occasionally result in vascular spasm, precluding infusion of chemotherapy. Kishi et al.[59] advocate the use of an occlusion-balloon infusion technique by which the nonfeeding arteries are occluded, and the chemotherapeutic agents are infused into the feeding arteries without the need for their catheterization, thereby avoiding catheterization or guidewire trauma or spasm of the feeding arteries. In their series of six patients with squamous cell carcinoma of the lower lip fed by the facial artery, a 4F, double-lumen balloon catheter was introduced through superficial temporal

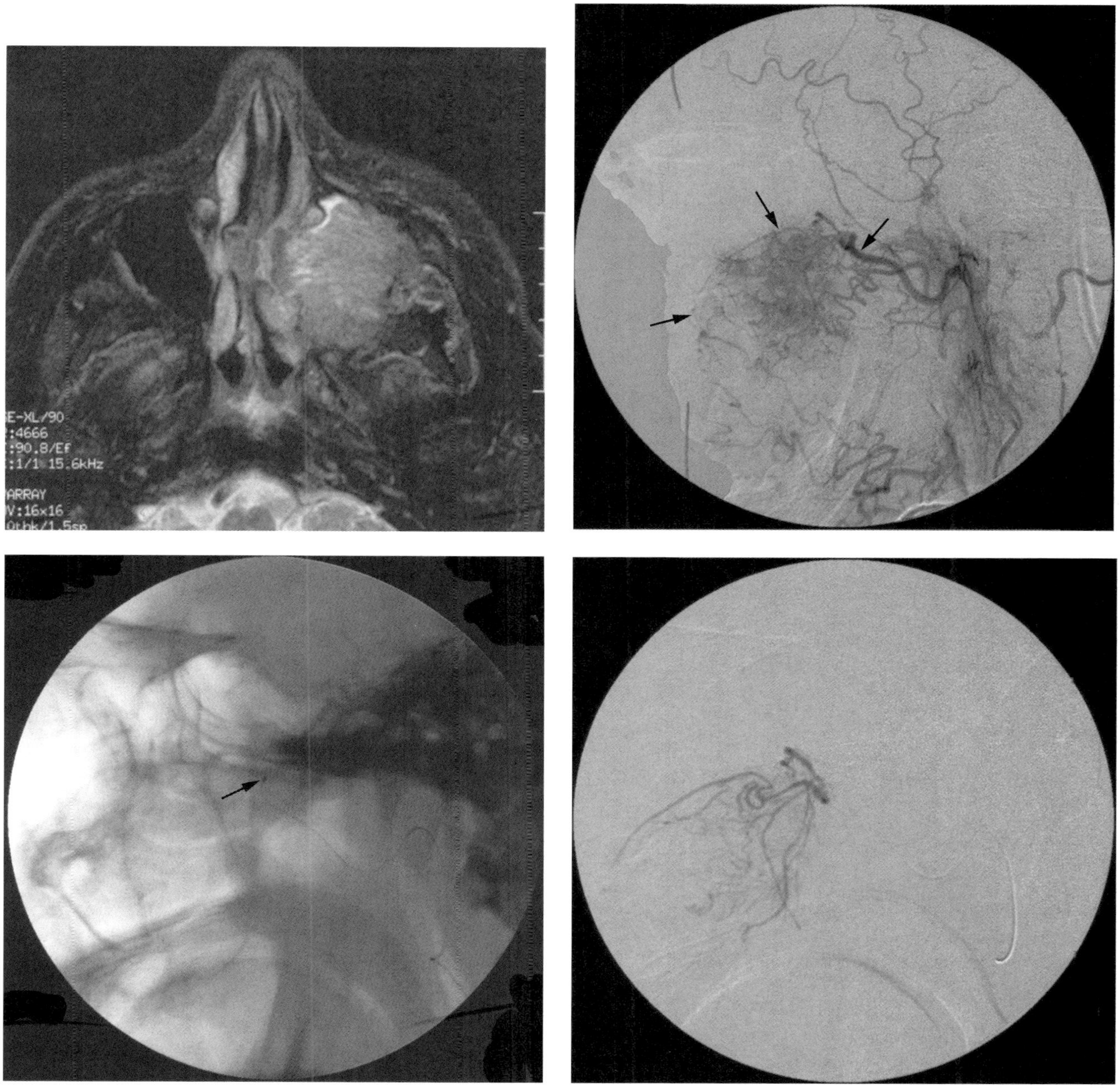

Figure 14-7. Intra-arterial chemotherapy for maxillary carcinoma. (A) Axial magnetic resonance image shows left maxillary tumor. (B) External carotid angiogram demonstrates hypervascular tumor supplied predominantly by internal maxillary artery (arrow). (C and D) A coaxially advanced microcatheter (arrow) was selectively placed in the internal maxillary artery for infusion of chemotherapy.

artery access, and the balloon was inflated in the external carotid artery just distal to the origin of the facial artery.

A tumor stain is not always seen on angiography in head and neck cancers, many of which are not vascular. Certain investigators have successfully used arterial infusion of indigocarmine dye to identify the feeding vessels for head and neck tumors that are located at a visible site.[56, 57] Intra-arterial infusion of corticosteroids immediately after infusion of cisplatin has been advocated to prevent local side effects.[57]

REFERENCES

1. Bakal CW, Cynamon J, Lakritz PS, et al. Value of preoperative renal artery embolization in reducing blood transfusion requirements during nephrectomy for renal cell carcinoma. *J Vasc Interv Radiol* 1993; 4:727–731.
2. Kalman D, Varenhorst E. The role of arterial embolization in renal cell carcinoma. *Scand J Urol Nephrol* 1999; 33:162–170.
3. Lanigan D, Jurriaans E, Hammonds JC, et al. The current status of embolization in renal cell carcinoma—a survey of local and national practice. *Clin Radiol* 1992; 44:176.
4. Mebust WK, Weigel JW, Lee KR, et al. Renal cell carcinoma angioinfarction. *J Urol* 1984; 131:231–235.

5. Wallace S, Chuang VP, Swanson DA, et al. Embolization of renal carcinoma: experience with 100 patients. *Radiology* 1981; 138:563.
6. Zielinski H, Szmiegielski S, Petrovich Z. Comparison of preoperative embolization followed by radical nephrectomy with radical nephrectomy alone for renal cell carcinoma. *Am J Clin Oncol* 2000; 23:6–12.
7. Wallace S, Charnsangavej C, Carrasco CH. Intra-arterial interventional therapy for malignant genitourinary neoplasms. In: Pollack HM, McClennan BL, eds. *Clinical Urography*. Philadelphia: WB Saunders; 2000:3380–3395.
8. Leinonen A. Embolization of renal carcinoma: comparison between the early results of Gelfoam and absolute ethanol embolization. *Ann Clin Res* 1985; 17:299–305.
9. Park JH, Kim SH, Han JK, Chung JW, Han MC. Transcatheter arterial embolization of unresectable renal cell carcinoma with a mixture of ethanol and iodized oil. *Cardiovasc Intervent Radiol* 1994; 17:23.
10. Klimberg I, Hunter P, Hawkins IF, Drylie DM, Wajsman Z. Preoperative angio-infarction of localized renal cell carcinoma using absolute ethanol. *J Urol* 1985; 133:21–24.
11. Richter GM, Rassweiler J, Kauffmann GW, et al. Experimental study on the effectiveness of capillary embolization using contrast-enhanced Ethibloc. *Invest Radiol* 1984; 19:36–44.
12. Cox GG, Lee KR, Price HI, et al. Colonic infarction following ethanol embolization of renal cell carcinoma. *Radiology* 1982; 145:343.
13. Lammer J, Justich E, Schreyer H, Pettek R. Complications of renal tumor embolization. *Cardiovasc Intervent Radiol* 1985;8:31–35.
14. Weber J, Dociu N, Zabel G. Gas without abscess in renal tumor embolization. *Ann Radiol* 1984; 27:305.
15. Sella A, Logothetis CJ, Fitz K, et al. Phase II study of interferon-α and chemotherapy (5-fluorouracil and mitomycin C) in metastatic renal cell cancer. *J Urol* 1992; 147:573.
16. Barton PP, Waneck RE, Karnel FJ, Ritschl P, Kramer J, Lechner GL. Embolization of bone metastases. *J Vasc Interv Radiol* 1996; 7:81–88.
17. Chatziioannou AN, Johnson ME, Pneumaticos SG, Lawrence DD, Carrasco CH. Preoperative embolization of bone metastases from renal cell carcinoma. *Eur Radiol* 2000; 10:593–596.
18. Chuang VP, Wallace S, Swanson D, et al. Arterial occlusion in the management of pain from metastatic renal carcinoma. *Radiology* 1979; 133:611–614.
19. Gellad FE, Sadato N, Numaguchi Y, Levine AM. Vascular metastatic lesions of the spine: preoperative embolization. *Radiology* 1990; 176:683–686.
20. Hemingway AP, Allison DJ. Complications of embolization: analysis of 410 procedures. *Radiology* 1988; 166:669–672.
21. Smith TP, Gray L, Weinstein JN, Richardson WJ, Payne CS. Preoperative transarterial embolization of spinal column neoplasms. *J Vasc Interv Radiol* 1995; 6:863–869.
22. Sun S, Lang EV. Bone metastases from renal cell carcinoma: preoperative embolization. *J Vasc Interv Radiol* 1998; 9:263–269.
23. Hare W, Lond F, Holland C. Paresis following internal iliac artery embolization. *Radiology* 1983; 146:47–51.
24. Spiro IJ, Rosenberg AE, Springfield D, et al. Combined surgery and radiation therapy for limb preservation in soft tissue sarcoma of the extremity: the Massachusetts General Hospital experience. *Cancer Invest* 1995; 13:86–95.
25. Stewart DJ, Benjamin RS, Zimmerman S, et al. Clinical pharmacology of intra-arterial cis-diamminedichloroplatinum (II). *Cancer Res* 1983; 43:917–920.
26. Benjamin RS, Chawla SP, Carrasco CH, et al. Preoperative chemotherapy for osteosarcoma with intravenous Adriamycin and intra-arterial cisplatinum. *Ann Oncol* 1992; 3 (suppl II):3–6.
27. Picci P, Bacci G, Ruggieri P, et al. The treatment of localized osteosarcoma of the extremities: the Italian experience. *Ann Oncol* 1992; 3(suppl II):13–18.
28. Benjamin RS. Regional chemotherapy for osteosarcoma. *Semin Oncol* 1989; 16: 323–327.
29. Winkler K, Bielack S, Delling G, et al. Effect of intraarterial versus intravenous cisplatin in addition to systemic doxorubicin, high-dose methotrexate, and ifosfamide on histologic tumor response in osteosarcoma (Study COSS 86). *Cancer* 1990; 66:1703–1710.
30. Jaffe N, Raymond AK, Ayala A, et al. Effect of cumulative courses of intra-arterial cisdiamminedichloroplatinum-II on the primary tumor in osteosarcoma. *Cancer* 1989; 63:63–67.
31. Azzarelli A, Quagliuolo V, Fissi S, et al. Intra-arterial induction chemotherapy for soft tissue sarcomas. *Ann Oncol* 1992; 3(suppl II):67–70.
32. Soulen MC, Weissmann JR, Sullivan KL, et al. Intraarterial chemotherapy and limb-sparing resection of large soft-tissue sarcomas of the extremities. *J Vasc Interv Radiol* 1992; 3:659–663.
33. Carrasco CH, Charnsangavej C, Richli WR, Raymond AK, Wallace S, Benjamin RS. Osteosarcoma: interventional radiology in diagnosis and management. *Semin Roentgenol* 1989; 24:193–200.
34. Carrasco CH, Charnsangavej C, Raymond AK, et al. Osteosarcoma: angiographic assessment of response to pre-operative chemotherapy. *Radiology* 1989; 170:839–842.
35. Soulen MC. Intraarterial chemotherapy for sarcomas. In: Baun S, Pentecost MJ, eds. *Abrams' Angiography: Vascular and Interventional Radiology*. 4th ed. Boston: Little Brown; 1997:1031–1036.
36. Homma H, Doi T, Mezawa S, et al. A novel arterial infusion chemotherapy for the treatment of patients with advanced pancreatic carcinoma after vascular supply distribution via superselective embolization. *Cancer* 2000; 89:303–313.
37. Muchmore JH, Preslan JE, George WJ. Regional chemotherapy for inoperable pancreatic carcinoma. *Cancer* 1996; 78:664–673.
38. Ohigashi H, Ishikawa O, Imaoka S, et al. A new method of intra-arterial regional chemotherapy with more selective drug delivery for locally advanced pancreatic cancer. *Hepato-Gastroenterol* 1996; 43:338–345.
39. Neyazaki T, Ikeda M, Seki Y, et al. Bronchial artery infusion therapy for lung cancer. *Cancer* 1969; 24:912–922.
40. Osaki T, Hanagiri T, Nakanishi R, Yoshino I, Taga S, Yasumoto K. Bronchial arterial infusion is an effective therapeutic modality for centrally located early-stage lung cancer: results of a pilot study. *Chest* 1999; 115:1424–1428.
41. Watanabe Y, Shimizu J, Murakami S, et al. Reappraisal of bronchial arterial infusion therapy for advanced lung cancer. *Jpn J Surg* 1990; 20:27–35.
42. Kigawa J, Minagawa Y, Ishihara H, Itamochi H, Kanamori Y, Terakawa N. The role of neoadjuvant intraarterial infusion chemotherapy with cisplatin and bleomycin for locally advanced cervical cancer. *Am J Clin Oncol* 1996; 19:255–259.
43. Nagata Y, Araki N, Kimura H, et al. Neoadjuvant chemotherapy by transcatheter arterial infusion method for uterine cervical cancer. *J Vasc Interv Radiol* 2000; 11:313–319.
44. Adachi S, Ogasawara T, Wakimoto E, et al. Phase I/II study of intravenous nedaplatin and intraarterial cisplatin with transcatheter arterial embolization for patients with locally advanced uterine cervical carcinoma. *Cancer* 2001; 91:74–79.
45. Motoyama S, Takeuchi S, Hamana S, et al. Super high-dose intraarterial cisplatin infusion under percutaneous pelvic perfusion with extracorporeal chemofiltration for advanced uterine cervical carcinoma, II: its impact on clinical response and subsequent surgery. *Am J Clin Oncol* 2001; 24:247–250.
46. Eapen L, Stewart D, Crook J, et al. Intraarterial cisplatin and concurrent radiation for locally advanced bladder cancer [abstract 625]. *Proc Am Soc Clin Oncol* 1995; 14: 238.
47. Mokarim A, Uetani M, Hayashi N, et al. Combined intraarterial chemotherapy and radiotherapy in the treatment of bladder carcinoma. *Cancer* 1997; 80:1776–1785.
48. Akimoto T, Matsumoto M, Mashimo T, Mitsuhashi N, Niibe H. Radiation therapy and concurrent daily intra-arterial infusion of low-dose cisplatin following alteration of pelvic blood flow for

invasive bladder cancer: a preliminary report. *Anticancer Res* 1998; 18:3731–3735.

49. Ganaha F, Yamada T, Ujita M, Irie T, Fukuda Y, Fukuda K. Intraarterial low-dose cisplatin via an indwelling port and concurrent radiotherapy for invasive bladder cancer. *J Vasc Interv Radiol* 2001; 12:379–384.
50. Arima K, Tochigi H, Sugimura Y, Kawamura J. Balloon-occluded arterial infusion as a useful neoadjuvant chemotherapy for bladder cancer. *Br J Urol* 1997; 80:417–420.
51. Sugimoto K, Hirota S, Imanaka K, Kawabe T, Nakayama Y, Takeuchi Y. Complications following balloon-occluded arterial infusion chemotherapy for pelvic malignancies. *Cardiovasc Intervent Radiol* 1999; 22:481–485.
52. Baker SR, Forastiere AA, Wheeler RH, Medvec BR. Intraarterial chemotherapy for head and neck cancer: an update of the totally implantable infusion pump. *Arch Otolaryngol Head Neck Surg* 1987; 113:1183–1190.
53. Lee YY, Wallace S, Dimery I, Goepfert H. Intraarterial chemotherapy of head and neck tumors. *Am J Neuroradiol* 1986; 7:343–348.
54. Robbins KT, Storniolo AMS, Hryniuk WH, Howell SB. Decadose effects of cisplatin on squamous cell carcinoma of the upper aerodigestive tract, part II: clinical studies. *Laryngoscope* 1996; 106:37–42.
55. Robbins KT, Kumar P, Wong FSH, et al. Targeted chemoradiation for advanced head and neck cancer: analysis of 213 patients. *Head Neck* 2000; 22:687–693.
56. Korogi Y, Toshinori H, Nishimura R, et al. Superselective intraarterial infusion of cisplatin for squamous cell carcinoma of the mouth: preliminary clinical experience. *Am J Roentgenol* 1995; 165:1269–1272.
57. Hirai T, Korogi Y, Hamatake S, et al. Stages III and IV squamous cell carcinoma of the mouth: three-year experience with superselective intraarterial chemotherapy using cisplatin prior to definitive treatment. *Cardiovasc Intervent Radiol* 1999; 22:201–205.
58. Nakasato T, Katoh K, Sone M, et al. Superselective continuous arterial infusion chemotherapy through the superficial temporal artery for oral cavity tumors. *Am J Neuroradiol* 2000; 21:1917–1922.
59. Kishi K, Matsunaka M, Sato M, Sonomura T, Sakurane M, Uede K. T1 and T2 lip cancer: a superselective method of facial arterial infusion therapy—preliminary experience. *Radiology* 1999; 213:173–179.

CHAPTER 15

MANAGEMENT OF DYSFUNCTIONAL CENTRAL VENOUS CATHETERS IN THE PATIENT WITH CANCER

KENT SATO, MD

CHARLES A. OWENS, MD

INTRODUCTION

First introduced by Broviac in 1973, central venous access devices (VADs) have played an ever-increasing role in the management of the cancer patient. Centrally placed catheters are frequently used for the infusion of chemotherapy, hyperalimentation, hemodialysis, and stem cell transfusion, as well as to provide dependable access for the delivery of antibiotics and hydration, for blood transfusions, and for frequent blood sampling (**Table 15-1**). Historically placed in an operating room, these tunneled and non-tunneled devices have increasingly fallen under the realm of the interventional radiology service. The reasons for this transference of responsibility are largely the safer and more proficient placement of central VADs enabled by ultrasound (US) and fluoroscopic guidance and the cost savings achieved by placing such devices in an angiography suite instead of the operating room. Interventional radiologists have provided unique and innovative approaches to the placement of central VADs in patients in whom routine central venous access is not available. With the exception of catheter-related venous thrombosis and infections, complications associated with central VADs are rare.[1] This tutorial focuses on catheter dysfunction and the more commonly encountered complication of catheter-related central venous thrombosis.

CATHETER DYSFUNCTION

Catheter-related dysfunction can be divided into *thrombotic* and *non-thrombotic* causes (**Table 15-2**).

TABLE 15-1
Uses for Central Venous Catheters in the Patient with Cancer

- Blood stem cell harvesting (apheresis)
- Chemotherapy
- Bone marrow transplantation
- Total parenteral nutrition
- Intravenous fluid and drug administration (i.e., antibiotics)
- Transfusion of blood products
- Hemodialysis

TABLE 15-2
Causes of Central Venous Catheter Dysfunction

Non-thrombotic catheter occlusion	Thrombotic occlusion
• Catheter kinking	Fibrin sheath
• Catheter fracture	Pericatheter thrombus
• Catheter misplacement	Vessel thrombosis
• Intraluminal precipitates	

Non-thrombotic causes include catheter misplacement, kinking, fracture, and occlusion from intraluminal precipitates. Thrombotic causes are on a continuum from obstruction of the catheter tip by a thin fibrin sheath to total thrombosis of the involved vessel. Once the central vein has become occluded, an important decision must be made: either to preserve the involved access or to abandon it for an alternate route. The life expectancy of the patient, associated symptoms (e.g., limb swelling, presence of infection), and the projected need for long-term central venous access will aid in this decision process.

NON-THROMBOTIC CATHETER OCCLUSION

Catheter Kinking, Malposition, or Fracture

Catheter malposition or kinking (**Fig. 15-1**) can readily be detected on a chest radiograph. Patients who are receiving potentially toxic chemotherapeutic agents should have routine (monthly) radiographs to avoid delivery of a toxic infusate through a misplaced catheter (**Fig. 15-2**). Patients who experience pain during chemotherapy should immediately have a chest radiograph followed by transcatheter venography if the radiograph proves inconclusive (**Fig. 15-3**). A simple venogram through each catheter port may disclose extravasation of contrast through a break (fracture) in the catheter, a catheter tip that has eroded the vessel wall, or reflux along a pericatheter thrombus or a fibrin sheath that exits at the venous entry site.[2]

The best technique for minimizing catheter dysfunction is the use of fluoroscopic guidance while placing the central VAD. The optimal position of the catheter tip, however, is somewhat controversial. Some authors warn against placement of the catheter tip too centrally (i.e., within the heart), for fear of eliciting malignant dysrhythmias or perforating the atrial wall.[3–5] Alternatively, others have recommended positioning the catheter tip at the junction of the right atrium and the superior vena cava

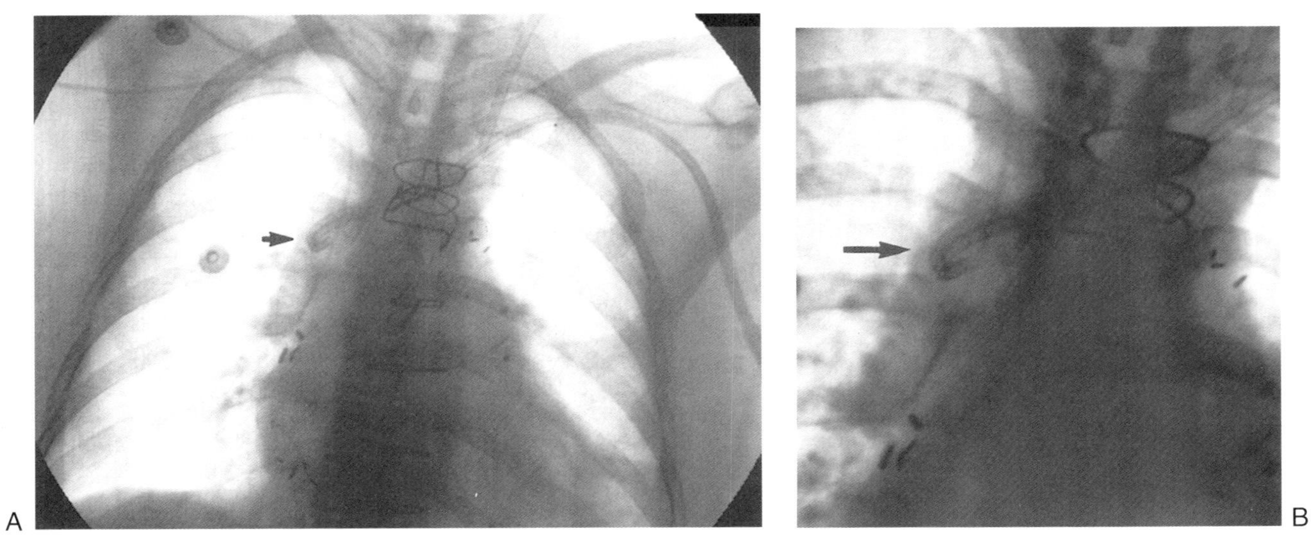

Figure 15-1. (A) Chest radiograph in a patient with dysfunctional left subclavian catheter reveals that the catheter tip (arrow) has migrated into the azygos vein and is kinked. (B) Magnified view of kinked catheter tip (arrow).

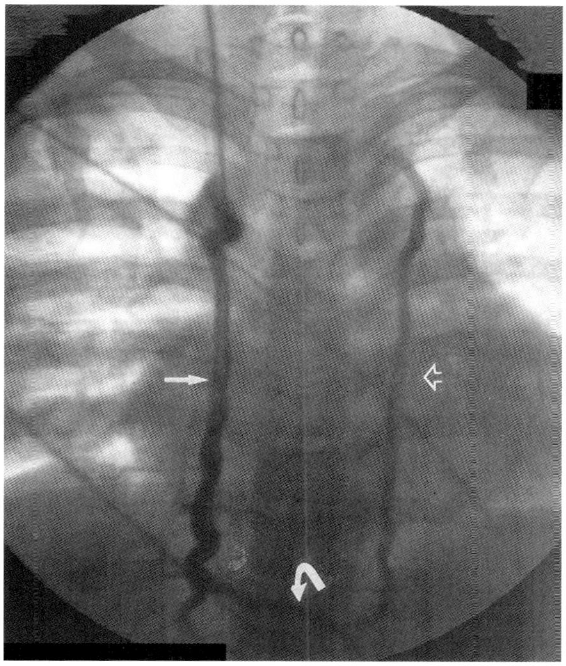

Figure 15-2. Venogram performed through a right internal jugular vein central venous catheter identifies the tip (arrow) misplaced into the right internal thoracic (mammary) vein. This was not discernable on the chest radiograph. Note the collateral filling of the left internal thoracic (mammary) vein (open arrow) via the retrosternal anastomosis (curved arrow).

(SVC) or within the proximal right atrium to preserve catheter function, especially when rapid catheter flow is required (e.g., hemodialysis).[6–8] Although most authors agree that the ideal catheter tip position would be at the cavoatrial junction, Kowalski et al. recommended that the initial placement of the catheter tip should be 3–4 cm more central than the desired final position to account for change of the chest wall when the patient is upright.[9]

Subcutaneously tunneled catheters placed via the internal jugular veins are prone to kinking at the venous insertion site where the catheter makes a sharp turn (**Fig. 15-4**). It is important that tunneled catheters be placed low enough in the neck so that the angle made by the catheter as it enters the vein is not too acute. Blunt dissection near the venous insertion site, particularly in areas scarred from previous catheterizations, may avoid tissue impingement on the catheter lumen. Occasionally, placing stiff guide wire(s) (stiff-shaft Glidewires, Boston Scientific Corp., Natick, MA) through the catheter lumen(s) and gently massaging the area of the neck where the kink is occurring can salvage the compromised catheter.

The pinched-off syndrome is a well-described complication of subclavicular central VADs. This mechanical obstruction is caused by compression of the catheter as it passes between the clavicle and first rib (**Fig. 15-5**). Narrowing of the catheter lumen can be seen on a chest radiograph; if it is ignored, the resulting shearing forces can cause transection and embolization of the distal catheter fragment.[10] Such catheters should be removed and placed more laterally within the subclavian vein, peripheral to the midclavicular line, or within an internal jugular vein.[11]

Intraluminal Precipitates

Various medications and mixtures of total parenteral nutrition (TPN) can occlude catheters by precipitating within the catheter lumen. Some authors have suggested that patency can be restored by dissolving the

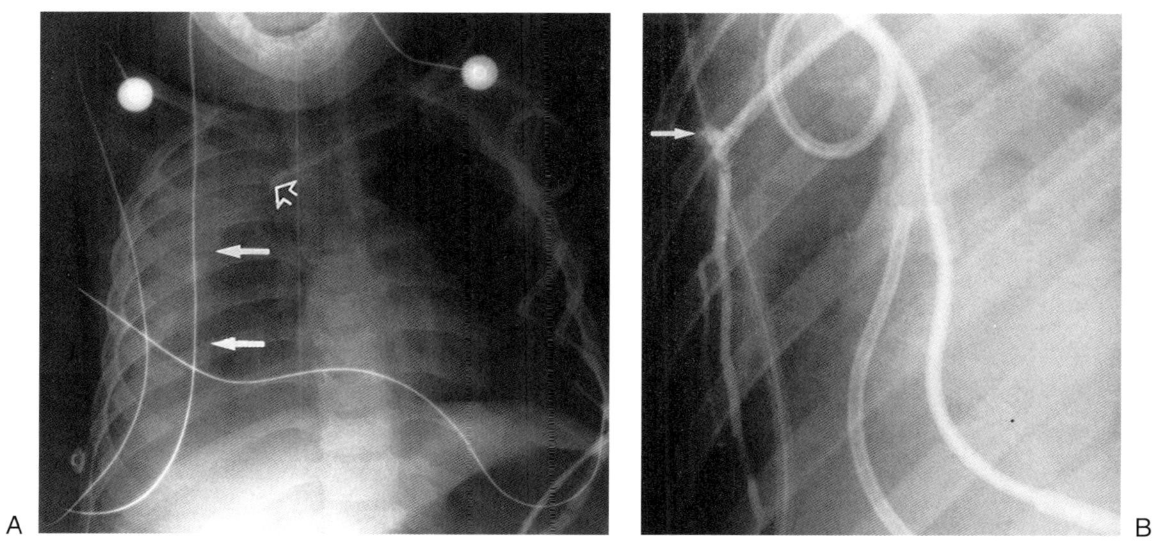

Figure 15-3. (A) After placement of a left subclavian vein tunneled catheter (open arrow) and after several chemotherapy treatments, a chest radiograph reveals a large right hydrothorax (solid arrows). Findings on the pretreatment chest radiograph were normal. (B) A venogram performed through the tunneled catheter reveals the catheter tip misplaced into the right internal thoracic (mammary) vein and an associated small pseudoaneurysm (arrow).

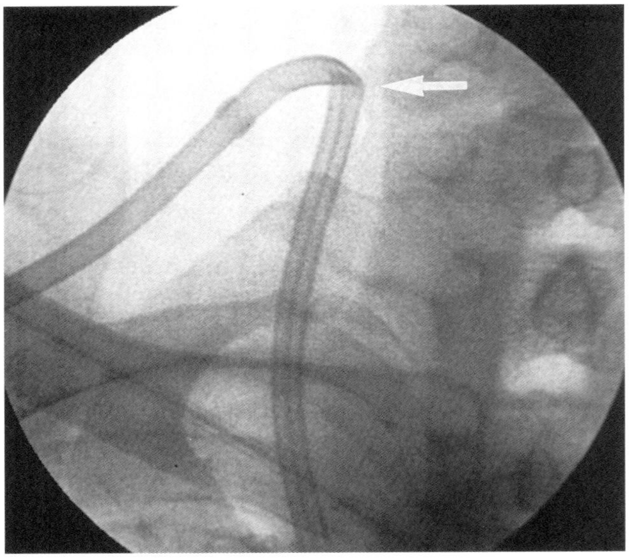

Figure 15-4. A tunneled right internal jugular vein catheter is placed too cephalad in the neck, causing kinking (arrow) of the catheter lumen.

precipitate with either a base or acidic solution.[12–16] Filling the catheter lumen with a solution of sodium bicarbonate (1 mEq/mL) has been reported to restore patency in catheters obstructed with medications soluble at a high pH (> 7.0).[12] A 0.1-M solution of hydrochloric acid (HCl) has also been used to dissolve medications soluble at a low pH (< 6.0).[13–15] After the appropriate estimated luminal volume of HCl or sodium bicarbonate has been infused into the catheter and left for 20 minutes, the contents are aspirated. The use of 3 mL of 70% alcohol, in a similar fashion, has been described to dissolve lipid protein complexes caused by the infusion of TPN.[16] It should be noted that the U.S. Food and Drug Administration (USFDA) has *not* approved the use of alcohol, HCl, or sodium bicarbonate to dissolve intraluminal catheter precipitates.

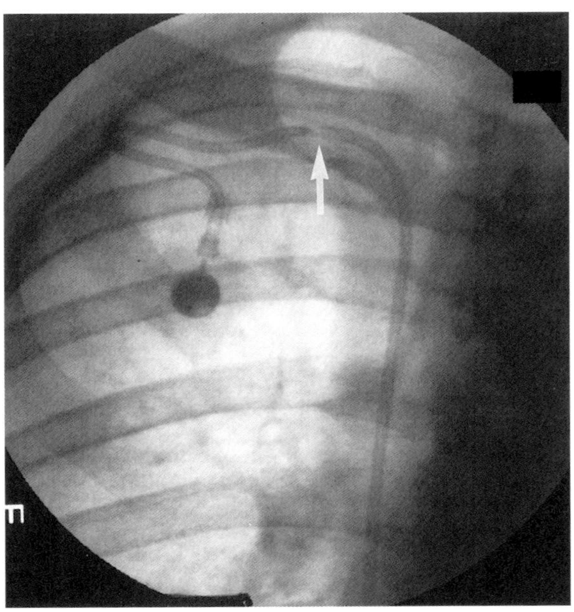

Figure 15-5. Tunneled right subclavian vein Portacath with fractured catheter (arrow) caused by compression from the clavicle and first rib (pinched-off syndrome).

THROMBOTIC CATHETER OCCLUSION

As a rule, catheter dysfunction in well-positioned catheters is due to the presence of a pericatheter fibrin sheath or a thrombus encompassing the catheter tip. Thrombotic occlusion is the most common noninfectious catheter complication and has been reported as occurring in up to 36% of central VADs and as being the underlying cause in 95% of catheter occlusions.[17] In one series of patients with cancer, the reported incidence of catheter-related thrombosis was 66%.[18] Symptomatic thrombosis, however, only occurred in 6% of the patients in this study. Thrombosis-associated catheter dysfunction can vary from pericatheter clot or fibrin to complete thrombosis of the catheterized vein.

There are many causes for catheter-related thrombosis in patients with cancer. The caustic nature of certain chemotherapeutic agents, TPN solutions, and antibiotics may damage the endothelial wall, leading to platelet adherence.[19] Catheter movement, from cardiac and respiratory motion, may also lead to wall abrasion.[20] Catheter composition and stiffness may affect vein patency; polyurethane and silastic materials are less traumatic to the vessel wall.[21] Hypercoagulability, often seen in patients with malignancies, and duration of catheterization contribute to central venous occlusion and catheter thrombosis.[22–24]

Fibrin Sheath

In 1973, Broviac et al. first described the occurrence of pericatheter fibrin sheaths. Fibrin sheath formation is thought to occur in 80%–100% of central VADs. Although it is a relatively benign process, it can be the underlying cause of major catheter dysfunction.[25–27] Fibrin sheath formation has been reported to occur as early as 24 hours after catheter placement, propagating from the venous insertion site until it envelops the catheter tip and obstructs flow.[25]

Intravascular US (**Fig. 15-6**) has been used to demonstrate fibrin sheaths[28]; however, transcatheter venography, with or without partial withdrawal of the catheter prior to injection, is the most widely used and accepted diagnostic modality (**Fig. 15-7**). During contrast injection, care must be taken to not disrupt the

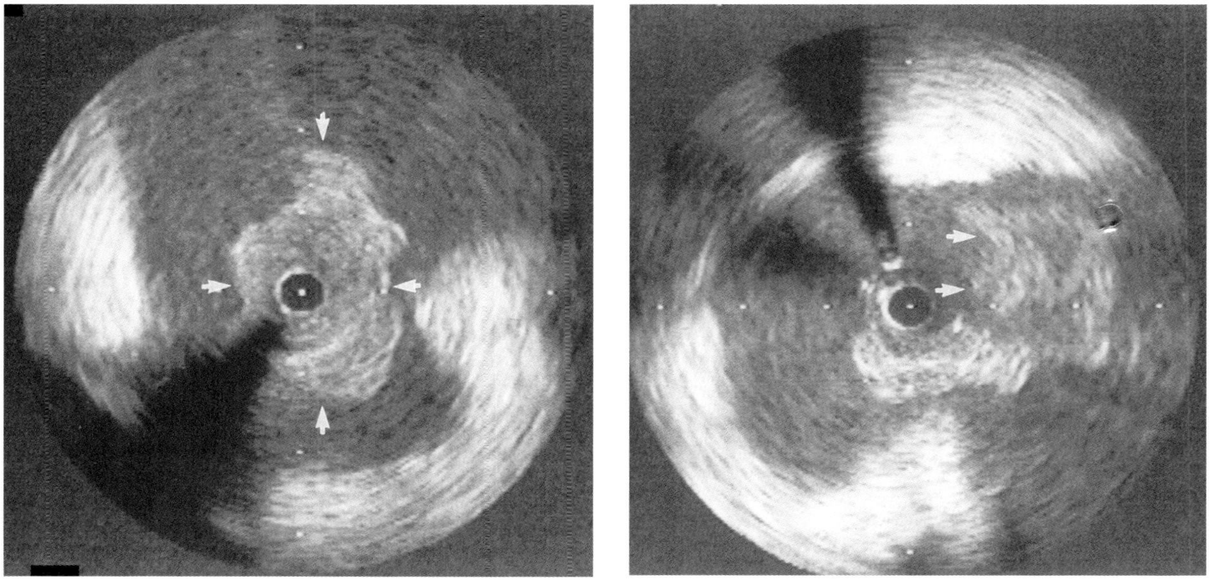

A B

Figure 15-6. (A) Dysfunctional central venous catheter in a patient with severe contrast allergy and limited venous access. The catheter was exchanged over a wire for an intravascular ultrasound catheter (IVUS), and a large pericatheter thrombus (arrows), extending into the right atrium, was identified. (B) The patient was too ill to undergo surgical thrombectomy. After an unsuccessful trial of thrombolysis, angioplasty was performed on the thrombus and a new central venous catheter was placed through the same venous access site. The new catheter functioned well after angioplasty fractured the pericatheter thrombus (arrows). There was no clinical evidence that the patient experienced a pulmonary embolic event. Case photos courtesy of Marc Borge, MD, of Loyola University Medical Center, Maywood, IL.

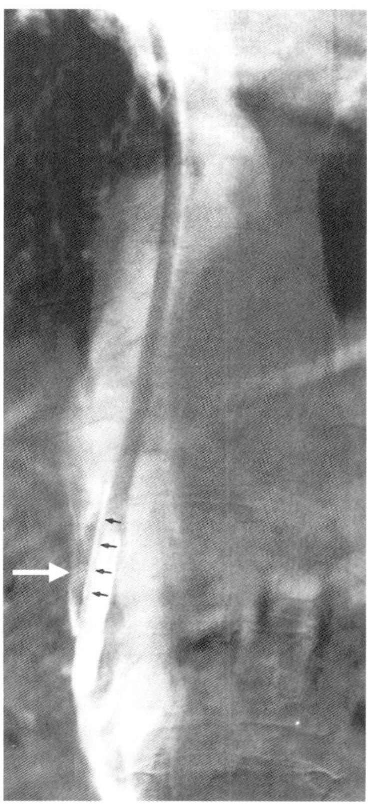

Figure 15-7. Venogram performed through a right internal jugular vein dysfunctional catheter positioned in the superior vena cava reveals pericatheter thrombus–fibrin sheath encasing the tip of the catheter (white arrow). Contrast can be seen tracking between the catheter and thrombus–fibrin sheath (black arrows).

fibrin sheath. Disruption of the sheath may obscure the correct diagnosis, interfere with planned thrombolytic treatment, or both.

The sensitivity of venographic detection is not known; major catheter dysfunction caused by radiographically undetectable fibrin sheaths has been described.[29,30] Partial occlusion of the catheter creates a ball–valve phenomenon that allows the infusion of fluids but occlusion during aspiration when negative pressure is applied.

Pericatheter and Mural Thrombus

Pericatheter thrombus may occur from the progression of a fibrin sheath or, more likely, from thrombus that originated from adjacent damaged endothelium. Untreated, the thrombus can progress to occlude the surrounding vessel (**Fig. 15-8**), be the source of a pulmonary embolic event, or both.[31–34]

The diagnosis of pericatheter thrombus can be confirmed by a variety of diagnostic tests including US, echocardiography (transthoracic or transesophageal), computed tomography (CT), magnetic resonance (MR) imaging, and venography. Venography performed through the dysfunctional catheter may underestimate the extent of the thrombus. Simultaneous venography, performed from both upper extremities, can better define vessel patency. The amount of pericatheter thrombus and availability of alternative venous access will determine what treatment will be undertaken.

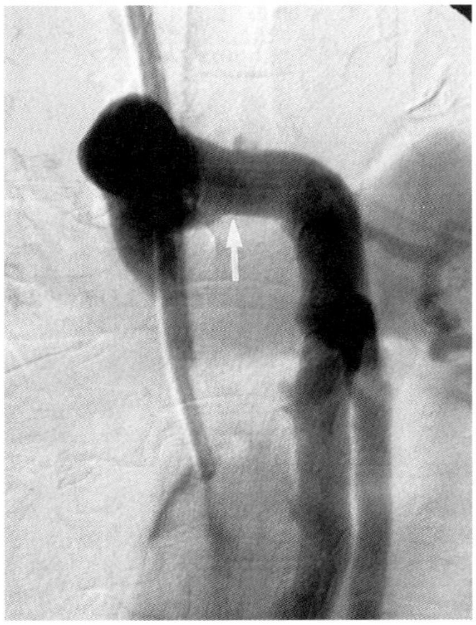

Figure 15-8. Venogram performed through both the proximal and distal ports of this right internal jugular vein catheter positioned within the superior vena cava (SVC) reveals that the SVC is completely occluded and thrombus has entirely encased the catheter tip. Note collateral venous flow via the azygos vein (arrow).

If only a small amount of pericatheter thrombus is present, then techniques used to treat fibrin sheaths would be appropriate (e.g., catheter stripping, thrombolysis, catheter exchange). If the amount of existing clot raises the potential for significant pulmonary emboli, then catheter-directed thrombolysis or surgical thrombectomy might prove to be the safest option. For situations in which surgery and thrombolysis are not reasonable, percutaneous thrombectomy has been suggested.[35]

Complete Venous Thrombosis

Almost 40% of upper-extremity deep vein thromboses (DVTs) can be attributed to long-term central venous catheterization.[36] The incidence of catheter-related central venous thrombosis has been reported to be anywhere between 0.7% and 74%.[8,37,38] Thrombotic catheter dysfunction can progress to complete vein occlusion with or without associated symptoms.[39]

The severity of the symptoms is related to the level of obstruction, acuteness of the occlusion, and sufficiency of collateral venous flow. Thrombosis of the innominate or subclavian vein may result in upper-extremity edema, pain, cyanosis, and paresthesia. Occlusion of the SVC can present with dyspnea, chest pain, cough, dysphagia, swelling, and symptoms related to increased intracranial pressure.[40,41] Physical signs include jugular vein distention, distended collateral veins of the upper extremities and neck, facial swelling, periorbital edema, and cyanosis.

Asymptomatic patients, in whom future central venous access is not required, can be treated by removal of the catheter followed by anticoagulation. Most upper-extremity swelling due to DVT will decrease with anticoagulation as additional venous collaterals enlarge to compensate for the altered venous drainage. The severity of related symptoms, the patient's clinical state, and the need for future venous access will direct which therapeutic approach is taken.[42] When long-term central venous access is expected or the patient is profoundly symptomatic, aggressive treatment of the underlying occlusion should be undertaken. Recanalization of the occluded vessel has been achieved with the use of mechanical or pharmacologic thrombolytics, angioplasty, and stenting.

TREATING CATHETER MALFUNCTION

Preventive Measures for Thrombotic Catheter Occlusion

Maintaining catheter function begins with optimizing catheter care provided by the service using the catheter and by the patient. Studies have demonstrated a correlation between catheter infection and thrombosis.[43,44] The routine prophylactic use of a small dose of a thrombolytic (urokinase) has been demonstrated to decrease the incidence of both catheter thrombosis and catheter-related infections. The weekly use of thrombolytics, in addition to routine heparin flushes, has been shown to be both safe and effective.[45,46] Other studies have demonstrated a reduction in catheter-induced thrombosis with the use of prophylactic low-dose warfarin (Coumadin).[22,47,48] At a dose of 1 mg of Coumadin per day, a reduction in clinically detectable thrombosis has been demonstrated in patients with cancer, without significantly altering their coagulation parameters.

Bolus (Injection) Thrombolysis

Approximately 5% to 25% of catheter occlusion is due to intraluminal thrombus.[49] Filling the lumen(s) of the dysfunctional catheter with a thrombolytic agent (e.g., urokinase [UK, Abbokinase, Abbott Lab., Abbott Park, IL], streptokinase, recombinant tissue-type plasminogen activator [rt-PA, Alteplase, Genentech, South San Francisco CA]) and allowing the agent to dwell within the catheter for a short time has been shown to be very effective at restoring patency.[50–52] Currently, rt-PA is the only agent used in the United States for simple catheter clearance and is routinely used in outpatient clinics. Before 1999, when the USFDA removed urokinase (UK, Abbokinase) from the U.S. market, a bolus injection of 5,000 U of UK was found to be effective at restoring dialysis catheter function in 74%–81% of cases.[53,54] Compared to rt-PA and UK, streptokinase is more likely to cause an anaphylactic reaction especially in patients with prior exposure to streptococcal infections; therefore, its use as a catheter-clearing agent has been discouraged.[55,56]

The first line of therapy begins with injecting 0.5–2 mg of rt-PA (1mg/mL) into the dysfunctional catheter and allowing the lytic agent to dwell within the catheter lumen(s) for 5–60 minutes[56–58] (**Fig. 15-9**). The risk of catheter rupture by forceful injection of the thrombolytic agent into an occluded lumen can be reduced by attaching an empty 10-mL syringe and a second syringe filled with 2 mg rt-PA to the catheter via a three-way stopcock. Negative pressure is created within the catheter lumen by aspiration with the empty 10-mL syringe. The stopcock is then turned to allow negative pressure to pull the thrombolytic agent into the occluded catheter lumen.[52]

Infusion Thrombolysis

When simple instillation of a thrombolytic agent proves unsuccessful, a continuous infusion (4–6 hours) of a higher dose of the agent has been shown to restore patency in most catheters (**Fig. 15-10**). Various dosages and infusion rates of thrombolytics have been described, but there is no evidence that any single protocol has proven superior. The overall success rates range from 76% to 97%, and associated complications are rare to nonexistent.[58–62] Lund et al. reported an 80% success rate at restoring patency of hemodialysis catheters using a 6-hour infusion of 20,000 U of UK per hour per lumen.[60] Alternatively, Saveder et al. reported success using a 3-hour infusion of rt-PA (2.5 mg in 50 mL of normal saline) at a rate of 17 mL/h per port.[63]

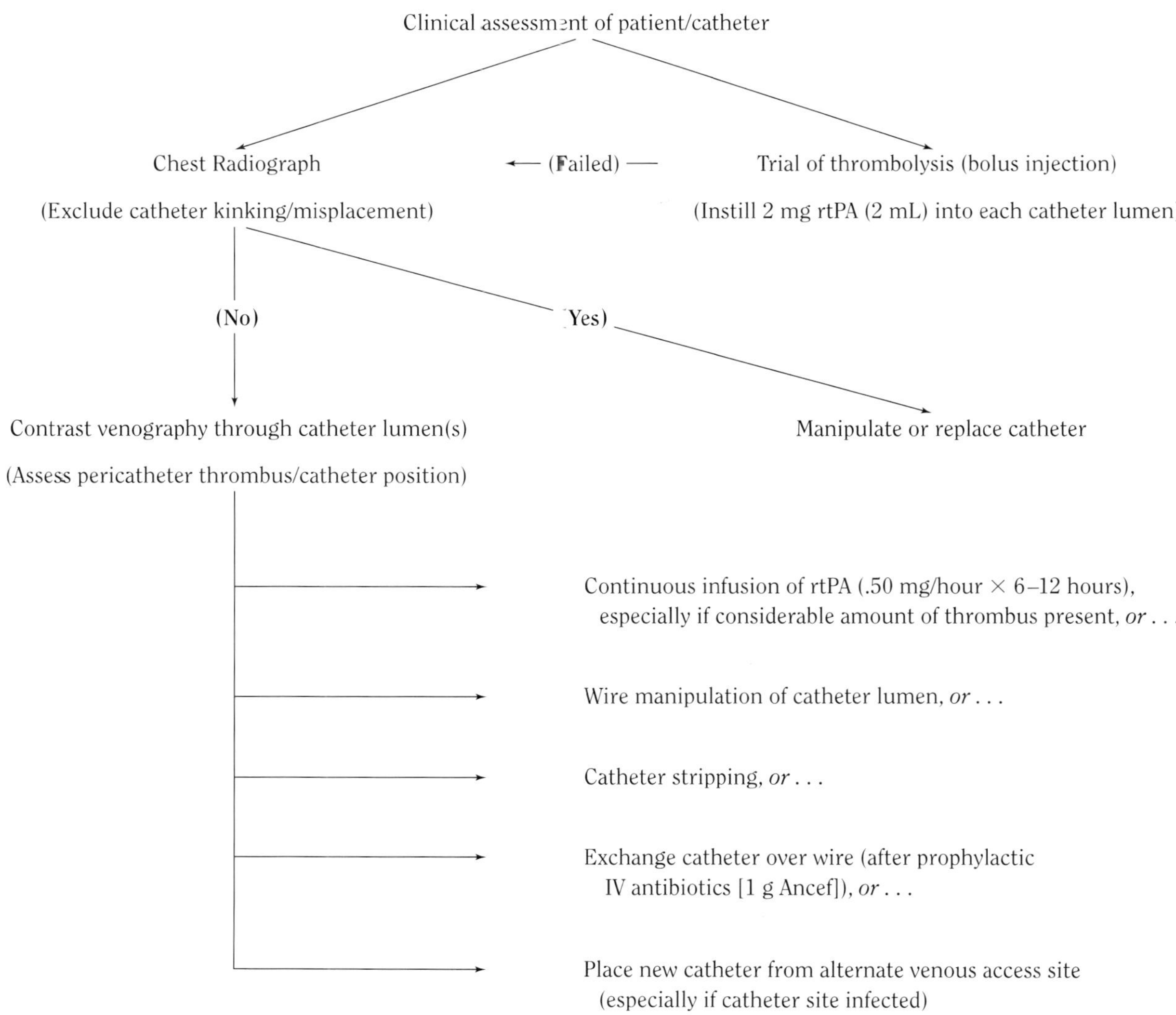

Figure 15-9. Flow diagram for the assessment and treatment of catheter dysfunction.

A

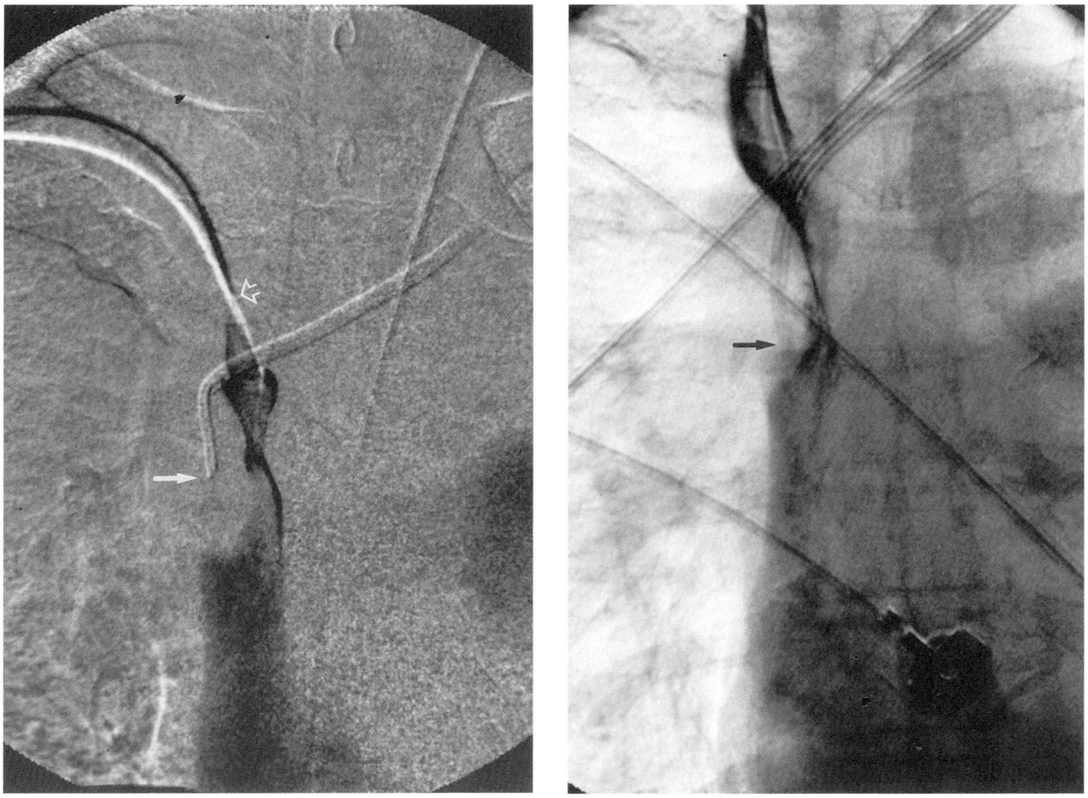

B

C

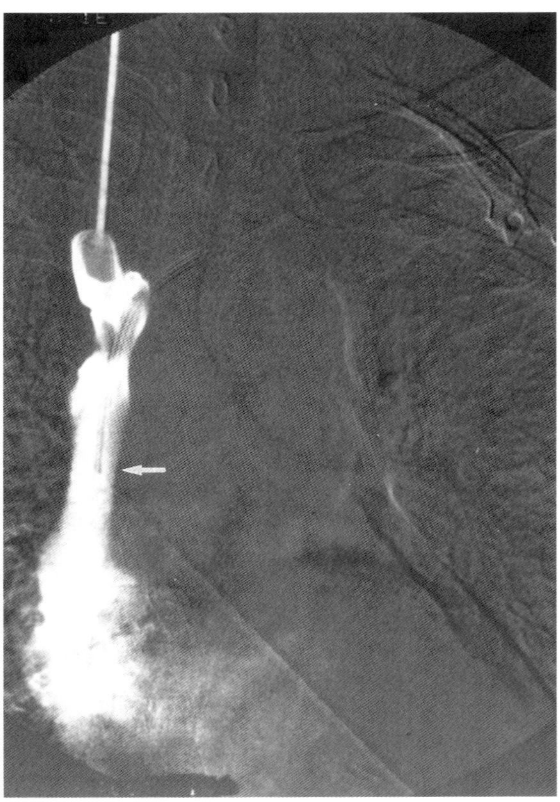

Figure 15-10. (A) Digital venogram of the superior vena cava (SVC) performed through a 5-F catheter (open arrow) placed from the right upper extremity. The dysfunctional left internal jugular vein central venous catheter abuts the lateral wall of the SVC and is encased in thrombus (solid arrow). The SVC is narrowed by thrombus but patent. (B) After 24 hours of thrombolytic therapy (.48 mg/h recombinant tissue-type plasminogen activator) delivered via the 5-F right upper-extremity catheter embedded in the thrombus, a follow-up venogram reveals minimal improvement, but the central venous catheter (arrow) has begun to migrate toward the right atrium. (C) After 48 hours of thrombolytic therapy, the now functioning left internal jugular vein catheter (arrow) has migrated back toward the right atrium and the SVC is open with minimal residual stenosis.

The advantages of infusion thrombolysis are that the process is relatively painless, the catheter and the primary access site are preserved, and the procedure can be performed in a monitored outpatient holding area. The disadvantage is the cost of monitoring the patient during therapy, especially if the treatment requires overnight hospitalization. Jones et al. reported the successful treatment of catheter-related sepsis and thrombosis with the use of thrombolytics and antibiotics in combination.[64,65] Others question the effectiveness of this approach and recommend catheter removal followed by appropriate antibiotic treatment.

Catheter Stripping

Percutaneous stripping to remove fibrin sheaths and pericatheter thrombus from central VADs was first described by Knelson et al.[66] This approach requires venipuncture, typically from a common femoral vein, through which a 15- or 25-mm diameter Amplatz nitinol Gooseneck snare (Microvena, White Bear Lake, MN) is advanced and looped over the dysfunctional catheter (**Fig. 15-11**). The snare is tightened and pulled along the catheter, stripping away the pericatheter fibrin sheath/thrombus. A wire, placed through one of the lumens of the dysfunctional catheter and into the inferior vena cava (IVC), can assist readvancement of the snare onto the catheter. The stripping is repeated until catheter function is restored.

Pericatheter stripping has been shown to lengthen catheter life; however, repeat interventions are typically required, and long-term patency is less than encouraging.[67,68] Crain et al. reported that the life of a dialysis catheter could be extended 2.8 months with a single intervention. The patency rate at 6 months, however, was only 28%.[67] In a prospective study comparing the patency rates of dialysis catheters that were mechanically stripped (n = 28) versus ones that were infused with urokinase, Gray et al. found the initial clinical success of pericatheter stripping to be 89%; however, they found the 15-, 30-, and 45-day primary patency rates to be 75%, 52%, and 35%, respectively.[69] Merport et al. reported the 1-, 2-, 3-, and 4-month patency rates of dialysis catheters after pericatheter stripping to be 31%, 16%, 7%, and 0%, respectively.[70]

Catheter Exchange

Exchanging a dysfunctional catheter over a guide wire for a new catheter has distinct advantages, such as maintenance of venous access,[71] high technical success rate, and short completion time. Prophylactic intravenous antibiotics (1 g Cephazolin) given 1 hour before the exchange will minimize catheter infections. The catheter and surrounding area are sterilely prepared and draped. After the catheter tunnel is infiltrated with a local anesthetic (2% lidocaine), a hydrophilic guide wire (Boston Scientific Corp., Natick, MA) is placed through the catheter lumen and positioned into the IVC. The indwelling catheter cuff is released with blunt dissection and the catheter is removed. Pressure is applied over the tunnel to minimize bleeding and avoid creating an air embolism. The new catheter is then placed on the wire, manipulated through the tunnel, and properly positioned in the SVC. Mechanical disruption of the pericatheter sheath can be achieved with twirling of a pigtail catheter, an angioplasty balloon, or an over-the-wire Fogarty embolectomy catheter (Baxter, Irvine, CA).[68,72,73] Performing such interventions through a flexible 8-F or 9-F introducer sheath can minimize bleeding. Pericatheter bleeding after catheter placement can be managed by placement of a purse-string suture where the catheter exits the tunnel.

Catheters replaced in such a manner have been reported to have the same life expectancy as those placed at a new access site.[71] Other researchers have suggested a higher rate of catheter colonization and catheter-related bacteremias when new catheters are placed through preexisting tunnels.[74] Merport et al. reported the patency rates of hemodialysis catheters after over-the-wire exchanges to be 71%, 33%, 27%, and 27% at 1, 2, 3, and 4 months, respectively.[70]

Alternative Venous Access

The internal jugular vein is the preferred approach for both tunneled and non-tunneled central venous access because of the associated lower rate of central venous thrombosis/stenosis[75] (**Table 15-3**). Image-guided placement of central VADs via the internal jugular vein has proven highly successful and is associated with a very low complication rate.[72,76] US-guided access to the internal jugular vein is technically easier than the subclavian veins, and the risk of brachial plexus injury is avoided.[77,78] The internal jugular vein approach also carries a lower incidence of symptomatic venous thrombosis.[79]

The right internal jugular vein is favored over the left because it provides a more direct route to the right atrium. A catheter placed from the left internal jugular vein must transverse the angle made by the left brachiocephalic vein and SVC, causing it to lie against the lateral wall of the SVC (Fig. 15-10). Respiratory and cardiac motion, along with the inherent stiffness of the catheter, can damage the caval wall.

After the internal jugular veins, the subclavian veins are the next most commonly preferred route despite a significantly high rate of subsequent venous stenosis.[80]

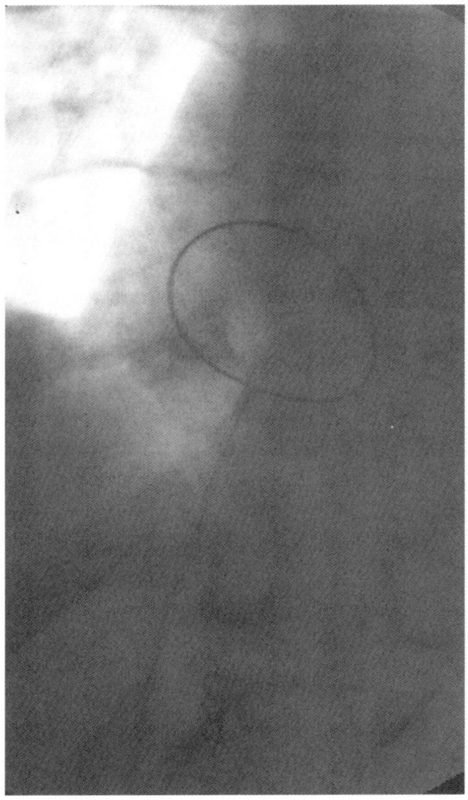

A

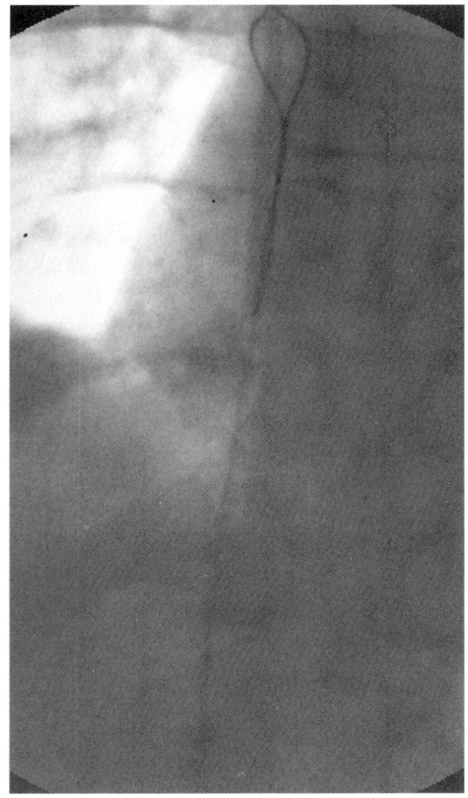

B

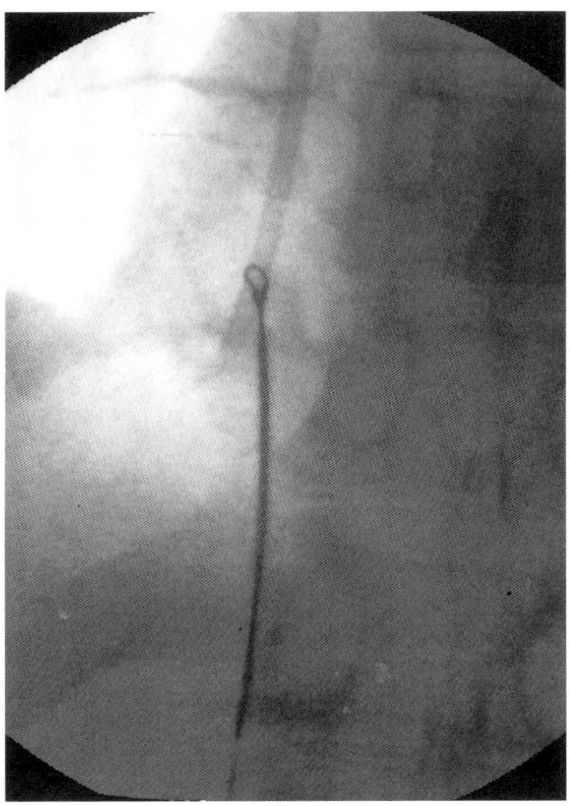

C

Figure 15-11. (A) Catheter stripping using a Amplatz nitinol Gooseneck snare. Approaching the dysfunctional superior vena cava (SVC) catheter from a femoral vein, the snare device is opened in the right atrium/SVC as it is looped over the catheter tip. (B) The Amplatz nitinol Gooseneck snare device is closed as it approaches the most cephalic aspect of the intravascular segment of the catheter. (C) With the snare held snuggly around the catheter, it is pulled toward the tip, stripping away pericatheter thrombus/fibrin sheath. This procedure is repeated until catheter function has been restored.

TABLE 15-3
Alternative Venous Access

1. Right internal jugular vein
2. Left internal jugular vein
3. Left subclavian vein
4. Right subclavian vein
5. Common femoral veins
6. Inferior vena cava (translumbar)
7. Hepatic vein (transhepatic)

The angle created by the subclavian vein makes as it joins the SVC is more acute on the right than the left, making an approach from the left subclavian vein more favorable and thereby reducing the risk of damage to the SVC.[81,82]

Atypical Approaches

Patients who require long-term central venous catheterization eventually develop occlusive complications of the commonly used access routes. Innovative and unique approaches to central VADs has allowed interventional radiologists to provide much-needed assistance to patients with central venous occlusions.

When central venous access from the neck and upper extremities is not available, then transfemoral, translumbar, and transhepatic approaches may provide useful and reliable alternatives.[83–87] Catheterization of the femoral vein is frequently used, although the incidence of catheter-related infection is high, approaching 30%.[87,88] The translumbar approach to the placement of IVC catheters has become an acceptable and important alternative route for patients requiring long-term central venous access.[89,90] The initial access to the IVC may be aided by CT or sonographic guidance, followed by positioning of the catheter tip under fluoroscopy. When the IVC is inaccessible, the transhepatic approach may prove to be lifesaving,[86,91] although catheter dislodgement from hepatic motion during respiration has the potential of causing life-threatening hemorrhage and peritonitis.[92] During catheter removal, the transhepatic tract should be embolized to avoid major intraperitoneal bleeding.[91,92] Both translumbar and transhepatic routes for central VAD placement should be reserved for those patients in whom other access options have been exhausted.

Innovative approaches to reach the central venous circulation have been described for when traditional access sites can no longer be used. Use of an intercostal vein for placement of a central VAD was described in two separate reports.[93,94] Engorged collateral veins have also been used to gain access into patent central vessels, bypassing occluded vein segments[95–98] (**Fig. 15–12**).

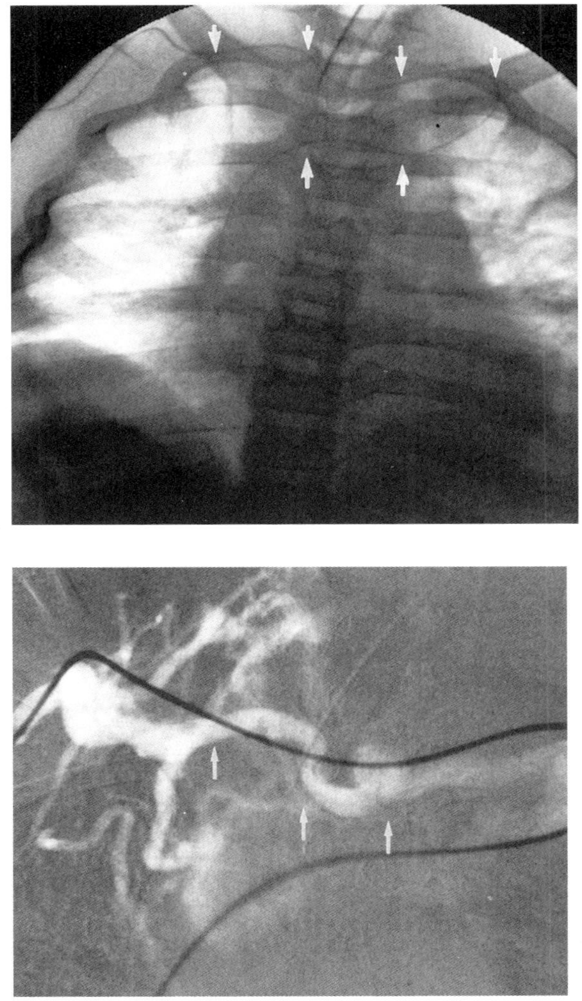

A

B

Figure 15-12. (A) In a patient with occluded internal jugular, left subclavian, and right brachiocephalic veins, a catheter and wire were negotiated from a patent segment of the right axillary vein, across the jugular arch (arrows) and into the superior vena cava via either a small but patent left brachiocephalic vein or superior intercostal vein. (B) Chest radiograph showing the course of the catheter (arrows).

RECANALIZATION OF CENTRAL VENOUS OCCLUSIONS

Venous recanalization with or without venous angioplasty or stenting is sometimes required to achieve successful central venous catheterization. Not only can patients with malignancies require frequent central venous catheterizations that can cause central venous thrombosis but also, the underlying malignancy itself can lead to SVC occlusion. Placement of a catheter through an occluded route preserves alterative patent veins for future access. This can be of vital importance in patients who may require long-term venous access and/or are prone to catheter-related infections and thromboses.

Direct Tunneling

Various catheters and wires can be used in combination to traverse venous occlusions (**Fig. 15-13**). An angled 5-F catheter and a 0.035-in stiff-shaft hydrophilic wire are frequently preferred. The wire is often looped on itself as it is negotiated across the occlusion. Once the catheter reenters a patent venous lumen, it is replaced with a stiffer wire to allow passage of dilators and a peel-away introducer sheath. Occasionally, performing an angioplasty in the tract will allow negotiation of the catheter past the occluded vein segment (**Fig. 15-14**). Care is taken, however, to not penetrate the vessel wall and to evade extravascular structures (e.g., the mediastinum). In such a case, the catheter is withdrawn and rerouted or the access is abandoned. Some authors have recommended placement of a through-and-through wire, from a femoral vein or contralateral axillary vein approach, to facilitate venous recanalization by stabilizing the wire during angioplasty and/or stent placement.[99] If the occluded vessel has been crossed from a femoral approach, a wire or the catheter itself may be snared and pulled across the obstruction.

Loop Snare Or Target Technique

When routine upper-extremity central venous access becomes difficult because of venous occlusions, placement of catheters through small venous collaterals in the neck or chest can be achieved from a femoral approach (**Fig. 15-15**). Ferral et al. described using a looped snare, placed from a femoral vein approach. The snare is opened within a neck vein and used as a target through which a needle is fluoroscopically placed.[100] The loop snare is then closed up on the needle and the needle is replaced with an exchange-length wire (0.018 in). The wire is then pulled through the femoral access in a through-and-through manner. Once the wire from the upper access is secured, the percutaneous tract in the neck can be dilated and an appropriate central VAD can be placed.[95]

Sharp Recanalization

Farrell et al. described the use of a Rösch–Uchida needle (Cook Inc., Bloomington, IN) or a coaxial sheathed needle with a 21-gauge stylet to puncture through short venous occlusions that are resistant to crossing with a standard guide wire and catheter.[101] The length of the obstruction can be accurately determined by simultaneously advancing two catheters to the points of occlusion, one from a femoral and another from an upper-extremity approach. Once the occlusion is crossed, the sharp needle is exchanged for a stiff wire, over which a balloon catheter is advanced. The tract is then dilated in preparation for placement of the central VAD (**Fig. 15-16**).

To minimize the risk of significant extravascular hemorrhage, Farrell et al. recommended advancement of the needle from the transfemoral approach in light of the lower venous pressure on the central side of the occlusion. Once the occlusion is crossed, the wire is then snared

A

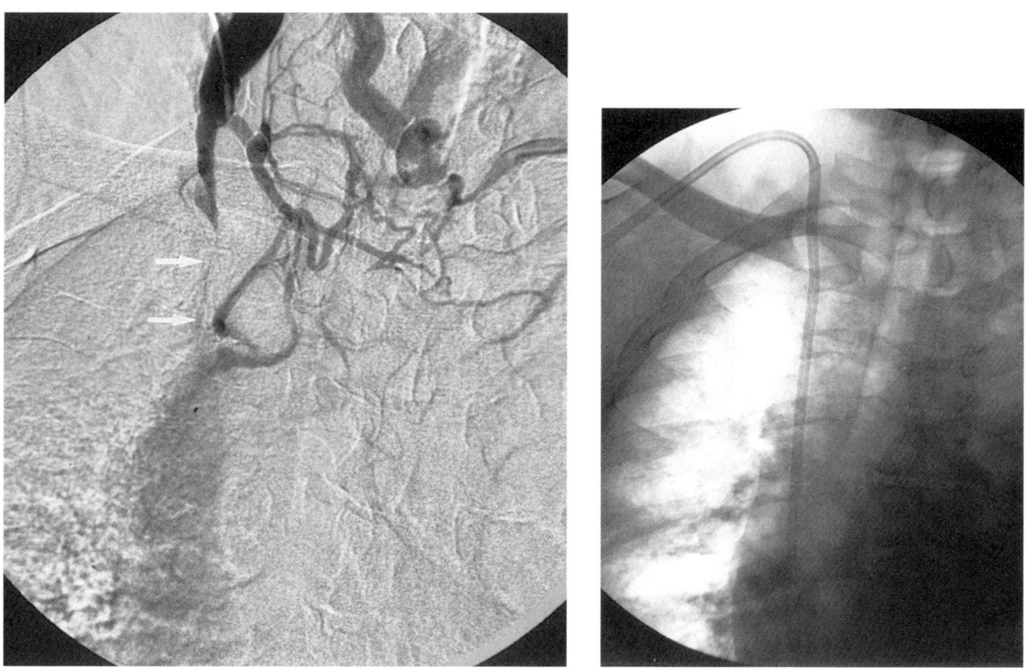

B

Figure 15-13. (A) Venogram from the right internal jugular vein demonstrates nearly complete occlusion of the right central internal jugular and brachiocephalic veins (arrows). The area was crossed using a catheter and Glide wire (Boston Scientific Corp; Natick, MA). After the Glide wire was exchanged for a stiffer wire, a peel away sheath was placed into the superior vena cava (SVC). (B) A tunneled catheter was positioned in the SVC.

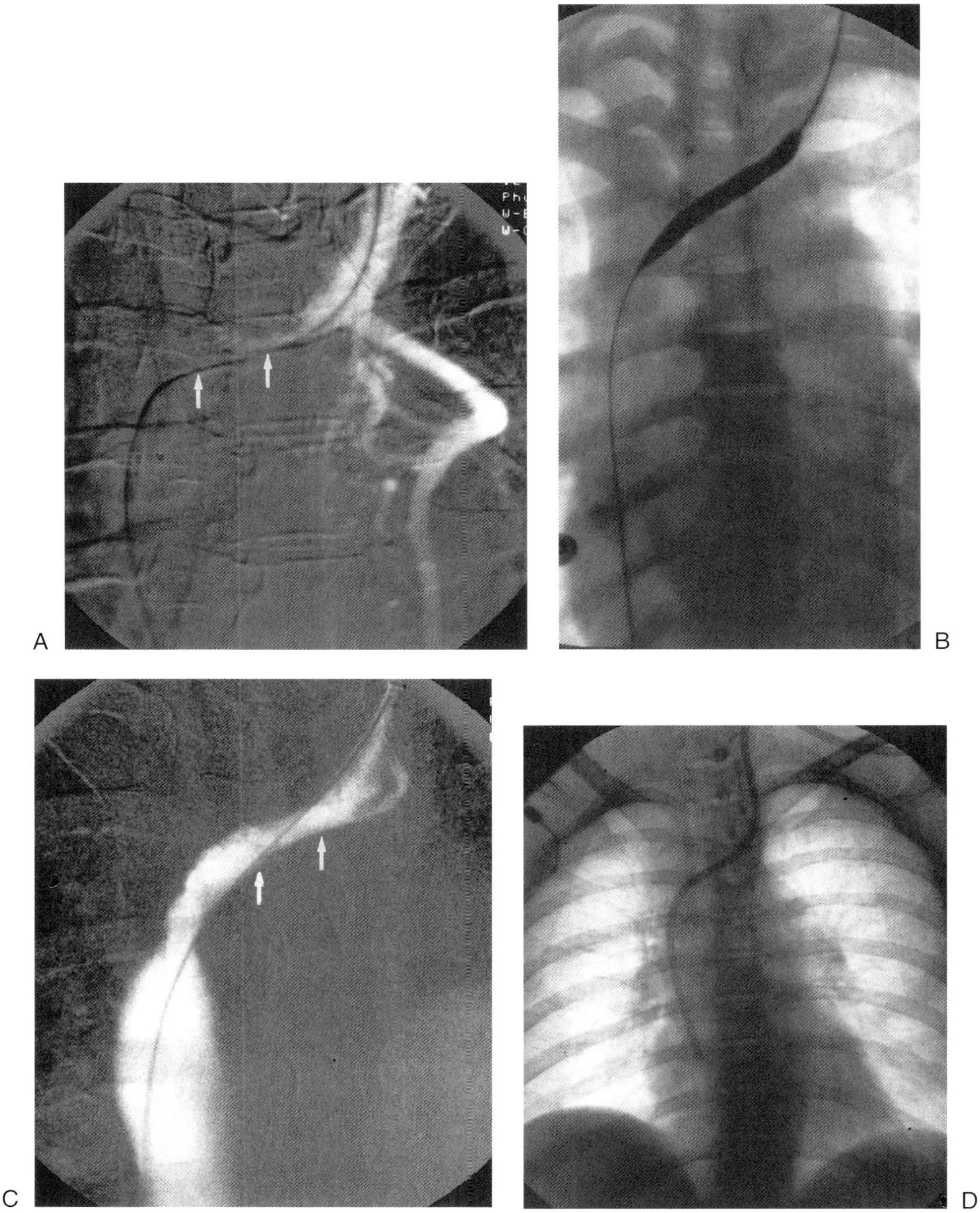

Figure 15-14. (A) In a patient with occlusion of both brachiocephalic and right internal jugular veins, a digital road map image was obtained after access was gained into the patent left internal jugular vein. With the use of a Glide wire (Boston Scientific Corp; Natick, MA) and 5-F catheter, access was gained across the occluded left brachiocephalic vein (arrows) and into the superior vena cava (SVC). (B) After positioning of a stiff wire into the inferior vena cava, angioplasty of the occluded vein segment is accomplished with a 6-mm × 4-cm balloon followed by a 10-mm × 4-cm balloon. (C) A postangioplasty venogram demonstrates restoration of blood flow through the left brachiocephalic vein (arrows). (D) A tunneled catheter is then placed across the newly revised vein segment and positioned in the SVC.

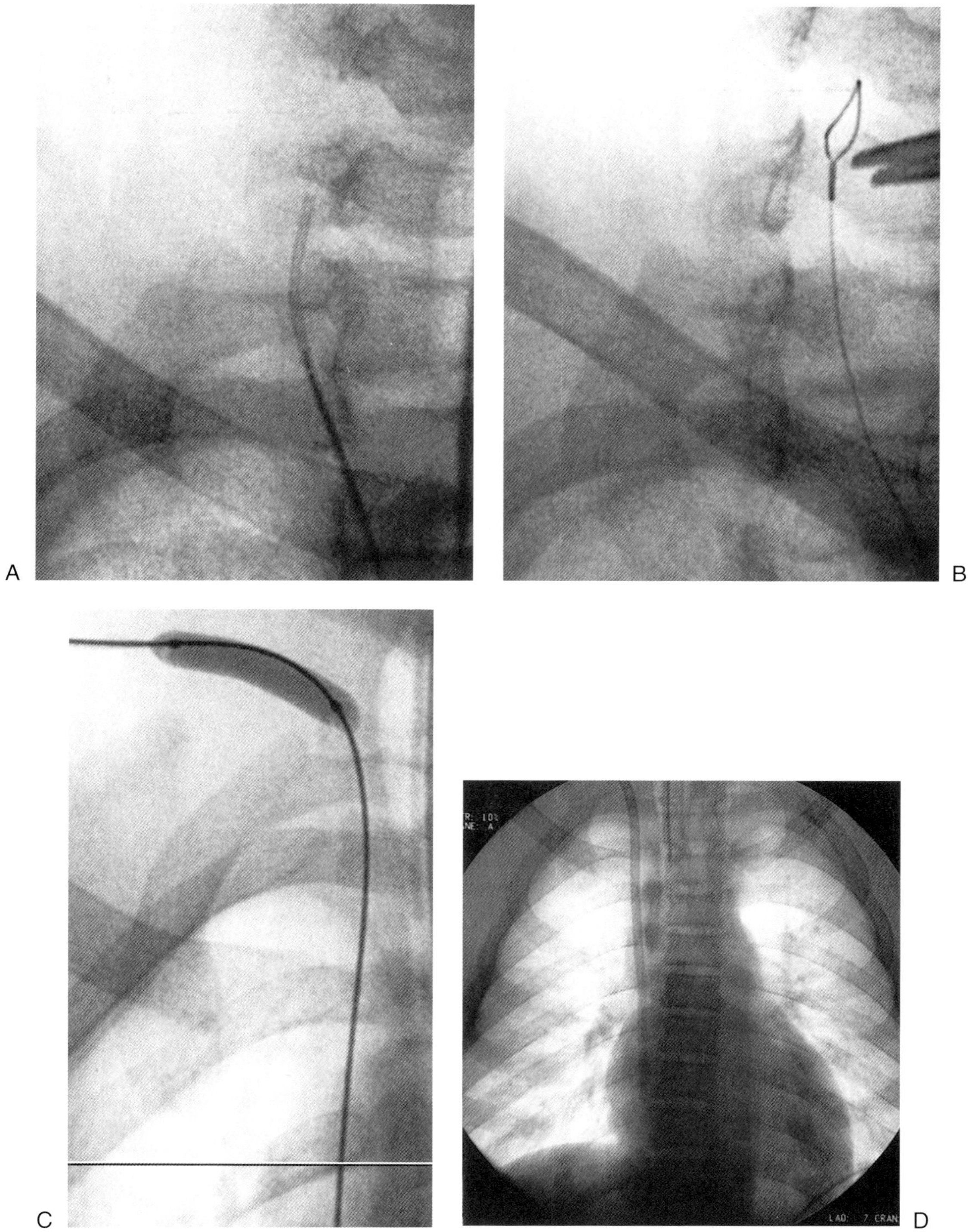

Figure 15-15. (A) In a patient with occluded bilateral internal jugular and subclavian veins, a catheter and wire are placed from the right femoral vein and negotiated into a small but patent neck vein. (B) The wire is replaced with a Amplatz nitinol Gooseneck snare. Under fluoroscopic guidance, the snare is used as a target and a needle is percutaneously placed through the snare loop. Ultrasound is used to verify the distance to the snare and direct the approach so that the needle will not transverse any major artery. Once the snare is closed around the needle, the needle is replaced with an 0.035-in, 260-cm-length guide wire. With the snare tightened around the guide wire, the wire is pulled from the percutaneous access in the neck, through the venous system, and out the femoral vein. A 4-F Glide cath (Boston Scientific Corp., Natick, MA) is then passed over the wire from the neck access and into the superior vena cava (SVC), where the guide wire is replaced with a stiff wire. (C) The percutaneous access is then dilated down to the SVC and a banana-peel catheter is placed over a stiff wire. (D) A tunneled catheter is then negotiated into the SVC.

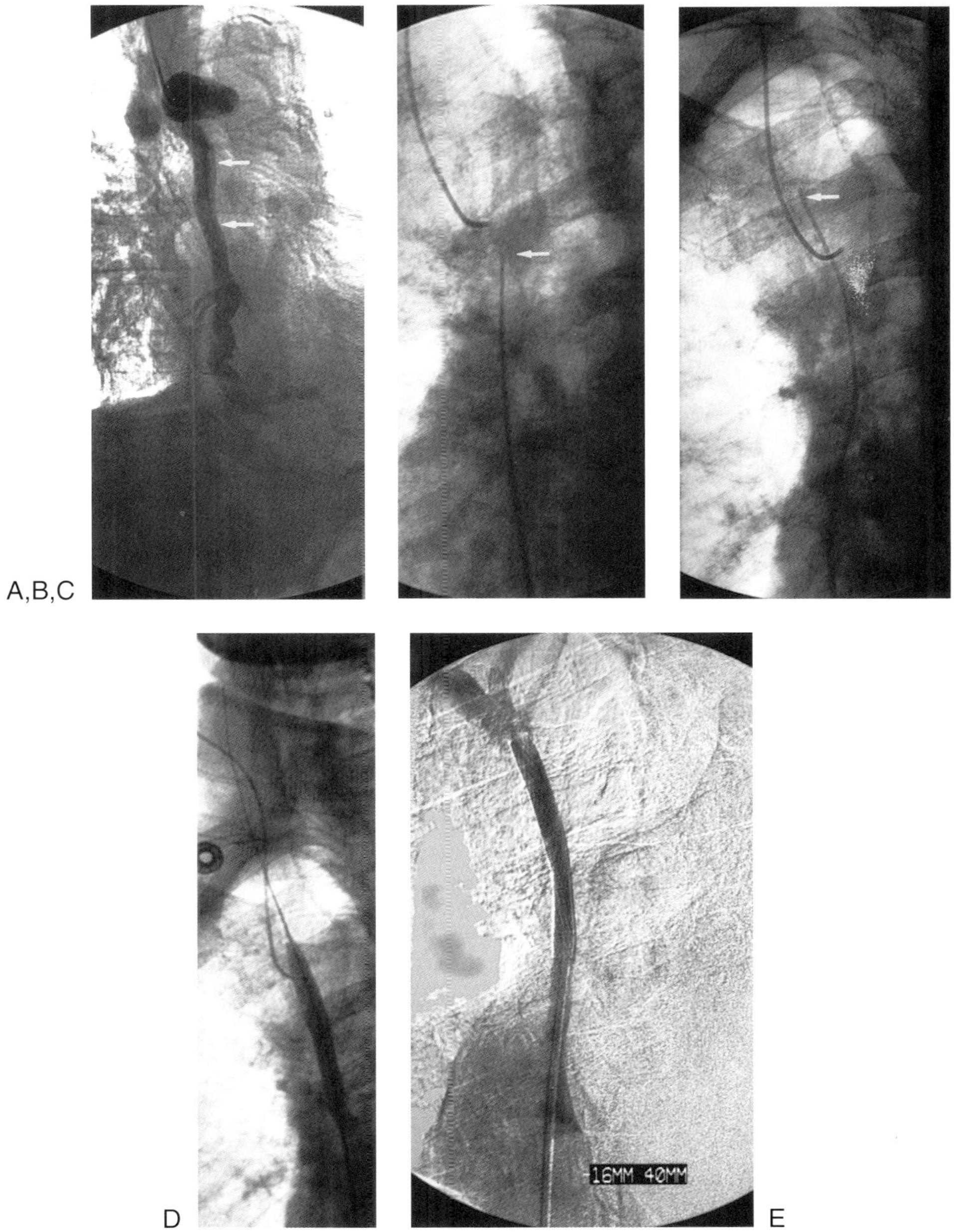

Figure 15-16. (A) Sharp recanalization of an occluded central vein. Venogram performed from a right internal jugular vein demonstrates occlusion of the superior vena cava (SVC) and collateral venous drainage via the azygos vein (arrows). (B) After several failed attempts to traverse the occluded SVC from the right internal jugular vein access site, a catheter and wire are positioned within the SVC from the femoral vein (arrow). (C) Using the stiff end of a stiff-shaft Glide wire (Boston Scientific Corp., Natick, MA) (arrow), supported by a long sheath and catheter from the femoral vein, the occluded SVC is successfully traversed. (D) Angioplasty of the occluded segment is performed using a 10-mm × 40-mm balloon. (E) A 16-mm × 40-mm Wallstent (Boston Scientific Corp.), is deployed across the recanalize segment. (Case photos courtesy of Tony Farrell, MD, of Evanston Memorial Hospital, Evanston, IL.)

from above and pulled through the percutaneous access. When extravasation occurs after recanalization, then prolonged inflation of an angioplasty balloon or prompt placement of a covered stent should be considered.

Pharmacologic Thrombolysis

Restoration of vascular patency may not be necessary in asymptomatic or minimally symptomatic patients, because developing venous collaterals will often manage the complications of venous hypertension. In patients with limited venous access or in those who require long-term catheterization, aggressive measures to maintain venous access are justified.

One approach to central venous thrombolysis is to begin with a venogram to define the extent of central vein occlusion. If the occlusion can be crossed with a catheter and wire, then a multiple side-hole infusion catheter is positioned within the thrombus and infusion of rt-PA is begun at a rate of 0.5–1.0 mg/h at a concentration of 4 mg rt-PA in 1000 mL normal saline (**Fig. 15-10**). Heparin can be infused via the introducer sheath at a rate of 500 U/h, delivering a higher concentration directly to the thrombus and minimizing systemic effects.

Thrombolysis can be augmented by angioplasty of the thrombus before and during thrombolysis. Mechanical disruption will increase the exposed surface area of the thrombus to the lytic agent; however, care must be taken to not dislodge large emboli into the pulmonary circulation. The infusion of rt-PA is continued until follow-up venography shows complete resolution or no interval change in the thrombus. When an underlying residual stenosis is found, the abnormality is typically dilated or stented, or both.

Mechanical Thrombectomy

Several devices have been developed to remove and/or macerate arterial and venous thrombus. Three of the more commonly used devices, approved in the United States, are

- Amplatz thrombectomy device (Microvena, White Bear Lake, MN)
- Hydrolyser (Cordis Corp., Miami, FL)
- AngioJet ([rheolytic thrombectomy catheter] Possis Medical, Minneapolis, MN)

Catheter-directed pharmacologic thrombolysis is considered the treatment of choice for the removal of thrombus during recanalization of central venous occlusions. In patients in whom surgery and thrombolytics are contraindicated or when faster recanalization is necessary, the use of a mechanical thrombectomy device may provide sufficient debulking of the thrombus. The ideal mechanical device should be effective at removing a large amount of thrombus without creating clinically significant pulmonary emboli or damage to the vessel wall. A review of these endovascular devices and their mechanism of action can be found in an article by Sharafuddin and Hicks.[102]

Although most clinical experience with the use of mechanical thrombectomy devices has been in the pulmonary arteries and deep venous system of the lower extremities, a few scattered reports have shown promising results in treating thrombosis of the upper central venous system.[103–107] Kasirajan et al. described the clinical use of the AngioJet rheolytic thrombectomy device (Possis) to recanalize both upper and lower central venous and lower-extremity DVT.[103] They found the device to be effective at removing greater than 50% of the thrombus in 59% of patients (n = 17). This device has been shown in in vitro studies to remove thrombi up to a diameter of 10 mm.[108]

Despite significant removal of thrombus, additional procedures (angioplasty, stenting, thrombolytic therapy) are commonly necessary to provide successful and complete recanalization. Uflacker found the Amplatz thrombectomy device (Microvena) to be effective at reducing the amount of thrombus; however, ancillary procedures were required in the majority of patients treated.[104] The initial debulking of the large clot increases the surface area exposed to a lytic agent and decreases the duration of thrombolytic therapy. Like pharmacologic thrombolysis, the mechanical devices were found to be more effective when the thrombus was not chronic and well organized.[104]

Recanalization of central venous occlusions with mechanical thrombectomy devices has been shown in animal studies to be safe.[108–110] Some of the limitations of the rheolytic devices, however, are the possibility of fluid overload in patients with congestive heart failure and the risk of renal damage from hemolysis, which becomes particularly important in patients with reversible renal failure.[111] Large multicenter clinical studies are needed to determine the safety and appropriate use of mechanical thrombectomy devices for the treatment of central venous thrombosis. New percutaneous devices using endovascular US to assist thrombolysis are currently under investigation and may prove to have a promising future.[112,113]

Percutaneous Venous Angioplasty and Stenting

Venous thrombolysis followed by angioplasty alone of subclavian vein thrombosis has been shown by Beygui et al. to have a poor patency rate.[114] Deployment of a stent followed by anticoagulation with warfarin is recommended especially when there is considerable thrombus present, slow venous blood flow, or incomplete opening of the stent.

The optimal stent diameter in the subclavian and brachiocephalic veins is between 6 and 10 mm, whereas the SVC typically requires a 14- to 16-mm-diameter stent.[101] Several reports have demonstrated respectable long-term patency of venous stenoses treated with the Gianturco-Rösch Z stent (Cook Inc., Bloomington, IN) (**Fig. 15-17**), Wallstent (Boston Scientific Corp., Natick, MA), and Palmaz stent (Cordis Corp., Miami, FL).[115–120] To achieve long-term clinical success, however, close surveillance and multiple reinterventions are typically necessary.[121–123]

Angioplasty of the stenosis prior to deployment of the stent is recommended to reduce the risk of stent migration during deployment. In the event the underlying stenosis cannot be dilated with a balloon, a stent should

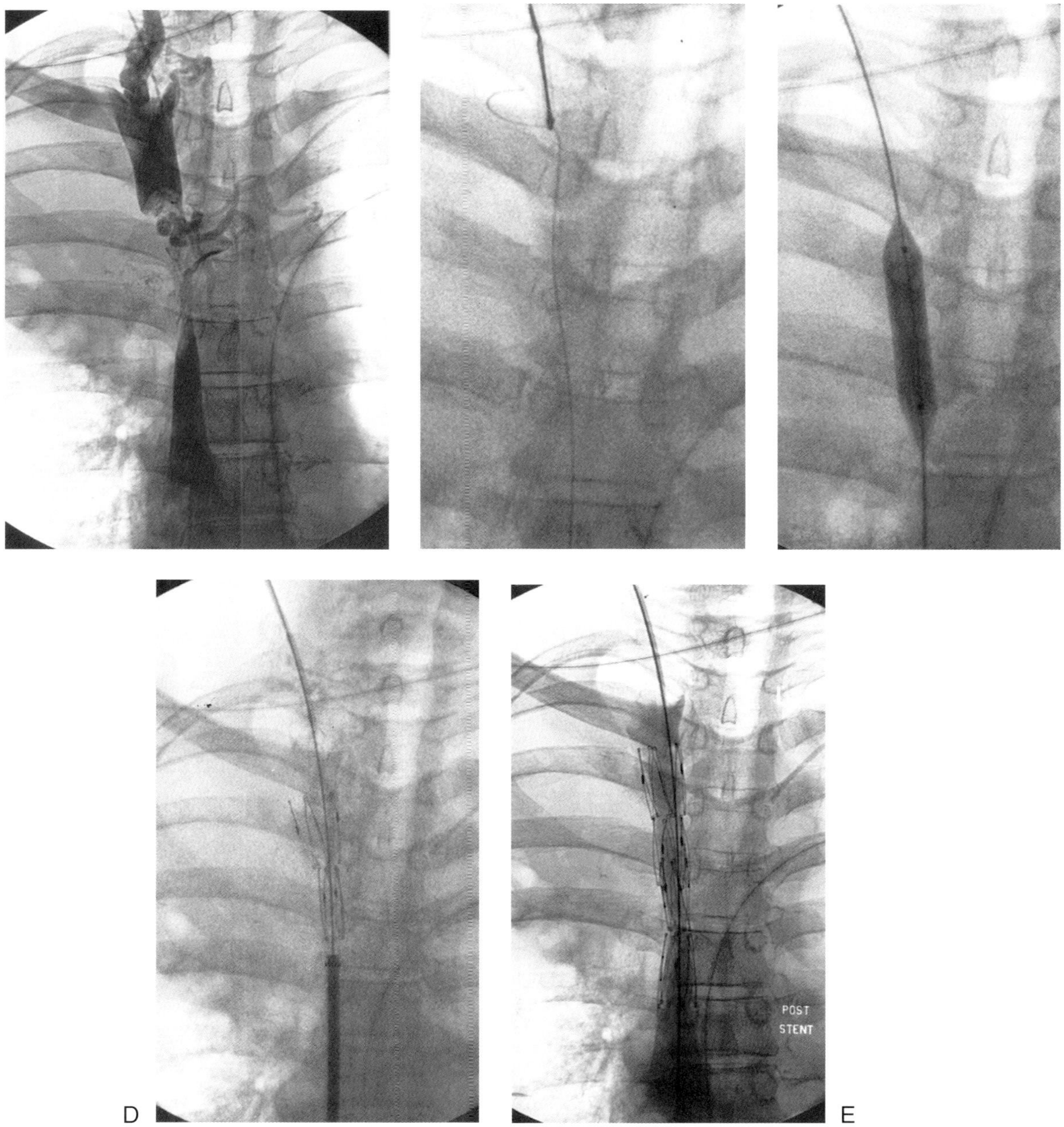

Figure 15-17. (A) Venogram demonstrating malignant occlusion of the superior vena cava. (B) A femoral wire is passed through the occlusion and snared within the right brachiocephalic vein. The wire is then pulled through a right internal jugular vein sheath. (C) Angioplasty of the occlusion is performed over a wire that is now secured from both the internal jugular and femoral venous sites. (D) A self-expanding Gianturco-Rösch Z stent (Cook, Inc., Bloomington, IN) is deployed across the occlusion from the femoral vein. (E) Venogram is performed after angioplasty of the deployed stent. (Case photos courtesy of William Rilling, MD, of Medical College of Wisconsin, Milwaukee, WI.)

not be deployed. Self-expanding stents, when properly sized, have an advantage over balloon-expandable stents because the diameter of the vein is known to vary during changes in the patient's position, respiratory variation, and hydration status. A properly placed balloon-expandable stent may become too small if the vein expands or if the stent is compressed by external forces, allowing it to migrate toward the right atrium.

CONCLUSION

Central venous catheters are indispensable in the day-to-day treatment of patients with malignancy; however, catheter dysfunction is a source of considerable patient morbidity. Well-designed, controlled studies are needed to identify the risk factors and best treatment options for the treatment of patients with dysfunctional central venous catheters. The possibility of newer catheter designs made from non-thrombogenic, infection-resistant materials are also needed.

The placement and care of central venous catheters has become, in large part, the responsibility of the interventional radiologist. Having a thorough knowledge of the causes of catheter malfunction and appropriate management options is essential in providing the best care for the patient with cancer who requires temporary or long-term central venous access.

REFERENCES

1. Freytes CO. Indications and complications of intravenous devices for chemotherapy. *Curr Opin Oncol* 2000;12:303–307.
2. Wickham R, Purl S, Welker D. Long-term central venous catheters: issues for care. *Semin Oncol Nurs* 1992;8:133–147.
3. Cooper RA, James RD, Taylor KJ. Cardiac perforation associated with continuous infusional chemotherapy. *Clin Oncol (R Coll Radiol)* 1996;8:404–405.
4. Collier PE, Goodman GB. Cardiac tamponade caused by central venous catheter perforation of the heart: a preventable complication. *J Am Coll Surg* 1995;181:459–463.
5. Curelaru I, Linder LE, Gustavsson B. Displacement of catheters inserted through internal jugular veins with neck flexion and extension. A preliminary study. *Intensive Care Med* 1980;6:179–183.
6. O'Farrell LO, Griffith JW, Lang CM. Histologic development of the sheath that forms around long-term implanted central venous catheters. *J Parenter Enteral Nutr* 1996;20:156–158.
7. Petersen J, Delaney JH, Brakstad MT, Rowbotham RK, Bagley CM. Silicone venous access devices positioned with their tips high in the superior vena cava are more likely to malfunction. *Am J Surg* 1999;178(1):38–41.
8. Pithie A, Souter JS, Pennigton CR. Catheter tip position in central vein thrombosis. *J Parenter Enteral Nutr* 1988;12:613–614.
9. Kowalski CM, Kaufman JA, Rivitz SM, Geller SC, Waltman AC. Migration of central venous catheters: implications for initial catheter tip positioning. *J Vasc Interv Radiol* 1997;8:443–447.
10. Andris DA, Krzywda EA. Catheter pinch-off syndrome: recognition and management. *J Intraven Nurs* 1997;20:233–237.
11. Hinke DH, Zandt-Stastny DA, Goodman LR, et al. Pinch-off syndrome: a complication of implantable subclavian venous access devices. *Radiology* 1990;177:353–356.
12. Akinwande KI, Keehn DM. Dissolution of phenytoin precipitate with Sodium bicarbonate in an occluded central venous access device. *Ann Pharmacother* 1995;29:707–709.
13. Shulman RJ, Reed T, Pitre D, Laine L. Use of hydrochloric acid to clear obstructed central venous catheters. *J Parenter Enteral Nutr* 1988;12:509–510.
14. Holcombe BJ, Forloines-Lynn S, Garmhausen LW. Restoring patency of long-term central venous access devices. *J Intraven Nurs* 1992;15:36–41.
15. Krzywda E. Central venous access: catheters, technology and physiology. *Medsurg Nurs* 1998;7:132–140.
16. Krzywda EA. Predisposing factors, prevention, and management of central venous catheter occlusions. *J Intraven Nurs* 1999;22:S11–S17.
17. Hoch JR. Management of the complications of long-term venous access. *Semin Vascular Surg* 1997;10:135–143.
18. De Cicco M, Matovic M, Balestreri L, et al. Central venous thrombosis: an early and frequent complication in cancer patients bearing long-term Silastic catheters: a prospective study. *Thromb Res* 1997;86:101–113.
19. Baglin TP, Boughton BJ. Central venous thrombosis due to bolus injections of anti-leukaemic chemotherapy. *Br J Haematol* 1986;63:606–607.
20. Eastridge BJ, Lefor AT. Complications of indwelling venous catheter devices in cancer patients. *J Clin Oncol* 1995;13:233–238.
21. Welch GW, McKeel DW Jr, Silverstein P, Walker HL. Role of catheter composition in the development of thrombophlebitis. *Surg Gynecol Obstet* 1974;138:421–424.
22. Bern MM, Lokich JJ, Wallach SR, et al. Very low doses of warfarin can prevent thrombosis in central venous catheters: a randomized prospective trial. *Ann Intern Med* 1990;112:423–428.
23. Devie-Hubert I, Carlier M, Pozzo Di Borgo C. Venous thrombosis on central catheters in oncology. *Rev Med Interne* 1996;17:821–825.
24. Horattas MC, Wright DJ, Fenton AH, et al. Changing concepts of deep venous thrombosis of the upper extremity: report of a series and review of the literature. *Surgery* 1988;104:561–567.
25. Hoshal VL Jr, Ause RG, Hoskins PA. Fibrin sleeve formation on indwelling subclavian central venous catheters. *Arch Surg* 1971;102:353–358.
26. Ahmed N, Payne RF. Thrombosis after central venous cannulation. *Med J Aust* 1976;1:217–220.
27. Brismar BO, Hardstedt C, Jacobson S. Diagnosis of thrombosis by catheter phlebography after prolonged central venous catheterization. *Ann Surg* 1981;194:779–783.
28. Bolz KD, Fjermeros G, Wideroe TE, Hatlinghus S. Catheter malfunction and thrombus formation on double-lumen hemodialysis catheters: an intravascular ultrasonographic study. *Am J Kidney Dis* 1995;25:597–602.
29. Rockall AG, Harris A, Wetton CWN, et al. Stripping of failing haemodialysis catheters using the Ampltaz gooseneck snare. *Clin Radiol* 1997;52:616–620.
30. Brady PS, Spence LD, Levitin A, Mickolich CT, Dolmatch BL. Efficacy of percutaneous fibrin sheath stripping in restoring patency of tunneled hemodialysis catheters. *Am J Roentgenol* 1999;173:1023–1027.
31. Kooij JD, van der Zant FM, van Beek EJ, Reekers JA. Pulmonary embolism in deep venous thrombosis of the upper extremity: more often in catheter-related thrombosis. *Neth J Med* 1997;50:238–242.
32. Mailloux RJ, DeLegge MH, Kirby DF. Pulmonary embolism as a complication of long-term total parenteral nutrition. *J Parenter Enteral Nutr* 1993;17:578–582.
33. Monreal M, Raventos A, Lerma R, et al. Pulmonary embolism in patients with upper extremity DVT associated to venous central lines—a prospective study. *Thromb Haemost* 1994;72:548–550.
34. Prandoni P, Bernardi E. Upper extremity deep vein thrombosis. *Curr Opin Pulm Med* 1999;5:222–226.
35. Beregi JP, Aumegeat V, Loubeyre C, et al. Right atrial thrombi: percutaneous mechanical thrombectomy. *Cardiovasc Intervent Radiol* 1997;20:142–145.
36. Horattas MC, Wright DJ, Fenton AH, et al. Changing concepts of deep venous thrombosis of the upper extremity: report of a series and review of the literature. *Surgery* 1988;104:561–567.
37. Barzaghi A, Dell'Orto M, Rovelli A, et al. Central venous catheter clots: incidence, clinical significance, and catheter care in patients with hematologic malignancies. *Pediatr Hematol Oncol* 1995;12:243–250.
38. Kee ST, Kinoshita L, Razavi MK, et al. Superior vena cava syndrome: treatment with catheter-directed thrombolysis and endovascular stent placement. *Radiology* 1998;206:187–193.
39. Balestreri L, DeCicco M, Matoure M, et al. Central venous catheter-related thrombosis in clinically asymptomatic oncology patients: a phlebographic study. *Eur J Radiol* 1995;20:108–111.
40. Fincher R. Superior vena cava syndrome: experience in a teaching hospital. *South Med J* 1987;80:1243–1245.
41. Markman M. Diagnosis and management of superior vena cava syndrome. *Cleve Clin J Med* 1999;66:59–61.

42. Whitman ED. Complications associated with the use of central venous access devices. *Curr Prob Surg* 1996;33:309–388.
43. Raad II, Luna M, Khalil SA, et al. Relationship between thrombotic and infectious complications of central venous catheters. *JAMA* 1994;271:1014–1016.
44. Press OW, Ramsey PG, Larson EB, Fefer A, Hickman RO. Hickman catheter infections in patients with malignancies. *Medicine* 1984;63:189–200.
45. Barrett N, Spencer S, McIvor J, Brown EA. Subclavian stenosis: a major complication of subclavian dialysis catheters. *Nephrol Dial Transplant* 1990;3:423–425.
46. Ray CE, Shenoy SS, McCarthy PL, Broderick KA, Kaufman JA. Weekly prophylactic urokinase instillation in tunneled central venous access devices. *J Vasc Interv Radiol* 1999;10:1330–1334.
47. Carr KM, Rabinowitz I. Physician compliance with warfarin prophylaxis for central venous catheters in patients with solid tumors. *J Clin Oncol* 2000;18:3665–3667.
48. Boraks P, Seale J, Price J, et al. Prevention of central venous catheter associated thrombosis using minidose warfarin in patients with haematological malignancies. *Br J Haematol* 1998;101:483–486.
49. Andris DA, Krzywda EA. Central venous access: clinical practice issues. *Nurs Clin North Am* 1997;32:717–740.
50. Hurtubise MR, Bottino JC, Lawson M, McCredie KB. Restoring patency of occluded central venous catheters. *Arch Surg* 1980;115:212–213.
51. Atkinson JB, Bagnall HA, Gomperts E. Investigational use of tissue plasminogen activator (t-PA) for occluded central venous catheters. *J Parenter Enteral Nutr* 1990;14:310–311.
52. Schneider TC, Krzywda E, Andris D, Quebbeman EJ. The malfunctioning Silastic catheter: radiologic assessment. *J Parenter Enteral Nutr* 1986;10:70–73.
53. Moss AH, Vasilakis C, Holley JL, et al. Use of a silicone dual-lumen catheter with a Dacron cuff as a long-term vascular access for hemodialysis patients. *Am J Kidney Dis* 1990;26:211–215.
54. Suhocki PV, Conlon PJ Jr, Knelson MH, Harland R, Schwab SJ. Silastic cuffed catheters for hemodialysis vascular access: thrombolytic and mechanical correction of malfunction. *Am J Kidney Dis* 1996;28:379–386.
55. Hohage H, Schulte B, Mehrens T, et al. Serum antibody titers in a systemic lytic therapy with streptokinase. *South Med J* 1998 91:1019–1023.
56. Davis SN, Vermeulen L, Banton J, Schwartz BS, Williams EC. Activity and dosage of alteplase dilution for clearing occlusions of venous-access devices. *Am J Health Syst Pharm* 2000;57:1039–1045.
57. Lawson M. Partial occlusion of indwelling central venous catheters. *J Intraven Nurs* 1991;14:157–159.
58. Haire WD, Lieberman RP, Lund GB, Edney J, Wieczorek BM. Obstructed central venous catheters: restoring function with a 12-hour infusion of low-dose urokinase. *Cancer* 1990;66:2279–2285.
59. Haire WD, Lieberman RP. Thrombosed central venous catheters: restoring function with 6-hour urokinase infusion after failure of bolus urokinase. *J Parent Enter Nutr* 1992;16:129–132.
60. Lund GB, Trerotola SO, Scheel PF Jr, et al. Outcome of tunneled hemodialysis catheters placed by radiologists. *Radiology* 1996;198:467–472.
61. Horne MK III, Mayo DJ. Low-dose urokinase infusions to treat fibrinous obstruction of venous access devices in cancer patients. *J Clin Oncol* 1997;15:2709–2714.
62. Northsea C. Using urokinase to restore patency in double lumen catheters. *Am Nephrol Nurses Assoc J* 1994;21:261–264.
63. Savader SJ, Haikal LC, Ehrman KO, Porter DJ, Oteham AC. Hemodialysis catheter-associated fibrin sheaths: treatment with a low-dose rt-PA infusion. *J Vasc Interv Radiol* 2000;11:1131–1136.
64. Jones GR, Konsler GK, Dunaway RP, Lacey SR, Azizkhan RG. Prospective analysis of urokinase in the treatment of catheter sepsis in pediatric hematology-oncology patients. *J Pediatr Surg* 1993;28:350–357.
65. Jones GR, Konsler GK, Dunaway RP. Urokinase in the treatment of bacteremia and candidemia in patients with right atrial catheters. *Am J Infect Control* 1996;24:160–166.
66. Knelson MH, Hudson BR, Suhocki PV, et al. Functional restoration of occluded central venous catheters: new interventional techniques. *J Vasc Interv Radiol* 1995;6:623–627.
67. Crain MR, Mewissen MW, Ostrowski GJ, et al. Fibrin sleeve stripping for salvage of failing hemodialysis catheters: technique and initial results. *Radiology* 1996;198:41–44.
68. Haskal ZJ, Leen VH, Thomas-Hawkins C, et al. Transvenous removal of fibrin sheaths from tunneled hemodialysis catheters. *J Vasc Interv Radiol* 1996;7:513–517.
69. Gray RJ, Levitin A, Buck D, et al. Percutaneous fibrin sheath stripping versus transcatheter urokinase infusion for malfunctioning well-positioned tunneled central venous dialysis catheters: a prospective, randomized trial. *J Vasc Interv Radiol* 2000;11:1121–1129.
70. Merport M, Murphy TP, Egglin TK, Dubel GJ. Fibrin sheath stripping versus catheter exchange for the treatment of failed tunneled hemodialysis catheters: randomized clinical trial. *J Vasc Interv Radiol* 2000;11:1115–1120.
71. Duszak R, Haskal ZJ, Thomas-Hawkins C, Baum RA, Shlansky-Goldberg RD, Cope C. Replacement of failing hemodialysis catheters through pre-existing subcutaneous tunnels: a comparison of catheter function and infection rates for de novo placements and over-the-wire exchanges. *J Vasc Interv Radiol* 1998;9:321–327.
72. Trerotola SO, Johnson MS, Harris VJ, et al. Outcome of tunneled hemodialysis catheters placed via the right internal jugular vein by interventional radiologists. *Radiology* 1997;203:489–495.
73. Mauro MA. Delayed complications of venous access. *Tech Vasc Intervent Radiol* 1998;1:158–167.
74. Timsit JF. Scheduled replacement of central venous catheters is not necessary. *Infect Control Hosp Epidemiol* 2000;21:371–374.
75. Schillinger F, Schillinger D, Montagnac R, Milcent T. Post-catheterization vein stenosis in haemodialysis: comparative angiographic study of 50 subclavian and 50 internal jugular accesses. *Nephrol Dial Transplant* 1991;6:722–724.
76. Silberzweig JE, Mitty HA. Central venous access: low internal jugular vein approach using imaging guidance. *Am J Roentgenol* 1998;170:1617–1620.
77. Gordon AC, Saliken JC, Johns D, Owen R, Gray RR. US-guided puncture of the internal jugular vein: complications and anatomic considerations. *J Vasc Interv Radiol* 1998;9:333–338.
78. Karakaya D, Baris S, Guldogus F, et al. Brachial plexus injury during subclavian vein catheterization for hemodialysis. *J Clin Anesth* 2000;12:220–223.
79. Trerotola SO, Kuhn-Fulton J, Johnson MS, et al. Tunneled infusion catheters: increased incidence of symptomatic venous thrombosis after subclavian versus internal jugular venous access. *Radiology* 2000;217:89–93.
80. Cimochowski GE, Worley E, Rutherford WE, et al. Superiority of the internal jugular over the subclavian access for temporary hemodialysis. *Nephron* 1990;54:154–161.
81. McBride KD, Fisher R, Warnock N, et al. A comparative analysis of radiological and surgical placement of central venous catheters. *Cardiovasc Intervent Radiol* 1997;20:17–22.
82. Bakker J, van Overhagen H, Wielenga J, et al. Infectious complications of radiologically inserted Hickman catheters in patients with hematologic disorders. *Cardiovasc Intervent Radiol* 1998;21:116–121.
83. Lund GB, Lieberman RP, Haire WD, et al. Translumbar IVC catheters for long-term venous access. *Radiology* 1990;174:31–35.
84. Denny DF Jr, Greenwood LH, Morse SS, Lee GK, Baquero J. Inferior vena cava: translumbar catheterization for central venous access. *Radiology* 1989;170:1013–1014.
85. Kaufman JA, Greenfield AJ, Fitzpatrick GF. Transhepatic cannulation of the inferior vena cava. *J Vasc Interv Radiol* 1991;2:331–334.

86. Azizkhan RG, Taylor LA, Jaques PF, Mauro MA, Lacey SR. Percutaneous translumbar and transhepatic inferior vena caval catheters for prolonged vascular access in children. *J Pediatr Surg* 1992;27:165–169.
87. Zaleski GX, Funaki B, Lorenz JM, et al. Experience with tunneled femoral hemodialysis catheters. *Am J Roentgenol* 1999;172:493–496.
88. Mathur MN, Storey DW, White GH, Ramsey-Stewart G. Percutaneous insertion of long-term venous access catheters via the external iliac vein. *Aust N Z J Surg* 1993;63:858–863.
89. Brooks M. Translumbar inferior vena cava access for Hickman line insertion. *Australas Radiol* 1998;42:383–384.
90. Rajan DK, Croteau DL, Sturza SG, Harvill ML, Mehall CJ. Translumbar placement of inferior vena caval catheters: a solution for challenging hemodialysis access. *Radiographics* 1998;18:1155–1167.
91. Bergey EA, Kaye RD, Reyes J, Towbin RB. Transhepatic insertion of vascular dialysis catheters in children: a safe, life-prolonging procedure. *Pediatr Radiol* 1999;29(1):42–45.
92. Putnam SG 3rd, Ball D, Cohen GS. Transhepatic dialysis catheter tract embolization to close a venous-biliary-peritoneal fistula. *J Vasc Interv Radiol* 1998;9:149–151.
93. Solomon BA, Solomon J, Shlansky-Goldberg R. Percutaneous placement of an intercostal central venous catheter for chronic hyperalimentation guided by transhepatic venography. *J Parenter Enteral Nutr* 2001;25:42–44.
94. Kaufman JA, Crenshaw WB, Kuter I, Geller SC. Percutaneous placement of a central venous access device via an intercostal vein. *Am J Roentgenol* 1995;164:459–460.
95. Funaki B, Zaleski G, Leef J, et al. Radiologic placement of tunneled hemodialysis catheters in occluded neck, chest, or small thyrocervical collateral veins in central venous occlusion. *Radiology* 2001;218:471–476.
96. Kaufman JA, Kazanjian SA, Rivitz SM, Geller SC, Waltman AC. Long-term central venous catheterization in patients with limited access. *Am J Roentgenol* 1996;167:1327–1333.
97. Forauer AR, Brenner B, Haddad LF, Bocchini TP. Placement of hemodialysis catheters through dilated external jugular and collateral veins in patients with internal jugular vein occlusions. *Am J Roentgenol* 2000;174:361–362.
98. Funaki B, Zaleski GX, Leef JA, Rosenblum JD. Radiologic placement of long-term hemodialysis catheters in occluded jugular or subclavian veins or through patent thyrocervical collateral veins. *Am J Roentgenol* 1998;170:1194–1196.
99. Dondelinger RF, Gofette P, Kurdziel JC, Roche A. Expandable metal stents for stenoses of the vena cava and large veins. *Semin Interv Radiol* 1991;8:252–263.
100. Ferral H, Bjarnason H, Wholey M, et al. Recanalization of occluded veins to provide access for central catheter placement. *J Vasc Interv Radiol* 1996;7:681–685.
101. Farrell T, Lang EV, Barnhart W. Sharp recanalization of central venous occlusions. *J Vasc Interv Radiol* 1999;10:149–154.
102. Sharafuddin MJ, Hicks ME. Current status of percutaneous mechanical thrombectomy. Part II. Devices and mechanisms of action. *J Vasc Interv Radiol* 1998;9:15–31.
103. Kasirajan K, Gray B, Ouriel K. Percutaneous AngioJet thrombectomy in the management of extensive deep venous thrombosis. *J Vasc Interv Radiol* 2001;12:179–185.
104. Uflacker R. Mechanical thrombectomy in acute and subacute thrombosis with use of the Amplatz device: arterial and venous applications. *J Vasc Interv Radiol* 1997;8:923–932.
105. Henry M, Amor M, Henry I, Tricoche O, Allaoui M. Thrombectomy with the hydrolysing catheter. Apropos of 50 cases. *Arch Mal Coeur Vaiss* 1997;90:797–804.
106. Yedlicka JW, Carlson JE, Hunter DW, Castañeda-Zuñiga WR, Amplatz K. Thrombectomy with the transluminal endarterectomy catheter (TEC) system: experimental study and case report. *J Vasc Interv Radiol* 1991;2:343–347.
107. Edwards RD, Jackson JE. Case report: superior vena caval obstruction treated by thrombolysis, mechanical thrombectomy and metallic stents. *Clin Radiol* 1993;48:215–217.
108. Sharafuddin MJA, Hicks ME, Jenson ML, et al. Rheolytic thrombectomy with the AngioJet F-105 catheter: preclinical evaluation of safety. *J Vasc Interv Radiol* 1997;8:939–945.
109. Tacke J, Vorwerk D, Bücker A, et al. Experimental treatment of early chronic iliac vein thrombosis with a modified hydrodynamic catheter: Preliminary animal experience. *J Vasc Interv Radiol* 1999;10:57–63.
110. Vicol C, Dalichau H. Recanalization of aged venous thrombotic occlusions with the aid of a rheolytic system: an experimental study. *Cardiovasc Intervent Radiol* 1996;19:255–259.
111. Uflacker R, Rajagopalan PR, Vujic I, Stutley J. Treatment of thrombosed dialysis access grafts: randomized trial of surgical thrombectomy versus mechanical thrombectomy with the Amplatz device. *J Vasc Interv Radiol* 1996;7:185–192.
112. Luo H, Nishioka T, Fishbein MC, et al. Transcutaneous ultrasound augments lysis of arterial thrombi in vivo. *Circulation* 1996; 94:775–778.
113. Shlansky-Goldberg RD, Cines DB, Sehgal CM. Catheter-delivered ultrasound potentiates in vitro thrombolysis. *J Vasc Interv Radiol* 1996;7:313–320.
114. Beygui RE, Olcott C, Dalman RL. Subclavian vein thrombosis: outcome analysis based on etiology and modality of treatment. *Ann Vasc Surg* 1997;11:247–255.
115. Stock KW, Jacob AL, Proske M, Bolliger CT, Rochlitz C. Steinbrich treatment of malignant obstruction of the superior vena cava with the self-expanding Wallstent. *Thorax* 1995;50:1151–1156.
116. Dyet JF, Nicholson AA, Cook AM. The use of the Wallstent endovascular prosthesis in the treatment of malignant obstruction of the superior vena cava. *Clin Radiol* 1993;48:381–385.
117. Hennequin LM, Fade O, Fays JG, et al. Superior vena cava stent placement: results with the Wallstent endoprosthesis. *Radiology* 1995;196:353–361.
118. Rosch J, Bedell JE, Putnam J, Antonovic R, Uchida B. Gianturco expandable wire stents in the treatment of superior vena cava syndrome recurring after maximum-tolerance radiation. *Cancer* 1987;60:1243–1246.
119. Gaines PA, Belli AM, Anderson PB, McBride K, Hemingway AP. Superior vena caval obstruction managed by the Gianturco Z stent. *Clin Radiol* 1994;49:202–206.
120. Elson JD, Becker GJ, Wholey MH, Ehrman KO. Vena caval and central venous stenoses: management with Palmaz balloon-expandable intraluminal stents. *J Vasc Interv Radiol* 1991;2:215–223.
121. Vesely TM, Hovsepian DM, Pilgram TK, Coyne DW, Shenoy S. Upper extremity central venous obstruction in hemodialysis patients: treatment with Wallstents. *Radiology* 1997;204:343–348.
122. Mickley V, Gorich J, Rilinger N, Storck M, Abendroth D. Stenting of central venous stenoses in hemodialysis patients: long-term results. *Kidney Int* 1997;51:277–280.
123. Oderich GS, Treiman GS, Schneider P, Bhirangi K. Stent placement for treatment of central and peripheral venous obstruction: a long-term multi-institutional experience. *J Vasc Surg* 2000;32:760–769.

CHAPTER 16

RADIOFREQUENCY TUMOR ABLATION

KENNETH D. MURPHY, MD

INTRODUCTION

Primary and secondary malignancies present complex challenges to practitioners of clinical medicine. In western nations, colorectal, lung, and breast cancers are the three leading causes of death.[1] The emphasis on minimally invasive techniques, accompanied by technological advances, has ushered in a new era of percutaneous and regional tumor management with sundry devices, probes, and energies. Techniques of local tumor ablation may be categorized into three classes—heat, freezing, and injectables. The technique of using heat includes radiofrequency (RF) ablation, microwave coagulation, laser treatment, and high-energy ultrasound (US).

The use of "heat" to treat malignancies was reported in 1930 in the *Edwin Smith Surgical Papyrus*, in which oils, cautery, and other heated tools were utilized to destroy tumors.[2] These seemingly crude techniques reflect practices dating 5000 years back to the Second Egyptian Dynasty. In 1909, Possi described ablating skin lesions with "fulguration heat" using the Oudin spark.[3] During the 20th century, the role of "heat" therapy evolved to encompass tumor ablation and hemostasis. In the 1970s, efforts focused on treating tumors with heat energy from alternative sources. Coley[4] recognized that tumor cells were sensitive to hyperthermia and attempted to treat them with toxin-induced febrile states. LeVeen and colleagues[5] investigated treatment of tumors with extracorporeal heat energy. McGahon and

Rossi and their associates[6, 7] first introduced the concept of percutaneous, localized thermal ablation of tumors using RF energy in the 1990s. Since these early reports, the clinical experience of RF tumor ablation has grown significantly with expanded indications and techniques. This chapter presents the current status of RF tumor ablation.

OPERATIONAL PRINCIPLE

Radiofrequency tumor ablation is a form of interstitial therapy, a treatment method in which the therapeutic stimulus is delivered directly within the tumor. In the case of RF ablation, the stimulus is thermal energy. The patient is essentially placed in a closed-loop electrical circuit composed of a generator, wiring, probe, and grounding pads (**Fig. 16-1**). The patient's tumor lesion essentially acts as a resistor in the circuit. High-frequency alternating current (400,000–1,250,000 Hz) is delivered via the probe, causing local ionic agitation within the target tissue as the ions attempt to align themselves with the directional changes of the current. The ionic agitation generates local frictional heating, resulting in heating of the target above 45°–50° Celsius. Studies have demonstrated that heating cells above 45° Celsius has cytotoxic effects.[8–10] The tissue surrounding the probe tip is heated rather than the electrode itself.[11] Cytotoxic injury results in conductive changes of the tumor characterized by diminished capacity to conduct electrical current, that is, increased tissue resistance or impedance. Impedance is an electrical marker of cellular death.

The zone of thermal injury is focal and is limited in size by the properties of heating. The discrepancy between the surface area of the probe and dispersive grounding pads results in a compact volume of heat surrounding the probe tip. Heating is proportional to the square of the alternating current multiplied by the tissue resistance ($I^2 \times R$).[12] Therefore, heating drops off as the inverse of the distance from probe tip, yielding a small, focal zone of tissue destruction.[13, 14] The "focality" of tissue destruction in RF ablation is ideal for small lesions, because normal adjacent tissue is spared; several strategies to increase the size of ablated tissue are under investigation. Raising the power does not necessarily increase the size of thermal injury, because higher wattage leads to (1) induction of near-field tissue "charring" and (2) increased impedance and decreased conduction of thermal energy through the charred tissue. Successful strategies include multiple-array probe configurations for larger tissue penetration and saline-cooled probes designed to minimize "charring" and promote a greater volume of thermal injury.

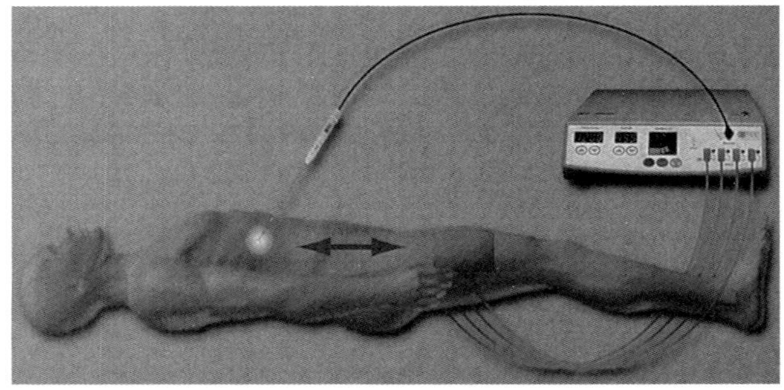

Figure 16-1. Radiofrequency ablation closed-loop electrical circuit consisting of generator, probe, patient, and grounding pads. (Courtesy of Boston Scientific/Medi-Tech®, Natick, MA.)

DEVICES

Table 16-1 outlines important characteristics for each of the currently available RF models.

RadioTherapeutics System

The LeVeen™ needle electrode is manufactured by RadioTherapeutics Corporation (Sunnyvale, CA) and marketed by Boston Scientific/Medi-Tech® (Watertown, MA). The LeVeen™ electrode is a 15-gauge insulated needle with a modified tip consisting of 8–12 wires (tines) arranged in a radial array (**Fig. 16-2**). The needle

TABLE 16-1
Currently Commercially Available RF Models

	Needle configuration			
Unit	Needle size	Needle configuration	Ablation zone	Endpoint
RadioTherapeutics	15-gauge	Radial array	2–4 cm	Impedance
RITA	14-gauge	Radial array	4–7 cm	Temperature
Radionics	17-gauge	Single	2–3 cm	Time
		Cluster	5 cm	

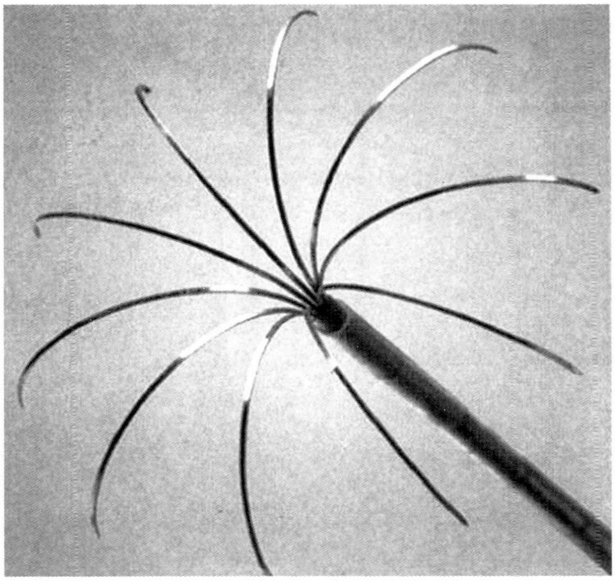

Figure 16-2. LeVeen™ electrode tip. (Courtesy of Boston Scientific/ Medi-Tech®, Natick, MA.)

is powered by a generator with a 200-W power supply, which delivers constant voltage to the needle.

The principles of Ohm's law dictate the course of the ablation, because the endpoint for this device is a rise in impedance. The RF energy is initially distributed into the tissue at the tips of tines. As that tissue desiccates, the zone of ablation travels back toward the center of the array, and then outward again until the interspaces between the tines are ablated. The tines sense tissue desiccation and rise in impedance, and then shift RF energy to unablated tissues. When all tissue is ablated, the rise in impedance is sensed by the tines, and the current delivered to the electrode drops, signaling completion of the ablation. The needle is available in two lengths (12-cm and 15-cm) and various array diameters (2.0–4.0 cm). A coaxial needle system is also available to facilitate pre-ablation biopsy, pre-ablation injection of agents,

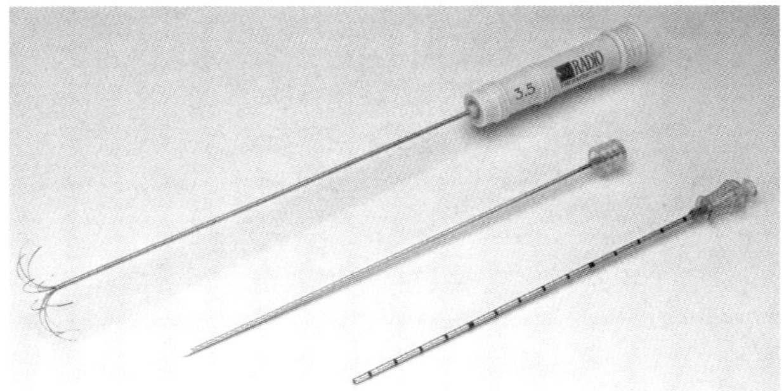

Figure 16-3. LeVeen™ coaxial needle system. (Courtesy of Boston Scientific/Medi-Tech®, Natick, MA.)

needle positioning, and post-ablation needle track embolization (**Fig. 16-3**).

RITA System

The RITA System is manufactured by RITA Medical Systems (Mountain View, CA). The RITA Starburst™ XLi probe is a 14-gauge needle with nine retractable tines, each composed of five active electrodes and four passive thermocouples, all arranged in an array (**Fig. 16-4**). The thermocouples monitor temperature, and the generator is activated to a maximum of 150 W for a target temperature of 70° Celsius. The active electrodes release hypertonic saline to promote shorter ablation times and minimize charring. The needle array diameters range from 4 to 7 cm. The system also allows for track ablation.

Radionics System

The Radionics System is manufactured Radionics, a Division of Tyco Healthcare (Burlington, MA). The Cool-tip® RF electrodes are 17-gauge needles that have single and cluster electrode designs (**Fig. 16-5**). The various designs also have saline-cooled and pulsed-energy features to minimize charring and maximize energy delivery for larger ablation zones. The zone of ablation for the single electrode is rated at 2–3 cm, and that of the cluster electrode at up to 5 cm. The Radionics System's

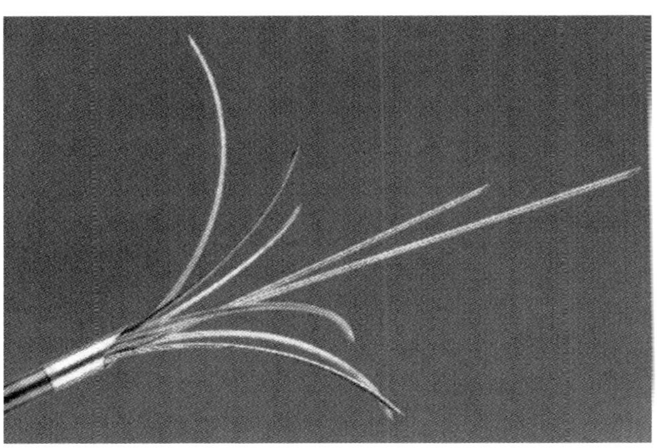

Figure 16-4. RITA Starburst™ XLi probe. (Courtesy of RITA Medical Systems, Mountainview, CA.)

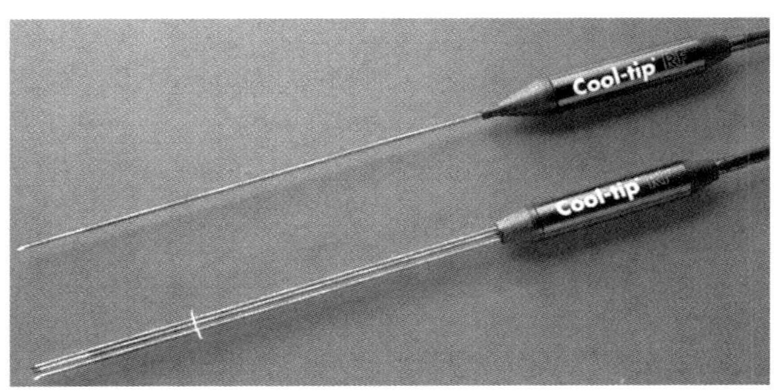

Figure 16-5. Cool-tip® RF electrode. (Courtesy of Radionics, Burlington, MA.)

endpoint is time, with treatment cycles of 12 minutes. This system also allows for track ablation.

PATHOLOGY

The pathologic changes associated with RF-induced thermal injury to soft tissues have been studied in animal and human models, principally in the liver and lung. The tissue response to thermal energy varies with the level of interstitial hyperthermia (temperature) and the duration of exposure (time). The tumor cell susceptibility to irradiation or chemotherapy is enhanced at 42° Celsius, a feature promoting combination therapy. Heating tumor cells at 45° Celsius for hours results in irreversible cellular destruction. The time to achieve irreversible cellular death is reduced to 5–6 minutes when temperatures are 50°–55° Celsius. There is near-spontaneous cell death at temperatures of 60°–100° Celsius, and vaporization at temperatures in excess of 100° Celsius. In the temperature range of RF ablation, the initial tissue response to heating above 50° Celsius is destruction of the lipid bilayers of cell membranes and intracellular protein denaturation, leading to localized tissue desiccation and cellular necrosis.

To demonstrate cellular necrosis by histopathologic examination, special stains are necessary. Conventional hematoxylin and eosin (H&E) stains inconsistently demonstrate the degree of tissue necrosis, particularly in the acute phase (<24 hours) of cellular death. The "vital" stain nicotinamide adenine dinucleotide–diaphorase (NADH-diaphorase) is more accurate for assessing cellular viability, because its uptake is based on the presence or absence of cellular metabolism. The histopathologic evaluation for RF-induced cellular death relies on this NADH technique (**Fig. 16-6**).

In one of the original preclinical animal studies, McGahan[9] evaluated the liver response to RF in the porcine model. He demonstrated that the zone of tissue injury was focal with a central area of "char" surrounded by pale hepatic tissue. Histologic examination showed a central cavity of "char" surrounded by a zone of shrunken hepatocytes with pyknotic nuclei that were in an early stage of necrosis. There was a thin, congestive layer at the junction with adjacent normal tissue.[9]

In the human model, secondary liver tumors treated with RF ablation and subsequently resected within 6 weeks were evaluated pathologically by means of the NADH technique.[15] Gross evaluation of the specimens demonstrated a pale yellow or orange appearance to ablated areas, with sharp demarcation from adjacent normal tissue. The lesions' shape was consistently oval or spherical. Microscopic examination revealed the ablated margins to be sharply circumscribed with no NADH staining. Conventional H&E stains demonstrated disrupted cell membranes, increased cytoplasmic eosinophilia, and preservation of nuclear staining.[15]

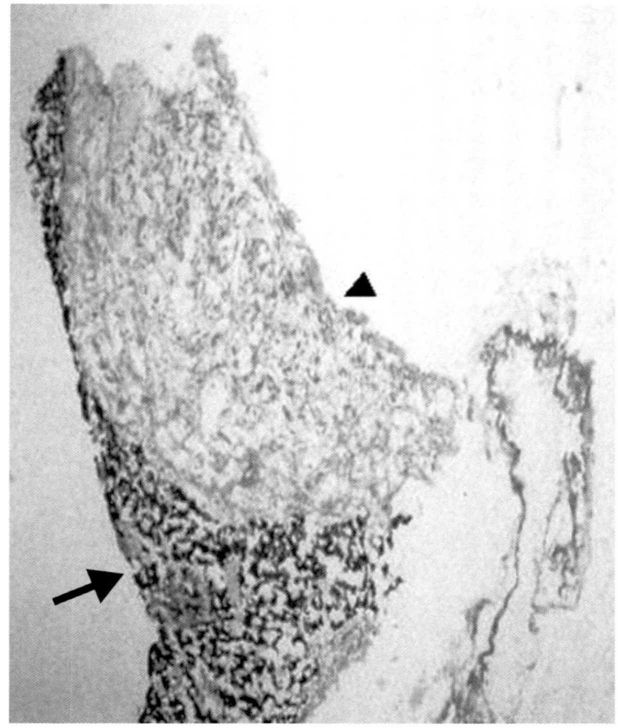

Figure 16-6. Microscopic section of a liver after RF ablation (NADH technique). Viable tumor outside the zone of ablation is represented by NADH-diaphorase uptake (arrow), and ablated tumor is devoid of NADH uptake (arrowhead).

RF ABLATION IN THE LIVER

Background

Primary and secondary hepatic malignancies are the leading causes of cancer death. Hepatocellular carcinoma (HCC) is one of the most common fatal malignancies, affecting more than 1 million people worldwide each year. Colorectal carcinoma is a leading cause of cancer death in the United States; death is usually attributable to metastatic hepatic disease.[16] The management of primary and metastatic diseases of the liver is a formidable challenge to medical and surgical oncologists. Less than half of all cases of metastatic colorectal cancer respond to systemic chemotherapy; hepatoma demonstrates minimal, if any, response to chemotherapy. Surgical excision has evolved as a viable therapeutic option, with 5-year survival rates of 30%–35% achieved for colorectal metastases.[17–19] In practice, however, the narrow selection criteria and the significant morbidity and perioperative mortality of 2%–10%

associated with metastasectomy limit its role.[17–19] As an alternative addressing the limitations of systemic chemotherapy and surgery, RF liver tumor ablation is emerging as a valid treatment option, with the goal of prolonged survival for patients with both unifocal and multifocal disease.

Technique

Today, with the refined imaging modalities computed tomography (CT), US, and magnetic resonance imaging (MRI), the role of percutaneous image-guided RF ablation has grown to complement and expand the original surgical experience. To maximize patient benefit, RF treatment of liver lesions should be a multidisciplinary effort involving the expertise of the interventional radiologist, oncologist, surgical oncologist, hepatologist, and radiation oncologist. The percutaneous procedure should be initiated by a consultation with a review of all pertinent data, including history, physical examination, laboratory results, pathologic findings, and imaging studies.

An accurate pre-procedure imaging evaluation is fundamental to the success of RF ablation. The patient selection criteria are listed in **Table 16-2**. Most interventionists prefer pre-procedure US and contrast-enhanced CT. US allows evaluation of the vascularity within and adjacent to tumor as well as of the potential for perfusion-mediated tissue cooling or probe-induced vessel injury (**Fig. 16-7**). Pre-procedure US also allows assessment of the feasibility of probe positioning under US guidance. Liver MRI is also helpful to further classify lesions with respect to size, number, and location (**Fig. 16-8**).

Positron emission tomography (PET) with fluoro-2-deoxy-D-glucose (FDG) is emerging as a tool to further identify and characterize hepatic malignancies (**Fig. 16-9**). FDG PET has an overall sensitivity of 95% in the identification of whole-body colorectal metastases[20] and a sensitivity of 90% for liver metastases.[21] Clearly, PET

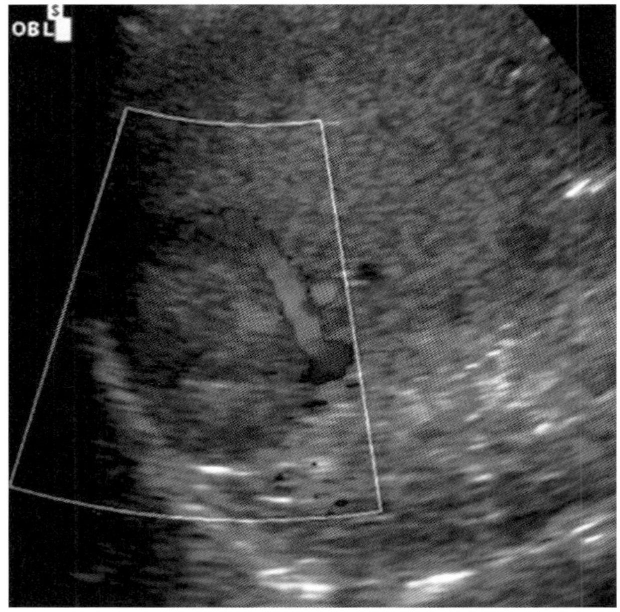

Figure 16-7. Pre-RF color Doppler US of a liver tumor demonstrates a prominent hepatic vein draped along the inferior margin of the lesion.

has a role in defining extrahepatic colorectal disease; however, the role of PET in identification of primary and secondary hepatic malignancies appears less defined, because false-positive and false-negative results are common.

The percutaneous RF ablation procedure is typically performed on an outpatient basis with the use of conscious sedation or general anesthesia. A peripheral intravenous (IV) catheter is placed, and the procedure is performed under CT or US guidance. Prophylactic an-

TABLE 16-2
Selection Criteria for RF Ablation in the Liver

- Four or fewer primary/secondary malignant hepatic tumors
- Tumors < 5 cm
- Patient not a candidate for liver resection
- No evidence of extrahepatic tumor
- Life expectancy > 6 months
- No coagulopathy
- No active hepatic infection

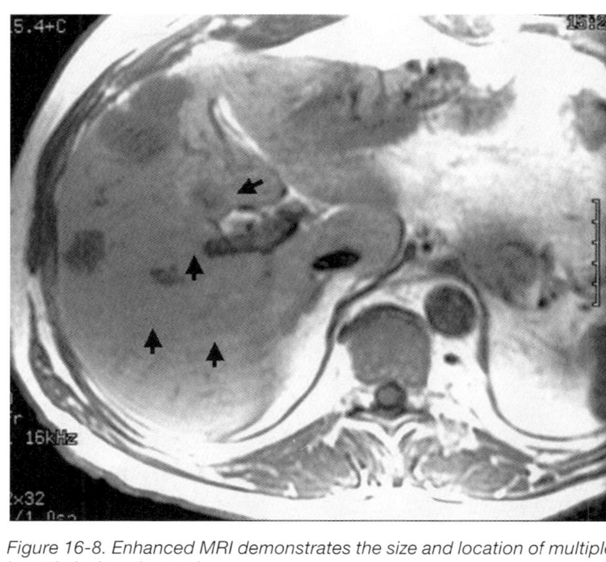

Figure 16-8. Enhanced MRI demonstrates the size and location of multiple hepatic lesions (arrows).

A

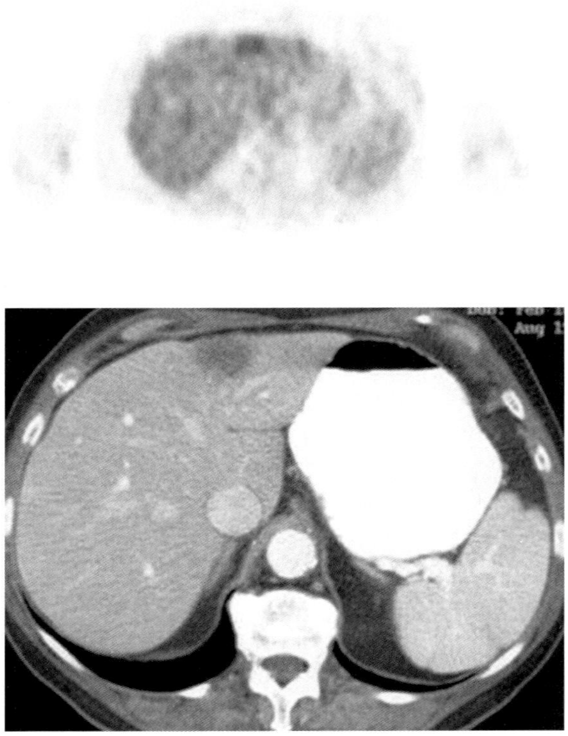

B

Figure 16-9. (A) PET images with focal uptake in the left hepatic lobe consistent with metastasis. (B) CT correlation of the liver lesion.

tibiotics are not routinely used, except in the presence of large tumors, necrotic tumors, immunosuppression, cirrhosis, concomitant infections, or biliary disease such as a biliary-enteric anastomosis. Grounding dispersive pads are typically placed on the thighs in a longitudinal orientation to minimize the risk of cutaneous burns (see Fig. 16-1). The probe is positioned within the lesion under CT or US guidance. US offers the advantages of real-time capability, vessel identification, availability, speed, and low cost. Its main disadvantage is the limited ability to assess the adequacy of RF ablation response because of the dense echogenic response in the tumor bed. CT guidance is limited by needle artifacts and axial-gantry angulation constraints.

The array-type probes are usually positioned 0.5–1.0 cm beyond the most distant tumor margin, whereas the single-tip or clustered-tip probes are positioned in a slightly more central position. A tumor-free margin of 1 cm is desirable and requires meticulous probe positioning. Probe activation is carried out according to the protocol of the specific device until the desired endpoint is achieved.

The lesion and probe size dictate the number and type of overlapping probe positions required for any

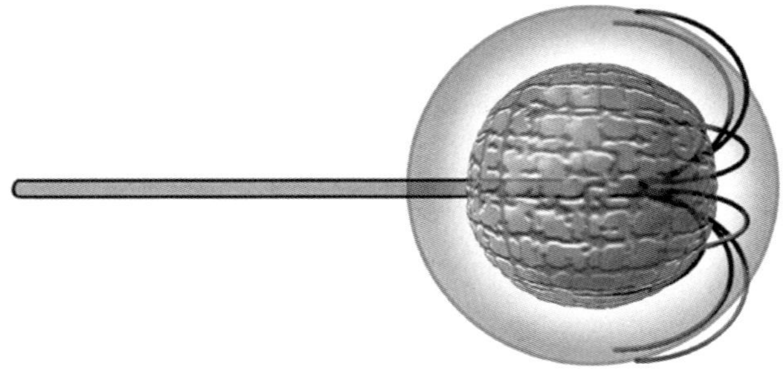

Figure 16-10. Single needle ablation: 1-cm lesion.

given tumor. For example, if a 3-cm probe diameter were used for a 1-cm lesion, a single station probe position would be sufficient to insure a 1-cm tumor-free margin (**Fig. 16-10**). Six overlapping ablations would be required for 2- to 3-cm lesions (**Fig. 16-11**), and significantly more overlapping ablations for lesions larger than 3 cm. Because overlapping of ablations in excess of six positions is burdensome, time-consuming, and essentially impractical, the technique of overlapping "cylinders" is used to ensure geometric coverage of lesions larger than 3 cm (**Fig. 16-12**).

After the needles are removed, the probe track can be managed by observation or dependent patient positioning without intervention. Given the relatively large probe size (14–17 gauge), track occlusion and/or ablation is attractive to minimize the risk of post-procedure bleeding. Strategies to occlude the track include "burning" with the RF probe during withdrawal (Radionics and RITA) and embolizing with absorbable gelatin sponge (Gelfoam). Embolization of the track requires a coaxial technique using a coaxial introducer needle (RadioTherapeutics) or a vascular sheath fabricated in a coaxial fashion around the probe. Track tumor seeding is a concern with any percutaneous procedure[22]; this complication is rarely documented, however, with RF ablation of liver tumors.[23]

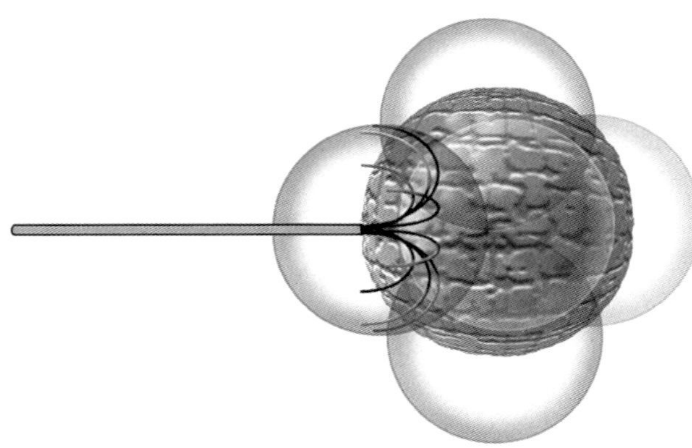

Figure 16-11. Overlapping sphere ablations: 2- to 3-cm lesion.

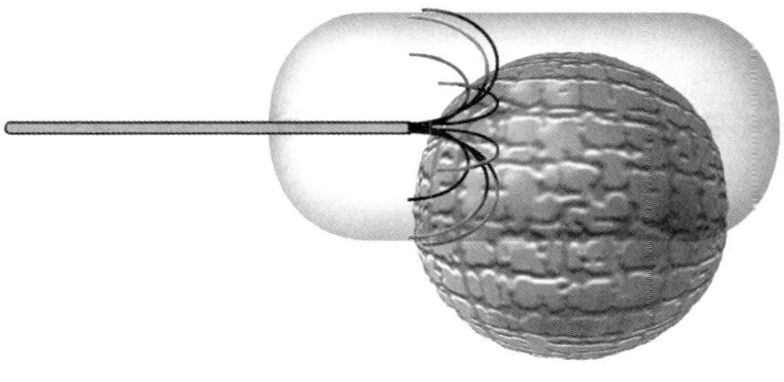

Figure 16-12. Overlapping cylinder ablations: > 3-cm lesion.

Complications

The complication rate for hepatic RF ablation is reported to be less than 2%.[24–26] The most common complication is focal pain. Tumors juxtaposed to the liver capsule, gallbladder, main portal vessels, or diaphragm are associated with greater peri- and post-procedure pain. The pain is usually adequately managed with liberal use of analgesics and local anesthetics. The perceived pain is maximum during probe activation and generally subsides once activation is complete. In 15% of patients the pain lingers, and such patients require analgesics or nonsteroidal antiinflammatory medications at discharge.[27]

Nausea is another common complication that rarely persists beyond 3 hours after the procedure. Ablation near the gallbladder can result in cholecystitis, which is usually managed conservatively. Other complications are parenchymal hemorrhage (**Fig. 16-13**), pleural effusion, ascites, thermal injury to adjacent bowel, tumor track seeding, burns from the grounding pad, thermal injury to bile ducts, and hepatic abscess formation.

Infectious complications are more common in patients with severe cirrhosis, immunosuppression, biliary obstruction, concomitant infection, and prior biliary duct surgery. Prophylactic antibiotics are indicated in such high-risk patients. Some patients experience a "flulike" syndrome 3–5 days after the procedure, with low-grade fever, occasional night sweats, and general malaise. This syndrome, which generally lasts up to 5 days, is managed with supportive analgesics and antipyretics. Fevers greater than 38.8° Celsius require evaluation to exclude an infectious complication.

Perfusion-Mediated Tissue Cooling

Perfusion-mediated tissue cooling describes the effect of "unheated" blood flowing into a zone of ablation, lowering the net temperature, and limiting the efficacy and size of the targeted burn. Animal in vivo studies have demonstrated that larger areas of RF-induced coagulation necrosis are obtained when the portal vein (i.e., the major potential source of "unheated" blood) is occluded during probe activation than when the portal vein is left open.[28] In a small in vivo human clinical study, greater coagulation diameter was observed for liver metastases ablated during portal inflow occlusion than for tumors treated with normal portal vein patency.[28] A separate study demonstrated an inverse, linear relationship of coagulation diameter and liver blood flow.[29]

Perfusion-mediated tissue cooling is likely due to the aggregate blood flow within the targeted volume as well as to the juxtaposition of larger hepatic vessels that act as a heat sink.[30] Hansen and associates[31] demonstrated that vessels more than 3 mm in diameter could prevent complete ablation of the targeted liver lesion, probably from a heat sink effect.

A

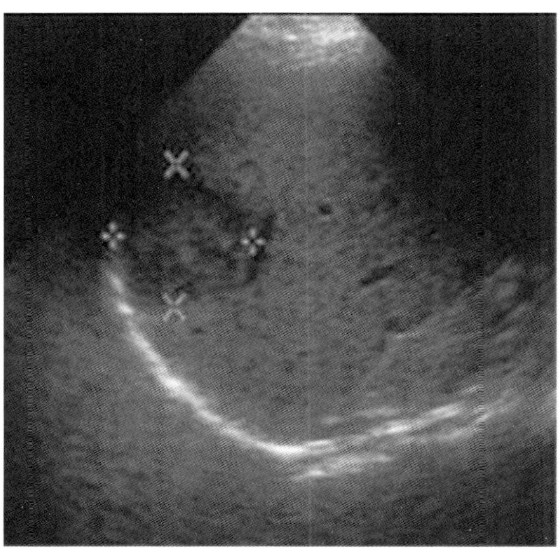

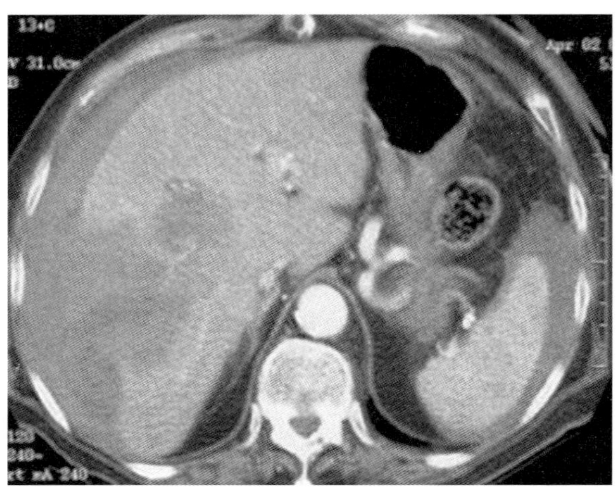

B

Figure 16-13. Hemorrhage as a complication of RF ablation. (A) Pre-RF US demonstrates four 1-cm metastases. (B) Post-ablation CT documents parenchymal, subcapsular, and intraperitoneal blood.

In an attempt to minimize the effects of perfusion-mediated tissue cooling, several strategies continue to be evaluated. The Pringle maneuver involves direct surgical occlusion of the main portal vein and proper hepatic artery, thus eliminating the entire potential source of unheated blood. The Pringle maneuver can involve an extensive surgical dissection and, therefore, may not be reasonable in all patients. The safety of clamping the liver hilum has not yet been established, reports of portal vein thrombosis being associated with this maneuver.[15]

Balloon occlusion of the hepatic artery, although technically feasible, would not affect the inflow of portal vein blood. Pre-RF arterial particulate embolization is an attractive alternative that is currently being evaluated.[32] The rationale is to facilitate blockade to limit perfusion-mediated tissue cooling as well as to deprive the tumor bed of oxygen and nutrients. Arata and coworkers found the rate of achievement of the desired RF endpoint to be higher and the rate of local recurrence to be lower when patients underwent pre-RF arterial embolization.[33] The role of RF ablation in combination with other therapies appears encouraging but requires further investigation (**Fig. 16-14**).

Follow-up Imaging

Follow-up surveillance is a critical component of RF ablation. The reliability of documenting residual or recurrent tumor remains a diagnostic challenge. Serum tumor markers are unreliable for assessing tumor response because their levels may be normal before treatment (small lesion) or may decrease or normalize even when necrosis is incomplete. Evaluation of tumor response is therefore based on imaging studies.

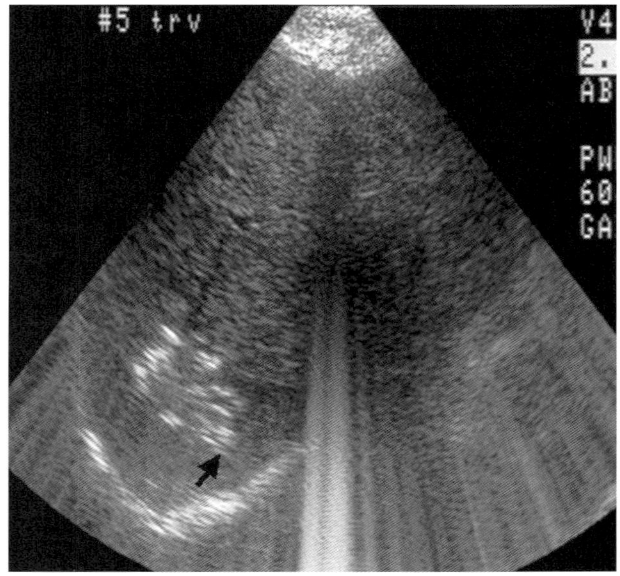

Figure 16-15. US with hyperechoic appearance of liver tumor after RF ablation (arrow).

The US appearance of the post-ablation liver lesion is a homogeneous, hyperechoic area around the probe. This appearance, however, is unreliable for accurately demonstrating response (**Fig. 16-15**). In cases of HCC, color and power Doppler US may help assess tumor response through demonstration of persistent intratumoral blood flow in cases of residual tumor[34]; colorectal

A 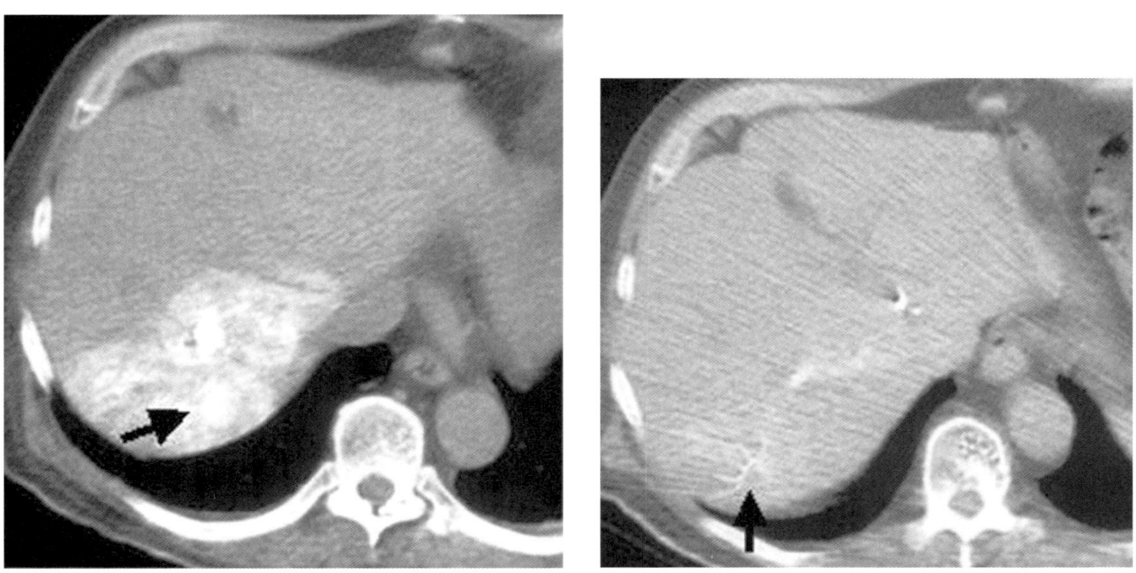 B

Figure 16-14. Combination therapy. (A) Lesion in the posterior segment of the right hepatic lobe after chemoembolization (arrow). (B) Post-chemoembolization RF ablation (probe is indicated by arrow).

metastases, which are typically hypovascular, are not adequately assessed by Doppler evaluation. Contrast-enhanced US has improved the diagnostic accuracy of tumor response evaluations.[35, 36] In practice, color and power Doppler as well as contrast-enhanced US may be useful for immediate assessment of residual HCC but are probably not adequate for the assessment of post-procedure metastatic disease.

Contrast-enhanced spiral CT is the mainstay of RF liver ablation follow-up. Successful tumor ablation is characterized by hypoattenuating areas that enhance during neither the arterial phase (HCC) nor the portal venous phases (colorectal metastases).[37, 38] Peripheral nodular enhancement is the CT finding most indicative of residual or recurrent tumor (**Fig. 16-16**). Post-procedure timing of the CT is critical to accurate assessment of response. In general, a characteristic hyperemic rim that surrounds the ablated tissue can be difficult to distinguish from nodular residual tumor. This hyperemic rim can appear within days of the procedure and can last for up to 1 month.[16] The recommended follow-up protocol for RF ablation of liver tumor consists of triple-phase contrast-enhanced spiral CT at 1 month; if it shows no evidence of recurrent or residual tumor, the same evaluation is performed at 3-month intervals thereafter.[16]

MRI is also an option for follow-up imaging. At least one study claims MRI to be more sensitive than CT for assessing tumor response.[39] Tumor necrosis is demonstrated as a change from a hyperintense signal to a hypointense signal on T_2-weighted images.[40] Some investigators have suggested that contrast-enhanced MRI with the use of hepatobiliary or reticuloendothelial system agents gives more accurate results than unenhanced MRI.[40]

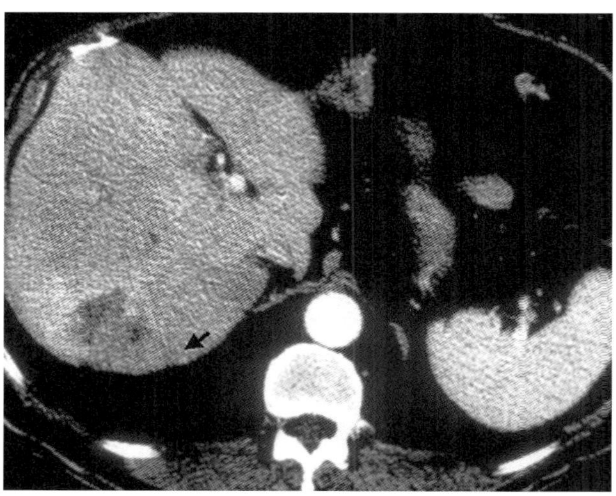

Figure 16-16. Nodular CT enhancement indicative of residual or recurrent tumor (arrow).

The role of PET in assessing tumor viability after RF treatment is not yet established. The sensitivity and specificity of PET detection of liver metastases depend on tumor size and type. In one study, PET demonstrated only 70% of liver metastases, with false-negative results attributed to small lesion size.[41] Given the rates of false-negative and false-positive results for PET in detection of hepatic metastases, the current role of PET may be complementary to that of CT or MRI; this modality is unlikely to replace either cross-sectional imaging modality. PET is very useful to evaluate for extrahepatic disease, however, and certainly remains important when a patient's candidacy for RF tumor ablation is being considered.

Regardless of the imaging modality, the depicted zone of necrosis must incorporate the entire lesion and a safety margin. The "surgical" margin of hepatic metastasectomy is at least 2–3 cm. Given the limits of probe design and the size of thermal ablation zones, a 0.5–0.7-cm safety margin of coagulation necrosis in the liver parenchyma on follow-up imaging is considered adequate for RF ablation.[40]

Outcomes

Analysis of the published literature on RF ablation in the liver reflects the evolving technology, probe design, and ablative techniques as well as the vast differences in tumor type and size. Several clinical series have documented the results of percutaneous RF therapy for HCC.[24, 37, 42, 43] Rossi and colleagues[37] reported the first HCC study using a conventional needle probe. Subsequently, the same group published a second study on the use of an umbrella-type probe,[24] after which Livraghi and associates[42] and Francica and Marone[43] reported on separate experiences with cooled-tip probes. In all four series, 90% tumor necrosis was observed at 6 months for lesions smaller than 3 cm.[24, 37, 42, 43] Livraghi and associates[42] reported complete necrosis in 47 of 52 (90%) HCC lesions measuring less than 3 cm. They also found the rate of complete response to be higher for RF ablation than that achieved in a comparable subset of patients treated with percutaneous ethanol instillation (PEI).[42] The number of treatment sessions was also significantly lower for RF than for PEI (1.2 versus 4.8 sessions/tumor). Lencioni and colleagues[44] reported results of a prospective, randomized trial comparing RF with PEI in patients with fewer than three HCC lesions, each measuring 5 cm or less.[44] At a mean follow-up of 2 years, those treated with RF ablation had a significantly lower local recurrence rate and a significantly higher disease-free survival rate.

Results of these small series suggest that percutaneous RF ablation for small (<3 cm) HCC lesions is successful. Unfortunately, treatment of larger HCC lesions remains problematic. Livraghi and associates,[45] using RF ablation to treat 126 HCC lesions larger than 3 cm (mean 5.4 cm) with RF, achieved a complete necrosis rate of only 47.6%. Therefore, combination strategies continue to be investigated, particularly for HCC lesions larger than 3 cm. Lencioni and colleagues[46]evaluated a combination strategy for large HCC. In their series, 62 patients with "large" HCCs (mean, 4.7 cm) were treated with RF ablation after occlusion of tumor arterial supply by either balloon occlusion or gelatin sponge embolization. The immediate complete response rate was 90%; partial response was more common in lesions larger than 5.5 cm. These investigators found no difference in response rate between balloon occlusion and gelatin sponge embolization of the arterial supply.[46]

RF ablation for colorectal metastases is evolving but until now has been less efficacious than RF ablation for HCC. Five separate studies of RF ablation for colorectal metastases using conventional probes with and without saline infusion have been reported.[37, 38, 47–49]Analysis of their results shows that a total of 99 patients were treated, with a mean follow-up of 10.4 months. The rate of complete necrosis ranged from 52% to 88%.[37, 38, 47–49] Rossi and associates[24] reported another series of 14 patients who had colorectal metastases and underwent treatment with the umbrella-type probe, in which the rate of complete necrosis was 93%. The rate of tumor-free survival after RF treatment varied in these series from 76% at 6 months[38] to 11% at 11 months.[37]

Curley and associates[50] reported RF treatment of 169 primary and secondary lesions, with local recurrence in 3 of 169 tumors; however, additional lesions (metastases) developed in 27.6% of cases.[50] Gillams and Lees[51] reported the survival impact of RF therapy for colorectal metastases in 69 patients, each with with an average of three lesions, in whom chemotherapy or surgery had failed. Rates of survival at 1, 2, 3, and 4 years were 90%, 60%, 34%, and 22%, respectively.[51] These figures are encouraging compared with those for systemic chemotherapy, which has a 1-year survival rate of 48% and a 3-year survival rate of 3%.[40]

Although these results for colorectal metastases are encouraging, the wide ranges for tumor necrosis and tumor-free survival rates remain problematic. The discrepancy in survival and tumor necrosis is likely due to the biology of metastatic disease, perfusion-mediated tissue cooling, and the limitations of accurate detection of complete hepatic tumor burden at the time of treatment. It is likely that many patients with small (2–3 cm) metastases have other, smaller tumor foci that are not detected with current imaging techniques. Diligent follow-up and surveillance are necessary to detect tumor recurrences and treat them accordingly.

RF ABLATION IN THE LUNG

Background

Lung cancer is the leading cause of cancer death in the United States and the leading type of cancer in men. The most common type of malignant lung cancer is non–small-cell lung cancer (NSCLC). Unfortunately, only a minority of lung malignancies are amenable to potentially curative resection because most cases are diagnosed at advanced stages.[52] Several features of lung malignancy suggest RF as a potentially therapeutic modality; they are the typical focal nature and limited size of lung cancer as well as the insulating effects of adjacent air. The experience of RF ablation of lung tumors has been limited to date, but early results are encouraging. As early as 1979, Sugaar and LeVeen[53] described the histopathologic changes caused by targeting lung lesions in three patients with external RF energy using disc-shaped skin electrodes. They found tumor cell degeneration, round cell infiltration, and obliteration of tumor vascularity.[53]

The use of RF ablation in the lung has been essentially dormant. The refinement of probes, coupled with the growing experience with RF in the liver, has now fueled investigation into the feasibility and efficacy of using this modality to treat lung tumors.

Technique

The technique of RF ablation in the lung is similar to that in the liver, except that the imaging modality is limited to CT. A successful lung RF program relies on collaborative communication among oncologists, thoracic surgeons, radiation oncologists, and interventional radiologists. All potential candidates should be carefully screened for potential curative resection prior to consideration for RF ablation. The selection criteria for RF ablation in the lung are listed in **Table 16-3**.

The lung RF ablation procedure is typically performed on an outpatient basis, with patients given conscious sedation. A single dose of prophylactic antibiotics is usually given. The needle probe is placed during shal-

TABLE 16-3
Selection Criteria for RF Ablation in the Lung

- Primary or secondary lung carcinoma < 4 cm
- Four or fewer lesions
- Lesions not invading pericardium or mediastinum
- Life expectancy > 6 months
- No coagulopathy
- No cardiac pacemaker

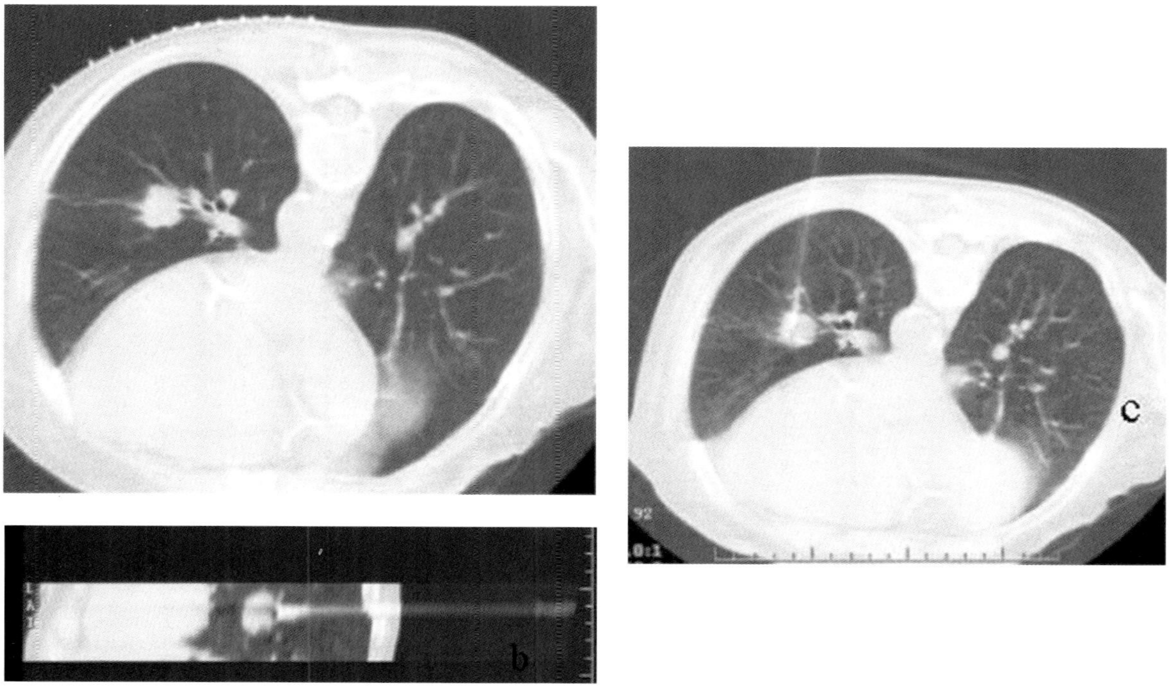

Figure 16-17. RF ablation technique in the lung. (A) CT localization of 2-cm tumor in the left lung. (B) Reformatted sagittal images confirm central needle position. (C) Deployed probe array within the lesion.

low breathing and with CT guidance, typically with CT gantry angulation. Thin-slice helical CT images are reformatted in sagittal and coronal planes to document accurate needle placement (**Fig. 16-17**). The patients are observed for 4–6 hours after the procedure, and radiographs are obtained immediately after the procedure and later. Follow-up consists of CT examination at 3-month intervals, and tumor response is represented by a decrease in lesion size (**Fig. 16-18**).

Outcomes and Observations

Despite the growing excitement about lung RF ablation, the body of published literature is scant. Dupuy and

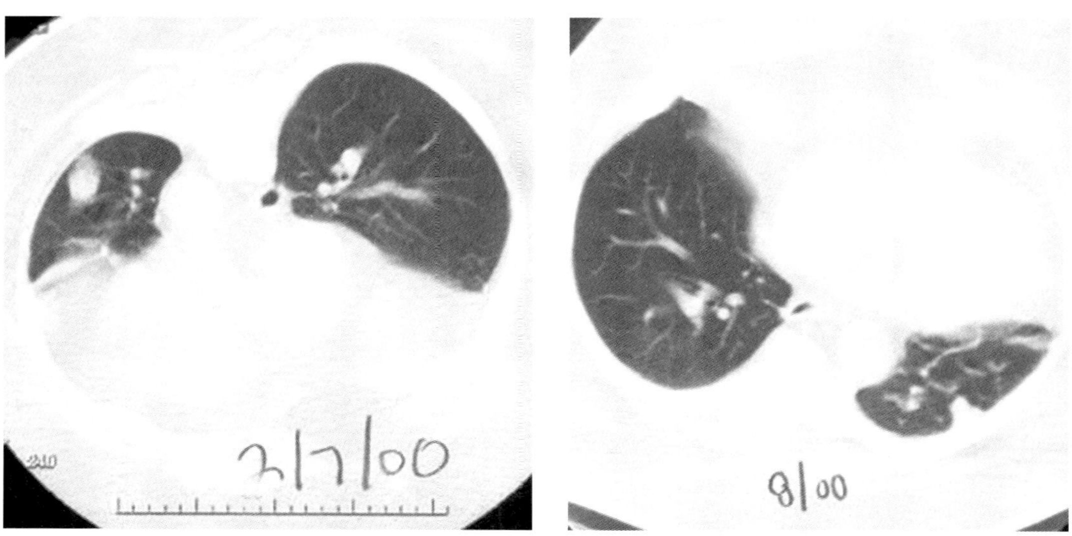

Figure 16-18. Follow-up of RF ablation of a lung tumor. (A) Pre-RF lesion is 2 cm. (B) Six months after RF ablation, the lesion is smaller (1.6 cm) and scarred to the pleura.

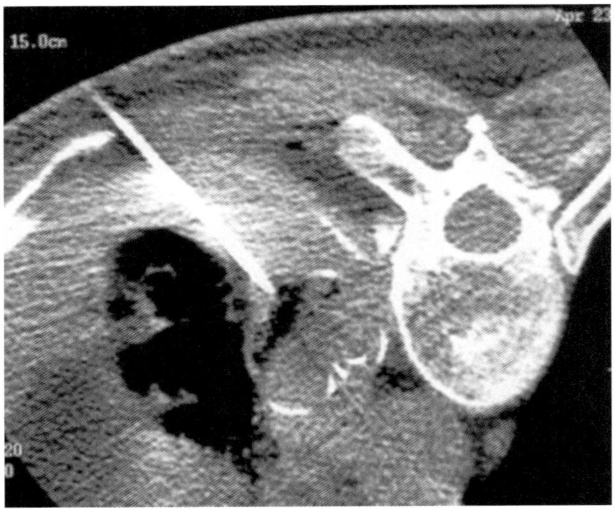

Figure 16-19. RF ablation of posterior mediastinal thymoma.

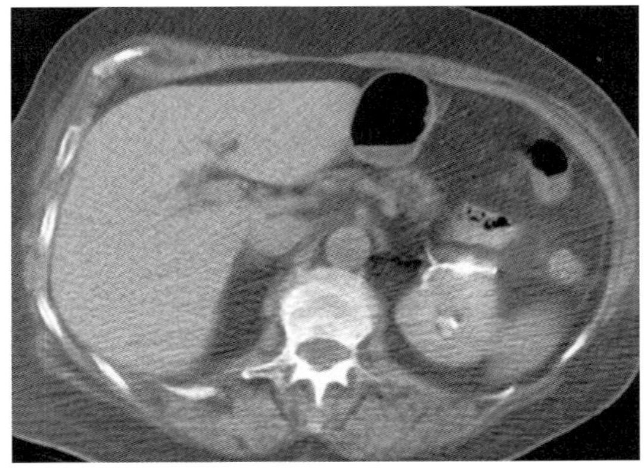

Figure 16-20. Exophytic renal cell carcinoma treated with CT-guided RF ablation via a retroperitoneal approach.

colleagues[54] reported treating three patients with primary lung cancer with single-electrode RF. There were no pneumothoraces, but all patients experienced pleural effusions. In follow-up, one lesion regressed, one lesion was PET-negative, and the remaining patient expired of an unrelated cause.[54] Unpublished clinical experiences, available mainly in abstract form, have documented treatment for primary and secondary lung cancers as well as some mediastinal lesions (**Fig. 16-19**). In addition, this author's center has observed the following complications in association with lung RF ablation: pleural effusions, pleurisy, myalgia, brown sputum, and low-grade fevers. RF ablation in the lung remains an exciting investigational procedure, awaiting further experience and literature-based safety and efficacy results.

RF ABLATION IN THE KIDNEY

Renal cell carcinoma accounts for 2% of new cancers diagnosed annually in the United States, leading to approximately 30,000 new cases per year.[55] Radical nephrectomy is the standard treatment, with smaller (<4 cm) lesions being amenable to partial nephrectomy. Advances in CT and MRI have resulted in detection of small, asymptomatic renal tumors, typically in the elderly population for whom conventional surgery poses a high risk. These renal cell cancers, often exophytic and slow growing, are easily targeted with CT (**Fig. 16-20**).

Published reports have described successful management of such small renal cell carcinomas with RF.[56, 57] In addition, RF ablation may be a kidney-sparing treatment option for patients with Von Hippel–Lindau disease and multiple, bilateral renal cell cancers. RF ablative therapy for renal cell cancer may also be attractive to the patient with a solitary kidney. The reported techniques for kidney RF ablation include percutaneous RF with CT[56] and US guidance[57] as well as surgical RF with US guidance or direct exposure.[58] Central and ventral lesions are problematic because of the close proximity of hilar vessels and the collecting system. The patient selection criteria for RF ablation in the kidney are listed in **Table 16-4**. Follow-up usually consists of CT or US, with size and enhancement pattern being used as markers for response.

The clinical experience and published literature for kidney RF are significantly less than for liver RF. Gervais and associates[57] reported on percutaneous RF ablation of nine renal cell carcinomas in eight patients with US or CT guidance. Both exophytic and central lesions were treated, with a mean tumor size of 3.3 cm. Treatment success was characterized by lack of contrast enhancement on follow-up CT. At 6-month follow-up with CT, all (100%) exophytic tumors did not enhance; however, only 33% of central lesions were free of enhancement.[57] Walther and coworkers[58] reported renal RF ablation to be free of adverse effects on kidney function.

The efficacy and recurrence rates of this modality remain to be defined. Kachura and colleagues[59] described

TABLE 16-4
Selection Criteria for RF Ablation in the Kidney

- Small renal tumors (<3–5 cm)
- Contraindications to complete/partial nephrectomy
- Solitary kidney with tumor
- Von Hippel–Lindau disease with multiple, bilateral renal cancers
- Elderly patient with small, exophytic tumor
- Peripheral lesions favored over central lesions

pathologic findings for five small renal cell tumors (mean, 2.6 cm) treated with percutaneous RF and resected within 1 week. In three of the five tumors, variable tumor cells composed 5%–10% of the tumor volume.[59] Given the vascularity of the kidney and renal cell tumors, the role of perfusion-mediated tissue cooling has been suggested as a factor accounting for residual tumor. In a porcine model, Mikityansky and associates[60] demonstrated a greater diameter of thermal injury in renal lesions after renal blood flow obstruction with vessel clamping and particulate embolization. Further long-term clinical follow-up and investigation into optimal technique for kidney RF ablation are needed to more clearly define the role of RF in managing renal lesions.

RF ABLATION IN BONE

RF ablation has been successful in the management of benign and malignant bone neoplasms. The greatest experience in skeletal RF has been with osteoid osteomas. Benign bone-forming tumors, osteoid osteomas characteristically affect the cortices of long bones in children and adolescents (**Fig. 16-21A**). The classic clinical presentation is nocturnal pain that is relieved by anti-inflammatory drugs. The lesions are typically small, with a central tumor nidus that produces prostaglandin, resulting in pain. Percutaneous or surgical biopsy can be challenging because of the small size of the central nidus and surrounding dense cortical bone. In some instances, biopsy can result in clinical improvement or cure, because the procedure effectively evacuates the nidus. Traditional treatment has been surgical resection by a cortical osteotomy.[61]

As an alternative to surgery, RF ablation has evolved as an effective treatment for osteoid osteoma (**Fig. 16-21B**). The RF procedure is performed with CT guidance using conscious sedation or general anesthesia. The dense bone surrounding the nidus is penetrated with a bone-cutting needle. The RF probe is placed through the entry channel into the nidus and activated. The "cure" rate with one session of RF is reported to be 90%.[61] Woertler and colleagues[62] reported treating 47 cases of osteoid osteoma with RF with a clinical success of 94%; the cases for which RF ablation failed were successfully managed with a second RF procedure. RF for osteoid osteomas can be performed as an outpatient procedure with minimal morbidity; this modality avoids the scars and wound healing complications associated with surgical treatment.

TABLE 16-5
Selection Criteria for RF Ablation in Bone

- Osteoid osteoma
- Bony metastases with refractory pain

RF ablation can also be performed for other primary benign and malignant bone lesions, although the experience in such lesions is smaller than in osteoid osteoma. There is, however, significant RF experience with metastatic bone disease (**Table 16-5**). Metastatic bone cancer is the most common skeletal neoplasm, with breast, lung, and prostate primaries accounting for more than 80% of cases.[63] The most common indication for RF treatment of metastatic bone disease is pain refractory to radiotherapy, hormonal therapy, systemic chemotherapy, and/or analgesic pumps (**Fig. 16-22**). Because the life expectancy of patients with osseous metastases is 3 to 6 months, expeditious palliation is important. The procedure is usually performed under CT guidance with conscious sedation. The pain relief from RF ablation of skeletal metastases is likely due to destruction of nerve endings, reduction in tumor volume

A
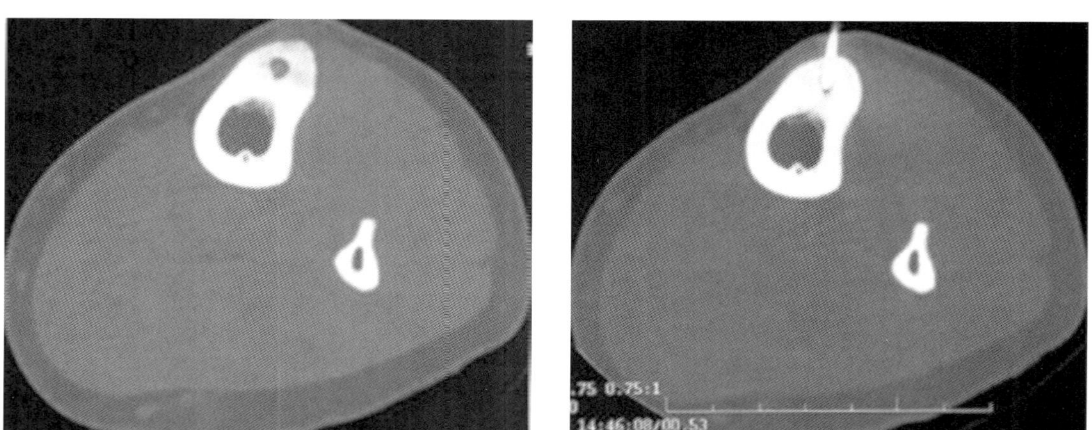
B

Figure 16-21. (A) Osteoid osteoma of the tibia. (B) Osteoid osteoma treated with single-tip RF probe.

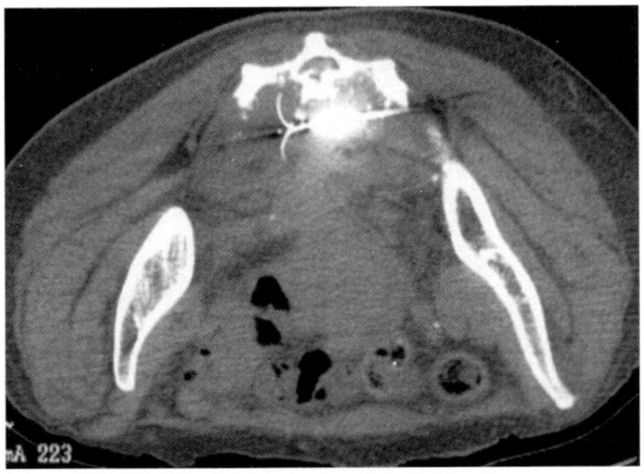

Figure 16-22. RF ablation of a painful sacral metastasis.

with decrease in production of painful inflammatory cytokines, and diminished pressure effect on adjacent bone or neural structures. Dupuy and coworkers,[64] using RF treatment for painful osseous metastases in 10 patients, reported pain relief in 90% of cases by 4 months.

RF ABLATION IN THE BREAST

RF application for breast carcinoma remains investigational, clinical experience still being limited. Current treatment methods for breast malignancy include breast-sparing excisional biopsy, axillary lymph node dissection, sentinel lymph node mapping, external beam irradiation, and chemotherapy. These therapies have proven success with encouraging cure rates. Such established treatment regimens have a relatively wide safety margin with acceptable morbidity rates; therefore, emphasis on RF techniques has been limited.

RF ablation in patients with early-stage (stage I or II) breast carcinoma may be an attractive alternative to excisional biopsy for cosmetic reasons if it can produce local control rates similar to those of resection. In 1999, Jeffrey and associates first reported the use of RF in breast cancer. A small series of patients was treated with RF prior to excisional biopsy for infiltrative carcinoma, and pathologic examination demonstrated coagulation necrosis in the treated tumor bed.[65] Preliminary work has demonstrated relative responsiveness of breast cancer to RF, which may be due to the insulating properties of the surrounding fibrofatty tissue. Izzo and colleagues[66] have reported on a pilot trial in which 26 invasive small breast cancers (mean diameter 1.8 cm) were treated with US-guided RF followed by immediate resection. All but one specimen demonstrated complete coagulation necrosis.[66] Thus, there may be potential for RF ablation in managing early-stage breast carcinomas as an adjunct to sentinel lymph node mapping and irradiation. The efficacy of RF ablation for breast cancer, its complication rates, and its effect on follow-up imaging and determination of tumor responsiveness remain exciting areas of investigation.

CONCLUSION

RF tumor ablation is an evolving treatment modality for solid tumors. To date, the largest experience has been in treating primary and secondary liver malignancies. Experience with this modality in other organs, including lung, bone, kidney, and breast, is growing. Image guidance and imaging follow-up, clearly the domain of the interventional radiologist, are critical to the success of the procedure. Future refinements and technological advancements in probe design, coupled with additional clinical experience and outcome assessment, should validate the current practice of RF ablation and serve to expand its indications.

REFERENCES

1. LeVeen RF. Laser hyperthermia and radiofrequency ablation of hepatic lesions. *Semin Intervent Radiol* 1997;14:313–324.
2. Breasted JH. *The Edwin Smith Surgical Papyrus*. Chicago, IL: Chicago University Press; 1930;54.
3. Kelly HA, Ward GE. *Electrosurgery*. Philadelphia, PA: WB Saunders; 1932:1–9.
4. Coley WB. The treatment of malignant tumors by repeated inoculations of erysipelas with a report of ten original cases. *Am J Med Sci* 1993;105:487.
5. LeVeen HH, Ahmed N, Piccone VA, Sugaar S, Falk G. Radiofrequency therapy: clinical experience. *Ann N Y Acad Sci* 1980;335:362–371.
6. McGahan JP, Browning PD, Brock JM, Tesluk H. Hepatic ablation using radiofrequency electrocautery. *Invest Radiol* 1990;25:267–270.
7. Rossi S, Fornari F, Pathies C, Buscarini L. Thermal lesions induced by 480 KH_2 localized current fields in guinea pig and pig liver. *Tumori* 1990;76:54–57.
8. Lounsberry W, Goldschmidt V, Linke C. The early histologic changes following electrocoagulation. *Gastrointest Endosc* 1995;41:68–70.
9. McGahan J, Brock J, Tesluk H. Hepatic ablation with use of radiofrequency electrocautery in the animal model. *J Vasc Interv Radiol* 1992;3:291–297.
10. McGahan J, Schneider P, Brock J. Treatment of liver tumors by percutaneous radiofrequency electrocautery. *Semin Intervent Radiol* 1993;10:143–149.
11. Organ LW. Electrophysiologic principles of radiofrequency lesion making. *Appl Neurophysiol* 1976/77;39:69–76.
12. O'Connor JL, Bloom DL, William T. Bovie and electrosurgery. *Surgery* 1996;119:390–396.
13. Haines DE, Watson DD. Tissue heating during radiofrequency catheter ablation: a thermodynamic model and observations in isolated perfused and superfused canine right ventricular free wall. *Pace* 1989; 12:962–976.
14. Gazelle GS, Goldberg SN, Solbiati L, Livraghi T. Tumor ablation with radio-frequency energy. *Radiology* 2000;217:633–646.
15. Scudamore CH, Lee SI, Patterson EJ, et al. Radiofrequency ablation followed by resection of malignant liver tumors. *Am J Surg* 1999; 177:411–417.

16. McGahan JP, Dodd GD. Radiofrequency ablation of the liver: current status. *Am J Roentgenol* 2001;176:3–16.
17. Petrelli N, Gupta B, Piedmonte M, Herrera L. Morbidity and survival of liver resection for colorectal adenocarcinoma. *Dis Colon Rectum* 1991;34:899–904.
18. Steele G, Bleday R, Mayer RJ, Lindblad A, Petrelli N, Weaver D. A prospective evaluation of hepatic resection for colorectal carcinoma metastases to the liver: gastrointestinal tumor study group protocol 6584. *J Clin Oncol* 1991;9:1105–1112.
19. Fong Y, Blumgart LH, Cohen AM. Surgical treatment of colorectal metastases to the liver. *CA Cancer J Clin* 1995;197:101–108.
20. Huebner RH, Park KC, Shepherd JE, et al. A meta-analysis of the literature for whole-body FDG PET detection of recurrent colorectal cancer. *J Nucl Med* 2000;41:1177–1189.
21. Kinkel K, Lu Y, Both M, Warren RS, Thoeni RF. Detection of hepatic metastases from cancers of the gastrointestinal tract by using noninvasive imaging methods (US, CT, MR Imaging, PET): a meta-analysis. *Radiology* 2002;224:748–756.
22. Llovet JM, Vilana R, Bru C, et al. Increased risk of tumor seeding after percutaneous radiofrequency ablation for single hepatocellular carcinoma *Hepatology* 2001;33:1124–1129.
23. de Baere T, Elias D, Risse O, et al. Complications of percutaneous and perioperative radiofrequency ablation of liver tumors (abstr). *J Vasc Interv Radiol* 2002;13(suppl): S63.
24. Rossi S, Buscarini E, Garbagnati F, et al. Percutaneous treatment of small hepatic tumors by an expandable RF needle electrode. *Am J Roentgenol* 1998;170:1015–1022.
25. Kainuma O, Asano T, Aoyama H, et al. Combined therapy with radiofrequency thermal ablation and intra-arterial infusion chemotherapy for hepatic metastases from colorectal cancer. *Hepatogastroenterology* 1999;46:1071–1077.
26. Livraghi T, Solbiati L, Meloni F, Ierce T, Goldberg SN. Complications after cool-tip RF ablation of liver cancer: initial report of the Italian Multicenter Cool-Tip RF Study Group. *Radiology* 2000;217(suppl):18.
27. Lees WR, Gillams AR. Complications of radiofrequency and laser ablation of liver metastases: Incidence and management (abstr). Radiology 1999;213:122.
28. Goldberg SN, Hahn PF, Tanabe KK, et al. Percutaneous radiofrequency tissue ablation: does perfusion-mediated tissue cooling limit coagulation necrosis? *J Vac Interv Radiol* 1998;9:101–111.
29. Goldberg SN, Hahn PF, Halporn E, Fogle R, Gazelle GS. Radiofrequency tissue ablation: effect of pharmacologic modulation of blood flow on coagulation diameter. *Radiology* 1998;209:761–767.
30. Rossi S, Garbagnati F, Lencioni R, et al. Percutaneous radiofrequency thermal ablation of nonresectable hepatocellular carcinoma after occlusion of tumor blood supply. *Radiology* 2000;217:119–126.
31. Hansen PD, Rogers S, Corless CL, Siperstein AE, Swanstrom LL. Radiofrequency ablation lesion in a pig model. *J Surg Res* 1999;87:114–121.
32. Fang D, Soulen MC, Nisenbaum HL, et al. Combined chemoembolization and radiofrequency ablation for mid-size hepatic malignancies. *J Vasc Interv Radiol* 2002;13 (suppl):S73.
33. Arata MA, Nisenbaum HL, Clark TW, Soulen MC. Percutaneous radiofrequency ablation of liver tumors with the LeVeen probe: is roll-off predictive of response? *J Vasc Interv Radiol* 2001;12:455–458.
34. Lencioni R, Caramella D, Bartolozzi C. Hepatocellular carcinoma: use of color Doppler US to evaluate response to treatment with percutaneous ethanol injection. *Radiology* 1995;194:113–118.
35. Bartolozzi C, Lencioni R, Ricci P, et al. Hepatocellular carcinoma treatment with percutaneous ethanol injection: evaluation with contrast-enhanced color Doppler US. *Radiology* 1998;209:387–393.
36. Cioni D, Lencioni R, Bartolozzi C. Therapeutic effect of transcatheter arterial chemoembolization on hepatocellular carcinoma: evaluation with contrast-enhanced harmonic power Doppler ultrasound. *Eur Radiol* 2000;10:1570–1575.
37. Rossi S, DiStasi M, Buscarini E, et al. Percutaneous RF interstitial thermal ablation in the treatment of hepatic cancer. *Am J Roentgenol* 1996;167:759–768.
38. Solbiati L, Goldberg SN, Ierace T, et al. Hepatic metastases: percutaneous radiofrequency ablation with cooled-tip electrodes. *Radiology* 1997;205:367–373.
39. Dromain C, DeBaere TJ, Elias D, Ducre M, Sabourin J, Vanel D. Follow-up imaging of liver tumors treated using percutaneous radiofrequency (RF) therapy with helical CT and MRI imaging [abstract]. *Radiology* 1999;213: 382.
40. Lencioni R, Cioni D, Bartolozzi C. Percutaneous radiofrequency thermal ablation of liver malignancies: techniques, indications, imaging findings, and clinical results. *Abdom Imaging* 2001;26:345–360.
41. Fong Y, Saldinger PF, Akhurst T, et al. Utility of ^{18}F- FDG position emission tomography scanning in selection of patients for resection of hepatic colorectal metastases. *Am J Surg* 1999;178:282–287.
42. Livraghi T, Goldberg SN, Lazzaroni S, Meloni F, Solbiati L, Gazelle GS. Radiofrequency ablation vs ethanol injection in the treatment of small hepatocellular carcinoma. *Radiology* 1999;210:655–661.
43. Francica G, Marone G. Ultrasound-guided percutaneous treatment of small hepatocellular carcinoma. *Eur J Ultrasound* 1999;9: 145–153.
44. Lencioni R, Cioni D, Donati F, et al. Percutaneous treatment of small hepatocellular carcinoma in cirrhosis: radiofrequency thermal ablation versus ethanol injection—a prospective, randomized trial. *Radiology* 1999;213:123.
45. Livraghi T, Goldberg SN, Lazzaroni S, et al. Hepatocellular carcinoma: radiofrequency ablation of medium and large lesions. *Radiology* 2000;214:761–768.
46. Lencioni R, Paolicchi A, Moretti M, et al. Combined transcatheter arterial chemoembolization and percutaneous ethanol injection for the treatment of large hepatocellular carcinoma: local therapeutic effect and long-term survival rate. *Eur Radiol* 1998;8:439–444.
47. Solbiati L, Ierace T, Goldberg SN, et al. Percutaneous US-guided RF tissue ablation of liver metastases: results of treatment and follow-up in 16 patients. *Radiology* 1997;202:195–203.
48. Livraghi T, Goldberg SN, Monti F, et al. Saline-enhanced radiofrequency tissue ablation in the treatment of liver metastases. *Radiology* 1997;202:205–210.
49. Lencioni R, Goletti O, Armillota N, et al. Radiofrequency thermal ablation of liver metastases with a cooled-tip electrode needle: results of a pilot clinical trial. *Eur Radiol* 1998;8:1205–1211.
50. Curley SA, Izzo F, Delrio P, et al. Radiofrequency ablation of unresectable primary and metastatic hepatic malignancies. *Ann Surg* 1999;230:1–8.
51. Gillams AR, Lees WR. Survival after percutaneous, image-guided, thermal ablation of hepatic metastases from colorectal cancer. *Dis Colon Rectum* 2000,43:656–661.
52. Schottenfeld D. Epidemiology of lung cancer. In: Pass HI, Mitchell JB, Johnson DH, Turrisi AT, eds. *Lung Cancer Principles and Practice.* Philadelphia, Pa: Lippincott-Raven; 1996:305–321.
53. Sugaar S, LeVeen HH. A histopathologic study on the effects of radiofrequency thermotherapy on malignant tumors of the lung. *Cancer* 1979;43:767–783.
54. Dupuy DE, Zagoria RJ, Akerley W, Mayo-Smith MW, Kavanaugh PV, Safran H. Percutaneous radiofrequency ablation of malignancies in the lung. *Am J Roentgenol* 2000;174:57–59.
55. Landis SH, Murray T, Bolden S, Wingo PA. Cancer statistics, 1999. *CA Cancer J Clin* 1999;49:8–31.
56. McGovern FJ, Wood BJ, Goldberg SN, McDougal WS, Mueller PR. Radiofrequency ablation of renal cell carcinoma via image-guided needle electrodes. *J Urol* 1999;161:599–600.
57. Gervais DA, McGovern FJ, Wood BJ, Goldberg SN, McDougal WS, Mueller PR. Radiofrequency ablation of renal cell carcinoma: early clinical experience. *Radiology* 2000;217:665–672.

58. Walther MM, Shawkes TH, Libutti SK, et al. A phase 2 study of radiofrequency interstitial tissue ablation of localized renal tumors. *J Urol* 2000;163:1424–1427.
59. Kachura JR, Rendon RA, Gertner MR, Sweet JM, Sherar MD, Jewett MA. Radiofrequency ablation (RFA) of renal cell carcinoma with post-RFA CT and pathologic correlations [abstract]. *J Vasc Interv Radiol* 2002;13(suppl):S62.
60. Mikityansky I, Chang I, Pritchard WF, et al. Perfusion effect on radiofrequency ablation in the kidneys [abstract]. *J Vasc Interv Radiol* 2002;13(suppl):S94.
61. Rosenthal DI, Hornicek FJ, Wolfe MW, Jennings LC, Gephart MC, Mankin HJ. Changes in the management of osteoid osteoma. *J Bone Joint Surg* 1998;80:815–821.
62. Woertler K, Vestring T, Boettnes F, Winkelmann W, Heindel W, Lindner N. Osteoid osteoma: CT-guided percutaneous radiofrequency ablation and follow-up in 47 patients. *J Vasc Interv Radiol* 2001;12:717–722.
63. Stoll BA, Parbhoo S, eds. *Bone Metastasis: Monitoring and Treatment.* New York, NY: Raven Press; 1983.
64. Dupuy DE, Safran H, Mayo-Smith WW, Goldberg SN. Radiofrequency ablation of painful osseous metastasis [abstract]. *Radiology* 1998;2000: 389.
65. Jeffrey SS, Bindwell RL, Ikeda DM, et al. Radiofrequency ablation of breast cancer: first report of an emerging technology. *Arch Surg* 1999;134:1064–1068.
66. Izzo F, Thomas R, Delrio P, et al. Radiofrequency ablation in patients with primary breast carcinoma. *Cancer* 2001;92:2036–2044.

CHAPTER 17

INTERSTITIAL TUMOR ABLATION

DHEERAJ K. RAJAN, MD, FRCPC
MURRAY ASCH, MD, FRCPC

INTRODUCTION

The incidence of both primary and metastatic tumors of the liver appears to be increasing. This is likely due to a combination of factors, including prolonged life expectancy, better imaging techniques, and an increase in the incidence of viral hepatitis. There are approximately 160,000 new cases of colorectal cancer per year in the United States and up to 1 million cases of hepatoma worldwide. It is well accepted that surgical resection (or transplantation) remains the standard first-line therapy; in appropriately selected patients, 5-year survival rates of 25%–40% are not unusual. Unfortunately, in less than 20% of patients is surgery appropriate. This is often because of technical aspects of tumor distribution or insufficient hepatic reserve.

There are other options for tumor control when surgery is not an option, including standard systemic chemotherapy, hepatic artery infusion (HAI), transarterial chemoembolization (TACE), gene therapy, radiofrequency ablation (RFA), and local interstitial tumor ablation (ITA). Transarterial chemoembolization and RFA are covered elsewhere in this text; therefore, this chapter focuses on ITA.

Although ITA techniques may be applied to tumors in virtually any organ, thus far, the majority of experience is within the liver. Such techniques are well suited to the population whose tumors are currently deemed unresectable for several reasons. The major effect is targeted at the tumor, so there is relative sparing of "normal" parenchyma. The majority of scientific literature on ITA has focused on the use of percutaneous ethanol

TABLE 17-1

General Classes of Interstitial Tumor Ablation Therapies

Thermal	Liquid
Cryotherapy	Alcohol
Radiofrequency	Acetic acid
Microwave	Boiling saline
Laser	Boiling contrast

injection (PEI), which has been used in the treatment of hepatocellular carcinomas (HCCs) without significant adverse effects on adjacent parenchyma and therefore can be performed in patients with advanced cirrhosis.[1] Studies investigating the clinical utility of PEI have shown that this method preserves more residual liver function than surgery and TACE, especially in patients with cirrhosis, with lower mortality and morbidity rates.[2,3] These findings are similar to those of other therapies discussed below.

These procedures can often be performed percutaneously, so they are truly minimally invasive, and may be repeated without significant requirement for lengthy hospitalizations or recovery. Many of these procedures may be combined with other procedures with the hope that each will potentiate the other. Most recently gaining popularity is the application of these techniques 1 day after TACE has been done. It is hypothesized that the relative devascularization produced by embolization will increase the effectiveness of these more local techniques, as recently demonstrated in an animal study.[4]

There are several different ITA modalities, which may be separated into two general classes: thermal and liquid (**Table 17-1**).

GENERAL PRINCIPLES

Science and Ethics

Given the relative novelty of these procedures, and the lack of true scientific data assessing survival rates when compared with accepted surgical techniques, these therapies should be reserved for patients who cannot undergo surgical resection. It should not be assumed that these interventions are equivalent to surgical resection at this time. ITA is best applied on the advice of a multidisciplinary tumor board, as part of the armamentarium available to best treat individual patients. Similarly, it should not be assumed that debulking tumors in asymptomatic patients would result in prolonged survival. There are many novel approaches to tumor therapy that should be offered as part of a clinical study with the approval of an institution's review board. The simple availability of a technique should not result in its indiscriminate use.

Patients should be carefully selected using general inclusion criteria. Standard practice includes patients with three or fewer tumors, each less than 3–5 cm in size.[5–10] When tumors become larger or more numerous than this, it is often a sign that there is systemic disease or that these local techniques will fail as a result of limitations with current equipment. These criteria are taken from the surgical literature, which has shown that these patients can benefit from surgical resection.

Contraindications

Contraindications to local tumor ablation therapy are generally those factors that would increase risk. As with any percutaneous hepatic intervention, the presence of gross ascites, uncorrectable coagulopathy, severe portal hypertension, and obstructive jaundice increases the risks of bleeding and bile peritonitis. The presence of a biliary-enteric anastomosis also increases the risk of infection/abscess, as the biliary tree is contaminated by gut organisms.[11] This risk factor may be minimized by using aggressive intravenous antibiotic therapy before and after intervention, possibly with associated oral antibiotics in an attempt to sterilize the gut.

The other class of relative contraindication includes a short-term expected survival as a result of extralesional factors. The presence of tumor thrombosis in the main portal trunk and/or extrahepatic disease suggests that local tumor ablation will not prolong survival. Recently, Meloni et al. included Child-Pugh class C patients as those for whom percutaneous ethanol injection is contraindicated because of poor hepatic reserve and a statistically significant difference in survival when compared with Child-Pugh class A and B patients.[12]

Imaging Guidance

These techniques share many factors in common. They all require state-of-the-art imaging equipment and operator expertise for safe and appropriate results. Imaging is important in several ways, and at different times, of local ablation therapy. First, the imaging technique must be good enough to identify and characterize lesions. Second, it must be possible to image the lesion during the course of the procedure. Finally, in follow-up treatment, the technique must allow identification of complications and assessment of local and/or distant tumor recurrence.

Most widely available, relatively inexpensive, and without ionizing radiation, real-time ultrasound (US) is an excellent modality for guiding these procedures. However, unlike with simple biopsies, there are artifacts generated as part of these procedures, which interferes with sonographic monitoring. A dense local echogenic cloud forms as a result of gas bubbles, ice crystals, or from an injected liquid; this cloud obscures the treated area. In some instances the negative effect can be minimized by starting the ablation toward the posterior aspect of the lesion and working toward the transducer. In patients treated with RFA, the microbubbles persist only for a short time, so waiting just a few minutes restores the ability to visualize local structures (and the needle). The availability of US contrast agents may help to better target residual tumor during the procedure itself, rather than waiting several weeks for follow-up computed tomography (CT) or magnetic resonance (MR) imaging to identify untreated tumor.

Intraoperative US should be available at all institutions where liver resections are performed. The availability of laparoscopic ultrasound (LAPUS) will allow for ITA to be performed without laparotomy when percutaneous access is impossible. A novel technique for US imaging and guidance to segments VII and VIII is production of an artificial hydrothorax.[13]

CT guidance is valuable for lesions not well seen sonographically or in locations that are technically difficult to access. The availability of CT fluoroscopy, or a magnetic guidance system, should further increase the value of this guidance modality. Still, there are a number of hepatomas that are visible on CT only during the arterial phase of contrast injection. Multiple investigators have found that the intra-arterial injection of Lipiodol several weeks preceding the ITA therapy results in persistent tumor stain, facilitating subsequent intervention with CT.[14,15]

MR may have the greatest potential for guidance in that it is a highly sensitive method to locate small lesions and that thermal mapping techniques may be the best way to identify complete tumor kill. Currently, there are few open magnets available, and much of the equipment used for these techniques is not compatible with the environment of MR imaging.

Follow-up imaging is an essential tool used in any local tumor ablation program. The interventional radiologist should take a strong lead in this area. Subsequent imaging appointments may be also used as a means to see the patient for follow-up assessment. It is advantageous to schedule an early imaging study to ensure that the entire lesion has been successfully ablated and that there are no complications. At our center, we perform follow-up triphasic CT (unenhanced, arterial, and portal venous phase) scans at 2 weeks and at 3 months, then at 3- to 6-month intervals as appropriate.

Evaluation of effect can be determined with US, CT, or MR imaging. CT scans are the most common method of evaluating the effects of local tumor ablation therapy. Necrotic lesions typically demonstrate uniform low density without any arterial contrast enhancement. However, early CT imaging within 1–2 weeks of the ablation often shows abnormal areas of enhancement in and around the treated lesion. These changes are due to local hyperemia, hemorrhage, and perfusion defects and may make it difficult to differentiate between residual neoplasm and artifact. These findings have been shown to be most marked after microwave therapy, where they may persist for up to 1 month.[16]

Routine sonography cannot reliably demonstrate residual tumor, but perfusion within residual viable tissue can be detected by color Doppler US.[17] Color Doppler and harmonic imaging using US contrast agents may be more sensitive than power Doppler for detection of untreated tumor.

MR imaging will show necrotic lesions as hypointense on T_2-weighted images, whereas active residual tumor will be seen as a hyperintense signal on T_2-weighted sequences and as an enhancing area on contrast-enhanced T_1-weighted images.[18,19]

Biopsies can also give false negative results because of sampling error if the area of residual disease is not biopsied. When serum alpha fetoprotein (AFP) or carcinoembryonic antigen (CEA) levels are elevated prior to treatment, monitoring them may provide an estimate of tumor control.

Liquid Versus Thermal

Given the wide variety of devices and techniques available, it becomes immediately apparent that there is no perfect modality for local tumor ablation. The advantages of the liquid agents are that they are typically readily available, inexpensive, and easy to administer percutaneously using a very small access (22-gauge) needle. Conversely, to be effective, they must diffuse throughout the lesion. In cases of fibrotic tumors (such as colorectal metastasis), this may not be possible, leading to incomplete local control. In the presence of a fibrotic capsule (hepatomas), local satellite tumors beyond the capsule may not be ablated. These treatments often have to be administered in multiple sessions, as it is usually impossible to inject the required volume in a single session. The thermal techniques, on the other hand, result in complete ablation within the volume of tissue that is exposed to the critical temperature. Satellite lesions are easily encompassed, and tumor type is unimportant. Thermal techniques have to be applied only once to

TABLE 17-2

Comparison of Various Characteristics of Different Interstitial Tumor Ablation Therapeutic Modalities

Modality	Size of needle probe	Maximum size of ablation zone	No. of treatment sessions required
Radiofrequency ablation	14 g	5 cm	1
Cryotherapy	3–10 mm	6 cm	1
Percutaneous microwave coagulation therapy	18 g	1.6–2.4 cm	1
Laser-induced thermotherapy	9 F	1.6 cm	1
Hot saline injection	21- to 22-gauge	Unlimited	Many
Percutaneous acetic acid injection	21- to 22-gauge	Unlimited	Many
Percutaneous ethanol injection	21- to 22-gauge	Unlimited	Many

achieve complete tumor kill. The negative aspect of thermal devices is the size of the access, which may be up to 1 cm in diameter for some cryotherapy units or 9 F for some sheaths requiring cooling. The application of energy while withdrawing the probe has been described as a method of reducing local hemorrhagic complications secondary to the large size of these devices. Microwaving the tract as been described to prevent bleeding during withdrawal of the probe.[20,21] Another consideration is the possibility of collateral damage to adjacent organs by transfer of heat through conduction. The basic differences between modalities are summarized in **Table 17-2**.

The Anatomy of Failure

There are several potential causes for failure of these therapies. The first is local tumor recurrence as a result of technical issues. With liquid agents, it may not be possible to completely ablate the tumor within the injected lesion or to penetrate beyond the lesion to kill small satellite lesions or micrometastases that would have been removed with a 1-cm margin using standard surgical techniques.

Although thermal techniques are more likely to result in a uniform local ablation, there is still a limitation of ablation size related to the diameter of devices. Even a device that yields a 4-cm ablation zone could effectively ablate only a tumor that is 2 cm in size (if the standard practice of obtaining a 1-cm surgical margin is adhered to). For ablation of a larger tumor, multiple overlapping probe placements are required. Although in theory this sounds fairly simple, in practice it is difficult to see the probe or be certain of the area already ablated to reposition for subsequent cycles, using current readily available image guidance. Specifically, in the case of cryosurgery, it may be impossible to place a new probe into a frozen area for up to 45 minutes after the initial freeze.

The second cause for failure is the development of new distant (intra- or extrahepatic) disease. The natural history of cirrhosis is to form new hepatic neoplasms. New lesions occur frequently in other areas of the liver after successful local tumor ablation and are believed to represent the nature of cirrhosis/HCC rather than failure of local tumor ablation.[22] Similarly, micrometastases may have been present and undetected prior to intervention and may grow, being visible only on follow-up imaging studies.

Complications

In spite of the different available techniques, the observed complications are similar. The specifics are discussed in each section, but an overview is given here. Common complications are those expected with any percutaneous hepatic intervention, including hemorrhage and abscess formation.

Pain is a common complaint referable to these procedures. Depending on the size of the tumor to be ablated, some form of the classic post-embolization syndrome can be expected. Tumor implantation along needle tracts has been shown as a complication of standard biopsies and even surgical intervention and has similarly been reported for these ablative techniques.[23–27] Probably one of the most important risks is that of acute liver failure if too much tissue is ablated in a patient with low liver reserve. This is particularly true if the lesion is in a position that results in associated hepatic infarction. Other systemic complications include adult respiratory distress syndrome and myoglobinuria. Transient hepatic encephalopathy may be seen in patients secondary to use of benzodiazepines and narcotics during the procedure.

Reactive pleural effusions are common and may be seen in up to 7.5% of patients after these procedures. Subcapsular hematomas may be observed in up to 4% of patients but are often asymptomatic. Intra-abdominal or hepatic abscess may be seen in 2% and is most often treated with percutaneous drainage. Bile duct injury has been reported in up to 6% and is due to damage to small or large biliary radicals adjacent to the treated areas. When very peripheral, this may not require treatment; for obstruction of the central ducts, percutaneous intervention may be required. Tumors treated in the vicinity of the hepatic hilum are particularly at risk.[28]

Major complications include intraperitoneal hemorrhage and hemobilia, both of which may be treated by transcatheter embolization. Small areas of hepatic infarction are common; however, massive infarction will result in death because of hepatic insufficiency.[11,24,25,29–33]

Additional Interventions

Thermal techniques (whether hot or cold) are adversely affected by local heat sinks. Heat sinks occur in the presence of a large vascular structure in the vicinity of the ablation, resulting in less efficient delivery of thermal effect. Although on one hand this protects the vessel from damage,[34] it may prolong the length of time of the ablation or prevent cells immediately adjacent to the vessel from being sufficiently injured to cause cell death. A number of interventions to decrease the heat sink effect have been suggested. The most well known is the Pringle maneuver. This surgical technique involves temporary cessation of all vascular inflow to the liver by clamping the vascular pedicle (hepatic artery, portal vein, and bile duct). This is commonly performed intraoperatively during hepatic resection to reduce blood loss. It is now commonly performed during intraoperative ITA. The goal now is to find a similar technique that can be performed percutaneously. Such techniques include bland hepatic arterial embolization, TACE, or balloon occlusion of the hepatic or portal venous system.[4,35] These techniques clearly increase the complexity of ITA and therefore need to be evaluated scientifically to establish their value.

Pain Control

When administered percutaneously, all these techniques are fairly similar in their ability to induce pain. A thorough knowledge of intraprocedural sedation and analgesia is required to keep patients comfortable. A close working relationship with the local anesthesiologist is very valuable. This is particularly true with the techniques that require multiple treatment sessions. Issues regarding pain management are discussed in Chapter 5.

ITA THERAPIES

Liquid

Acetic Acid

Acetic acid (AA) has a stronger necrotizing effect than ethanol. It has the ability to penetrate cells, where it extracts collagen and lipids.[36,37] A concentration of 15% AA induces the same degree of necrosis as does absolute alcohol (99.5%) in equal volumes. The effect reaches a plateau at 50% concentration[37,38] for hepatocyte necrosis. Cytologic changes seen with percutaneous AA injection (PAI) are decreased cell number, reduced cellular aggregation, and degeneration of the cytoplasm and nucleus.[39] The first reported use of AA for treating HCC was in 1993.[38] To date, reports of some 100 cases using this method have been published in the literature. In PAI, AA penetrates the septa through dissociation of cross-links of collagen, theoretically making it more effective in completeness of ablation than with other liquid agents that lack this effect.[36,40]

A 22-gauge needle is inserted into the deep portion of the lesion with US guidance. AA is then slowly injected while the needle is withdrawn to the more superficial portion of the tumor. The injection is stopped when a hyperechoic area, covering the length of the tumor, appears immediately after injection or resistance is met. The endpoint of treatment is when the tumor changes to a hyperechoic mass and contrast-enhanced CT does not demonstrate any residual viable tumor. If residual tumor is detected, PAI may be administered for one or two more sessions. Total volume injected is based on the formula suggested by Shiina et al.,[41] with modification for AA because only one third of the volume for AA is required for the same degree of necrosis, compared with ethanol[37]:

$$\text{PEI:}\quad \text{volume} = (4/3)(\pi)(r + 0.5)^3;$$

where r is the radius of the lesion

$$\text{PAI:}\quad \text{volume} = [(4/3)(\pi)(r + 0.5)^3] \times 1/3$$

The recommended therapeutic regimen administered is 1.4 mL of 50% AA for 1- to 2-cm nodules and 2.4 mL for 2- to 3-cm nodules, over multiple sessions. Typically, one injection per session—with there being two sessions per week—are administered, with an average of four sessions for HCCs measuring approximately 3 cm. Ohnishi et al. reported that they deposit Gelfoam powder along the hepatic tract to prevent leakage.[37]

A second recommended protocol is single high-dose AA injection.[42] In one report, this method was attempted in 18 patients with 22 treated HCC nodules. Seventeen (77%) of the treated nodules showed no local recurrence after a mean follow-up period of 15.6 months.[42] It has been suggested that multiple sidehole needles (Cliny, Yokohama, Japan) may allow for a more even distribution of AA to cover the whole nodule in a single injection.[42]

On US, tumors appear hyperechoic after treatment; on CT, they appear as an area of low attenuation. On follow-up imaging studies, treated tumors demonstrate a volume reduction of approximately 50% after 6 months.

After undergoing PAI, most patients feel transient local pain; this is especially prominent during the first treatment session. Pain is also more common and intense during treatment of a subcapsular lesion. Major complications described in case reports include separate single published incidents of unexplained acute renal failure and liver perforation.[43,44] Ohnishi et al. reported a higher cytotoxic effect with PAI than with ethanol, with liquefactive necrosis, a lower recurrence rate (8% versus 37%), and better survival rate (92% versus 63%) for small HCCs.[37,45] Hepatomas larger than 3 cm have also been treated with AA concentrations ranging from 15% to 50%. For hypervascular tumors, recurrence rates from the primary treated tumor were 0%, 20%, and 20% at 1, 2, and 3 years, respectively.[46] A local recurrence rate of 8% at 3 years for 3- to 4-cm HCCs was also noted.[46] In this study, reimaging and needle biopsy were performed at 2 weeks to assess the need for further treatment. In a separate study, 91 patients were treated for HCCs smaller than 3 cm; there was no regrowth of treated lesions and no serious complications.[46] The 1- and 2-year cancer-free survival rates were 83% and 54%, respectively.

The number of treatment sessions required for PAI compared with PEI for HCCs of similar sizes is smaller (PAI, 2.5 ± 0.9; PEI, 3.9 ± 1.6).[37] It has also been suggested that recurrence rates for new HCCs in the remaining liver were lower with PAI (42%) than with PEI (66%–74%) for similar-size lesions at 3 years (P = NS).[37,47–49] This may be related to the smaller number of treatment sessions required for PAI. One-, 3-, and 5-year cancer-free survival rates for HCCs smaller than 3 cm after PAI was suggested to be comparable to those for hepatic resection; these results are similar to results found for PEI.[46,49] When comparing PAI with PEI for HCCs smaller than 3 cm in a prospective randomized controlled trial, Ohnishi demonstrated an 8% local recurrence for PAI versus 37% for PEI ($P > 0.001$), with 1- and 2-year survival rates of 100% and 92%, respectively, with PAI versus 83% and 63%, respectively, with PEI.[50] Multivariate analysis revealed that treatment was an independent predictor of survival. With PAI, complete necrosis of intracapsular cancer foci has also been demonstrated.[46,49] A deficiency of this study is an unexplained survival rate for PEI that is much lower in this study than in others.[1,2,41,47,49,51–54]

In a study by Ohnishi et al., 25 patients were treated with PAI; routine follow-up fine-needle biopsy did not demonstrate any viable tumor cells.[45] In addition, 2 patients underwent resection of PAI-treated lesions that demonstrated complete coagulative necrosis encapsulated with a thick fibrous band with no viable cancer cells. Also, in the animal portion of the study, 50% AA was found to cause a larger necrotic area than absolute (99.5%) ethanol.

In two studies, AA injection has also been proposed as a one-time treatment method for hyperfunctioning adrenal nodules. Three patients were treated percutaneously and remained symptom-free after 1 year, with a follow-up period of 5–27 months.[55,56]

Ethanol

First introduced by Sugiura et al. in 1983, PEI has now become accepted as an alternative method of treating HCC for patients who cannot undergo surgery.[57] Some other applications outside the liver have been described. Absolute ethanol diffuses into tumor cells and causes coagulation necrosis by protein denaturation and dehydration of the cytoplasm. This necrosis is followed by occlusion of small vessels due to necrosis of the vascular endothelium and subsequent platelet aggregation, thereby causing ischemic tissue necrosis.[58,59] Histopathologic examinations of surgically resected HCCs have revealed almost complete necrosis after PEI.[60]

Ethanol is injected into or along the margin of lesion, and injection is repeated once or twice a week for a total of four to six sessions, depending on tumor size. The use of glass syringes and special attention to needle type are important, as the alcohol has a tendency to melt many types of plastics, including needle hubs, on contact. A 21- or 22-gauge multiple-sidehole Chiba needle (Cook, Inc., Bloomington, IN) is introduced into the tumor percutaneously under US guidance, and absolute ethanol (99.5%) is slowly injected. Ethanol should be injected through the entire lesion for maximum effect. Multiple needles can be placed into the lesion prior to injection.[61] During injection, the needle is slowly withdrawn through the lesion. If ethanol is seen to leak into the portal veins, hepatic veins, or the bile ducts, the injection should be stopped to prevent injury to these structures. It is common to see vascular intravasation of alcohol during the initial portion of the first injection. This is likely due to the highly vascular nature of hepatomas. Some authors report that they leave the needle in the tract for a few minutes to prevent reflux of alcohol along the tract, whereas others report that they place Gelfoam powder in the tract to prevent reflux.[54,59,62] Simply allowing the pressure within the tumor to decompress alcohol back into the syringe reduces the subsequent reflux of alcohol along the tract; this reflux is the major cause of peritoneal irritation. Injection is done under US or CT guidance to allow visualization of the distribution of ethanol. Absolute ethanol has a low CT attenuation value (approximately −240 HU), allowing for easy identification.[59] Direct correlation between volume of ethanol used and area of necrosis has been reported.[53] The volume to be injected can be determined by the formula:

$$\text{volume} = (4/3)(\pi)(r + 0.5)^3;$$
where r = radius of lesion in centimeters

The intent should be to inject as much alcohol as possible during each session. This may be limited either by pain or by extralesional extravasation. If the lesion is large enough, it seems safe to inject up to 60 mL per session. When there are multiple sessions, the treatment course should be complete within a short period of time to ensure that the resultant devascularization and fibrosis does not interfere with subsequent diffusion of the alcohol. Single large-volume injections with the patient under general anesthesia (to avoid pain) have been described as a method of avoiding the nearly 15 treatment sessions required for large lesions.[64,65] This method appears to have higher complication rates and increased mortality,[65–67] although this finding is not consistent.[68] In the largest study regarding single-session PEI,[67] for single lesions smaller than 5 cm, survival at 1 and 4 years was 90% and 82%, respectively. One- and 4-year survival rates of 97% and 59%, respectively, were attained for lesions larger than 5 cm. With multiple nodules, 1- and 5-year survival rates of 97% and 60%, respectively, were observed, which are comparable to rates for traditional treatment methods.[67] Advantages to single-session PEI include less pain, the ability to place multiple needles simultaneously, the need for only one treatment session, and a theoretic decreased risk of tract seeding. One should be concerned, however, about a dose-dependent effect of the alcohol; it has been recommended that the volume be limited to 60 mL.[67] Single-session PEI is performed with the patient under general anesthesia, with or without endotracheal intubation.[12,64] Meloni et al. described administering 7500 mg fructose 1,6-diphosphonate and 1200 mg glutathione-SH intravenously to quicken the metabolism of alcohol.[12]

Common complications of PEI are pain, fever, and alcohol intoxication.[2,41,47] The latter complication depends on the amount of alcohol injected and is transient. Major complications include intraperitoneal hemorrhage, hemobilia, hepatic infarction, liver abscess formation, and tract implantation. The overall complication rate is reported to be approximately 1.3%–2.4%.[11,24,25,31–33,49] The rate of needle tract seeding after PEI has been reported to be as high as 1.1% for HCCs larger than 2 cm.[24] PEI is extremely safe and has a low mortality, compared with surgery's mortality of 1.4%–11% and morbidity of 58%.[2,60,69]

Rates of complete tumor necrosis after PEI for HCC range from 60% to 100%, with best results observed in lesions smaller than 3 cm.[62] Reported 5-year recurrence rates after PEI range from 64% to 100%, which is comparable to curative surgical resection in comparable patients.[41] Reported 1- and 5-year survival rates range from 46% to 96% and 0% to 72%, respectively.[1,2,49,51–54] The effect of PEI on prognosis for HCCs smaller than 3 cm is comparable to the prognosis after surgical resection.[3,41,47,48,70] The efficacy of PEI for HCCs smaller than 3 cm is high, with complete necrosis ranging from 70% to 90%.[2,60] However, to date there have been no prospective randomized trials comparing PEI to hepatic resection for HCC. Percutaneous ethanol ablation is considered to be less effective for HCCs larger than 3 cm because it is difficult to inject ethanol throughout the entire tumor volume because of varying texture, the tumor's resistance to perfusion of ethanol, or the existence of intratumoral septa. This results in a higher local recurrence rate for larger lesions because the frequency of capsule and septum formation increases with increasing tumor size.[2,41,62,71,72] When there is incomplete necrosis after PEI, residual cancer cells remain in small nodules surrounding the main tumor, in regions isolated by septa or in the periphery of the lesion.[60] Local recurrence is seen in approximately 10% of PEI-treated nodules. PEI has been found to be ineffective when there is intra- or extra-capsular invasion, because ethanol is blocked by the fibrous capsule and fails to reach the tumor cells.[62,71,73] Injected ethanol may flow into the vessels surrounding the tumor instead of into the tumor itself, particularly when the surrounding liver is normal.[59] HCCs with a capsule supposedly provide an ideal local environment for ablation using a liquid agent.

Generally, three or fewer HCC nodules, each less than 3 cm in diameter, are considered suitable for PEI. This is particularly true for an encapsulated tumor where distribution is relatively homogeneous. Nodules less than 2 cm in diameter are completely ablated, whereas larger tumors are only partially destroyed.[62] Because of this, larger lesions require follow-up imaging. The incidence of recurrence is particularly high in HCCs with intratumoral septa, which limits the intratumoral spread of alcohol.[74] It has been reported that the local recurrence rate is higher with PEI for smaller HCCs with fibrous septa than in tumors without septa.[60] The local recurrence rate after PEI is 10.5% to 26%.[2,48,74] Uneven distribution of the ethanol in intralesional injection is a drawback of this method.[59] In a series of 108 patients treated for HCCs larger than 5 cm, 1- and 3-year survival rates for single encapsulated HCCs were 72% and 57%, respectively, and 73% and 42% in single infiltrating tumors between 5 and 10 cm or multiple tumors.[66]

In randomized trials comparing RFA and PEI in the treatment of small (< 3 cm) HCCs, RFA obtained better results in terms of local efficacy, local recurrence, and treatment duration. In a study by Livraghi et al., complete necrosis was obtained in 90% of RFA-treated lesions and in 80% of PEI-treated lesions; the difference between treatments, however, was not statistically significant (P = 0.13). All lesions treated were HCCs smaller than 3 cm and had limited follow-up monitoring. The main advantage of PEI in this study was a lower rate of complications when compared with RFA treatments.[75]

For large inoperable HCCs, a combination of TACE with PEI has been proposed as an alternative treatment that may be more effective than TACE alone.[76–79] It has also been suggested that TACE combined with PEI before transplantation may improve disease-free survival (DFS) rates.[80] In those studies, PEI was initiated approximately 2–4 weeks after a single TACE treatment. Combination therapy resulted in a higher response rate and a lower rate of primary tumor recurrence than for TACE alone.[76,77] Although isolated reports exist regarding use of PEI therapy for metastatic disease and cholangiocarcinoma, the fibrotic nature of these lesions compared with HCCs causes incomplete local ablation. Thus, PEI does not appear to have a role here.[25,81–85]

Intra-arterial administration of absolute ethanol has been described for ablation of renal arterial tumor supply and for ablation of the kidneys for uncontrolled hypertension in the setting of end-stage renal disease. Initial damage occurs in the glomerular capillaries and the glomerular endothelial, epithelial, and mesangial cells.[86] In a study of 20 patients, absolute ethanol was injected into the renal artery after balloon occlusion. No patients developed hypertension, and gross hematuria resolved completely in 9 patients.[87] In a separate study by Onishi et al., 24 patients underwent transarterial alcohol ablation, delivered by balloon catheter, of renal cell carcinomas. There was a significant difference in median survival for treated versus untreated patients (229 days and 116 days, respectively).[88] A single patient with an aldosterone-producing adenoma has been successfully treated with a 4-mL injection of absolute alcohol.[89]

Percutaneous ethanol ablation has been used in head and neck tumors, particularly in the treatment of hyperfunctioning thyroid nodules and parathyroid adenomas as an alternative to surgical resection. Basic principles and techniques are similar to those for ablation in the liver. Approximately 0.5–1 mL of absolute ethanol is injected percutaneously until the tumor becomes hyperechoic. Success rates are as high as 80%.[90–94] Morbidity has been limited to transient pain and transient or permanent (3%) vocal cord paralysis; there has been one described case of Horner's syndrome.[95,96]

RFA after PEI in a rat breast model suggests that this combination therapy may provide greater areas of coagulation necrosis than either therapy alone.[97] PEI has also been used successfully to treat a mesenteric lymphangioma.[98]

Hot Saline Injection

Hot saline injection (PHot) directly into intrahepatic malignant lesions has been proposed as an alternative to ethanol ablation. Benefits include reduced cost and the physiologic non-toxic nature of the agent.

Boiling physiologic saline is heated to the maximum possible temperature and injected using a glass syringe directly into the tumor through a 21-gauge Chiba needle (Cook Inc., Bloomington, IN). This has been found to cause complete coagulation necrosis of tumor tissue and the capsule for HCCs. The mechanism of action is heat-induced coagulation necrosis of the tumor. Because this particular agent is physiologic saline, when the solution cools after it is injected, it has no toxic effects. Research in this area is very limited, with the largest series being that conducted by Honda et al.[99] Given the nontoxicity of the solution, larger lesions can theoretically be treated with a larger injection volume per session and in fewer sessions than PEI. No serious complications have been reported,[99–101] although some patients have reported local pain with injection of 10 mL.[99]

More recently, Yoon et al.[101] treated 29 patients with large HCCs (mean tumor diameter, 7 cm) when TACE was not feasible. He found a median survival of 10 months (range, 3–36 months) in his series. Still, it remains to be proven that it is efficacious to treat large tumors and that a nontoxic agent will provide adequate cell necrosis on the basis of heat alone.

Thermal

Microwave Therapy

The microwave tissue coagulator was initially developed for hemostasis and liver transection during liver surgery, showing reduced blood loss and less morbidity than with conventional hepatectomies.[102,103] The first described percutaneous use was by Tabuse and Katsumi in 1979 to stop bleeding in four ruptured HCCs.[104] Percutaneous use with US guidance for treatment of

HCCs was first described by Seki et al. in 1999.[21] Application of this modality has been primarily described for treatment of focal HCCs and metastases to the liver.[105,106]

Percutaneous microwave coagulation therapy (PMCT) heats tissue by molecular vibration of dipoles, particularly of water in tissue, and induces thermal coagulation in the target area.[107] The microwaves are emitted from a needle electrode inserted directly into the tumor. Multiple treatments are required for lesions larger than 2 cm because the coagulated area formed by PMCT is small. Large lesions are likely not amenable to this treatment modality because PMCT requires multiple treatment sessions and because the possibility of incomplete ablation of portions of the tumor exists. There are, however, reports of lesions of up to 5 cm being treated successfully.[28]

The microwave generator applies energy through an electrode that can have a diameter of 1–2 mm, with a variable shaft length (Microtaze, Nipon Shoji, Osaka, Japan). Treatment power is between 70 and 90 W for a duration of 30–60 seconds. The frequency of the microwave generators most commonly used is 2450 MHz, with a wavelength of 12 cm. In a rabbit model, 60 seconds has been described as the optimal time for necrosis, with no significant change in the size of the necrotic area with increased burn time.[21] Similar to RFA, in PMCT for large lesions, multiple overlapping placements of the antennae with multiple irradiations must be performed to ablate the entire tumor volume.

Early CT imaging within 1 month often shows an area of enhancement of normal hepatic parenchyma adjacent to the treated area. This may be caused by the treatment itself (hyperemia, local inflammatory changes) or regional arterioportal shunting.[16] This area of enhancement disappears in 97% of patients after 1 month.

Most patients report feeling localized heat sensation during microwave therapy; however, this is well tolerated with conscious sedation and local anesthesia.[16] No significant complications have been noted in many small studies.[20,21,107] Complications described with open surgical microwave coagulation therapy (MCT) include biloma formation (5%), intrahepatic abscess (14%), hepatic failure (2%), and implantation of cancer (5%).[106]

Seki et al. found that with moderately to poorly differentiated HCCs, 5-year survival after PMCT was 78%, versus rates for survival after PEI of 35% ($P = 0.03$).[21] No significant difference between the two methods was found for well-differentiated HCCs. This was a retrospective, nonrandomized study; no other study to date has reproduced a similar 5-year survival rate for patients undergoing PMCT. In a series of patients receiving either open MCT (n = 27) or wedge resection (n = 23) for HCC, the overall 3-year survival rate was 86% versus 75%, respectively. DFS after 3 years with open MCT was 44%, versus 14% for wedge resection, with less blood loss and lower morbidity rates in patients treated with open MCT.[103]

Tumor cell differentiation and AFP concentration prior to treatment have been found, by univariate analysis, to influence local recurrences with PEI. Under multivariate analysis, tumor size influenced local recurrence with PMCT.[108] Specifically, PEI therapy was effective with well-differentiated HCCs and PMCT was effective against lesions smaller than 1.5 cm. No significant difference was found between PMCT (70%) and PEI (78%) in overall 5-year survival rates for HCCs smaller than 2 cm that were well differentiated. Other applications of open MCT that have been described in brief reports include local ablation of adrenal tumors in a dog model, followed by successful treatment of primary hyperaldosteronism in a single patient and renal tumor ablation in a rabbit model.[109,110]

Interstitial Laser Therapy or Interstitial Laser-Induced Thermotherapy

Interstitial laser therapy (ILT) is based on the delivery of electromagnetic energy in the spectrum of visible light through thin, flexible fibers to tumors. This type of energy causes tissue coagulation, with protein denaturation and subsequent tissue necrosis. Neodymium yttrium-aluminum-garnet (Nd:YAG) lasers and diode light (wavelength, 890 nm) are the two most common systems in use.[29]

Nd:YAG laser fibers provide good tissue penetration with high power (50–80 W), producing vaporization at the tip of the fibers. Low power (1–2 W), administered over 500–1000 seconds, results in deeper penetration and greater coagulation necrosis.[111] This causes destruction of the tumor by directly applying thermal energy, substantially limiting damage to surrounding structures such as nerves and vessels; local tissue charring may result in a smaller zone of ablation. Histologic findings confirm cell degeneration and coagulative necrosis of both normal and tumor cells.[112] Current use of cylindrical diffusing fiber tips increases diffusion of photoenergy, which results in treatment to a larger tissue area.[113] However, a single fiber cannot produce an area of coagulation exceeding 1.6 cm diameter.[114] Multiple fibers can be applied to treat areas larger than 2 cm.

Fibers are placed through needles placed percutaneously. Most commercial systems come with a cannulation needle (length, 20 cm; diameter, 1.3 mm) with a tetragonal beveled tip and stylet, a 9-F sheath with stylet, and a 7-F double-tube thermostable protective catheter that allows internal cooling via a mechanically pumped cooled saline solution (Dornier MediLas 5060, Germering, Germany). Internal cooling of the surface of the laser fiber modifies the radial temperature distribution so that deeper tissue layers are treated.

An alternative system uses US guidance to position the laser application kit (SOMATEX, Berlin, Germany) into the tumor. This kit has an outer 9-F sheath. Laser fibers (400 μm) are then passed through the inner protective catheter, attached to the laser, and excited at 2–4 W for 5–15 minutes. Beam splitters are necessary to activate many fibers simultaneously.

US is poor at monitoring thermal lesions during ILT; recently, however, MR monitoring of ILT during treatment of liver metastasis has been performed.[115] Online thermography during MR guidance allows exact monitoring of the interventional procedure.[116] The advantage of MR guidance and monitoring over CT and US lies in the thermosensitivity of MR sequences, which allows for real-time documentation of ILT effects and topographic accuracy because of excellent soft-tissue contrast and high spatial resolution. The laser-generating equipment is located outside the MR suite, with passage of light energy into the room via an optical fiber.

Amin et al. used ILT to treat 55 liver metastases in 21 patients.[113] Tumor necrosis of more than 50% was achieved in 82% of tumors, and 100% necrosis was seen in 38%. Metastases smaller than 4 cm were treated more effectively and required fewer treatments. Nolsoe et al. treated 16 colorectal metastases, of which 12 had a mean diameter of 2.4 cm, and found complete necrosis in those 12 lesions.[117] The remaining 4 had lesser degrees of necrosis. In another study by Vogl et al., ILT was used to treat 1914 metastatic liver lesions and various primary lesions.[30] Lesions larger than 5 cm were excluded. An outer sheath (9 F) was placed under CT guidance. During the treatment within an MR suite that followed, formations of ellipsoid hypointense areas were visualized. In 95% of cases, complete necrosis with a 5-mm safety margin was obtained, with a mean survival time of 35 months.[30] In a study by Mack et al., 1981 lesions were treated, with 1- and 3-year survival rates for colorectal metastases of 93% and 50%, respectively. For breast-cancer metastasis, the mean survival was 4.3 years.[118]

Laser-induced thermotherapy (LITT) has also been investigated as a tool for ablation of thyroid cancer devoid of cystic areas. In a study by Pancella et al.,[119] 18 resected thyroid glands were treated with 2 *in vivo* tests on volunteers. The researchers found that large colloid or fluid collections did not allow for uniform heat diffusion. Formation of a hyperechoic zone on US served as a rough guide to extent of necrosis. This study was conducted to test feasibility of use of LITT in thyroid tissue; the researchers concluded that this modality could be used effectively for highly selected thyroid tumors.

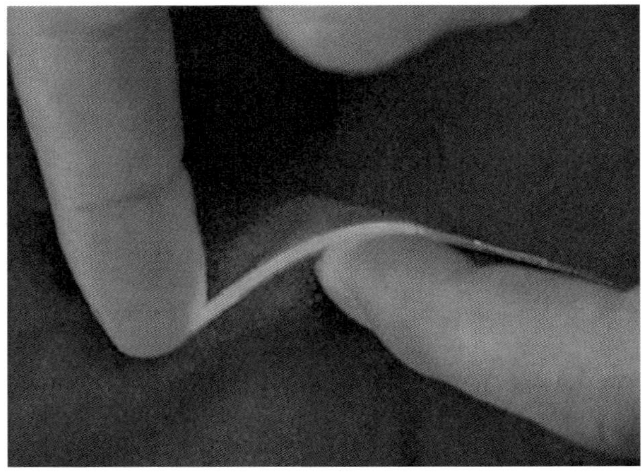

Figure 17-1. Laser fiber that is introduced through an inner protective catheter. (Photo courtesy of SOMATEX, Berlin, Germany).

Fig. 17-1 demonstrates the size of a laser fiber that can be placed percutaneously in a coaxial fashion.

Cryotherapy

Cryotherapy originated in 1845 when James Arnott of England described the benefits of local application of cold as a method of treatment of a variety of conditions, including freezing of advanced cancers such as breast and uterine cervical cancer. He found that this resulted in improvement in pain and a reduction in the size of the tumor.[120] An automated cryosurgical apparatus cooled by liquid nitrogen was first introduced in 1961 and used clinically in 1985 for the treatment of hepatic neoplasms.[122]

Cryotherapy causes non-specific tissue necrosis as a result of freezing and microvascular thrombosis. This is performed by applying extremely low temperatures (–196° Celsius) to the tissue from a probe cooled with circulating liquid nitrogen or argon gas–based systems (Cryocare; Endocare, Irvine, CA). The agent is used to cool a vacuum-insulated cryoprobe that is inserted into the tumor under imaging guidance. As a result of the large size of many of the probes, these procedures are often performed during a laparotomy. Recent advances have allowed the probe size to be decreased, so that some surgeons are performing this procedure percutaneously. Although most literature to date describes an approach with laparotomy, more recently both laparoscopic and percutaneous techniques have been described.[123–127] Multiple lesions and bilobar disease can be treated percutaneously because there is no removal of tissue. However, treatment of tumors occupying more than 50% of the total liver volume and lesions larger than 6 cm in diameter are associated with high morbidity. Ice balls larger than 8 cm cannot be formed with current technology.[128]

Cell injury and cell death result from a combination of physiologic mechanisms: intracellular ice crystal formation, osmotic dehydration during cooling, denaturation of cellular enzymes, rupture of the cell membrane, microcirculatory arrest, and anoxia resulting in cellular necrosis.[129,130] Cellular destruction is more effective with more than one freeze–thaw cycle and with slow thawing.[131] Both absolute temperature and rate of temperature change are important factors in achieving total cell death, particularly at the periphery of the freeze front. Tumoricidal temperatures are reported to be between −20° and −50° Celsius for different tissues,[132] with *in vivo* destruction of colorectal metastasis occurring at −38° Celsius.[133] Thermal gradients of up to 10° Celsius can occur per millimeter of tissue, with a temperature of 0° to −5° Celsius at the edge of the ice ball. For this reason, a 1-cm margin is recommended.

Principles for maximizing tumoricidal effect are as follows[134–137]:

1. Rapid freezing to temperatures at or below −35° Celsius
2. Maintaining the ice ball frozen state for several minutes
3. Slow rethawing
4. Completing more than one freeze cycle

Large vessels are protected from cryogenic damage from the heat-sink effect of flowing blood.[131] For treatment of liver lesions, intraoperative US has been described as the most effective modality for precise localization of the tumor and surrounding structures. On US, the extent of freezing is identified as a hyperechoic rim

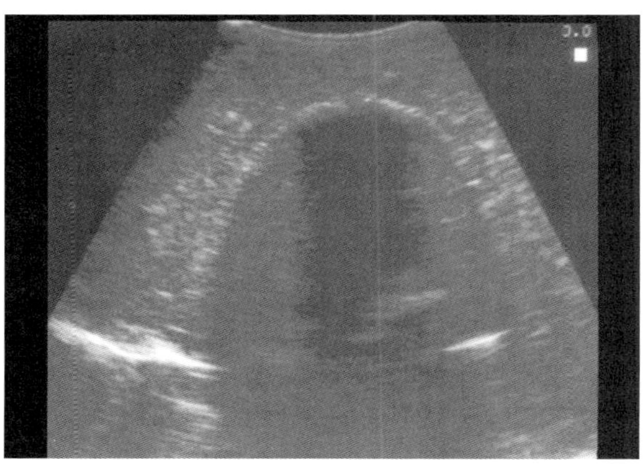

Figure 17-2. Intraoperative ultrasound image of a focal lesion being treated with cryotherapy. The hyperechoic rim correlates with the border of the ice ball formed.

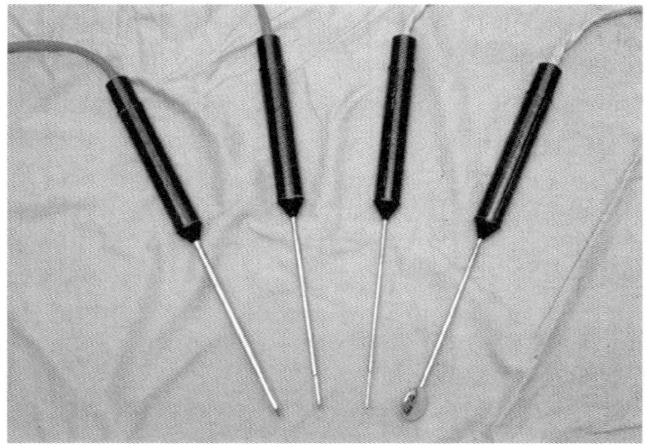

Figure 17-3. Four different cryoprobes. Each probe has a different diameter that correlates with the size of ice ball formed.

with posterior acoustic shadowing[138] (**Fig. 17-2**). On CT during freezing, the ice ball appears as an area of decreased attenuation (1.0 HU ± 20.7 HU).[127] Percutaneous MR guidance has recently been described using an open 0.5T MR imaging system; MR has the advantage of demonstrating the entire ice ball.[139]

Cryoprobe selection is based on the size and location of the lesion. The area frozen depends on the diameter and shape of the cryoprobe (**Fig. 17-3**). In general, 3-mm probes produce a 3-cm ice ball and 5-mm probes produce an ice ball approximately 4 cm in diameter. Larger zones of ablation can be obtained with new argon gas–based systems, allowing the use of smaller probes to produce equivalent ice ball sizes as their nitrogen-system counterparts. Combining several probes allows larger effective treatment zones. Circulating liquid nitrogen creates a probe tip temperature of −196° Celsius, with adjacent tissue temperatures of −100° to −160° Celsius.

Within a few weeks of treatment, the treated lesion appears hypodense on CT, with possible areas of hemorrhage and/or air, representing nitrogen gas from necrotic tissue. There may be some temporary rim enhancement, representing regenerating liver tissue (**Fig. 17-4**).

It has been suggested that there may be enhanced antitumor immunity after cryotherapy.[140] Further confirmatory studies are necessary.

Zhou and Tang reported a 40% 5-year survival for 235 patients undergoing cryotherapy for primary liver cancer and 55% for 80 patients with HCCs smaller than 5 cm.[141] Wong et al. reported a 30% survival at 2 years.[131] For metastatic liver disease, a number of recent studies have been completed. Seifert et al. treated 49 patients with metastatic disease; those patients had a median survival of 23 months and 1- and 2-year survival rates of 78% and 50%, respectively. Limitations of that

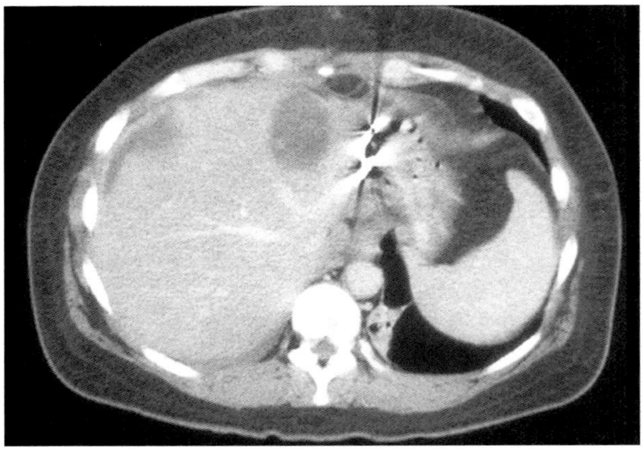

Figure 17-4. Computed tomography image taken after cryotherapy of a focal lesion. The low-density area represents an area of necrosis. No surrounding enhancement is seen to suggest residual tumor.

study were the short follow-up time (median, 13 months) and that some patients also underwent concurrent wedge resection.[142] Local tumor recurrence has been observed in 7%–44% of patients.[129,142–145] In a report by Shapiro et al., five patients were treated with carcinoid metastases; all obtained immediate symptomatic relief. Eighty percent survived at 6 months, and 60% survived at 1 year. Four of 5 (80%) patients had symptomatic relief exceeding 3 months.[146] In the largest published study of patients with metastatic neuroendocrine tumors, 13 patients were treated and reportedly remained mostly asymptomatic after a median follow-up period of 13.5 months; there was 1 unrelated death.[147] Two of the remaining 12 patients (17%) with initial complete tumor ablation have evidence of tumor recurrence.[147] A retrospective comparison of cryotherapy versus RFA for hepatic primary and metastatic malignancies demonstrated a local recurrence rate of 14% after cryotherapy versus 2% after RFA.[148]

Salvage prostate cryotherapy for patients in whom initial radiotherapy fails, who have a prostate-specific antigen (PSA) level higher than 10 ng/mL and a Gleason score of 9 or higher is unlikely to produce DFS.[149] This study also demonstrated that after failed prostate radiotherapy, hormonal therapy, and/or systemic chemotherapy, a double freeze–thaw cycle was more effective than a single cycle for achieving negative biopsy results.[149] Salvage cryotherapy compared with salvage prostatectomy has significantly less morbidity and mortality, with a negative biopsy results rate of 82%.[149] Regarding local treatment of prostate cancer, many studies define treatment success on the basis of PSA values and negative biopsy results after treatment. A PSA level of less than 0.4 ng/mL after treatment is suggested, as there is significant risk of continued PSA elevation and high likelihood of residual disease.[150] Pretreatment PSA levels have also been found to be predictive of subsequent treatment failure, with a PSA level of less than 20 ng/mL equating to fewer biochemical failures.[151] Recurrences are more common in the apex of the gland and the seminal vesicles.[151] Prostate cryotherapy is advocated as a therapeutic option for clinically localized disease. Pretreatment androgen ablation therapy has been advocated to shrink the prostate to a manageable size prior to cryotherapy.[126] In a retrospective outcomes analysis of treatment of 975 patients who underwent cryosurgical ablation of the prostate, the 5-year biochemical-free survival was comparable to that for conventional radiotherapy. Impotence was reported in 93% of patients.[152]

Cryotherapy of soft-tissue sarcomas of the extremities has also been described using intraoperative US guidance for local control prior to surgical resection. The degree of necrosis ranged from 50% to 100% on pathologic examination.[153] A recently described application of cryotherapy is in the treatment of small renal tumors (< 4 cm) with a percutaneous approach using MR imaging guidance. In one study in which 22 tumors were treated and in which the mean follow-up period was 9 months, no radiographic evidence of disease recurrence or new tumor development was observed.[154] An advantage of this modality is the ability to measure temperature gradients within the ice ball.[155] In another study, 34 renal tumors (mean size, 2.3 cm) were treated laparoscopically, and there was no evidence of local or port-site recurrence during a mean follow-up period of 16.2 months.[156] Application of cryotherapy for breast cancer has also been investigated in an animal model.[157]

No randomized trials comparing cryotherapy alone to cryotherapy in conjunction with other treatments have been performed to date.

In addition to the common complications seen with other local tumor ablation techniques, there are a few that appear to be specific to cryotherapy: post-procedure renal dysfunction related to acute tubular necrosis secondary to myoglobinuria and myoglobinemia, coagulopathy secondary to thrombocytopenia, and intraprocedural hypothermia. It is essential to perform these procedures using a warming blanket and to closely monitor the patient's core temperature to prevent systemic hypothermia. Hemorrhage from liver parenchyma is a very serious complication that may lead to delayed bleeding after the liver thaws. Hemorrhage is complicated by the associated thrombocytopenia. This is a problem particularly in patients with cirrhosis.[129,130,131,138] A survey of the complications of hepatic cryotherapy recorded a 1.5% perioperative mortality in 2173 patients. Eighteen percent were related to a syndrome of multiorgan failure, severe coagulopathy, and diffuse intravascular coagulopathy, a syndrome called cryoshock.[158]

CONCLUSION

The selection of an appropriate treatment strategy for patients with primary or metastatic liver malignancies relies on careful clinical and imaging assessment. With such a diversity of new modalities available for treatment, a careful assessment of expected outcome is necessary. In addition, many of the aforementioned studies often present promising results when compared with surgery outcomes. These results should be interpreted with some reservation, however, because many conclusions are based on retrospective, noncontrolled studies in small patient populations.

The above modalities, however, all provide palliative options, with the possibility of potential cure, for patients for whom surgical approaches are contraindicated. If long-term randomized studies validate the utility of these modalities, the gold standard of surgical treatment may be challenged. Furthermore, future validation of the effectiveness of these modalities may lead to applications outside the liver, as preliminary reports have already indicated.

REFERENCES

1. Lencioni R, Bartolozzi C, Caramella D, et al. Treatment of small hepatocellular carcinoma with percutaneous ethanol injection. Analysis of prognostic factors in 105 Western patients. *Cancer* 1995;76(10):1737–1746.
2. Livraghi T, Giorgio A, Marin G, et al. Hepatocellular carcinoma and cirrhosis in 746 patients: long-term results of percutaneous ethanol injection. *Radiology* 1995;197(1):101–108.
3. Livraghi T, Bolondi L, Lazzaroni S, et al. Percutaneous ethanol injection in the treatment of hepatocellular carcinoma in cirrhosis. A study on 207 patients. *Cancer* 1992;69(4):925–929.
4. Takamura M, Murakami T, Shibata T, et al. Microwave coagulation therapy with interruption of hepatic blood in- or outflow: an experimental study. *J Vasc Interv Radiol* 2001;12(5):619–622.
5. Bismuth H, Chiche L, Adam R, Castaing D, Diamond T, Dennison A. Liver resection versus transplantation for hepatocellular carcinoma in cirrhotic patients. *Ann Surg* 1993;218(2):145–151.
6. Mazzaferro V, Regalia E, Doci R, et al. Liver transplantation for the treatment of small hepatocellular carcinomas in patients with cirrhosis [see comments]. *N Engl J Med* 1996;334(11):693–699.
7. Pichlmayr R, Weimann A, Ringe B. Indications for liver transplantation in hepatobiliary malignancy. *Hepatology* 1994;20(1 Pt 2):33S–40S.
8. Scheele J, Stang R, Altendorf-Hofmann A, Paul M. Resection of colorectal liver metastases. *World J Surg* 1995;19(1):59–71.
9. Hughes K, Scheele J, Sugarbaker PH. Surgery for colorectal cancer metastatic to the liver. Optimizing the results of treatment. *Surg Clin North Am* 1989;69(2):339–359.
10. Taylor M, Forster J, Langer B, et al. A study of prognostic factors for hepatic resection for colorectal metastases. *Am J Surg* 1997;173(6):467–471.
11. Okada S, Aoki K, Okazaki N, et al. Liver abscess after percutaneous ethanol injection (PEI) therapy for hepatocellular carcinoma. A case report. *Hepatogastroenterology* 1993;40(5):496–498.
12. Meloni F, Lazzaroni S, Livraghi T. Percutaneous ethanol injection: single session treatment. *Eur J Ultrasound* 2001;13(2):107–115.
13. Shimada S, Hirota M, Beppu T, et al. A new procedure of percutaneous microwave coagulation therapy under artificial hydrothorax for patients with liver tumors in the hepatic dome. *Surg Today* 2001;31(1):40–44.
14. Sato M, Watanabe Y, Tokui K, et al. CT-guided treatment of ultrasonically invisible hepatocellular carcinoma. *Am J Gastroenterol* 2000;95(8):2102–2106.
15. Takayasu K, Moriyama N, Muramatsu Y, et al. The diagnosis of small hepatocellular carcinomas: efficacy of various imaging procedures in 100 patients. *Am J Roentgenol* 1990;155(1):49–54.
16. Ohmoto K, Tsuduki M, Kunieda T, Mitsui Y, Yamamoto S. CT appearance of hepatic parenchymal changes after percutaneous microwave coagulation therapy for hepatocellular carcinoma. *J Comput Assist Tomogr* 2000;24(6):866–871.
17. Lencioni R, Caramella D, Bartolozzi C. Hepatocellular carcinoma: use of color Doppler US to evaluate response to treatment with percutaneous ethanol injection. *Radiology* 1995;194(1):113–118.
18. Sironi S, Livraghi T, DelMaschio A. Small hepatocellular carcinoma treated with percutaneous ethanol injection: MR imaging findings. *Radiology* 1991;180(2):333–336.
19. Bartolozzi C, Lencioni R, Caramella D, Mazzeo S, Ciancia EM. Treatment of hepatocellular carcinoma with percutaneous ethanol injection: evaluation with contrast-enhanced MR imaging. *Am J Roentgenol* 1994;162(4):827–831.
20. Murakami R, Yoshimatsu S, Yamashita Y, et al. Treatment of hepatocellular carcinoma: value of percutaneous microwave coagulation. [see comments]. *Am J Roentgenol* 1995;164(5):1159–1164.
21. Seki T, Wakabayashi M, Nakagawa T, et al. Percutaneous microwave coagulation therapy for patients with small hepatocellular carcinoma: comparison with percutaneous ethanol injection therapy. *Cancer* 1999;85(8):1694–1702.
22. Pompili M, Rapaccini GL, de Luca F, et al. Risk factors for intrahepatic recurrence of hepatocellular carcinoma in cirrhotic patients treated by percutaneous ethanol injection. *Cancer* 1997;79(8):1501–1508.
23. Smith EH. The hazards of fine-needle aspiration biopsy. *Ultrasound Med Biol* 1984;10(5):629–634.
24. Ishii H, Okada S, Okusaka T, et al. Needle tract implantation of hepatocellular carcinoma after percutaneous ethanol injection. *Cancer* 1998;82(9):1638–1642.
25. Cedrone A, Rapaccini GL, Pompili M, et al. Neoplastic seeding complicating percutaneous ethanol injection for treatment of hepatocellular carcinoma. *Radiology* 1992;183(3):787–788.
26. Zerbey AL, Mueller PR, Dawson SL, Hoover HC Jr. Pleural seeding from hepatocellular carcinoma: a complication of percutaneous alcohol ablation. *Radiology* 1994;193(1):81–82.
27. Hamazaki K, Matsubara N, Mori M, et al. Needle tract implantation of hepatocellular carcinoma after ultrasonically guided needle liver biopsy: a case report. *Hepatogastroenterology* 1995;42(5):601–606.
28. Sato M, Watanabe Y, Ueda S, et al. Microwave coagulation therapy for hepatocellular carcinoma. *Gastroenterology* 1996;110(5):1507–1514.
29. Heisterkamp J, van Hillegersberg R, Ijzermans JN. Interstitial laser coagulation for hepatic tumours [see comments]. *Br J Surg* 1999;86(3):293–304.
30. Vogl TJ, Eichler K, Straub R, et al. Laser-induced thermotherapy of malignant liver tumors: general principals, equipment(s), procedure(s)—side effects, complications and results. *Eur J Ultrasound* 2001;13(2):117–127.
31. Isobe H, Fukai T, Iwamoto H, et al. Liver abscess complicating intratumoral ethanol injection therapy for HCC. *Am J Gastroenterol* 1990;85(12):1646–1648.
32. Seki T, Wakabayashi M, Nakagawa T, et al. Hepatic infarction following percutaneous ethanol injection therapy for hepatocellular carcinoma [see comments]. *Eur J Gastroenterol Hepatol* 1998;10(11): 915–918.
33. Fujimoto T. The experimental and clinical studies of percutaneous

ethanol injection therapy (PEIT) under ultrasonography for small hepatocellular carcinoma. *Acta Hepatol Jpn* 1988;29:52–59.
34. Weber SM, Lee FT Jr., Chinn DO, et al. Perivascular and intralesional tissue necrosis after hepatic cryoablation: results in a porcine model. *Surgery* 1997;122(4):742–747.
35. Shibata T, Murakami T, Ogata N. Percutaneous microwave coagulation therapy for patients with primary and metastatic hepatic tumors during interruption of hepatic blood flow. *Cancer* 2000;88(2):302–311.
36. Miller EJ, Rhodes RK. Preparation and characterization of the different types of collagen. *Methods Enzymol* 1982;82(Pt A):33–64.
37. Ohnishi K, Yoshioka H, Ito S, Fujiwara K. Prospective randomized controlled trial comparing percutaneous acetic acid injection and percutaneous ethanol injection for small hepatocellular carcinoma. *Hepatology* 1998;27(1):67–72.
38. Ohnishi K, Chin N, Ito S. Ultrasound guided intratumor injection of acetic acid for the treatment of small hepatocellular carcinoma. *Acta Hepatol Jpn* 1993;34:504–516.
39. Lin SM, Kuo SH, Lin DY, et al. Cytologic changes in hepatocellular carcinoma after percutaneous acetic acid injection. Correlation with helical computed tomography findings. *Acta Cytol* 2000;44(1):1–6.
40. Timpl R, Wiedemann H, van Delden V, Furthmayr H, Kuhn K. A network model for the organization of type IV collagen molecules in basement membranes. *Eur J Biochem* 1981;120(2):203–211.
41. Shiina S, Tagawa K, Niwa Y, et al. Percutaneous ethanol injection therapy for hepatocellular carcinoma: results in 146 patients. *Am J Roentgenol* 1993;160(5):1023–1028.
42. Liang HL, Yang CF, Pan HB, et al. Small hepatocellular carcinoma: safety and efficacy of single high-dose percutaneous acetic acid injection for treatment. *Radiology* 2000;214(3):769–774.
43. Van Hoof M, Joris JP, Horsmans Y, Geubel A. Acute renal failure requiring haemodialysis after high doses percutaneous acetic acid injection for hepatocellular carcinoma. *Acta Gastroenterol Belg* 1999;62(1):49–51.
44. Koda M, Tanaka H, Murawaki Y, et al. Liver perforation: a serious complication of percutaneous acetic acid injection for hepatocellular carcinoma. *Hepatogastroenterology* 2000;47:1110–1112.
45. Ohnishi K, Ohyama N, Ito S, Fujiwara K. Small hepatocellular carcinoma: treatment with US-guided intratumoral injection of acetic acid. *Radiology* 1994;193(3):747–752.
46. Ohnishi K, Nomura F, Ito S, Fujiwara K. Prognosis of small hepatocellular carcinoma (less than 3 cm) after percutaneous acetic acid injection: study of 91 cases. *Hepatology* 1996;23(5):994–1002.
47. Ebara M, Ohto M, Sugiura N, et al. Percutaneous ethanol injection for the treatment of small hepatocellular carcinoma. Study of 95 patients. *J Gastroenterol Hepatol* 1990;5(6):616–626.
48. Tanikawa K, Majima Y. Percutaneous ethanol injection therapy for recurrent hepatocellular carcinoma. *Hepatogastroenterology* 1993;40(4):324–327.
49. Castells A, Bruix J, Bru C, et al. Treatment of small hepatocellular carcinoma in cirrhotic patients: a cohort study comparing surgical resection and percutaneous ethanol injection. *Hepatology* 1993;18(5):1121–1126.
50. Ohnishi K. Comparison of percutaneous acetic acid injection and percutaneous ethanol injection for small hepatocellular carcinoma. *Hepatogastroenterology* 1998;45(suppl 3):1254–1258.
51. Shiina S, Imamura M, Obi S, et al. [Percutaneous ethanol injection therapy for small hepatocellular carcinoma]. *Gan To Kagaku Ryoho [Japanese Journal of Cancer & Chemotherapy]* 1996;23(7):835–839.
52. Lencioni R, Pinto F, Armillotta N, et al. Long-term results of percutaneous ethanol injection therapy for hepatocellular carcinoma in cirrhosis: a European experience. *Eur Radiol* 1997;7(4):514–519.
53. Livraghi T, Benedini V, Lazzaroni S, et al. Long term results of single session percutaneous ethanol injection in patients with large hepatocellular carcinoma. *Cancer* 1998;83(1):48–57.
54. Shiina S, Teratani T, Obi S, et al. Percutaneous ethanol injection therapy for liver tumors. *Eur J Ultrasound* 2001;13(2):95–106.
55. Liang HL, Pan HB, Lee YH, et al. Small functional adrenal cortical adenoma: treatment with CT-guided percutaneous acetic acid injection—report of three cases. *Radiology* 1999;213(2):612–615.
56. Minowada S, Enomoto Y, Korenaga T, et al. CT-guided acetic acid injection therapy for aldosterone-producing adrenocortical adenoma: a preliminary report of three cases. *Endocr J* 2000;47(2):185–189.
57. Sugiura N, Takara K, Ohto M, Okuda K, Hirooka N. Percutaneous intratumoral injection of ethanol under ultrasound imaging for treatment of small hepatocellular carcinoma. *Acta Hepatol Jpn* 1983;24:920–923.
58. Kawano M. An experimental study of percutaneous absolute ethanol injection therapy for small hepatocellular carcinoma: effects of absolute ethanol on the healthy canine liver. *Gastroenterologia Japonica* 1989;24(6):663–669.
59. Lee MJ, Mueller PR, Dawson SL, et al. Percutaneous ethanol injection for the treatment of hepatic tumors: indications, mechanism of action, technique, and efficacy. *Am J Roentgenol* 1995;164(1):215–220.
60. Shiina S, Tagawa K, Unuma T, et al. Percutaneous ethanol injection therapy for hepatocellular carcinoma. A histopathologic study. *Cancer* 1991;68(7):1524–1530.
61. Shiina S, Hata Y, Niwa Y, et al. Multiple-needle insertion method in percutaneous ethanol injection therapy for liver neoplasms. *Gastroenterologia Japonica* 1991;26(1):47–50.
62. Vilana R, Bruix J, Bru C, et al. Tumor size determines the efficacy of percutaneous ethanol injection for the treatment of small hepatocellular carcinoma. *Hepatology* 1992;16(2):353–357.
63. Shiina S, Tagawa K, Unuma T, Terano A. Percutaneous ethanol injection therapy for the treatment of hepatocellular carcinoma. *Am J Roentgenol.* 1990;154(5):947–951.
64. Giorgio A, Tarantino L, Mariniello N, et al. Percutaneous ethanol injection under general anesthesia for hepatocellular carcinoma: 3 year survival in 112 patients. *Eur J Ultrasound* 1998;8(3):201–206.
65. Livraghi T, Lazzaroni S, Pellicano S, et al. Percutaneous ethanol injection of hepatic tumors: single-session therapy with general anesthesia. *Am J Roentgenol* 1993;161(5):1065–1069.
66. Livraghi T. Percutaneous ethanol injection in the treatment of hepatocellular carcinoma in cirrhosis. *Hepatogastroenterology* 2001;48(37):20–24.
67. Giorgio A, Tarantino L, de Stefano G, et al. Ultrasound-guided percutaneous ethanol injection under general anesthesia for the treatment of hepatocellular carcinoma on cirrhosis: long-term results in 268 patients. *Eur J Ultrasound* 2000;12(2):145–154.
68. Elgindy N, Lindholm H, Gunven P. High-dose percutaneous ethanol injection therapy of liver tumors. Patient acceptance and complications. *Acta Radiol* 2000;41(5):458–463.
69. Livraghi T, Bolondi L, Buscarini L, et al. No treatment, resection and ethanol injection in hepatocellular carcinoma: a retrospective analysis of survival in 391 patients with cirrhosis. Italian Cooperative HCC Study Group. *J Hepatol* 1995;22(5):522–526.
70. Makuuchi M, Kosuge T, Takayama T, et al. Surgery for small liver cancers. *Semin Surg Oncol* 1993;9(4):298–304.
71. Ishii H, Okada S, Nose H, et al. Local recurrence of hepatocellular carcinoma after percutaneous ethanol injection. *Cancer* 1996;77(9):1792–1796.
72. Nakajima O. Pathological study on early hepatocellular carcinoma—a study of capsule and septum formation. *Acta Hepatol Jpn* 1989;30:28–34.
73. Seki T, Nonaka T, Kubota Y, Mizuno T, Sameshima Y. Ultrasonically guided percutaneous ethanol injection therapy for hepatocellular carcinoma. *Am J Gastroenterol* 1989;84(11):1400–1407.
74. Hirata M, Nishimura N. Hepatocellular carcinoma recurrence after percutaneous ethanol injection therapy: comparisons of tumors with or without a septum. *Jpn J Med Ultrasonics* 1993;20:548–554.

75. Livraghi T, Goldberg SN, Lazzaroni S, et al. Small hepatocellular carcinoma: treatment with radio-frequency ablation versus ethanol injection [see comments]. *Radiology* 1999;210(3):655–661.
76. Bartolozzi C, Lencioni R, Caramella D, et al. Treatment of large HCC: transcatheter arterial chemoembolization combined with percutaneous ethanol injection versus repeated transcatheter arterial chemoembolization. *Radiology* 1995;197(3):812–818.
77. Tanaka K, Nakamura S, Numata K, et al. Hepatocellular carcinoma: treatment with percutaneous ethanol injection and transcatheter arterial embolization. *Radiology* 1992;185(2):457–460.
78. Lencioni R, Vignali C, Caramella D, et al. Transcatheter arterial embolization followed by percutaneous ethanol injection in the treatment of hepatocellular carcinoma. *Cardiovasc Interv Radiol* 1994;17(2):70–75.
79. Ishii H, Okada S, Sato T, et al. Effect of percutaneous ethanol injection for postoperative recurrence of hepatocellular carcinoma in combination with transcatheter arterial embolization. *Hepatogastroenterology* 1996;43(9):644–650.
80. Troisi R, Defreyne L, Hesse UJ, et al. Multimodal treatment for hepatocellular carcinoma on cirrhosis: the role of chemoembolization and alcoholization before liver transplantation. *Clin Transplant* 1998;12(4):313–319.
81. Livraghi T, Festi D, Monti F, Salmi A, Vettori C. US-guided percutaneous alcohol injection of small hepatic and abdominal tumors. *Radiology* 1986;161(2):309–312.
82. Livraghi T, Vettori C, Lazzaroni S. Liver metastases: results of percutaneous ethanol injection in 14 patients. *Radiology* 1991;179(3):709–712.
83. Suyama Y, Horishi M, Shizumi Y, et al. [Clinicopathological effects of US-guided intratumoral ethanol injection to small liver cancer with special references to its adequate injected volume]. *Nippon Can Chiryo Gakkai Shi [Journal of Japanese Society for Cancer Therapy]* 1988;23(8):1727–1731.
84. Mazzotti A, Grazi GL, Gardini A, et al. An appraisal of percutaneous treatment of liver metastases. *Liver Transplant Surg* 1998;4(4):271–755.
85. Ryan JM, Dupuy DE, Pitman M, et al. Metastases to the liver from extraskeletal myxoid chondrosarcoma and successful treatment with percutaneous ethanol injection. *Clin Radiol* 2000;55(4):314–317.
86. Buchta K, Sands J, Rosenkrantz H, Roche WD. Early mechanism of action of arterially infused alcohol U.S.P. in renal devitalization *Radiology* 1982;145(1):45–48.
87. Ekelund L, Ek A, Forsberg L, et al. Occlusion of renal arterial tumor supply with absolute ethanol. Experience with 20 cases. *Acta Radiol Diagn* 1984;25(3):195–201.
88. Onishi T, Ohishi Y, Goto H, Tomita M, Abe K. An assessment of the immunological status of patients with renal cell carcinoma based on the relative abundance of T-helper 1- and -2 cytokine-producing CD4+ cells in peripheral blood. *BJU Int* 2001;87(9):755–759.
89. Rossi F, Savastano S, Tommaselli AP, et al. Percutaneous computed tomography–guided ethanol injection in aldosterone-producing adrenocortical adenoma [see comments]. *Eur J Endocr* 1995;132(3):302–305.
90. Karstrup S, Holm HH, Glenthoj A, Hegedus L. Nonsurgical treatment of primary hyperparathyroidism with sonographically guided percutaneous injection of ethanol: results in a selected series of patients. *Am J Roentgenol* 1990;154(5):1087–1090.
91. Giangrande A, Castiglioni A, Solbiati L, Allaria P. Ultrasound-guided percutaneous fine-needle ethanol injection into parathyroid glands in secondary hyperparathyroidism. *Nephrol Dial, Transplant* 1992;7(5):412–421.
92. Takeda S, Michigishi T, Takazakura E. Successful ultrasonically guided percutaneous ethanol injection for secondary hyperparathyroidism. *Nephron* 1992;62(1):100–103.
93. Verges B, Cercueil JP, Pfitzenmeyer P, et al. Percutaneous ethanol injection of parathyroid adenomas in primary hyperparathyroidism [letter; comment]. *Lancet* 1991;337(8754):1421–1422.
94. Solbiati L, Giangrande A, De Pra L, et al. Percutaneous ethanol injection of parathyroid tumors under US guidance: treatment for secondary hyperparathyroidism. *Radiology* 1985;155(3):607–610.
95. Karstrup S, Hegedus L, Holm HH. Ultrasonically guided chemical parathyroidectomy in patients with primary hyperparathyroidism: a follow-up study. *Clin Endocrinol* 1993;38(5):523–530.
96. Khafif A, Halperin D, Marshak G. Ethanol injection to parathyroid tissue: indications and limitations. *Ear Nose Throat J* 1998;77(7):538–540.
97. Goldberg SN, Kruskal JB, Oliver BS, Clouse M, Gazelle GS. Percutaneous tumor ablation: increased coagulation by combining radio-frequency ablation and ethanol instillation in a rat breast tumor model. *Radiology* 2001;217(3):827–831.
98. Stein M, Hsu RK, Schneider PD, Ruebner BH, Mina Y. Alcohol ablation of a mesenteric lymphangioma. *J Vasc Interv Radiol* 2000;11(2 Pt 1):247–250.
99. Honda N, Guo Q, Uchida H, Ohishi H, Hiasa Y. Percutaneous hot saline injection therapy for hepatic tumors: an alternative to percutaneous ethanol injection therapy [see comments]. *Radiology* 1994;190(1):53–57.
100. Honda N, Guo Q, Uchida H, et al. [Percutaneous hot water injection therapy (PHoT) for hepatic tumors: a clinical study]. *Nippon Igaku Hoshasen Gakkai Zasshi [Nippon Acta Radiologica]* 1993;53(7):781–789.
101. Yoon HK, Song HY, Sung KB, et al. Percutaneous hot saline injection therapy: effectiveness in large hepatocellular carcinoma. *J Vasc Interv Radiol* 1999;10(4):477–482.
102. Zhou XD, Tang ZY, Yu YQ, et al. Microwave surgery in the treatment of hepatocellular carcinoma. *Semin Surg Oncol* 1993;9(4):318–322.
103. Yamanaka N, Tanaka T, Oriyama T, et al. Microwave coagulonecrotic therapy for hepatocellular carcinoma. *World J Surg* 1996;20(8):1076–1081.
104. Tabuse K, Katsumi M. Application of a microwave tissue coagulator to hepatic surgery: the hemostatic effects on spontaneous rupture of hepatoma and tumor necrosis. *Nippon Geka Hokan [Archiv für Japanische Chirurgie]* 1981;50(4):571–579.
105. Seki T, Wakabayashi M, Nakagawa T, et al. Percutaneous microwave coagulation therapy for solitary metastatic liver tumors from colorectal cancer: a pilot clinical study [see comments]. *Am J Gastroenterol* 1999;94(2):322–327.
106. Shimada S, Hirota M, Beppu T, et al. Complications and management of microwave coagulation therapy for primary and metastatic liver tumors. *Surg Today* 1998;28(11):1130–1137.
107. Seki T, Wakabayashi M, Nakagawa T, et al. Ultrasonically guided percutaneous microwave coagulation therapy for small hepatocellular carcinoma. *Cancer* 1994;74(3):817–825.
108. Horigome H, Nomura T, Saso K, Itoh M. Standards for selecting percutaneous ethanol injection therapy or percutaneous microwave coagulation therapy for solitary small hepatocellular carcinoma: consideration of local recurrence. *Am J Gastroenterol* 1999;94(7):1914–1917.
109. Kigure T, Harada T, Satoh Y, Fujieda N, Wakayama Y. Microwave ablation of the adrenal gland: experimental study and clinical application. *Br J Urol* 1996;77(2):215–220.
110. Kigure T, Harada T, Satoh Y, et al. Percutaneous microwave coagulation therapy on small renal tumors: an experimental study. *J Microw Surg* 1994;12:71–79.
111. Thomsen S. Pathologic analysis of photothermal and photomechanical effects of laser-tissue interactions. *Photochem Photobiol* 1991;53(6):825–835.
112. Matthewson K, Coleridge-Smith P, O'Sullivan JP, Northfield TC, Bown SG. Biological effects of intrahepatic neodymium:yttrium-aluminum-garnet laser photocoagulation in rats. *Gastroenterology* 1987;93(3):550–557.
113. Amin Z, Donald JJ, Masters A, et al. Hepatic metastases: interstitial laser photocoagulation with real-time US monitoring and dynamic CT evaluation of treatment. *Radiology* 1993;187(2):339–347.

114. Bosman S, Phoa SS, Bosma A, van Gemert MJ. Effect of percutaneous interstitial thermal laser on normal liver of pigs: sonographic and histopathological correlations. *Br J Surg* 1991;78(5):572–575.
115. Vogl TJ, Muller PK, Hammerstingl R, et al. Malignant liver tumors treated with MR imaging–guided laser-induced thermotherapy: technique and prospective results. *Radiology* 1995;196(1):257–265.
116. Jolesz FA, Bleier AR, Jakab P, et al. MR imaging of laser–tissue interactions. *Radiology* 1988;168(1):249–253.
117. Nolsoe CP, Torp-Pedersen S, Burcharth F, et al. Interstitial hyperthermia of colorectal liver metastases with a US-guided Nd-YAG laser with a diffuser tip: a pilot clinical study. *Radiology* 1993;187(2): 333–337.
118. Mack MG, Straub R, Eichler K, et al. Percutaneous MR imaging–guided laser-induced thermography of hepatic metastases. *Abdom Imaging* 2001;26:369–374.
119. Pacella CM, Bizzarri G, Guglielmi R, et al. Thyroid tissue: US-guided percutaneous interstitial laser ablation—a feasibility study. *Radiology* 2000;217(3):673–677.
120. Arnott J. Practical illustrations of the remedial efficacy of a very low or anaesthetic temperature. *Lancet* 1850;2:257–259.
121. Cooper IS, Lee A. Cryostatic congelation: a system for producing a limited controlled region of cooling or freezing of biologic tissues. *J Nerv Ment Dis* 1961;133:259–263.
122. Onik G, Gilbert J, Hoddick W, et al. Sonographic monitoring of hepatic cryosurgery in an experimental animal model. *Am J Roentgenol* 1985;144(5):1043–1047.
123. Cuschieri A, Crosthwaite G, Shimi S, et al. Hepatic cryotherapy for liver tumors. Development and clinical evaluation of a high-efficiency insulated multineedle probe system for open and laparoscopic use. *Surg Endosc* 1995;9(5):483–489.
124. Adam R, Majno P, Castaing D, Giovenardi R, Bismuth H. Treatment of irresectable liver tumours by percutaneous cryosurgery. *Br J Surg* 1998;85(11):1493–1494.
125. Lezoche E, Paganini AM, Feliciotti F, et al. Ultrasound-guided laparoscopic cryoablation of hepatic tumors: preliminary report. *World J Surg* 1998;22(8):829–835; discussion, 835–836.
126. Lee F, Bahn DK, McHugh TA, Onik GM, Lee FT Jr. US-guided percutaneous cryoablation of prostate cancer. *Radiology* 1994;192(3):769–776.
127. Lee FT, Jr., Chosy SG, Littrup PJ, et al. CT-monitored percutaneous cryoablation in a pig liver model: pilot study. *Radiology* 1999;211(3):687–692.
128. Weaver ML, Atkinson D, Zemel R. Hepatic cryosurgery in treating colorectal metastases. *Cancer* 1995;76(2):210–214.
129. Ravikumar TS, Kane R, Cady B, et al. A 5-year study of cryosurgery in the treatment of liver tumors. *Arch Surg* 1991;126(12):1520–1523; discussion, 1523–1524.
130. McCarty TM, Kuhn JA. Cryotherapy for liver tumors. *Oncology* 1998;12(7):979–987; discussion, 990.
131. Wong WS, Patel SC, Cruz FS, Gala KV, Turner AF. Cryosurgery as a treatment for advanced stage hepatocellular carcinoma: results, complications, and alcohol ablation. *Cancer* 1998;82(7):1268–1278.
132. Gage AA, Guest K, Montes M, Caruana JA, Whalen DA Jr. Effect of varying freezing and thawing rates in experimental cryosurgery. *Cryobiology* 1985;22(2):175–182.
133. El-Shakhs SA, Shimi SA, Cuschieri A. Effective hepatic cryoablation: does it enhance tumor dissemination? *World J Surg* 1999;23(3):306–310.
134. Dutta P, Montes M, Gage AA. Large volume freezing in experimental hepatic cryosurgery. Avoidance of bleeding in hepatic freezing by an improvement in the technique. *Cryobiology* 1979;16(1):50–55.
135. Bischof J, Christov K, Rubinsky B. A morphological study of cooling rate response in normal and neoplastic human liver tissue: cryosurgical implications. *Cryobiology* 1993;30(5):482–492.
136. Ravikumar TS, Steele G, Kane R, King V. Experimental and clinical observations on hepatic cryosurgery for colorectal metastases. *Cancer Research* 1991;51(23 Pt 1):6323–6327.
137. Dilley AV, Dy DY, Warlters A, et al. Laboratory and animal model evaluation of the Cryotech LCS 2000 in hepatic cryotherapy. *Cryobiology* 1993;30(1):74–85.
138. Onik G, Rubinsky B, Zemel R, et al. Ultrasound-guided hepatic cryosurgery in the treatment of metastatic colon carcinoma. Preliminary results. *Cancer* 1991;67(4):901–907.
139. Silverman SG, Tuncali K, Adams DF, et al. MR imaging–guided percutaneous cryotherapy of liver tumors: initial experience. *Radiology* 2000;217(3):657–664.
140. Hamad GG, Neifeld JP. Biochemical, hematologic, and immunologic alterations following hepatic cryotherapy. *Semin Surg Oncol* 1998;14(2):122–128.
141. Zhou XD, Tang ZY. Cryotherapy for primary liver cancer. *Semin Surg Oncol* 1998;14(2):171–174.
142. Seifert JK, Achenbach T, Heintz A, Bottger TC, Junginger T. Cryotherapy for liver metastases. *Int J Colorectal Dis* 2000;15(3):161–166.
143. Seifert JK, Morris DL. Prognostic factors after cryotherapy for hepatic metastases from colorectal cancer. *Ann Surg* 1998;228(2):201–208.
144. Adam R, Akpinar E, Johann M, et al. Place of cryosurgery in the treatment of malignant liver tumors. *Ann Surg* 1997;225(1):39–38; discussion, 48–50.
145. Crews KA, Kuhn JA, McCarty TM, et al. Cryosurgical ablation of hepatic tumors. *Am J Surg* 1997;174(6):614–617; discussion, 617–618.
146. Shapiro RS, Shafir M, Sung M, Warner R, Glajchen N. Cryotherapy of metastatic carcinoid tumors. *Abdom Imaging* 1998;23(3):314–317.
147. Seifert JK, Cozzi PJ, Morris DL. Cryotherapy for neuroendocrine liver metastases. *Semin Surg Oncol* 1998;14(2):175–183.
148. Pearson AS, Izzo F, Fleming RY, et al. Intraoperative radiofrequency ablation or cryoablation for hepatic malignancies. *Am J Surg* 1999;178(6):592–599.
149. Pisters LL, Perrotte P, Scott SM, Greene GF, von Eschenbach AC. Patient selection for salvage cryotherapy for locally recurrent prostate cancer after radiation therapy. *J Clin Oncol* 1999;17(8):2514–2520.
150. Shinohara K, Rhee B, Presti JC, Carroll PR. Cryosurgical ablation of prostate cancer: patterns of cancer recurrence. *J Urol* 1997;158(6):2206–2209; discussion, 2209–2210.
151. Bahn DK, Lee F, Solomon MH, et al. Prostate cancer: US-guided percutaneous cryoablation. Work in progress. *Radiology* 1995;194(2):551–556.
152. Long JP, Bahn D, Lee F, et al. Five-year retrospective, multi-institutional pooled analysis of cancer-related outcomes after cryosurgical ablation of the prostate. *Urology* 2001;57(3):518–523.
153. Menendez LR, Tan MS, Kiyabu MT, Chawla SP. Cryosurgical ablation of soft tissue sarcomas: a phase I trial of feasibility and safety. *Cancer* 1999;86(1):50–57.
154. Shingleton WB, Sewell PE Jr. Percutaneous renal tumor cryoablation with magnetic resonance imaging guidance. *J Urol* 2001;165(3):773–776.
155. Gilbert JC, Rubinsky B, Wong ST, et al. Temperature determination in the frozen region during cryosurgery of rabbit liver using MR image analysis. *Magn Reson Imaging* 1997;15(6):657–667.
156. Gill IS, Novick AC, Meraney AM, et al. Laparoscopic renal cryoablation in 32 patients. *Urology* 2000;56(5):748–753.
157. Staren ED, Sabel MS, Gianakakis LM, et al. Cryosurgery of breast cancer [see comments]. *Arch Surg* 1997;132(1):28–33; discussion, 34.
158. Seifert JK, Morris DL. World survey on the complications of hepatic and prostate cryotherapy. *World J Surg* 1999;23(2):109–113; discussion, 113–114.

CHAPTER 18

INTRATUMORAL GENE THERAPY

MARSHALL E. HICKS, MD

INTRODUCTION

There are more than 500,000 cancer deaths annually in the United States, including a 50% mortality rate from solid tumors.[1, 2] Given these facts, it is probably not surprising that more than half of the phase 1 trials for gene therapy in the United States are cancer-related. Gene-based therapies may provide more effective means of treating or preventing cancers than previous, more conventional, types of therapy such as surgery, radiation, and pharmacologic therapies.[3]

Existing strategies involve tumor suppression, antiangiogenesis, inhibition of oncogene expression, induction of drug sensitivity (including suicide genes), increased immune response (via cytokines and activation of T lymphocytes), and protection of the host from toxicities associated with other cancer therapies with associated toxicities.[3]

Direct in vivo intratumoral therapy is one means of delivering the genetic vector. Image-guided direct intratumoral vector delivery provides advantages similar to those of other imaged-guided therapies: maximized efficiency of tumor therapy and documentation of physical position. Interventional radiology can play a critical role in the development of this new therapy, because a combination of imaging skills and interventional techniques is important for successful vector delivery.

A number of ongoing preclinical and clinical trials utilize direct in vivo intratumoral therapy. Most of the clinical trials are in phase 1 or phase 2 of development.

Some of these therapies are not utilizing image guidance currently, but it is important to understand the principles of therapy because a transition to image-based therapy is occurring. The most common utilizations of direct tumor therapy involve only a few general categories, which are addressed here. In addition, application of the techniques to image-guided therapy, limitations of direct intratumoral therapy, and updates of pertinent examples of preclinical and clinical trials are discussed.

PRINCIPLES OF INTRATUMORAL GENE THERAPY

General principles of cancer gene therapy are listed in **Table 18-1**. These principles apply to all methods of gene therapy for oncologic treatment, including those designed to alter (1) regulatory pathways, (2) tumor cells themselves, (3) the immune response, and (4) the response to other therapies. Specific modes of intratumoral therapy are listed in **Table 18-2**; these are precise mechanisms designed to effect the alterations listed in Table 18-1. Finally, detailed intratumoral therapies are listed in **Table 18-3**; these are examples of ongoing clinical trials utilizing explicit strategies for intratumoral therapy and are discussed here.

p53 Gene Transfer

Normal p53 genes are required for normal cell cycle kinetics and regulated growth. Mutations of p53 in cancer cells disturb the normal kinetics and growth. The addition of normal p53 genes via direct intratumoral injection restores normal cell growth, or even apoptosis, as has been demonstrated in several studies.[4–7] It is important to remember, however, that this restoration is not a cytotoxic effect.[8] It may explain the predominance of disease stabilization, as opposed to responses, seen in many studies.

The p53 gene has also been used as a marker for prognosis, with a predictably worse outcome in tumors with p53 deficiency.[9] However, the response to therapy is independent of endogenous p53 status.[10] A prototype image-guided intratumoral injection study is the phase 1 trial for small cell lung cancer reported by Swisher et al.[6] Twenty-eight patients were treated with monthly intratumoral injections of an adenovirus containing a normal p53 gene. Most injections were performed using CT guidance, although a few were injected via bronchoscopy. Biopsies were performed at the time of repeat intratumoral injection of the vector. Vector-related toxicity was minimal, and transgene expression was documented in biopsy specimens. Although only 2 patients (8%) had a partial response, disease stabilization was reported in 16 patients (64%). Disease progression was reported in 7 patients (28%). Additional benefit in the treatment of lung cancer patients may be derived from a radiosensitizing effect of gene therapy, as demonstrated in patients treated with a combination of p53 and irradiation or chemoradiation. **Figure 18-1** shows a dramatic response to therapy with direct intratumoral p53 injection in combination with radiation therapy.

Replication-Selective Oncolytic Adenovirus

Oncolytic virotherapy is another example of intratumoral gene therapy. This strategy involves a direct cytotoxic effect on the tumor. One example involves another use of p53 gene status. Cells deficient in the p53 tumor suppression activity are targeted for destruction. An attenuated human group C adenovirus is injected, which selectively replicates in cells deficient in p53 activity. The result is lysis and destruction of the cell. A clinical example of this type of study is the ONYX-015 study reported by Kirn.[11, 12] Although the therapy was well tolerated, the overall response rate was poor in these studies. Kirn noted, however, "A favorable and potentially synergistic interaction with chemotherapy was discovered in multiple tumor types and by multiple routes of administration." This study is, a demonstration of both a pitfall and a promise of gene therapy. Results of gene therapy alone

TABLE 18-1
General Principles of Cancer Gene Therapy

Shut down pathways that allow unrestricted growth
Direct action on tumor cells
Improve immune response
Improve response to other therapies

TABLE 18-2
Specific Modes of Cancer Gene Therapy

Tumor suppression and/or angiogenesis
Inhibition of oncogene expression
Induction of drug sensitivity (e.g., "suicide genes")
Increased immune response (e.g., cytokines, T lymphocytes)
Protection of host from cancer therapies

TABLE 18-3
Specific Intratumoral Therapies

p53 gene transfer
Replication-selective oncolytic adenovirus
Proactivating enzymes
Reintroduction of tumor antigenicity

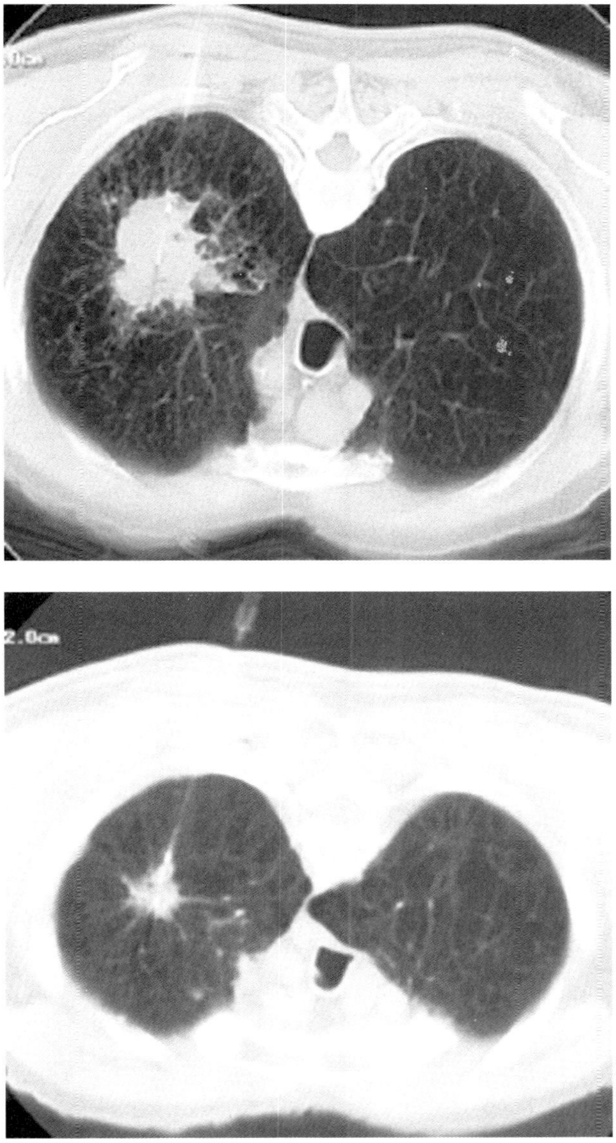

A

B

Figure 13-1. A 73-year-old man with adenocarcinoma of the left upper lobe. The patient was not deemed to be a surgical candidate because of poor pulmonary reserve. (A) Image from the biopsy at the time of initiation of p53 direct injection therapy demonstrates a large left upper lobe mass. (B) Four months after the initiation of p53 gene therapy, there is a marked decrease in the size of the mass. A 20-gauge core biopsy demonstrated fibrous tissues with no residual tumor. The patient was doing well at 3-year follow-up.

were disappointing, but those of combination therapy were beyond results expected with conventional (chemotherapy) alone. One might postulate that the "disease stabilization" achieved by gene therapy could provide an opportunity for adjunctive therapies to be effective.

Proactivating Enzymes

The intratumoral injection of a gene that encodes a specific enzyme has the potential to be an effective antitumor strategy. Theoretically, larger local drug dosages can be delivered with avoidance of dose-limiting toxicity. The principle involves the systemic introduction of a prodrug, with local conversion to an active form after intratumoral injection of an enzyme that converts the prodrug to an active metabolite. Thus, drugs that have documented antitumor effect but whose efficacy is limited by side effects from systemic therapy dosages can be "delivered" at higher dosages locally. The prototype example is a study reported by Miller et al.[13] They used 5-fluorocytosine (5-FC) as a systemically injected prodrug. A nontoxic antifungal drug, 5-FC can be deaminated to the anticancer agent 5-fluorouracil (5-FU). After local injection of a gene that encodes for enzymatic conversion of 5-FC to 5-FU, they observed a remarkable response in mice and in human glioma cells. The response was equivalent to that seen from gastrointestinal tumors.

Reintroduction of Tumor Antigenicity

Immunotherapy as a form of cancer treatment has long held promise, on the basis of the theory that tumor cells contain surface markers identifying them as "foreign" cells. Although tumor-specific antigens may play an important role in immunosurveillance, the majority of tumors arise in immunocompetent hosts. Some tumor cells, including melanoma cells, have reduction or absence of tumor antigens on their cell surface. The loss of these antigens, such as the major histocompatibility complex (MHC), may be one method by which tumor cells avoid natural host detection and destruction. So, cancerous cells must first be modified in order for the host immune system to recognize them as foreign and subsequently destroy them.

The phase 2 study reported by Stopeck et al.,[14] who used local injection of Allovectin-7, is one such effort. Allovectin-7 is a plasmid DNA encoding for two MHC class I proteins. It acts by several mechanisms, including expression of an immunogenic cell surface protein and enhancement of the host immune system by replacement of β_2-microglobulin, a stimulant for increased surface expression of the host MHC class I proteins. Local injection of Allovectin in phase 1 studies with varying dosage schedules demonstrated the safety of this therapy, with local regression of tumor in 28% of patients; 2 more of 28 patients experienced regression of tumor at sites remote from the injections. In the phase 2 study reported by Stopeck et al.,[14] who used an established dose of six injections of 10 micrograms each over a nine-week period, results were similar. A local response was observed in 18% of patients, with a median maximum tumor response at 11 weeks. However, the response was not homogeneous throughout the entire cohort. Patients with smaller tumor burden and with disease limited to cutaneous and/or nodal involvement were most likely to have a response, a finding consistent with preclinical studies demonstrating tumor burden to correlate negatively with response. Response was seen in 30% of patients with disease limited to cutaneous and/or nodal involvement; in 15% of these patients, an overall disease response developed, perhaps owing to the mechanisms discussed previously. The injections were well tolerated, with no toxicity-related discontinuations or delays of treatment.

REGULATORY AND SAFETY ISSUES

Currently, all gene transfer therapies in humans are investigational. Oversight for human gene transfer studies is performed at the federal and the institutional level. At the federal level, the Office of Biotechnology Activities (OBA), in the National Institutes of Health and Disease Prevention (NIH), is responsible for monitoring scientific progress in human genetics research in federally funded studies in order to anticipate future developments, including ethical, legal, and social concerns, in basic and clinical research involving recombinant DNA, genetic testing, and xenotransplantation. The OBA also manages the operation of the NIH Recombinant DNA Advisory Committee (RAC), which oversees federally funded research involving recombinant DNA, including protocol review. The *NIH Guidelines for Research Involving Recombinant DNA Molecules* can be found online through selection of information about the RAC at the OBA Web site (http://www4.od.hih.gov/oba/). Failure to comply with the requirements set forth in the *NIH Guidelines*, including reporting and responding to adverse serious events, can result in the limitation, suspension, or withdrawal of NIH support to an institution.

Other oversight at the federal level occurs through regulatory control by the U.S. Food and Drug Administration (FDA). Approval for gene therapy vectors must be obtained via the Investigation New Drug mechanism. Monitoring by clinical trials by the FDA helps to ensure the safety and protection of research subjects participating in these trials. At the institutional level, review by an institutional review board approval by an institutional biosafety committee is also mandatory before recombinant DNA research is undertaken.

Safety concerns are paramount, for both patients and institutional personnel.[15, 16] Joint Commission on Accreditation of Healthcare Organization guidelines are a framework for individual institutions to determine specific policies and procedures. Examples of these requirements are respiratory isolation for specific genetic vectors, negative-pressure rooms for introduction of genetic vectors, and the use of particulate respirators for personnel involved in delivery of recombinant gene therapy. Resources for individual institutional requirements include the environmental health and safety office, the biosafety committee, and nursing policy and procedure manuals.

REFERENCES

1. Welch HG, Schwartz LM, Woloshin S. Are increasing 5-year survival rates evidence of success against cancer? *JAMA* 2000; 283:2975–2978.
2. Feldman AL, Libutti SK. Progress in antiangiogenic gene therapy of cancer. Cancer 2000; 89:1181–1194.
3. Roth JA, Cristiano RJ. Gene therapy for cancer: what have we done and where are we going? *J Natl Cancer Inst* 1997; 89:21–39.
4. Lang FF, Yung WK, Sawaya R, Tofilon PJ. Adenovirus-mediated p53 gene therapy for human gliomas. *Neurosurgery* 1999; 45:1093–1104.
5. Clayman GL, Liu TJ, Overholt SM, et al. Gene therapy for head and neck cancer: comparing the tumor suppressor gene p53 and a cell cycle regulator WAF1/CIP1 (p21). *Arch Otolaryngol Head Neck Surg* 1996; 122:489–493.
6. Swisher SG, Roth JA, Nemunaitis J, et al. Adenovirus-mediated p53 gene transfer in advanced non-small-cell lung cancer. *J Natl Cancer Inst* 1999; 91:763–771.
7. Ramondetta L, Mills GB, Burke TW, Wolf JK. Adenovirus-mediated expression of p53 or p21 in a papillary serous endometrial carcinoma cell line (SPEC-2) results in both growth inhibition and apoptotic cell death: potential application of gene therapy to endometrial cancer. *Clin Cancer Res* 2000; 6:278–284.
8. Swisher SG, Roth JA. Gene therapy for human lung cancers. *Surg Oncol Clin N Am* 1998; 7:603–616.
9. Quinlan DC, Davidson AG, Summers CL, Warden HE, Doshi HM. Accumulation of p53 protein correlates with a poor prognosis in human lung cancer. *Cancer Res* 1992; 52:4828–4831.
10. Wolf JK, Mills GB, Bazzet L, Bast RC Jr, Roth JA, Gershenson DM. Adenovirus-mediated p53 growth inhibition of ovarian cancer cells is independent of endogenous p53 status. *Gynecol Oncol* 1999; 75:261–266.
11. Kirn D. Clinical research results with dl1520 (Onyx-015), a replication-selective adenovirus for the treatment of cancer: what have we learned? *Gene Ther* 2001; 8:89–98.
12. Kirn D. Replication-selective oncolytic adenoviruses: virotherapy aimed at genetic targets in cancer. *Oncogene* 2000; 19:6660–6669.
13. Miller CR, Williams CR, Buchsbaum DJ, Gillespie GY. Intratumoral 5-fluorouracil produced by cytosine deaminase/5-fluorocytosine gene therapy is effective for experimental human glioblastomas. *Cancer Res* 2002; 62:773–780.
14. Stopeck AT, Jones A, Hersh EM, et al. Phase II study of direct intralesional gene transfer of allovectin-7, an HLA-B7/beta2-microglobulin DNA-liposome complex, in patients with metastatic melanoma. *Clin Cancer Res* 2001; 7:2285–2291.
15. Noguchi PD. From Jim to gene and beyond: an odyssey of biologics regulation. *Food Drug Law J* 1996; 51:367–373.
16. Noguchi P. Risks and benefits of gene therapy. *N Engl J Med* 2003; 348:193–194.

CHAPTER 19

INTRACAVITARY THERAPY

ROBERT K. RYU, MD
ALBERT A. NEMCEK, JR., MD

The accumulation of fluid within various potential third-space compartments is a common and troublesome manifestation of disseminated cancer. Although pericardial tamponade from malignant effusion can be life threatening, ascites and pleural effusions tend to be less immediately threatening. However, dyspnea and severe abdominal distention can be debilitating symptoms and significantly diminish the quality of the patient's life. Effective, compassionate management of these troubling and ubiquitous manifestations of disease is an important component of the comprehensive care of the patient with cancer. Although surgical options may exist, techniques commonly used in everyday interventional radiology practices offer efficacy with minimal invasiveness, with little or no immediate adverse impact on quality of life.

DIAGNOSIS AND MANAGEMENT OF MALIGNANT ASCITES

Malignant ascites is a common manifestation of intra-abdominal tumors. Almost half of all cases of malignant ascites are related to ovarian carcinoma; other primary tumors associated with malignant ascites formation include those of the colon, stomach, pancreas, breast, lung, and uterus. Often, the primary tumor is never identified. Malignant ascites is generally a poor prognostic sign, with average survival depending on the tumor type but often being less than 6 months.

The peritoneum is very active from a physiologic standpoint, with the ability to constantly produce and reabsorb fluid within the abdominal cavity. Normally, approximately 50 mL of ascites is present within the peritoneum, with normal physiologic production and reabsorption of 4–5 mL/h.[1]

The accumulation of malignant ascites is, as one might expect, given the preponderance of physiologic factors involved, dependent on numerous variables. The major efflux pathway for ascites has been shown to be the diaphragmatic lymphatics,[2] with little or no contribution from mesenteric or omental lymphatics, or the thoracic duct. With malignant infiltration of the diaphragmatic lymphatics, accumulation of ascites occurs.

Creation or influx of ascites also has several potential contributing factors. Malignant ascitic fluid is largely exudative, with high levels of albumin. Albumin apparently accumulates as a result of leakage from tumor microvasculature. This is not believed to be related to actual leakage from endothelium; it is thought more likely that a vasoactive factor, such as vascular endothelial growth factor (VEGF), mediates this phenomenon.[3] Increased levels of VEGF have been found in malignant ascites, when compared with cirrhotic ascites.[4] Intraperitoneal tumor cells can also independently increase the amount of ascitic fluid produced, even in the absence of lymphatic obstruction.[5] Neoplastic angiogenesis appears to play a role in ascites development, as evidenced by the reduction of malignant ascites formation after administration of antiangiogenesis factors, at least in an experimental model.[6]

Elevation of the hepatic venous pressure has also been correlated with elevated plasma renin levels in patients with cirrhosis, ultimately resulting in fluid retention and accumulation of ascites.[7] Interestingly, in patients with large hepatic metastases with hepatic vein obstruction, spironolactone, an aldosterone antagonist, has been shown to be effective in reducing accumulation of ascites.[8]

Physical findings associated with ascites include abdominal distention, flank distention, fluid wave, and shifting dullness. Symptoms include abdominal pain, nausea, vomiting, dyspnea, lower-extremity edema, and weight gain. The diagnosis of ascites can be confirmed with abdominal ultrasound (US), which can be used for imaging guidance for therapeutic or diagnostic paracentesis. Of all malignant ascites specimens sent for cytologic evaluation, only 60% have positive findings.[9]

Given the poor prognosis associated with malignant ascites, failing systemic administration of chemotherapy, treatment should be tailored to minimally invasive therapies with improved quality of life as the main goal. The mainstay of therapy for malignant ascites is symptomatic paracentesis. Uncorrectable coagulopathy, extensive adhesion formation, and very small volume collections are generally considered the only relative contraindications to therapeutic paracentesis. We routinely perform paracentesis with US guidance, to decrease the risk of a bleeding complication and also to increase the yield by selecting the largest collection of ascites. The Yueh sheathed needle (Cook Inc., Bloomington, IN) is a 5-F multiple-sidehole straight Teflon cannula with a hollow sharp stylet within it (**Fig. 19-1**). The needle and cannula are advanced while aspiration is done with a syringe under US guidance. When there is free return of fluid through the needle, the cannula is advanced over the needle and into the peritoneal cavity. The cannula is connected to a vacuum bottle for drainage. When large-volume paracentesis is anticipated, use of a 6- or 8-F pigtail catheter may be more expeditious. Loculations, tumor foci, and adhesions can make paracentesis more technically difficult. US guidance is particularly helpful in these instances.

Local and systemic infection, bleeding, and hypotension from rapid intravascular to extravascular fluid shifts are potential complications of paracentesis. Complications are generally rare, particularly if care is

A

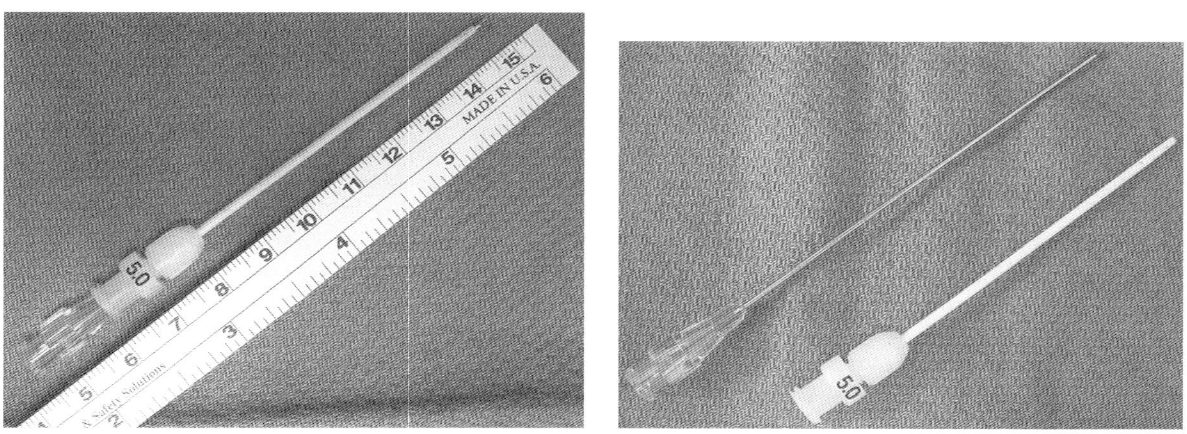

B

Figure 19-1. (A) The Yueh sheathed needle is made of Teflon. (B) The inner stylet is hollow, whereas the 5-F catheter has multiple sideholes.

taken to avoid the inferior epigastric artery that courses along the lateral margin of the rectus sheath. Careful color Doppler US usually reveals significant vascular structures that are to be avoided. We routinely administer albumin intravenously whenever the effluent volume exceeds 3 L during a therapeutic paracentesis. During routine paracentesis, drainage eventually decreases in rate. Often, gentle manual manipulation of the abdomen and decubitus positioning can help maximize the total volume yield.

Pleurx catheters (Denver Biomaterials, Boulder, CO; **Fig. 19-2**) are designed for chronic fluid drainage on an outpatient basis. Although they were originally described for use in pleural effusions, there are early reports describing their efficacy in the management of malignant ascites as well.[10,11]

Administration of systemic chemotherapy can decrease overall tumor burden and thus alleviate accumulation of ascites. Whether through direct effect on intraperitoneal tumor foci, with attendant decrease in VEGF levels, or by affecting the diaphragmatic lymphatic tumor involvement and improving lymphatic flow, chemotherapy may result in significant decrease or resolution of ascites. Unfortunately, associated systemic toxicity can limit the desired effect.

Intraperitoneal administration of chemotherapy has several limitations. Anatomically, the presence of adhesions and loculations may prevent the even distribution of chemotherapeutic agent over the entire peritoneal surface. This problem limits this treatment method to those patients with cancer who have not undergone previous surgical exploration, resection, or tumor debulking. Penetration of the agent into viable tumor cells is on the order of millimeters, which means that residual intraperitoneal tumor foci in excess of 1–2 cm may not respond because of inadequate penetration. Finally, if the tumor has been shown to be unresponsive to systemic administration of a particular chemotherapeutic agent, it is unlikely to respond to intraperitoneal infusion of the same drug.

The achievable concentration of chemotherapeutic agent within the peritoneum is estimated to be 10–20 times higher than sustainable systemic levels when administered intraperitoneally. This, in conjunction with significantly decreased systemic absorption and toxicity, makes the intraperitoneal route of administration an attractive one. Of course, complications are not entirely avoided: Neutropenia from marrow suppression, chemical peritonitis, infusion catheter–related problems, and intra-abdominal adhesions can occur, with significant associated morbidity.

In a randomized trial involving patients with stage III ovarian carcinoma with a median follow-up period of 4 years, a statistically significant improved survival rate was found in the patients who received intraperitoneal cisplatin and systemic cyclophosphamide versus systemic cisplatin and cyclophosphamide.[12] In a small study of patients undergoing resection of gastric carcinoma with serosal involvement, Hagiwara et al. demonstrated a survival advantage for those who received perioperative intraperitoneal mitomycin versus those who did not.[13]

Intraperitoneal photodynamic therapy relies on the selective absorption of high concentrations of a

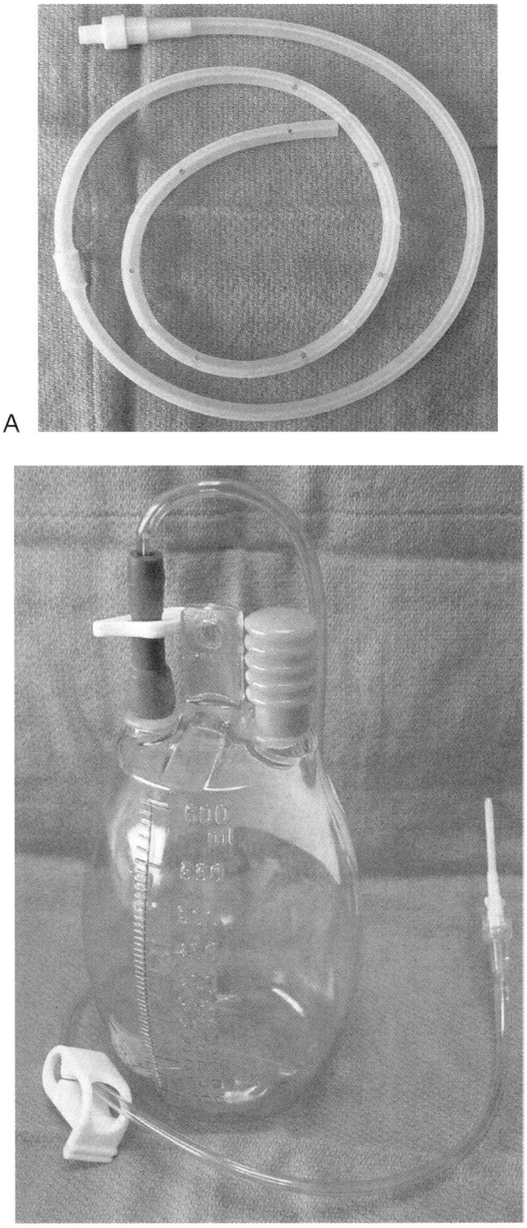

A

B

Figure 19-2. (A) The 15.5-F Pleurx catheter is designed to be tunneled under the skin. (B) The vacuum bottles come in a kit designed for use by either the patient or a visiting nurse at the patient's home.

photosensitizer drug by tumor cells. When exposed to oxygen and a particular light wavelength, oxygen free radicals are formed by the photosensitizer drug, resulting in tumor cell damage and subsequent death. Intraperitoneal photodynamic therapy is currently under investigation as an adjunctive measure combined with debulking of tumors with intraperitoneal spread. Results of a recently completed phase II trial are encouraging: a median survival of 21 months was achieved with acceptable systemic toxicity, including anemia (38%), liver function abnormalities (26%), and gastrointestinal toxicity (19%). One patient suffered a fatal myocardial infarction.[14]

Surgical options for the treatment of intractable ascites are limited. Le Veen, or peritoneovenous, shunts connect the peritoneal space with the central venous circulation. Le Veen shunts provide symptomatic relief in about 66% of patients. Unfortunately, the complication rate associated with peritoneovenous shunts is as high as 25%. Although most complications are related to catheter occlusion, more serious complications, including fluid overload and heart failure, as well as coagulopathy, can occur. Given the current plethora of safe, minimally invasive treatment options for intractable ascites, indications for surgical construction of peritoneovenous shunts are increasingly rare.

DIAGNOSIS AND MANAGEMENT OF MALIGNANT PLEURAL EFFUSIONS

Malignant pleural effusions are common. An estimated 50% of all patients with cancer will develop a malignant effusion sometime during the course of their disease. In fact, over half of all newly diagnosed pleural effusions are subsequently found to be related to an underlying malignancy. Breast and lung primary tumors account for almost 66% of these effusions, whereas the remainder is largely accounted for by gastrointestinal, genitourinary, and hematologic malignancies.

Like the peritoneal surface, the pleural surface is a remarkably active membrane, with exchange of 5–10 L per day across it. In patients without cancer, a scant 10–20 mL of fluid may actually be within the pleural space at any given time, despite the overall volume of fluid that is constantly exuded and reabsorbed. Reabsorption is predominantly mediated by pulmonary venous capillaries, whereas 10%–20% of pleural fluid is drained through lymphatic channels. The accumulation of a pleural effusion, therefore, may be caused by lymphatic infiltration and resultant obstruction, a pathophysiologic mechanism similar to that of malignant ascites. In addition, systemic hypoalbuminemia with a resultant decrease in osmotic pressure can play an important role in the formation of a pleural effusion.

Clinical symptoms of pleural effusion include shortness of breath, cough, pleuritic chest pain, and a sensation of chest fullness or heaviness. Clinical examination will reveal decreased breath sounds as well as dullness to percussion. Standard frontal chest radiographs will reveal effusions that are > 300 mL, whereas decubitus and lateral views are more sensitive because of the layering effect of the fluid. Computed tomography (CT) is highly sensitive for detecting pleural fluid and can help distinguish between fluid and pleural thickening or tumor. US is routinely used for imaging guidance during thoracentesis. It is particularly useful in cases of significant fluid loculation.

Laboratory analysis of the pleural fluid can provide valuable information. Cytologic evaluation is positive in 50%–80% of cases. Most malignant effusions are bloody and exudative in nature. A transudate should prompt a search for an alternative cause, such as congestive heart failure. Low pH (< 7.3) and glucose (< 60 mg/dL) tend to occur together and are associated with a poorer response to pleurodesis, poorer survival, and higher yield of malignant cells on fluid examination. Elevated lactate dehydrogenase (LDH) levels (> 600 IU/L) have also been associated with a poor prognosis and diminished response to pleurodesis. None of these laboratory findings, however, are contraindications to an attempt at pleurodesis.

Thoracentesis is performed in a fashion similar to paracentesis. US guidance is routinely used in conjunction with a Yueh needle. Care is taken to pass the needle over the superior surface of the rib to avoid the neurovascular bundle. The routine use of vacuum bottles during thoracentesis is to be avoided. Creation of excessively negative intrapleural pressure, particularly when the underlying lung parenchyma is trapped by tumor or adhesion, can result in damage to the lung itself, with pneumothorax formation or bronchopleural fistula. The extracted volume of fluid during a therapeutic thoracentesis should rarely exceed 1000–1200 mL, particularly in the outpatient setting. Re-expansion pulmonary edema, the physiology of which is poorly understood, occurs after rapid evacuation of excessive pleural fluid volume, usually more than 1 L, and can present dramatically. Emergency administration of oxygen and diuretics is required, but adjunctive use of steroids, inotropes, and ventilatory support are rarely indicated.

Few contraindications to thoracentesis exist other than intractable coagulopathy. Mechanical ventilation, once felt to be a contraindication, can be safely performed, particularly with US guidance in the hands of an experienced operator. Bleeding, infection, pneumothorax, and re-expansion pulmonary edema are potential complications of thoracentesis.

The 15.5-F Pleurx catheter is made of soft silicone and has multiple large sideholes designed to be placed into the thorax for long-term management of intractable pleural effusions[10]. It is placed through a subcutaneous tunnel to help decrease the rate of catheter-related infections. The catheter is valved, preventing inadvertent pneumothorax. It also requires little maintenance other than insertion-site care. The device and its attendant supplies are specifically designed for use by patients at home, even in the absence of home nursing assistance. The catheter has the unintended benefit of spontaneous pleurodesis, presumably caused by a local inflammatory reaction. In our experience, the incidence of spontaneous pleurodesis is as high as 65%.

Pleurodesis is a chemically induced inflammatory process that results in adherence of the visceral and parietal pleural surfaces, eliminating a potential space for fluid accumulation. It is a purely palliative treatment. Effusion-related dyspnea is a debilitating, troubling symptom amenable to treatment with pleurodesis. However, establishment of the effusion as the cause of dyspnea is vital to successful patient selection. Cross-sectional imaging is very helpful in assessing other potential causes of dyspnea, including pericardial effusions, pulmonary embolism, or pulmonary lymphangitic spread of tumor. Another approach is to proceed with therapeutic thoracentesis without prospective CT imaging. If thoracentesis does not produce significant symptomatic relief, pleurodesis is not offered and a search for other causes of dyspnea is initiated. Alternatively, if a patient has a large effusion but is completely asymptomatic, there is no indication for pleurodesis.

Numerous agents have been described for pleurodesis, the most common being talc, doxycycline, and bleomycin. Four grams of talc in a sterile saline slurry is the usual dose. Overall success is generally over 90%, but significant side effects are associated with talc usage. Pain, pneumonitis, and, rarely, respiratory distress syndrome and respiratory failure have been reported. After tetracycline became no longer available in the United States, doxycycline has been used as an alternative. It is usually given in 500–1000 mg doses, in a total volume of 50–100 mL. Somewhat less effective than talc, with success rates between 70% and 80%, doxycycline is better tolerated, with less pain and fewer complications. However, doxycycline must often be administered more than once for successful pleurodesis. Bleomycin has an effectiveness similar to that of doxycycline but is significantly more expensive on a per-dose basis. The usual dose is 1 mg/kg.

Pleurodesis requires tube thoracostomy placement. Tube sizes of 12-F to 14-F are preferred because they allow for better drainage and have larger sideholes. Pleurodesis may be attempted after tube output has decreased to less than 100 mL per day. Chest radiographs should be obtained to document reexpansion of the adjacent lung with good apposition of the pleural surfaces. In the setting of excessively negative intrapleural pressure, resulting lung injury and pneumothorax may occur. Often in this setting, the injury is explained by trapped, noncompliant lung parenchyma or intrabronchial lesions preventing adequate reexpansion. Persistently collapsed lung parenchyma and high tube outputs generally portend a poor response to pleurodesis. Before sclerosis, a long-acting local anesthetic, bupivacaine, is administered through the thoracostomy and allowed to dwell for 15–20 minutes. Conscious sedation is also administered. Evacuation of the local anesthetic is followed by instillation of the sclerosant through the thoracostomy, with approximately 1–2 hours of dwell time. Rolling the patient to help evenly distribute both the local anesthetic and sclerosant may be helpful, although this is debatable. Normal respiratory motion appears to be entirely adequate for this purpose. The thoracostomy is reopened to low suction for 24 hours and surveillance chest radiographs are obtained. The thoracostomy is removed when output is less than 100 mL per day. Readministration of sclerosant may be necessary before removal of the thoracostomy.

The use of intracavitary lytic therapy for complicated pleural fluid collections has been well described; however, most reports refer to the use of urokinase, which is no longer commercially available in the United States. Published reports on the use of tissue-type plasminogen activator (tPA) for this clinical application are scant.[15] At our institution, we use 5 mg of tPA in 25–50 mL of sterile saline, depending on the size of the cavity. After administration of the lytic agent through the thoracostomy, the tube is capped for approximately 1 hour, then reattached to water seal or suction, depending on the viscosity of the effluent. This treatment is typically performed two or three times daily, for 1–3 days, depending on the size of the cavity and fluid viscosity. After drainage decreases, follow-up cross-sectional imaging is routinely obtained to assess the result. Intracavitary lytics can also play a role in complex but sterile pleural fluid collections. After lytic treatment, more complete pleural drainage allows for better apposition of the pleural surfaces. This in turn increases the likelihood of successful pleurodesis.

DIAGNOSIS AND MANAGEMENT OF MALIGNANT PERICARDIAL EFFUSIONS

Symptomatic malignant pericardial effusions (MPEs) are probably underdiagnosed. In approximately half of all patients with pericardial effusions, pleural effusions are evident. Progressive dyspnea may be mistakenly attributed to the presence of pleural effusion, or progressive lung parenchymal disease. Therefore, the exact incidence of MPE is not known. Lung and breast primary malignancies are most commonly associated with MPE.

The proposed causes of MPE formation are similar to those associated with malignant pleural or peritoneal fluid accumulation. They include increased creation of fluid by the visceral pericardium in response to the presence of tumor deposits, as well as lymphatic invasion and obstruction.

The classic clinical presentation of MPE is a dyspneic patient with evidence of jugular venous distention, with cough and pleuritic chest pain, and a pericardial friction rub appreciated on auscultation. Electrocardiographic findings include decreased voltage and ST segment elevations and T-wave inversion. Pulsus paradoxus is associated with pericardial tamponade and is defined by a decrease in systolic blood pressure by at least 10 mm Hg during normal inspiration.

The classic chest radiograph finding is globular enlargement of the cardiac silhouette. Elevation of the pericardial fat pad is a subtle finding best identified on the lateral view. In the acute setting, however, chest radiographs may appear nearly normal. Rapidity, and not overall volume, of fluid accumulation has the most impact on cardiac hemodynamics. Highly sensitive and specific, echocardiography is the most widely used imaging test for the diagnosis of MPE. In addition to quantification of fluid within the pericardial sac, the hemodynamic effect of the MPE on the cardiac chambers can be appreciated using echocardiography and correlated with the clinical findings. Collapse of the right atrium and, to a lesser degree, the right ventricle can be seen. Acute elevations in pulmonary artery pressure, as seen in pulmonary embolism, can mimic the clinical presentation of MPE. Because MPE can essentially be ruled out with echocardiography, the diagnosis of pulmonary embolism must be excluded with other tests. CT can identify as little as 50 mL in the pericardial space; CT scans can also evaluate the pleural space and lung parenchyma, whereas US cannot. However, given the physiologic parameters that ultrasound can provide, echocardiography remains the test of choice for the diagnosis and evaluation of MPE.

Numerous treatment alternatives have been proposed. Simple therapeutic pericardiocentesis is a safe and effective approach to symptomatic relief as well as diagnosis. The diagnostic yield for cytologic specimens obtained from pericardiocentesis has been reported to be between 70% and 100%. Unfortunately, the incidence of recurrent fluid accumulation is high, necessitating more definitive therapy.

Systemic chemotherapy has been shown to be effective for the treatment of MPE, particularly in patients who have tumors that are responsive to the chemotherapeutic agent. Systemic toxicity and resistance to therapy are the limiting factors. External beam irradiation is also effective in reducing MPE symptoms. Unfortunately, pericarditis and myocarditis are rare but serious side effects that limit the applicability of radiotherapy.

Traditional surgical therapy is composed of three different approaches. Pericardiectomy requires a thoracotomy and has an associated mortality rate of up to 30%. However, when successfully performed, it is highly effective and the results are durable. Subxiphoid pericardiotomy, or creation of a pericardial window, can be performed with conscious sedation and is less invasive. It is also effective but still has a significant complication rate in a patient population that has a limited life expectancy. Because of that limited life expectancy, it is all the more important that whatever treatment is chosen, the patient's quality of remaining life be carefully considered. Video-assisted thoracoscopic surgical (VATS) pericardiotomy has the advantage of being less invasive but equally effective compared with the open surgical approach. However, technical expertise is required, and success rates, when compared with those for percutaneous treatment alternatives, are not significantly better.

Image-guided placement of small-bore drainage catheters followed by sclerosant instillation has been reported in several series.[16–18] US is most commonly used for guidance during drainage catheter placement, although CT guidance has also been reported.[19] A subxiphoid approach is commonly used. Pericardiodesis technique is similar to that of pleurodesis. After infusion and removal of a local anesthetic into the pericardial drainage catheter, the sclerosant is injected. The tube is clamped, then later opened to drainage. Hospital admission is required because several daily treatments are typically necessary to achieve the desired result. Tetracycline was the most widely used agent, but it is no longer available in the United States. Doxycycline, as an alternative to tetracycline, seems to be associated with more postprocedural pain and fever. It is usually administered in a dose of 500–1000 mg in 20 mL of sterile saline. When prospectively compared with bleomycin, doxycycline seems to be equally effective but to have a higher complication rate.[20] Dose for dose, bleomycin is also significantly more expensive than doxycycline; however, the cost difference is reduced by the prolonged hospitalization and repeated treatments associated with doxycycline. The reported doses of bleomycin range between 5 and 60 mg.[21–23] The most common side effects observed during pericardiodesis are chest pain, fever, transient dysrhythmias, infection, and recurrent effusion. Overall, successful treatment is achieved in approximately 75%–85% of cases with an overall complication rate of between 4% and 18%.

Percutaneous balloon pericardiotomy has also been reported as an effective, minimally invasive treatment alternative for MPE. The technique involves accessing the pericardial sac with US guidance, after which standard catheter and guide wire techniques are used to advance an angioplasty balloon across the parietal pericardium under fluoroscopic guidance. Balloon insufflation results in the creation of a pleuropericardial window, allowing for egress of pericardial contents into the pleural space. In a series of eight patients, seven of whom had malignancies, Di Segni et al. reported clinical success in five, with a mean survival of 70 days.[24] MPE recurred in two patients. Three patients developed pleural effusions after successful pericardiotomy.

REFERENCES

1. Hirabayashi K, Graham J. Genesis of ascites in ovarian carcinoma. *Am J Obstet Gynecol* 1970;106:492–497.
2. L Raybuck HE. The effects of obliteration of the diaphragmatic lymphatic plexus on serous fluid. *Anat Rec* 1960;137:25–32.
3. Yeo KT, Wang H, Nagy JA, et al. Vascular permeability factor levels in ascites, tumors, and human fluids [abstract]. *J Cell Biol* 1991;115:421a [abstract]
4. Zebrowski BK, Liu W, Ramirez K, et al. Markedly elevated levels of vascular endothelial growth factor in malignant ascites. *Ann Surg Oncol* 1999;6:373–378.
5. Nagy JA, Herzberg KT, Dvorak JM, Dvorak HF. Pathogenesis of malignant ascites formation: initiating events that lead to fluid accumulation. *Cancer Res* 1993;53:2631–2643.
6. Heuser LS, Taylor SH, Folkman J. Prevention of carcinomatosis and bloody malignant ascites in the rat by an inhibitor of angiogenesis. *J Surg Res* 1984;26:244–250.
7. Bosch J, Arroyo V, Betriu A, et al. Hepatic hemodynamics and the renin-angiotensin-aldosterone system in cirrhosis. *Gastroenterology* 1980;78:92–99.
8. Pockros PJ, Esrason KT, Nguyen C, Duque J, Woods S. Mobilization of malignant ascites with diuretics is dependent on ascitic fluid characteristics *Gastroenterology* 1992;103:1302–1306.
9. Runyon BA, Hoefs JC, Morgan TR. Ascitic fluid analysis in malignancy-related ascites. *Hepatology* 1988;8:1104–1109.
10. Pollak JS, Burdge CM, Rosenblatt M, et al. Treatment of malignant pleural effusions with tunneled long-term drainage catheters. *J Vasc Interv Radiol* 2001;12:201–208.
11. Richard HM, Coldwell DM, Boyd-Kranis RL, Murthy R, Van Echo DA. Pleurx tunneled catheter in the management of malignant ascites. *J Vasc Interv Radiol* 2001;12:373–375.
12. Alberts DS, Liu PY, Hannigan EV, et al. Phase III study of intraperitoneal cisplatin/intravenous cyclophosphamide versus IV cisplatin/IV cyclophosphamide in patients with optimal disease stage III ovarian cancer: a SWOG-GOG-ECOG intergroup study. *N Engl J Med* 1996;335:1950–1955.
13. Hagiwara A, Takahashi T, Kojima O, et al. Prophylaxis with carbon-absorbed mitomycin against peritoneal recurrence of gastric cancer. *Lancet* 1992;339:629–631.
14. Hendren SK, Hahn SM, Spitz FR, et al. Phase II trial of debulking surgery and photodynamic therapy for disseminated intraperitoneal tumors. *Ann Surg Oncol* 2001;8:65–71.
15. Sugimoto K, Kee ST, Semba CP, et al. Safety and efficacy of tissue plasminogen activator to treat loculated pleural effusions [abstract]. *J Vasc Interv Radiol* 2001;12:S107. [abstract]
16. Shepard FA, Morgan C, Evans WK. Medical management of malignant pericardial effusion by tetracycline sclerosis. *Am J Cardiol* 1987;60:1161–1166.
17. Davis S, Rambotti P, Grignani F. Intrapericardial tetracycline sclerosis in the treatment of malignant pericardial effusions. *J Clin Oncol* 1984;2:631–636.
18. van Belle SJ, Volckaert A, Taeymans Y, Spapen H, Block P. Treatment of malignant pericardial tamponade with sclerosis induced by instillation of bleomycin. *Int J Cardiol* 1987;16:155–160.
19. Bellon RJ, Wright WH, Unger EC. CT-guided pericardial drainage catheter placement with subsequent pericardial sclerosis. *J Comput Assist Tomogr* 1995;19:672–673.
20. Liu G, Crump M, Goss PE, Dancey J, Shepherd FA. Prospective comparison of the sclerosing agents doxycycline and bleomycin for the primary management of malignant pericardial effusion and cardiac tamponade. *J Clin Oncol* 1996;14:3141–3147.
21. Maher ER, Buckman R. Intrapericardial installation of bleomycin in malignant pericardial effusion. *Am Heart J* 1986;111:613–614.
22. Cormican MC, Nyman CR. Intrapericardial bleomycin for the management of cardiac tamponade secondary to malignant pericardial effusion. *Br Heart J* 1990;63:61–62.
23. Wei JY, Taylor GJ, Achuff SC. Recurrent cardiac tamponade and large pericardial effusions. *Am J Cardiol* 1978;42:281–282.
24. Di Segni E, Lavee J, Kaplinsky E, Vered Z. Percutaneous balloon pericardiostomy for treatment of cardiac tamponade. *Eur Heart J* 1995;16:184–187.

CHAPTER 20

IMAGE-GUIDED BRACHYTHERAPY: "INTERVENTIONAL BRACHYTHERAPY"

JAMES M. HEVEZI, PHD, FACR, FAAPM
CHARLES R. THOMAS, JR., MD

INTRODUCTION

Brachytherapy is a viable method of radiation delivery used to control many solid tumor systems, either as the primary mode of treatment or as a boost dose-delivery system after an initial course of external-beam radiotherapy. This chapter provides a brief history of this viable delivery system and describes the more recent three-dimensional characterization of dose distributions, based on the patient's own anatomic features, using computed tomography (CT), ultrasound (US), and magnetic resonance (MR) imaging. Finally, the chapter discusses the method we have dubbed interventional brachytherapy, which uses a three-dimensional stereotactic arm to localize needle tracks for radioactive seed delivery in the CT suite at the Cancer Therapy and Research Center (CTRC) in San Antonio, Texas.

In its early history, brachytherapy was the chief mode of delivering tumoricidal doses to targets using radium 226 sources,[1] but it has been supplanted by afterloading applicator techniques using modern radionuclide sources.[2] Nevertheless, the imaging techniques used to determine source positions in the body in the radium era were not perceptibly changed for many years of use of afterloading techniques. Even though the hand calculations of the Quimby[3] and Patterson–Parker[4] methods were replaced by computer-based calculations, the methodology remained similar for determining radiation dose to tumor/normal tissue sites via this delivery method. That is, localization radiographs were typically obtained with nonradioactive "dummy" sources in place to localize the sources for computer entry of position and activity data. Orthogonal-projection planar radiographs through the implanted area allowed computer identification of source positions such that a valid radiation dose distribution based on source positions could be calculated. Anatomic information, however, was considered secondary to the planning information provided by these images. Bony landmarks were frequently the only anatomic indicators by which correct placement of the sources and resulting dose distributions could be confirmed.

Currently, brachytherapy is practiced in several ways. Temporary (removable) sealed radioactive sources may be placed in and around the target volume in applicators, then removed when the target total dose reaches the prescribed level. Conversely, permanent sources may be placed in and around the target volume, and are the activity/source and source position in the target chosen such that at complete decay the total prescribed dose to the target is delivered. These brachytherapy procedures are typically low-dose-rate (LDR) procedures (dose rates around 10–100 cGy/hr), with the temporary implants placed while the patient is hospitalized as the dose reaches the prescribed level (typically over 24–72 hours). Most LDR gynecologic implants follow this temporary implantation procedure. Some permanent implants may require the patient to remain confined to the hospital for a time if high-energy sources are used that may produce higher levels of radiation exposure outside of the patient. The patient must therefore remain in a controlled and monitored setting until the sources decay sufficiently to allow the patient to be released. Fortunately, the radiation sources used in these cases have short half-lives, so the patient may require only a day or so of hospitalization. **Table 20-1** shows typical characteristics of brachytherapy sources used in LDR procedures, both temporary and permanent.

Another method to deliver brachytherapy is through the use of high-dose-rate (HDR) sources (dose rates around 100–500 cGy/min).[5] HDR brachytherapy consists in moving a high-activity source (normally 10 Ci of Iridium 192) along applicators previously placed in the treatment area by the radiation oncologist. Its advantage is that the radiation can be remotely delivered to the targets within the patient, without the concomitant radiation exposure to personnel attendant to non-HDR brachytherapy procedures. These dose-rate levels approach those typically experienced in external-beam procedures and, like them, require a fractionated schedule to achieve the tumoricidal effect on the target while allowing normal tissue recovery between delivered fractions. HDR brachytherapy is planned and performed using planar radiographs to localize the source dwell positions and times, much as with the LDR temporary implants discussed above. More recent HDR procedures are accomplished with the use of CT image–based planning, relating the source dwell positions to patient anatomy.

All of the sources used in contemporary brachytherapy are generally treated as point sources of radiation because they are small in physical dimensions compared with their dose-deposition distances. Cesium 137 tube source used in LDR gynecologic implant applicators is the exception to this statement. Their longer dimensions (approximately 2 cm long) require an integration of source activity along the length of the source to produce an accurate dose profile description. Current computer-based treatment planning systems carry out this integration easily or use look-up tables based on this integration to specify dose around each source implanted.

A task group report[6] of the American Association of Physicists in Medicine describing the emission of radiation from the point sources used in brachytherapy forms the basis for contemporary treatment planning systems used to calculate dose distributions around these point sources.

TABLE 20-1

Physical Characteristics of Radionuclides Used in Brachytherapy

Radionuclide	Half-life	Photon energy (MeV)	Half-value layer (mm lead)	Exposure rate constant (Rcm^2/miCi-h)
Radium 226	1600 y	0.047–2.45	8.0	8.25*Υ (Rcm^2/mg-h)
Cesium 137	30.0 y	0.662	8.0	3.26*f*
Iridium 192	74.2 days	0.38 average	2.5	4.69*f*
Gold 198	2.7 days	0.412	2.5	2.38*f*
Iodine 125	60.2 days	0.028 average	0.025	1.46*f*
Palladium 103	17.0 days	0.021 average	0.008	1.48*f*

In equilibrium with daughter products
Υ = *filtered by 0.5 mm. platinum; f = unfiltered.*

TEMPORARY VERSUS PERMANENT IMPLANTS

What differentiates temporary from permanent implant brachytherapy? As discussed above, temporary implants are left in place until the requisite dose is delivered to the appropriate point or isodose line. **Figure 20-1** depicts a typical isodose distribution for an iridium 192 ribbon template implant. The units of dose rate for this implant graph are in centigray per hour. The radiation oncologist chooses an isodose line that treats the peripheral volume at a particular dose rate, and the implant dwell time is determined by dividing the total prescribed dose by the isodose line's dose rate. Other higher or lower isodose lines will treat smaller (higher dose rate) or larger (lower dose rate) volumes of tissue than the prescription dose rate isodose line (volume) chosen.

Permanent implants rely on the activity and position of each source (seed) placed permanently in and around the target volume. The sources irradiate the volume surrounding the seeds until total decay of the sources is reached. As with any brachytherapy source or applicator in contact with body tissues, the sealed housings of the sources are constructed of biocompatible materials so that no untoward chemical reactions are experienced for the long indwelling times of these permanent implants. Because they are sealed, the actual radioactive material does not come in contact with patient tissues. To calculate the total dose to a treatment volume in this case, however, the average lifetime of the implanted source is used, rather than the dose rate as in temporary implants. An isodose distribution is calculated as in the case of the temporary implant, but the units depicted on isodose lines is *total dose* in centigray rather than the dose rate. In the calculation algorithm, the dose rate to a particular isodose line is multiplied by the average lifetime of the source implanted, in appropriate units. For example, the average life of iodine 125 is 2073.6 hours, so that the total dose to the 10 cGy/h isodose line in a typical iodine 125 prostate implant is 20,736 cGy. **Figure 20-2** shows an isodose distribution pattern through a typical plane of a prostate iodine 125 seed implant.

There are only a few radionuclides that lend themselves to permanent implantation into tumor targets. The chief determinants are the half-life of the radionuclide and, to a lesser extent, the energy of the emitted radiation. Iodine 125 and palladium 103 have half-lives that are relatively short and photon energies in the 20–30 keV range, making them good candidates for permanent seed implants. While gold 198 has a higher emitted photon energy (> 400 keV), its half-life is so short (approximately 3 days) that it, too, is a good candidate for permanent implants and has been used in such applications.

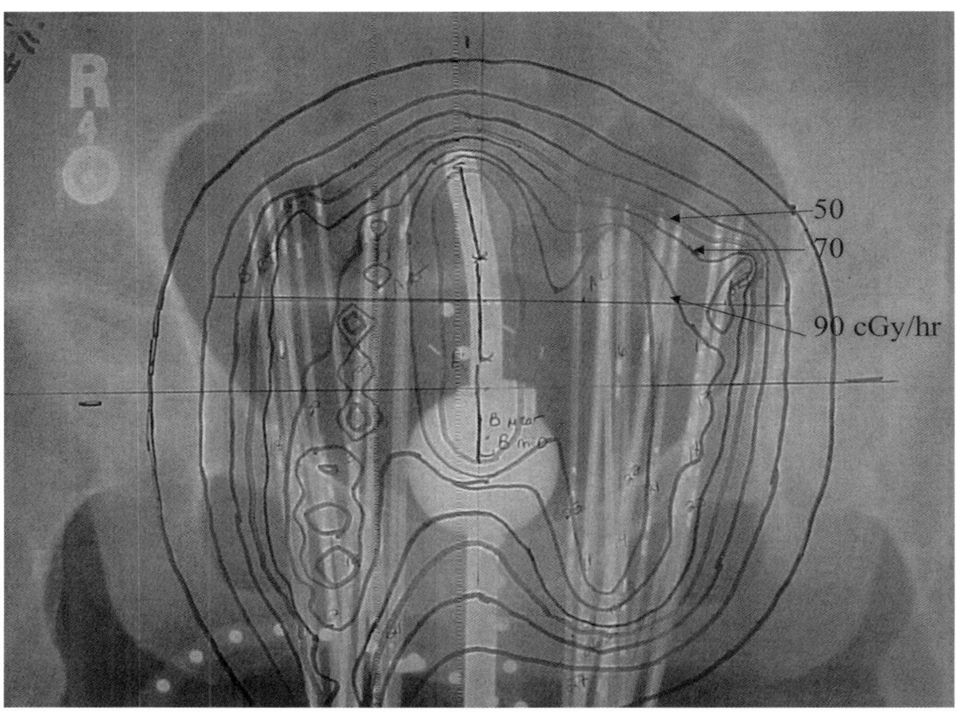

Figure 20-1. Typical isodose distribution for an iridium 192 ribbon/seed temporary implant. The visible needles will have the radioactive sources inserted at patient's bedside. Only bony anatomy indicated correct placement of applicators for this method of treating advanced cervical cancer.

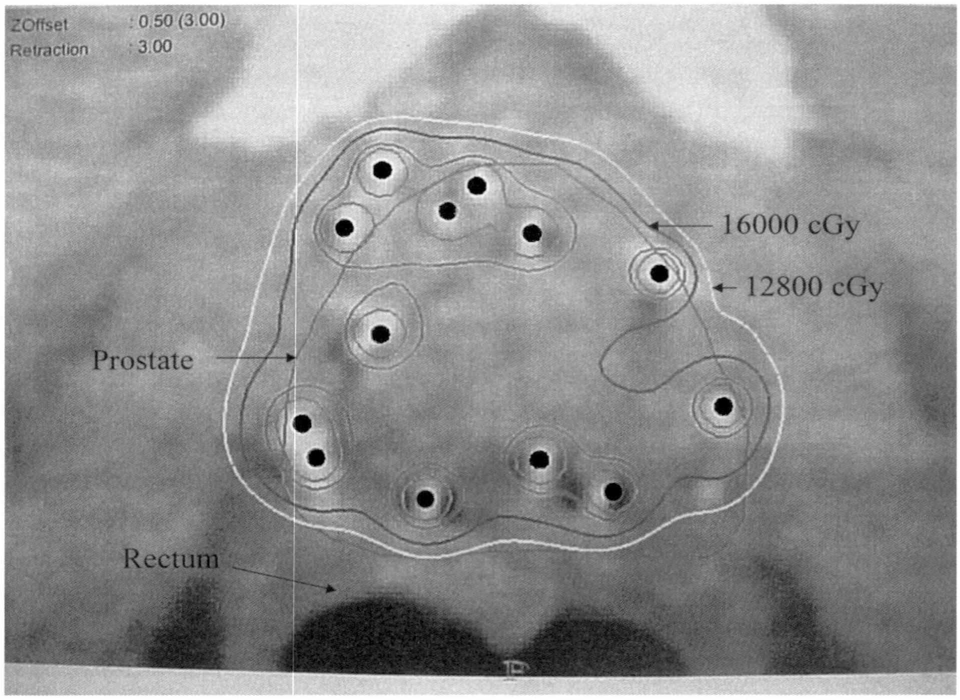

Figure 20-2. A typical computed tomography image demonstrating a permanent iodine 125 prostate implant isodose distribution. Black dots are seed positions in this plane, and the lines of equal dose surrounding the seeds diminish in value as the distance from the seeds increases. The prostate contour in this plane given the prescription dose, whereas the rectum is spared by the dose gradients in this area.

An advantage of using the permanent seed implant is that this procedure is most often performed on an outpatient basis and can be performed in an office or clinic setting, if appropriate sterile procedures and anesthesia delivery are available.

BEFORE THE ADVENT OF IMAGE-BASED PROCEDURES

Before image-based brachytherapy was prevalent, implant placement was preplanned in the following fashion: The radiation oncologist estimated the volume (height, width, breadth) of the tumor volume to be implanted from diagnostic images (CT, US, MR imaging, etc.) and provided these dimensions to the medical physicist. If a permanent implant was planned, the medical physicist chose source positions in and around the proposed volume (*x, y, z* coordinate system) and calculated the isodose distribution on the basis of the placed source positions. Sources were moved and edited to achieve a uniform dose distribution covering the target volume proposed by the radiation oncologist. The radiation oncologist could easily change the prescribed dose value by choosing more active or less active sources. Although for any given implant all of the radioactive seeds are generally chosen to have the same activity, sources of differing activity could be chosen for the same implantation procedure. A problem with using different sources is that identification of seed pairs of differing activity on the orthogonal localization radiographs can prove challenging. The final preplan was then used to obtain the requisite activity sources from the vendor, plus a few more for wastage. This calculation approach is the so-called preplan.

At implant time, the radiation oncologist would attempt to reproduce the source positions in the tumor as closely as possible to that determined by the preplan. There would inevitably be some deviation from the preplan, so a post-plan dose distribution was calculated to accurately portray the actual dose distribution in the implanted volume. Orthogonal localization films were taken through the implanted volume, and sources were identified on each, allowing the actual isodose distribution to be calculated. For use of a large number of seeds in an implant, identifying the same seed on each localization film many times proved difficult, so auto-sort algorithms were developed to aid seed identification.[7]

The success of permanent seed implantation in the prostate, based on transrectal US (TRUS)–guided imagery,[8] attests to the fact that this method of radiotherapy planning and delivery is very viable for attacking some solid tumors. Ten-year survival rates of up to 98% have been achieved.[9] The use of iodine 125, palladium 103, and occasionally gold 198 can control prostate cancer when used either as the primary treatment modality (monotherapy) or as a boost to external-beam radiotherapy. Indeed, although the highly conformal technique of intensity-modulated radiotherapy (IMRT) has become more common at some centers to treat prostate cancer with external-beam methods, the use of the low-energy photon emitters like iodine 125 or palladium 103 has made monotherapy an important option. The dose gradients at the periphery of prostate targets rival those of any of the IMRT external-beam conformality indices while allowing some interesting radiobiologic advantages that IMRT may not possess.

RADIOBIOLOGIC CONSIDERATIONS

Linear energy transfer (LET) has been implicated in the reduction of the oxygen effect[10] and, as the LET of the emitted radiations increases, anoxic cell populations are more meaningfully damaged by these low-energy, high-LET emissions. The average photon energies for iodine 125 and palladium 103 are in the 20- to 30-keV region and hence possess LET values well above the LETs attendant to the higher photon energies of megavoltage external-beam delivery systems. There is a paucity of objective data showing this positive effect for iodine 125 and palladium 103 emissions, but the success rates for tumors irradiated with these radionuclides certainly portends their effectiveness.

There appear to be three advantages of low-energy, permanent seed implant brachytherapy: (1) dose gradients at tumor–normal tissue interfaces can be made rather high; (2) continuous radiation insult to tumor cells allows malignant cells to pass into the sensitive phase of the cell cycle for damage; (3) high LET radiation from the low-energy sources used in this mode of brachytherapy effectively attacks hypoxic cell components frequently found in rapidly dividing cell populations of malignant solid tumors. The first advantage may have beneficial effects in addition to a high dose gradient between normal and malignant tissues. In prostate implants, for example, the radioactive seeds may be anatomically placed such that the course of the urethra through the gland is kept below some threshold dose, whereas the remainder of the gland receives the appropriately high prescribed dose. Finally, as mentioned earlier, an outpatient procedure may have some advantage over a procedure requiring several days of hospitalization or a protracted course of external-beam radiotherapy. Moreover, the low energy emissions provide a safety margin for staff involved with these permanent implants.

IMAGE-BASED BRACHYTHERAPY

With the advent of CT virtual simulation for external-beam radiotherapy, an image-based tool became available for brachytherapy for the determination of both preplanned implant dose distributions and planning these dose patterns after implantation, based on patient anatomy. Although use of the TRUS image–based system for permanent seed prostate brachytherapy is common practice in radiation oncology now, permanent seed brachytherapy based on CT or MRI imaging is in its infancy. **Figure 20-3** shows the anatomic detail available with the new, dedicated CT virtual-simulation scanners in use in many radiation oncology departments today. Contours through tumor volumes to be treated are superimposed on axial slices; these contoured images will be sent to the treatment planning computers to have dose distributions calculated for the treatment volumes prescribed by the radiation oncologist.

A number of articles have described temporary gynecologic implants based on CT imagery.[11,12] Indeed, HDR implants are increasingly being positioned on the basis of patient anatomy as shown on CT.

Placement of permanent seed implants on the basis of CT geometry has been reported.[13] In the CTRC in San Antonio, preplanned seed positions were based on CT axial slices through the tumor volume. At implant time, the patient was positioned in the preplanned position and a CT data set was obtained that mimicked the preplan CT study. Needle tracks to implant the target volume were determined and, after local needle track anesthesia was applied, seeds were dropped as close to the preplanned source coordinates as possible, consistent with anatomic availability.

Completing the procedure took a long time, however, tying up a diagnostic CT scanner. This procedure proved to not be the most efficient use of time for a scanner, because many diagnostic scans could have been performed in the same time frame. Only rarely would patients be referred for the procedure, and only those with few other therapeutic options.

Fortunately, a new device was being developed by a medical imaging equipment manufacturer, in cooperation with the radiation oncology department at the CTRC, that greatly streamlined the procedure. Marconi Medical Systems (now Philips Medical Systems) developed a stereotactic arm (PinPoint) whose tip position is correlated in three-dimensional space with the CT data set of a patient scanned on the CT scanner (Philips PQ5000). When this fully articulated arm is touched to the patient's skin, the image displays the patient's anatomy, on CT, under the touchpoint. Although not a real-time display, the image nonetheless contains a plethora of anatomic information, and as the touchpoint is moved along the patient's skin, the image display is automatically updated with new anatomic information under the new touchpoint. In addition to creating the ability to manually "scan" the patient's

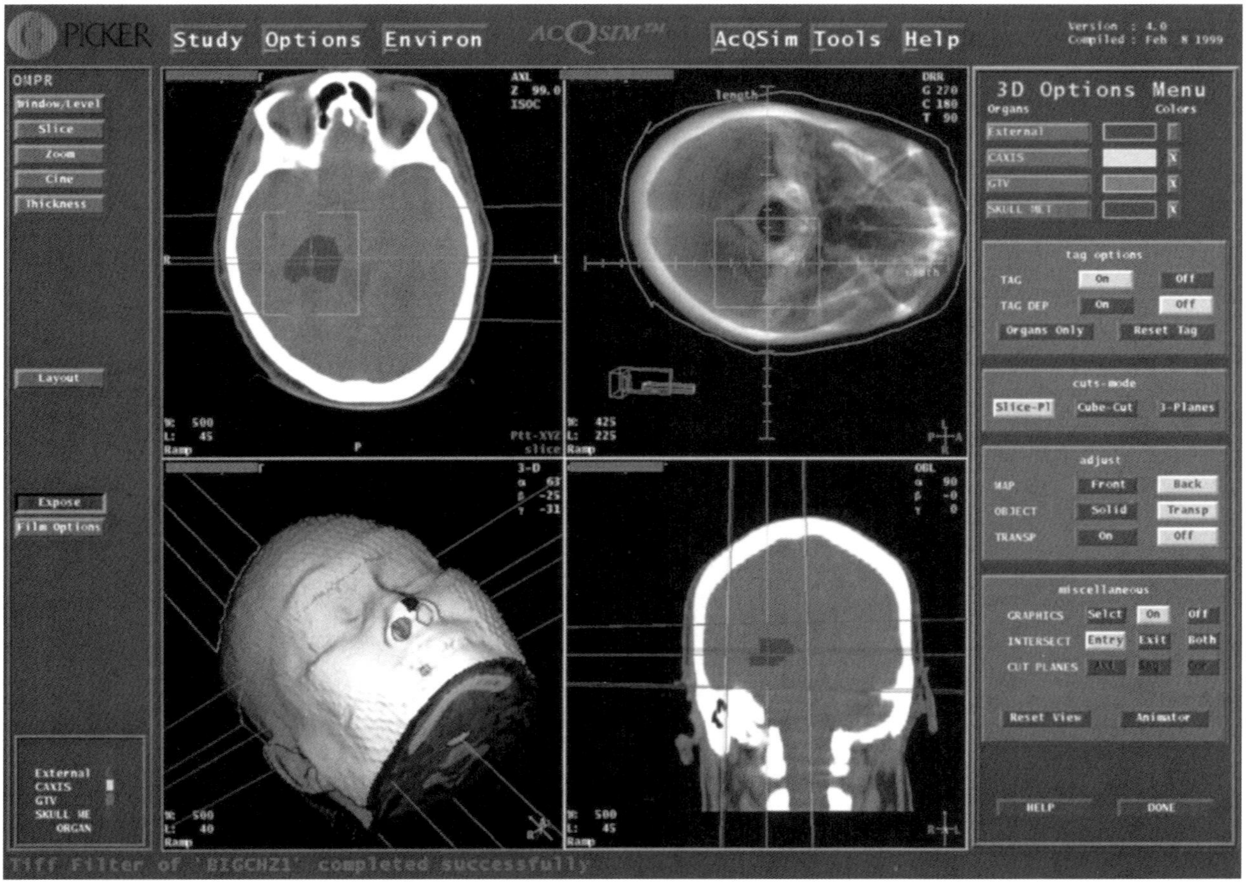

Figure 20-3. The anatomic detail available on CT simulators for external-beam treatment planning. Note the virtual vertex field depicted in the upper right panel. This field could not have been visualized with planar radiography, used to establish radiotherapy fields before the advent of these scanners and virtual-simulation software.

anatomy by CT in this way, the arm has another unique feature that allows use of the system in brachytherapy applications. From the arm's tip, the company has designed a "virtual needle" image projection along a vector direction from the arm's needle guide. This projection is adjustable in depth in the images (with a manually adjusted shaft encoder on the arm) and allows an array of virtual directions to be viewed in the patient's CT data set. When positioned for a particular approach to the target, the arm is used as a physical needle guide. **Figure 20-4** shows the arm in place on a patient. **Figure 20-5** shows the corresponding PinPoint image display with four panels. The upper left image is the axial CT slice immediately under the arm's touchpoint (arrow); the upper right image is the axial CT slice at the virtual needle's tip (cross). If the virtual needle projects at some arbitrary compound angle to the body axis, the path through anatomic tissues will not be evidenced on these axial images. They contain only the virtual needle entry point (arrow) and exit point (cross) axial images in the body. Fortunately, the company has reformatted the axial images into the two lower image panels such that the lower left panel always contains the plane of the virtual needle in an oblique axial image and the lower right image panel shows the complementary orthogonal view (oblique sagittal, in this case). Again, the complementary orthogonal view always contains the virtual needle, such that full three-dimensional information is presented to the operator regarding actual tissues being "pierced" by the virtual needle track.

The original intent of the company was to market the system as a solution to performing CT-guided needle biopsies in interventional radiology. We have actually used this system to perform several core biopsy procedures, but it is the use of the system to deliver radioactive seeds to precise coordinates that makes it a powerful adjunct to a radiotherapy program. **Figure 20-6** shows the setup in our radiotherapy department during a PinPoint-guided biopsy procedure. Because the PinPoint stereotactic arm system is not a real-time imaging system, the addition of a digital fluoroscopic

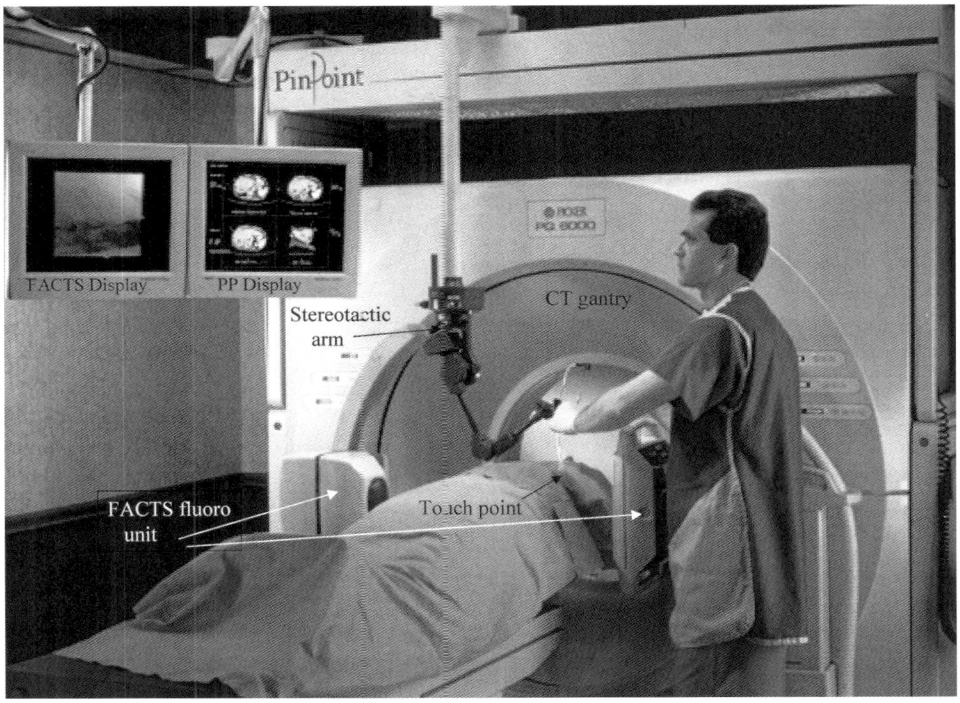

Figure 20-4. The Marconi (Philips) PinPoint stereotactic arm in use on a patient. The PinPoint display is continuously updated as the touchpoint of the PinPoint finger at the end of the arm is moved over the patient's skin. Both the computed tomography scanner (PQ6000) and the attached flat-plate fluoroscopy unit (FACTS [Fluoro Assisted Computed Tomography System]) are visible, along with the FACTS and PinPoint display screens.

unit to the CT scanner completes the loop in allowing outpatient brachytherapy to be performed in the department. This requirement is not much different than that requiring a real-time fluoroscopic image to guide seed deposits in TRUS-guided prostate implants. Once a needle track has been accessed and a real needle placed to the precise depth using the PinPoint arm, the digital fluoro unit (called FACTS, or Fluoro Assisted Computed Tomography System by Philips Medical Systems) is brought into place to allow real-time visualization of seed drops in preplanned positions along the needle track.

The medical team required for these outpatient implants performed on the radiation oncology CT planning scanner for external-beam procedures consists of an interventional radiologist, a radiation oncologist, and a clinical medical physicist. Other staff participating in these procedures include CT technologists, dosimetrists, a radiation safety officer, and nursing staff. Initially, CTRC patients presented for interventional brachytherapy because they had a solid tumor recurrence and had undergone full-course therapy with little "dose room" for further external-beam therapy in the affected area. All regions of the body accessible for transcutaneous needle insertion were considered candidates for the procedure. Additionally, patients were required to be ambulatory (outpatient) and have no frank evidence of other recurrences. We have placed implants in a host of anatomic areas, including submandibular nodal recurrences in head and neck cancers, paraspinal tumor recurrences, lung nodules in accessible pleural regions, and pelvic recurrences accessible transperineally and through abdominal punctures, avoiding bowel transit of the needle track.

PROCEDURAL METHODS USED AT THE CANCER THERAPY AND RESEARCH CENTER

A typical vignette of a paraspinal recurrence is presented here to identify the steps in an interventional brachytherapy procedure as practiced at the CTRC. The patient presented to the radiation oncologist for follow-up examination with CT evidence of a recurrent paraspinal sarcoma after a full course of external-beam radiotherapy was delivered to the chest. The spinal cord received tolerance doses, so it was thought that no additional dose to the cord could be given safely with external-beam radiotherapy. The patient was referred for interventional brachytherapy for a permanent iodine 125 implant to the involved site.

In the CT planning suite, the patient was placed in the prone position using an alpha cradle immobilization system. Patients undergoing interventional

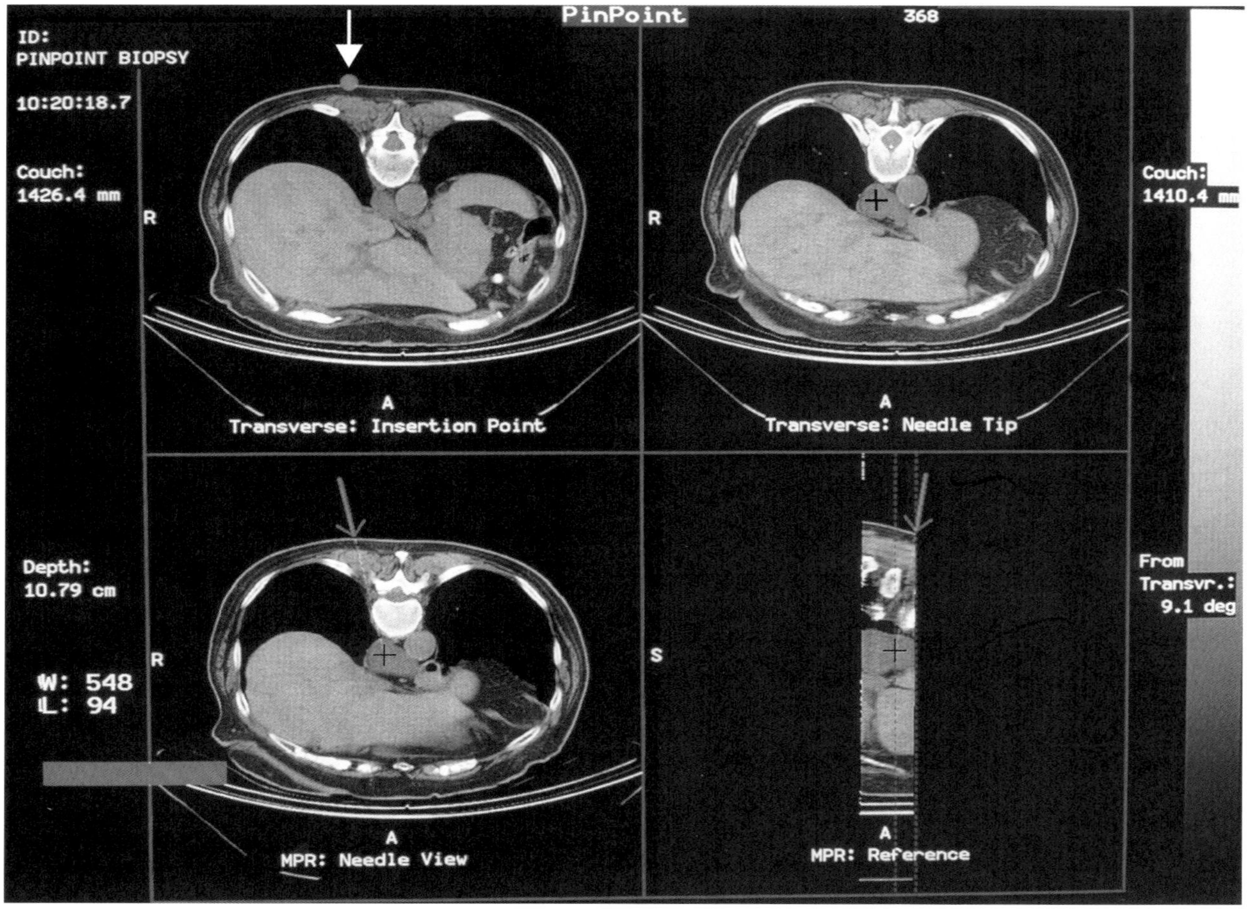

Figure 20-5. The four-panel PinPoint display screen. See text for complete description. The display image is continuously updated as the stereotactic arm's touchpoint on the patient's skin is moved from point to point, providing the operator with a plethora of anatomic information concerning the virtual, and subsequent physical, needle trajectories.

brachytherapy are immobilized in this way, as for CT planning for external-beam therapy. Because the PinPoint stereotactic arm system is not a real-time imaging system, it is crucial that the patient not move during the entire procedure of seed implantation, which can take 2 to 3 hours, depending on the number of seeds to be delivered. The alpha cradle immobilization device is a thermoplastic setting system that conforms to the patient's resting position and is used to define patient position from CT planning to treatment unit positioning during daily external-beam treatment. This immobilization has proven invaluable for interventional brachytherapy as well.

A preplan CT data set was obtained for this patient through the involved area of the chest. The PinPoint arm was positioned on the patient to begin determining virtual needle tracks that could be used in the implant procedure. A posterior approach was chosen to avoid the vertebral bodies, adjacent to which the main recurrent tumor lay. Additionally, needle tracks were chosen to minimize the necessity of traversing lung tissue. Fortunately, both requirements were met in this planning session, so the data set was sent to CTRC's brachytherapy planning system (Prowess, Alliant Inc.) for dose calculation. Iodine 125 seeds were inserted, image by image, on the data set and preplan dose distributions were calculated. The radiation oncologist called for an additional 4000–5000 cGy to the recurrent tumor volume, without giving an additional dose to the spinal cord. A total of nine iodine 125 seeds at 0.5 mCi per seed were planned along three needle tracks determined on PinPoint examination. With several extra seeds ordered, the implant procedure was scheduled and the interventional radiologist, radiation oncologist, and medical physicist prepared the patient for the interventional procedure.

After placing the patient in the preplanned immobilization device (prone), a CT data set on which the PinPoint system would operate was obtained. In a nonsterile setting, the arm was brought to the preplanned

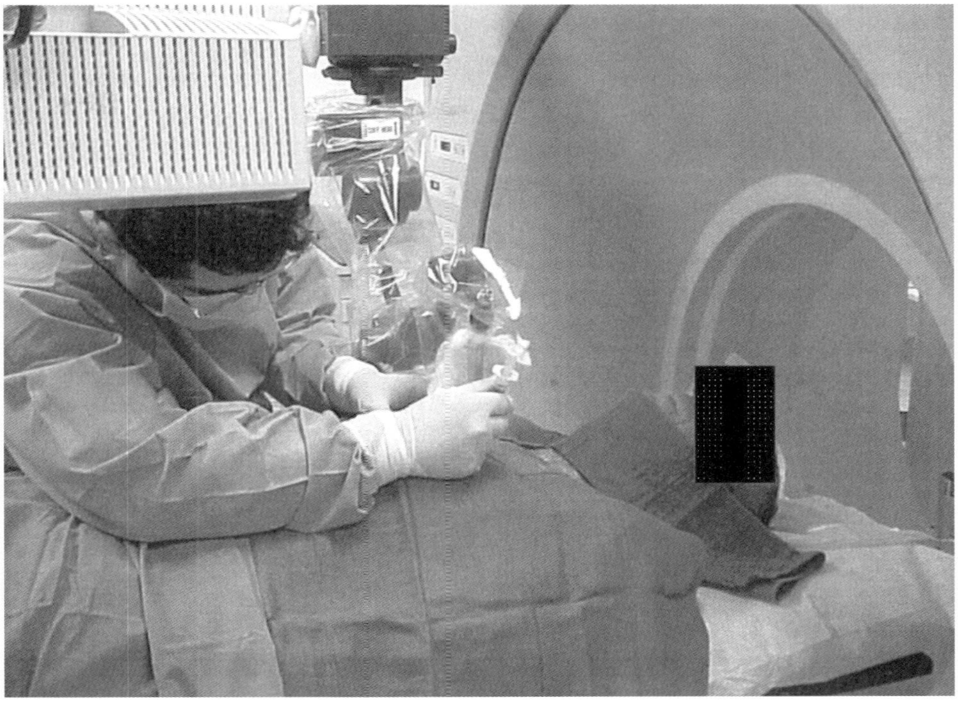

Figure 20-6. PinPoint setup in the radiation oncology department at the Cancer Therapy and Research Center in San Antonio, Texas, during a biopsy procedure. Note the interventional radiologist using the stereotactic arm (sterile field established) to guide local needle-track anesthesia application in preparation for the core biopsy to follow.

configuration to ensure our approach was appropriate to the CT data set obtained. The preplanned dose-distribution images were posted in the room for reference; when convinced that all needle tracks were accessible for approaching the preplanned targets, the interventional radiologist established a sterile field in the area where the actual needle punctures would be made. The PinPoint arm was wrapped with a sterile drape, allowing an opening to attach the PinPoint needle guide, also used in sterile fashion. The PinPoint arm may be used in a variety of positions to access the preplanned needle tracks. Locks on the "wrist" of the arm are available to constrain movement of the arm in only axial planes, or, when unlocked, the arm may be manipulated at compound angles to the body axis. This allows bony structures to be bypassed or critical structures to be avoided in the needle's passage to the target point. Because the preplanned anatomic images were available, we could be assured that the needle was approaching the target coordinate correctly through the match of current PinPoint images with the preplanned data set. When the correct position of the virtual needle was established for the first needle stick, the interventional radiologist used the PinPoint guide to anesthetize the needle track, using a 20-gauge needle with 2% lidocaine injected as the needle approached the correct depth as determined by the virtual needle. Subsequently, the interventionalist placed the seeding needle (18 gauge, 20-cm length) along the same track to the correct depth.

Once the seeding needle was in place, the radiation oncologist attached the Mick applicator (**Figure 20-7**) to the seeding needle, and the digital fluoro unit was brought into place to image the seed drops. Drops were made according to the preplanned arrangement, and then the needle was removed. In some instances, the first needle is placed under PinPoint guidance and left in place as a reference for subsequent needle placement. In this case, three iodine 125 seeds were positioned at 0.5-cm intervals along the needle track. The next PinPoint track was set up, and a similar procedure ensued until all tracks had been accessed and seeds deposited.

Figure 20-8 shows the FACTS image of the last seed being dropped for the last PinPoint needle position. **Figure 20-9** shows one of the axial post-planning images with its corresponding isodose distribution. Other plane-dose distributions indicated that the prescribed dose was delivered as intended. As a boost to the external-beam dose delivered previously to this area, the radiation oncologist prescribed an additional dose of 4000–5000 cGy to the periphery of the recurrent tumor adjacent to the vertebral body evidenced on the CT images. Although our brachytherapy treatment planning system cannot correct for heterogeneities (bone, lung, etc.) in the irradiated volume, the target volume was

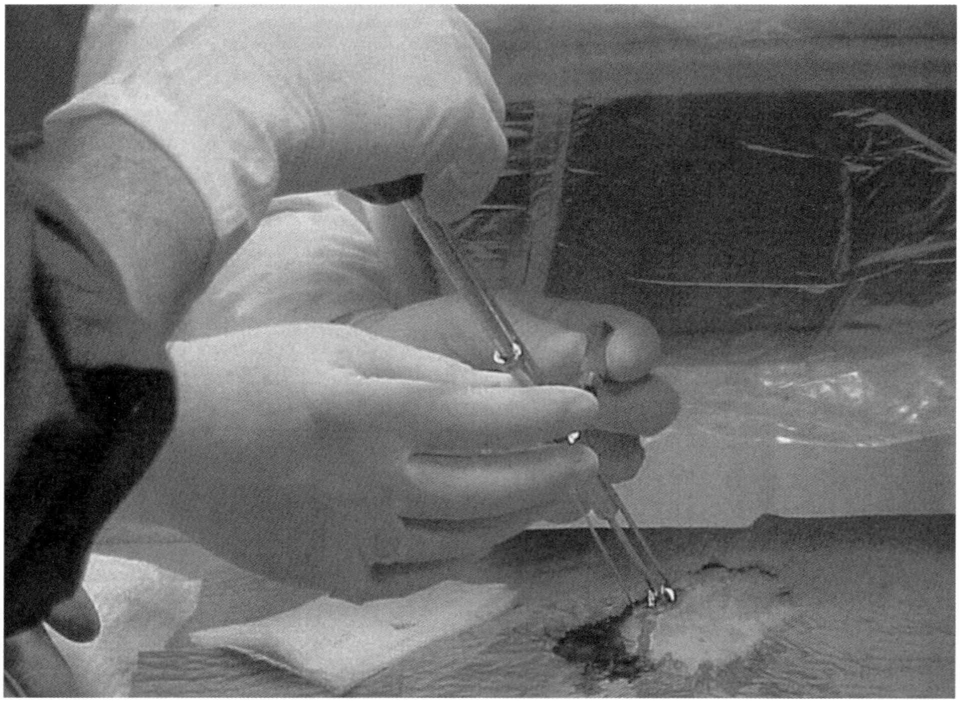

Figure 20-7. The seed applicator (Mick Radio-Nuclear Instruments, Inc.) being attached to the needle with seed cartridge positioned for seed deposition along the preplanned track.

well covered by the iodine 125 seed distribution. The usual 0.3–0.35 mCi seed activity that most prostate seed implanters use is increased to around 0.5 mCi per seed for PinPoint implants. The reason for this choice is to minimize the number of needle tracks necessary while preserving an adequate dose distribution to the prescribed volume.

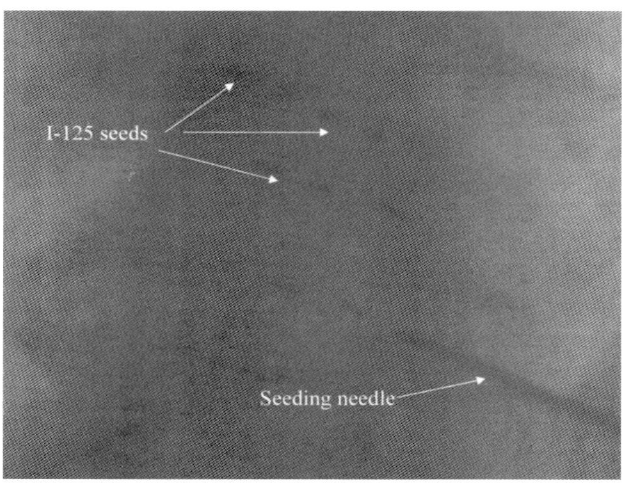

Figure 20-8. The appearance of the FACTS ([Fluoro Assisted Computed Tomography System] flat-plate fluoroscopic unit) image with the last of three needle insertions for the patient. The iodine 125 seeds dropped by previous insertions are indicated by arrows, because the contrast of the image against the vertebral bodies is low.

CT-guided implants take an average of 2 hours to place, depending on the number of seeds and the anatomic location of the implants. Because the PinPoint images are not real-time, periodic scans through the implanted seed volume may be obtained to assess coverage compared with preplanned distributions. As experience is obtained with the procedure, however, these interval scans become less necessary and the operator can rely on the real-time seed-drop images available with the solid-state fluoro unit to confirm correct placement of seeds.

As mentioned previously, the availability of the multiplanar reformatted (MPR) images available on the PinPoint display allows a large amount of anatomic information to be displayed to the interventional team. As the compound angle that the arm makes with the body axis approaches 90°, for example, the MPR plane containing the plane of the virtual needle becomes a coronal plane in the CT data set, whereas the corresponding MPR orthogonal plane is a normal sagittal plane of CT anatomy containing the plane of the virtual needle. **Figure 20-10** shows the PinPoint display panel in a planning session for a patient being evaluated for a prostate seed implant. The images illustrate the anatomic data available for the prone approach. The virtual needle entry point is displayed (red circle) as an axial slice, whereas the adjustable-depth virtual needle tip (red cross) pierces equivalently adjustable axial slices.

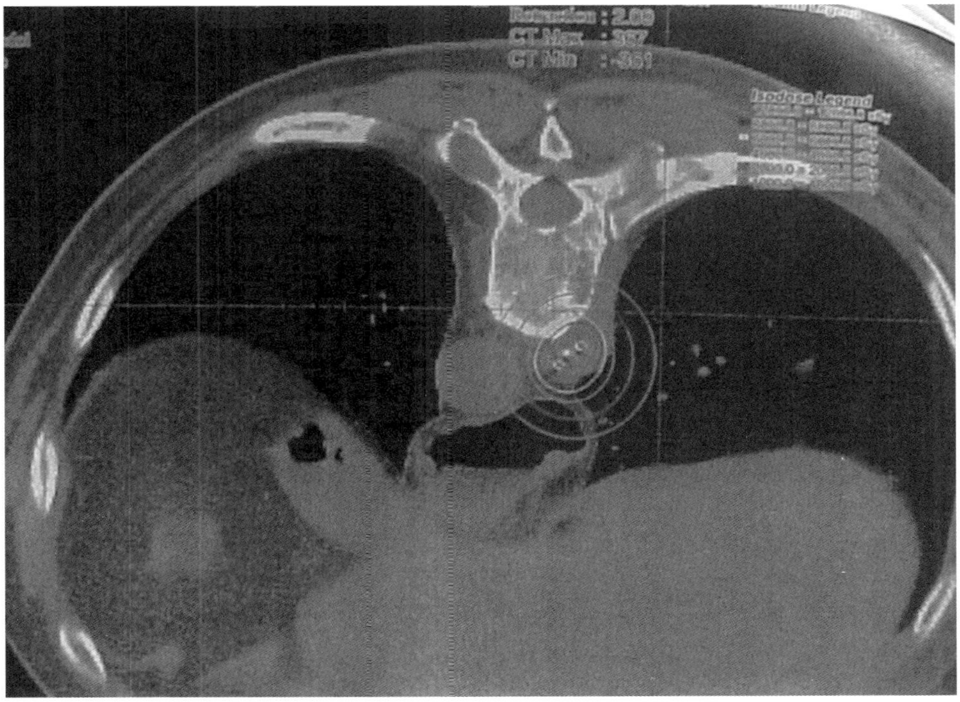

Figure 20-9. Post-plan view of one of the axial planes through the PinPoint-implanted volume. Seeds appear as isolated densities, allowing easy identification on the post-plan isodose distribution.

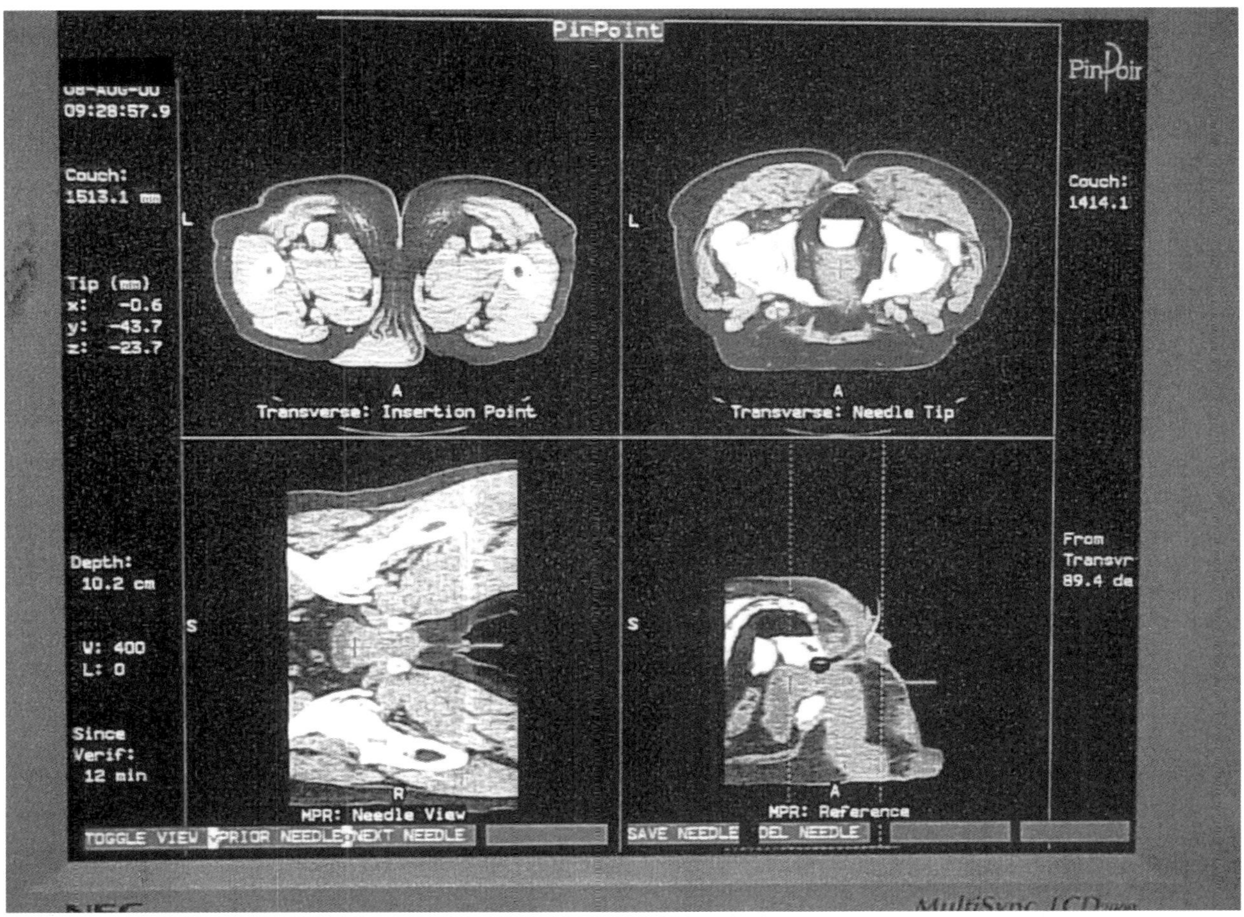

Figure 20-10. View of the PinPoint four-panel display when the stereotactic arm is positioned at the perineum along the body axis. Note that the multiplanar reformatted (MPR) images in the lower panels become a coronal plane containing the virtual needle (left panel, red line) and complementary sagittal plane (right panel, red line) containing the virtual needle.

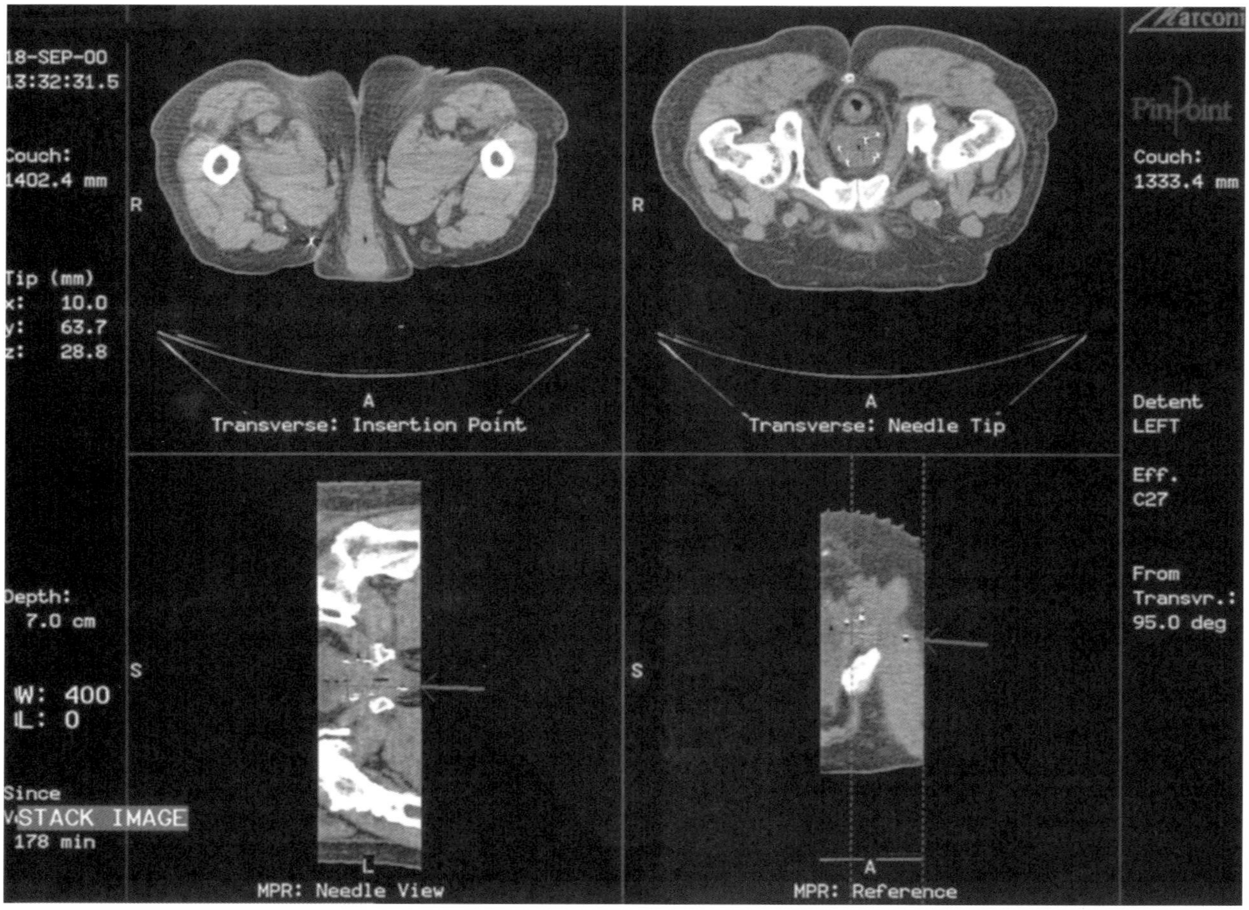

Figure 20-11. Screen capture of PinPoint screen showing a prostate seed implant in process. The upper right panel shows the tip of the virtual needle guiding the next needle direction into the gland, adjacent to iodine 125 seeds already deposited from previous needle insertions and drops with the Mick applicator.

Figure 20-11 shows the PinPoint four-panel image with the PinPoint touchpoint arm on a patient's perineum. This patient is in the process of receiving a permanent seed prostate implant with the PinPoint arm technology. Note the top two axial cuts as described above; the lower two panels illustrate the coronal (left, lower) and sagittal (right, lower) images containing the plane of the virtual needle (red dotted line). Further information on the left and right margins of the four panels is presented to the operator. At the top left and right margin are the positions of the axial cuts (needle entry and depth) relative to the origin at the CT aperture center.

On the left margin below the couch position indicator, coordinates of the virtual needle tip are displayed relative to an arbitrary origin chosen at scan time. Because point source distributions rely solely on source position to portray dose distribution patterns, these coordinates (rooted in the PinPoint-displayed anatomy) will be used to determine real-time dose distributions as seeds are dropped under this guidance system. The group in San Antonio is working closely with engineers at Philips Medical Systems to implement this important step in the process.

Finally, the current virtual needle depth from the touchpoint is displayed in the lower left margin in the PinPoint display. One can appreciate some of the seed positions around the periphery of the prostate gland in the upper right axial image. The full procedure for placing prostate implants with the technology has not been established as yet, but it appears that this type of guidance provides more information for the operator than does the TRUS approach. Further work is ongoing.

As mentioned previously, most of our patients referred for PinPoint brachytherapy have had full-course radiotherapy, and the implants have been used chiefly for recurrent solid tumors. We believe the approach is now well established, and we plan to apply the technique to de novo solitary lesions in the liver and pleural lung areas.

CONCLUSIONS

Permanent seed implant brachytherapy has been shown to be a viable method of treating some solid tumors, either as the sole treatment modality or as a boost to external-beam radiotherapy. CT-guided brachytherapy, especially those methods using a stereotactic arm and real-time fluoroscopy, have the potential of being more precise at delivering seeds to preplanned coordinates and using the CT planning scanner in the radiation oncology department to a greater extent. The ability to perform these procedures on an outpatient basis may make this procedure a part of the new technology armamentarium of modern radiation oncology departments.

ACKNOWLEDGMENTS

CT-guided placement of brachytherapy implants truly requires a team effort. New members of our team are our interventional radiologists, Robert Vasquez, MD, and Shailendra Chopra, MD. Many of our radiation oncologists at CTRC treated their patients with this method, including James C. Marbach, MD, Tony Eng, MD, Ardow Ameduri, MD, Keith Eyre, MD, and Joaquin Mira, MD. Charles Thomas, MD, suggested summarizing our work for this publication. The CTRC staff was instrumental in ensuring that the procedures went smoothly. Staff members include Art Escobedo, RT, and Shan Buxton, RTT, our CT technologists; Beth Dodge, CMD, our brachytherapy dosimetrist; and Kathy James, BS, our radiation safety officer.

We owe a special thanks to our excellent nursing staff members, who became adept at keeping our patients comfortable during the procedures. We also thank the staff of what was then called Marconi, especially Dave Hoffmeyer, BS, who personally worked with us on many of the procedures, and engineering staff members Jeff Yanof, PhD (PinPoint implementer), and Paul Klahr, MS, who developed much of the software magic, allowing us to progress as we have.

Lastly, we thank Melissa Blough, PhD, one of our medical physicists at CTRC, who took over when J. Hevezi could not make a scheduled appointment and who helped develop the pre- and postimplantation plans for our patients, along with Bret Heintz, MS, who made the Prowess planning software work for us.

REFERENCES

1. Mould RF. Radium brachytherapy: historical review. In: Mould RF, Batterman JJ, Mattinez AA, Speiser BL, eds. *Brachytherapy from Radium to Optimization*. The Netherlands: Nucletron International B.V.; 1994:1–8.
2. Pierquin B, Wilson JF, Chassagne D. *Modern Brachytherapy*. New York: Masson Publishing; 1987.
3. Quimby EH. Dosage table for linear radium sources. *Radiology* 1944;43:572.
4. Paterson R, Parker HM, Spiers FW. A system of dosage for cylindrical distributions of radium. *Br J Radiol* 1936;9:487.
5. O'Connel D, Joslin CAF, Howard N, Ramsey NW, Liversage WE. The treatment of uterine carcinoma using the Cathetron 1 technique. *Br J Radiol* 1967;40:882–887.
6. Nath R, Anderson LL, Luxton, et al. Dosimetry of interstitial brachytherapy sources: Recommendation of the AAPM Radiation Therapy Committee Task Group No. 43. *Med Phys* 1995;22:209–233.
7. Rosenthal MS. An automatic seed identification technique for interstitial implants using three isocentric radiographs. *Med Phys* 1983;10:475–479.
8. Grimm, PD, Blasko JC, Ragde H. Ultrasound-guided transperineal implantation of Iodine-125 and Palladium-103 for the treatment of early-stage prostate cancer. *Atlas Urol Clin North Am* 1994;2:113–125.
9. Ragde H, Elgamal A, Snow P, et al. Ten-year disease free survival after transperineal sonography-guided Iodine-124 brachytherapy with or without 45-Gray external beam irradiation in the treatment of patients with clinically localized, low to high Gleason grade prostate carcinoma. *Cancer* 1998;83:989–1001.
10. Hall E. *Radiobiology for the Radiologist*. Philadelphia: Lippincott Williams & Wilkins; 2000:120–123.
11. Christensen GE, Carlson B, Chao KS, et al. Image-based dose planning of intracavitary brachytherapy: registration of serial-imaging studies using deformable templates. *Int J Radiat Oncol Biol Phys* 2001;51:227–243.
12. Weeks KJ, Montana GS. A 3D applicator system for carcinoma of the uterine cervix. *Int J Radiat Oncol Biol Phys*. 1997;37:455–463.
13. Brinkman DH, Kline RW. Automated seed localization from CT datasets of the prostate. *Med Phys* 1998;25:1667–1672.

CHAPTER 21

MALIGNANT BILIARY OBSTRUCTION

JAMES H. TURNER, MD

GUIDO M. SCATORCHIA, MD

INTRODUCTION

Obstruction of the biliary system can be caused by a number of tumors, including hepatocellular carcinoma, cholangiocarcinoma, pancreatic tumors, ampullary carcinomas, and carcinoma of the gallbladder. Metastatic lymphadenopathy from other primary tumors, such as those of the stomach or colon, can also lead to biliary obstruction. Each of these tumors causes obstruction at different levels of the biliary system; for example, pancreatic carcinoma leads to distal biliary obstruction at the level of the common bile duct (CBD), whereas Klatskin tumors occur at the confluence of the main right and left biliary ducts.[1] Hepatocellular carcinoma occurs anywhere in the hepatic parenchyma, which can lead to isolated segmental duct obstruction. Most frequently, obstruction from metastatic sources occurs at the porta hepatis because of portal adenopathy. Regardless of the level of obstruction, similar clinical manifestations occur. There are, however, some important diagnostic and therapeutic differences depending on the level of obstruction. For instance, in unresectable pancreatic carcinoma, relief of biliary obstruction is often more easily achieved with endoscopic stent placement, rather than percutaneous stent placement. With a Klatskin tumor, the opposite is true, owing to the isolated ductal obstruction.

Clinical manifestations of biliary obstruction include hyperbilirubinemia leading to jaundice and pruritus, hepatic dysfunction with elevated hepatocellular enzymes, pain, and cholangitis. Curative resection offers the best hope of a good long-term outcome. However, the majority of patients with cholangiocarcinoma or hepatocellular carcinoma, for instance, initially present with disease that has progressed too far for resection. When the tumors involve vascular structures or metastasize beyond their primary organ, therapeutic options become limited, with poor long-term prognoses for many patients.[2–5] Pancreatic cancer, hepatocellular carcinoma, and gallbladder cancer also frequently present late in their natural history, making curative resection impossible. Depending on the type of tumor, the relief of obstructive symptoms becomes the main therapeutic goal and is a means to offer palliation during the remaining weeks or months of a patient's life.

HISTORICAL PERSPECTIVE

Prior to the early 1970s, relief of biliary obstruction was achieved through surgical means.[6] Pancreaticoduodenectomy with hepaticojejunostomy or choledochojejunostomy carries high surgical morbidity and mortality (10%–20%), with patients' mean survival being 5–8 months.[7] As an alternative to resection, surgical intubation of the biliary tract was first reported in the 1950s. Intubation of the bile ducts using a silastic stent was performed during surgery either in conjunction with an attempt at curative resection or for palliation alone if resection was not possible. A surgical mortality of 7% was reported with this procedure.[8]

Alternatives to surgery were conceived through established percutaneous methods. Percutaneous transhepatic cholangiography (PTC) had been an established diagnostic procedure since the 1950s. Placing a catheter across an obstructed duct during PTC was obviously the next logical step. Molnar and Stockum first reported placing a percutaneous catheter across a biliary obstruction in 1974.[9] Others, including Ring, Oleaga, Ferrucci, Mueller, and vanSonnenberg, expanded the technique and modified equipment to make the percutaneous placement of transhepatic catheters a safe and effective means of palliating malignant biliary obstruction.[10–12] The technique has evolved from external drainage only[6–9] to placing purely internal catheters[13–16] to what is the most widely accepted procedure today—placing internal–external drains.[17–20]

With stenting of the bile ducts to relieve obstruction, one of the objectives is to maintain stent patency for as long as possible. In addition, making the stent purely internal has also been a goal with percutaneous methods. Unfortunately, stents become obstructed with sludge and debris, making routine catheter exchange or some other reintervention necessary. The tendency of internal silastic stents to become obstructed with biliary sludge was noted, which prompted the use of expandable metal stents. The first report of an expandable metal stent for malignant biliary obstruction appeared in the literature in 1989.[21] This report, from a European trial, was followed by reports comparing plastic versus metal stents in both benign and malignant obstruction.[22–35] The metal stents had longer patency rates than did plastic stents, but the former still had a tendency to occlude with sludge. Several series have reported longer patency rates for metallic stents versus plastic stents. Davids reported a median patency of 273 days for metallic stents versus 126 days for polyethylene stents.[20]

Reintervention prolonged patients' useful lives, but at the expense of repeated procedures and additional hospitalizations. This form of disease management is acceptable for patients with a limited prognosis, such as seen in the types of malignancies discussed previously; however, permanent metallic stents are not acceptable with benign strictures where the life span of the patient far exceeds the primary and secondary patency rates of the stent. Consequently, surgical resection of benign biliary strictures is considered first-line therapy, with prolonged percutaneous stenting with a plastic internal–external drain reserved for surgery failures.

BILIARY DUCT ANATOMY

Bile is produced in hepatocytes and excreted into biliary radicles lying within the hepatic parenchyma. Biliary radicles coalesce to form subsegmental and segmental biliary ducts. At the subsegmental and segmental levels, the ducts lie within the hepatic segmental parenchyma. Paralleling the bile ducts are the segmental hepatic arteries and portal veins; the three structures together constitute the portal triad. This is in contrast to the hepatic venules (central veins) and hepatic veins, which lie between the hepatic segments. After the segmental level, the bile ducts combine to form main right and left ducts. The main right and left ducts join to form the common hepatic duct. After a short segment and at the level of the porta hepatis, the cystic duct joins the common hepatic duct to form the CBD. The CBD enters the pancreas and runs through the pancreatic head. Within the pancreas, the pancreatic duct joins the CBD to empty into the duodenum through a common orifice known as the sphincter of Oddi. There are a number of normal anatomic variations to this pattern of ductal branching. There is a common orifice with the pancreatic duct in 60% of patients. The remaining 40% have separate orifices. There are a number of additional normal anatomic variations to this pattern of ductal branching. Variations are seen in 5%–10% of cholangiograms, with the most common variation being an aberrant intrahepatic duct joining the common hepatic duct or CBD. The cystic duct entering the right hepatic duct instead of the common hepatic duct is the next most common variation.

TOOLS AND TECHNIQUES

Percutaneous transhepatic drainage (PTD) usually begins with a PTC. In a patient with biliary obstruction from an undetermined cause, other imaging studies (computed tomography [CT], ultrasound [US]) may establish the presence of biliary obstruction but may not be able to show the level of obstruction. A pancreatic head mass may impinge on the distal CBD, causing obstruction, but the mass may not be visible by imaging. Owing to the pronounced desmoplastic reaction caused by pancreatic carcinoma, a very small primary tumor may cause complete biliary obstruction. Another example might be a Klatskin tumor, where the obstruction may be visible by CT or US but the tumor itself is occult by conventional imaging. In such cases, PTC becomes extremely useful in determining the level of obstruction and consequently may offer a pathologic diagnosis (**Fig. 21-1**).

PTC begins by accessing either the right or left segmental or subsegmental bile ducts. The technique differs depending on which side the procedure is begun. For a right-sided approach, a 22-gauge Chiba (Cook, Inc., Bloomington, IN) or other small-gauge needle is inserted in the 9th or 10th intercostal space at the midaxillary line. Aiming slightly ventral and cephalad, the needle is advanced under fluoroscopic guidance to just lateral to the vertebral column. Contrast is injected slowly as the needle is withdrawn. Contrast flowing into the bile ducts indicates successful needle placement (**Fig. 21-2**). Remember, there are other "tubular" structures in the liver, and identifying which of the structures (bile duct, hepatic artery, hepatic vein, or portal vein) the needle tip is in is the first crucial step. Contrast should not flow away quickly from the needle tip; if it does, that indicates arterial or venous placement. Contrast flowing toward the hepatic periphery only, and not toward the porta hepatis, would indicate entry into the portal or arterial system. Contrast in the biliary system appears under fluoroscopy as a static contrast column extending toward the peripheral liver margin and toward the porta hepatis. Once entry into the bile ducts is confirmed, enough contrast is injected to outline both the right and left ducts, and an adequate volume of contrast should be injected to flow centrally to identify the level of obstruction. Obstruction from malignancy may appear either as an intraluminal-filling defect or as an extrinsic compression abnormality with a short, typically irregular transition ("shoulders") (**Figs. 21-1C** and **21-2A**).

On the left, access to the biliary system is usually gained with the aid of US guidance. The dilated biliary ductal system is confirmed by US, and access is gained with a small-gauge needle. Usually, the duct in Couinord segment II (anterolateral segment) is chosen, as the placement provides for a straighter course to the hepatic hilum than does segment III. Contrast is injected to confirm placement, and diagnostic cholangiography is continued as on the right side (**Fig. 21-2**).

Regardless of where the needle was placed for the cholangiogram, entry into the biliary system for the purposes of drainage should ensure adequate catheter placement; that is, the sideholes of the catheter should reside in the peripheral ductal branches to ensure adequate internal or external drainage. However, the sideholes should not reside too far in the periphery, which would allow bile to leak to the subcapsular space or to the skin surface, nor should they be placed too centrally, which would not allow significant sideholes in the intrahepatic ducts and would result in inadequate drainage of bile from the peripheral ducts. Ensuring adequate placement of the catheter to meet these needs might require placement of a second needle once the ducts are opacified with contrast. Frequently, the first needle is placed in a small subsegmental branch, which is fine for the diagnostic portion of the procedure. The second needle, however, requires placement in a midsegmental branch, typically either segment III on the left or segments V or VI on the right (**Fig. 21-1C**).

Once access into a midsegmental branch is obtained, the Seldinger technique is used to advance either a vascular sheath or a peel-away sheath into the biliary system. Placement of the sheath makes subsequent catheter and guide wire exchanges much simpler and less traumatic. Through the sheath, angled catheters and hydrophilic wires are helpful in traversing the obstruction, with the objective of placing a wire into the duodenum (**Fig. 21-1D**). Frequently, the obstruction cannot be traversed on the initial attempt. When this is the case, the patient should undergo external biliary drainage for a 24-hour period and another attempt at crossing the obstruction should be made. An obstruction can cause inflammation of the ducts at the level of the obstruction; relief of the obstruction by external drainage will allow the inflammation to subside and potentially decrease the degree of obstruction. Once a wire is placed into the duodenum, an internal–external drainage catheter is placed with the pigtail in the duodenum. Frequently, an 8-F catheter is placed initially and the catheter is upsized to 12 F or larger a few days later once the percutaneous tract has begun to mature (**Fig. 21-1E**). Once placed, the catheter should be set for external drainage for 24 hours to facilitate drainage and the clearing of any procedure-related hemobilia. A trial of internal drainage, with the

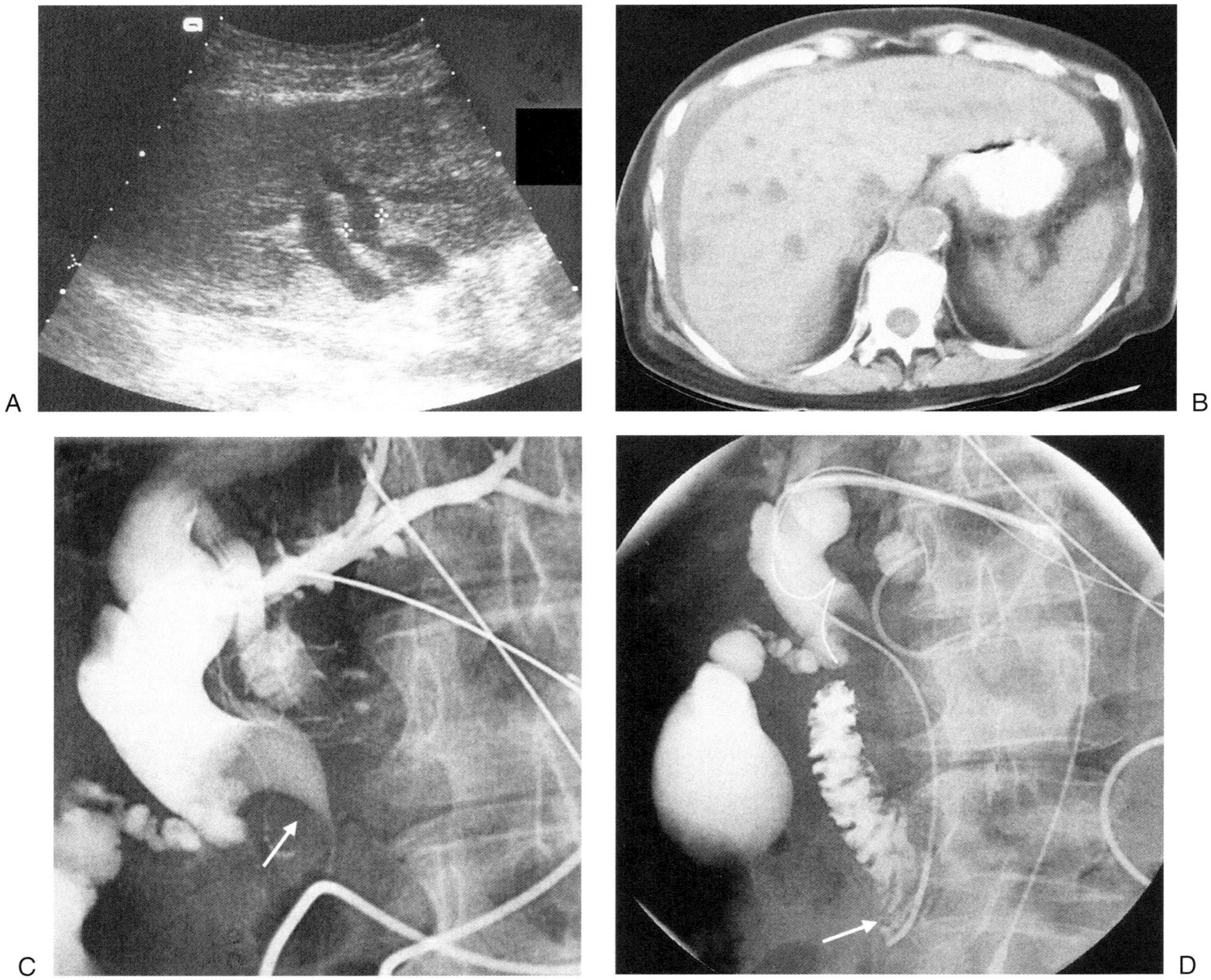

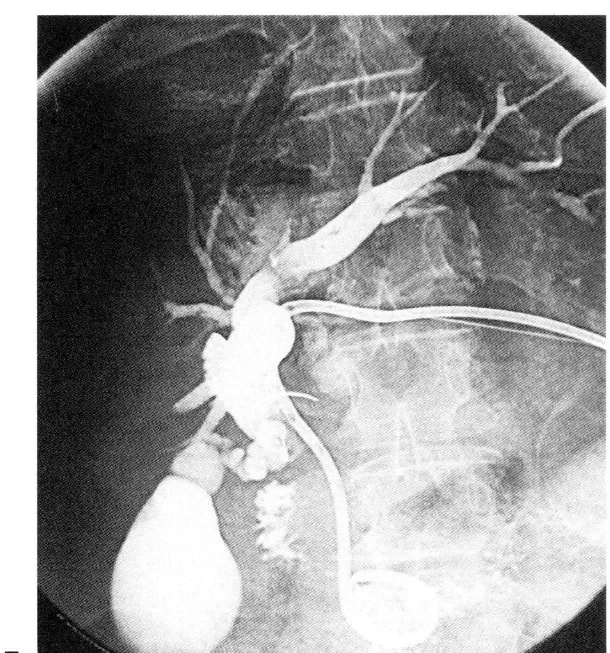

Figure 21-1. A 74-year-old woman presented with jaundice and abdominal pain. (A) Ultrasound of the right upper quadrant demonstrated intra- and extra-hepatic biliary ductal dilation. (B): Computed tomography of the abdomen confirmed the biliary ductal dilation but did not reveal the source or the level of the obstruction. (C) Percutaneous transhepatic cholangiogram was performed, with the initial needle placed in a peripheral biliary branch in the left hepatic lobe. A second needle was placed more centrally after opacification of the biliary system with contrast. Note the rounded, abrupt cutoff of contrast in the common bile duct (arrow). (D) The obstruction was passed using a hydrophilic wire and an angled angiographic catheter. Injection of contrast through the catheter confirmed placement in the duodenum (arrow). (E) Using standard over-the-wire exchange techniques, a 12-F internal–external biliary drainage catheter was placed, with the pigtail of the catheter in the duodenum. The intraluminal mass was later confirmed to be a cholangiocarcinoma.

A 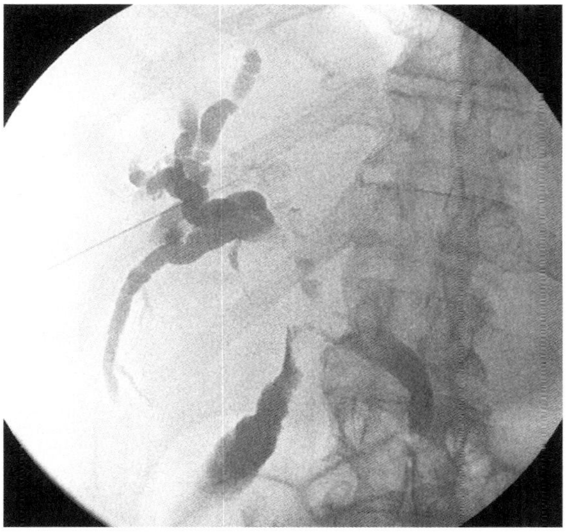

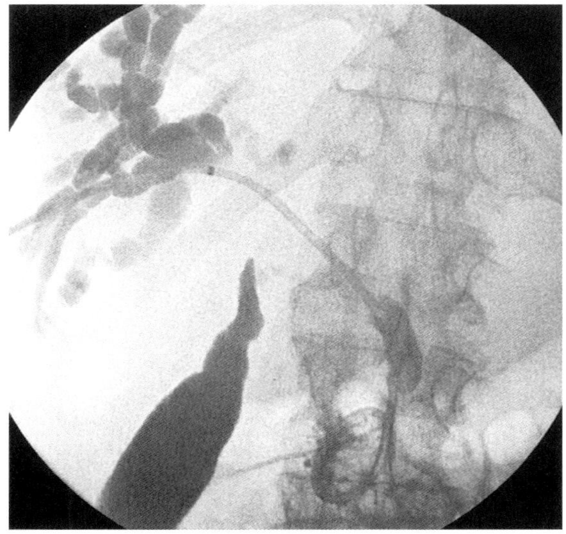 B

C 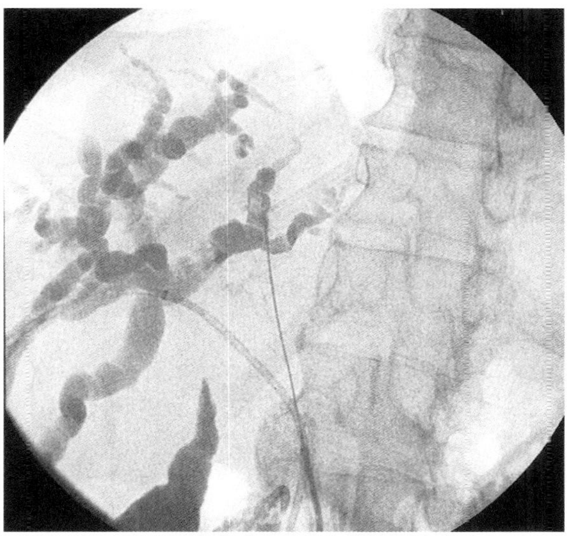

Figure 21-2. A 75-year-old woman presented with a history of metastatic colon cancer. Imaging studies (not shown) revealed biliary dilation and metastases to the liver as the source of obstruction. (A) Percutaneous transhepatic cholangiography (PTC) was performed via a right-sided approach; biliary dilation was confirmed. (B) An internal–external biliary drain was placed using standard technique. (C) Because the left-sided biliary ducts had not opacified, left-sided PTC was performed under ultrasound. The left-sided procedure demonstrated dilated ducts, similar to the right. (Case photos courtesy of Janette Durham, MD, from University of Colorado Health Sciences Center, Denver, CO.)

external portion of the catheter capped, should be attempted before the patient is discharged or other intervention is contemplated.

CHOLANGIOGRAPHIC APPEARANCE OF OBSTRUCTION

As a diagnostic test, PTC is most often used to confirm biliary obstruction. Moreover, the level of obstruction is more accurately defined with cholangiography than with other radiographic examinations. Most often, a three-dimensional imaging modality such as US or CT has already established the presence of biliary obstruction, but it may not have revealed the level or origin of the obstruction. Cholangiography is then performed to confirm the obstruction and establish the level of obstruction.

In cholangiography, obstruction appears as dilated intrahepatic ducts, extrahepatic bile ducts, or both (**Figs. 21-1–21-5**). As a general rule, the CBD should not exceed 10 mm in diameter in adults; however, in patients who have undergone cholecystectomy, the CBD may measure up to 15 mm in diameter. Moving more peripherally, the common hepatic duct, main right and left ducts, and segmental ducts become progressively more tapered with a smooth, even appearance.

A malignant obstruction may appear as an abrupt cut-off of contrast within the lumen of the bile duct (**Fig. 21-1C**) Alternatively, an intraluminal-filling defect may be present. With masses lying solely within the hepatic parenchyma, there may be non-filling of the intrahepatic ducts in that portion of the liver involved by the mass, owing to more peripheral obstruction of the segmental or subsegmental ducts.

ESTABLISHING THE DIAGNOSIS OF MALIGNANCY

The results of laboratory tests and imaging studies can often suggest the diagnosis of the mass causing the biliary obstruction. For instance, CA 2220 is a serum marker for pancreatic adenocarcinoma. An elevated serum CA 2220 level, along with an enlarged pancreatic head and biliary dilation, as identified by CT or US, is highly suggestive of the diagnosis of pancreatic carcinoma. Another example would be an elevated serum CEA (chorioembryonic antigen) level in the face of biliary obstruction from hilar adenopathy; this would be highly suggestive of metastatic lymphadenopathy from colorectal carcinoma. However, treatment decisions are typically based on a histologic identification of the mass, typically requiring either an open surgical biopsy or an image-guided percutaneous needle biopsy. In recent years, image-guided percutaneous needle biopsy has supplanted open surgical biopsy in most instances. With an obvious mass in the hepatic parenchyma or in the pancreatic head, image-guided needle biopsy is less invasive and typically yields good results. When the source of obstruction is less clear, as in the case of biliary obstruction with normal findings on imaging studies, the presumption is an occult mass in either the pancreatic head or the biliary tract. Bile cytology or brush biopsy obtained by endoscopic retrograde cholangiopancreatography (ERCP) can be helpful in these instances. The sensitivity of these tests for detecting occult malignancy in the biliary tract has been shown to be relatively low, on the order of 20%–30%. Other diagnostic options include PTC to identify the level of biliary obstruction with a forceps biopsy of an intraluminal mass. This has a higher sensitivity than bile cytology or brush biopsy, on the order of 80%–90%.[36] In the case of distal biliary obstruction without an identified mass detected by imaging studies or an intraluminal defect detected by PTC, blind forceps biopsy of the pancreatic head through the intrapancreatic portion of the CBD has been used with some success. The alternative is intraoperative US, which has a very high sensitivity for detecting pancreatic masses not visualized by other imaging methods.[37] A newer but less invasive procedure is intraluminal US performed during PTC or ERCP. This method is not widely available and is extremely operator dependent, meaning the operator must have a lot of experience with its use for it to be effective. Again, with the newer means of identifying occult masses (intraductal or intraoperative US), effective treatment is dependent on obtaining tissue for a histologic diagnosis.

POST-PROCEDURE CARE OF CATHETERS AND STENTS

Once placed, both internal–external and purely internal stents require some form of maintenance. Catheters and stents are subject to occlusion from accumulated biliary sludge and debris. Internal–external catheters require daily (sometimes two or three times daily) flushing with 10 mL of sterile saline to keep the sideholes from occluding. Even with routine flushing, the catheters become encrusted with bile salts, which build up over days to weeks. For long-term maintenance, over a period of months to years, the catheter is exchanged for a similar-size catheter over a guide wire in the interventional suite. As a starting point, catheter changes every 6 weeks is standard; the time interval can be adjusted for individual patients.

As stated previously, metallic stents are placed in patients whose life expectancy is limited (**Fig. 21-3**). The patency rate of the stent should be longer than the life expectancy of the patient, on the order of 4–5 months. In a series involving 100 patients, Dick et al. reported an average survival of 5 months after metallic stent placement. Of the metallic stents, 86% were patent at 5 months; 12% of the stents required some form of reintervention.[24] In a separate series of 50 patients, Gordon et al. reported an average patency of 5.8 months and survival of 7.5 months. In that study, 24% of the stents required reintervention.[25]

Should the metallic stent become occluded, reintervention may be required. Most frequently, percutaneous access to the biliary system must be made. Angioplasty or repeat stenting (i.e., placing a stent within the lumen of the pre-existing stent) is required. Another possibility is placing an internal–external catheter through the lumen of the metallic stent to provide drainage. Secondary patency rates are about the same as the primary patency rates (**Figs. 21-4 and 21-5**).

COMPLICATIONS

As with any percutaneous procedures, bleeding and infection are the most frequently encountered complications. Complications specific to PTC and PTD include

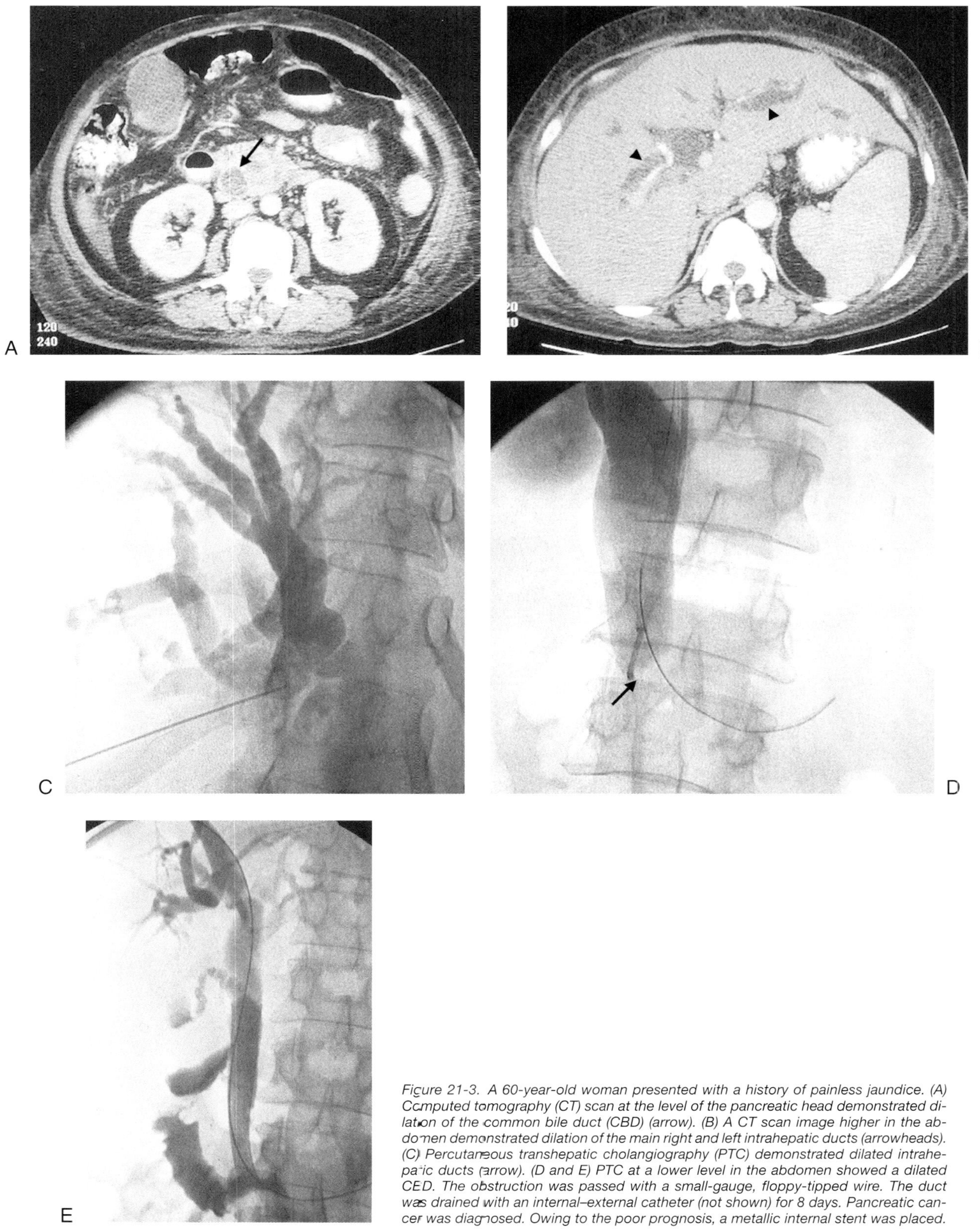

Figure 21-3. A 60-year-old woman presented with a history of painless jaundice. (A) Computed tomography (CT) scan at the level of the pancreatic head demonstrated dilation of the common bile duct (CBD) (arrow). (B) A CT scan image higher in the abdomen demonstrated dilation of the main right and left intrahepatic ducts (arrowheads). (C) Percutaneous transhepatic cholangiography (PTC) demonstrated dilated intrahepatic ducts (arrow). (D and E) PTC at a lower level in the abdomen showed a dilated CBD. The obstruction was passed with a small-gauge, floppy-tipped wire. The duct was drained with an internal–external catheter (not shown) for 8 days. Pancreatic cancer was diagnosed. Owing to the poor prognosis, a metallic internal stent was placed.

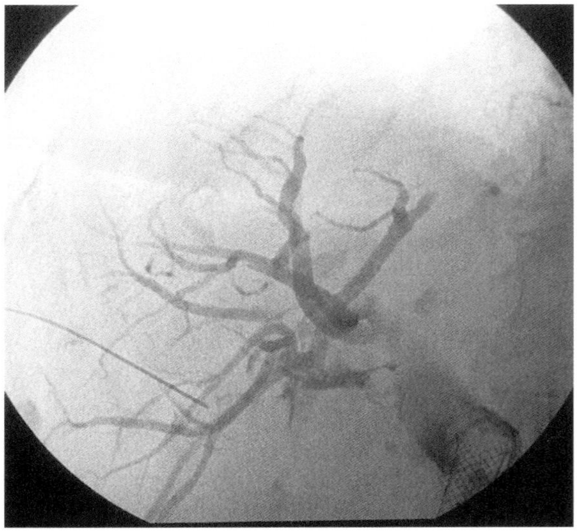

A

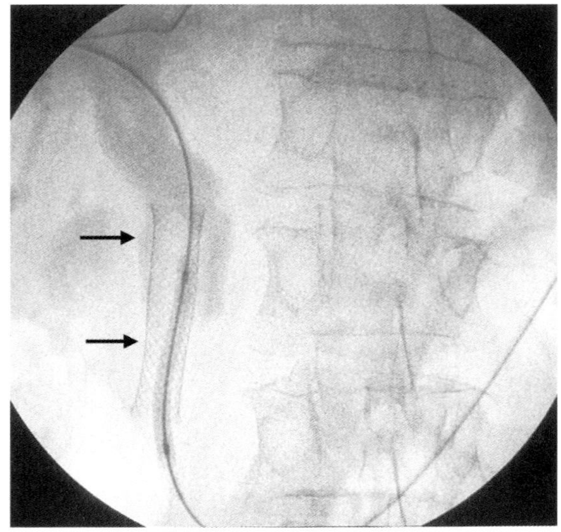

B

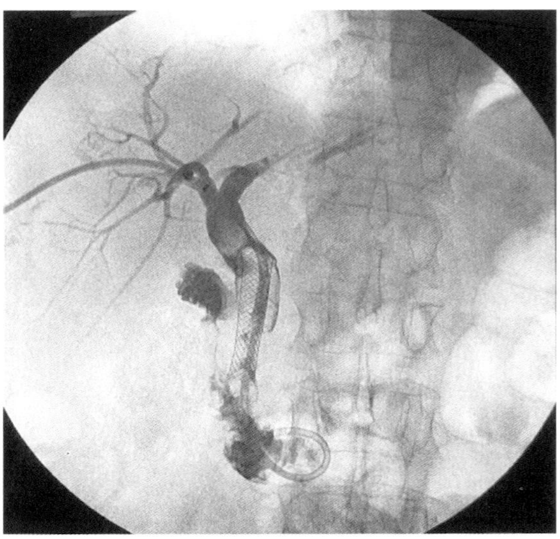

C

Figure 21-4. An 82-year-old woman presented with a history of ampullary pancreatic cancer. The patient had been given an internal metallic stent as part of palliative treatment. The patient returned with a complaint of pain and jaundice. (A) Percutaneous transhepatic cholangiography demonstrated mild dilation of the intrahepatic ducts and an occluded internal metallic stent. (B) The occluded metallic stent (arrows) was successfully crossed with a wire. Angioplasty of the stent was done in an attempt to restore patency, but it was not successful. (C) Through the occluded stent, an internal–external drain was placed for continued palliation. (Case photos courtesy of David Kumpe, MD, of University of Colorado Health Sciences Center, Denver, CO.)

hemobilia and bile fistula. During the initial puncture for PTC or subsequent manipulations, a branch of the hepatic artery may inadvertently be crossed. The lacerated artery may bleed into the biliary duct, causing hemobilia. Often, some bloody drainage may be present after catheter placement that will clear over a matter of hours. Copious bleeding or bleeding that continues past 24 hours represents hemobilia. Treatment options for hemobilia include increasing the size of the percutaneous catheter in an attempt to tamponade the bleeding vessel, removing the catheter and performing a percutaneous embolization along the tract, and performing a diagnostic hepatic arteriogram and arterial embolization.

ASSOCIATED TREATMENT OF MALIGNANCY

Some of the associated treatment modalities mentioned in this chapter are more fully discussed in other parts of the book, such as catheter-directed chemoembolization of unresectable hepatocellular carcinoma and radiofrequency ablation. However, external-beam radiation and intraluminal brachytherapy, combined with percutaneous drainage of the biliary tract, are important adjuncts in the treatment of unresectable cholangiocarcinoma. Palliation with intraluminal placement of an iridium-192 wire and external-beam radiation can maintain the patency of the internal metallic stent.[38,39]

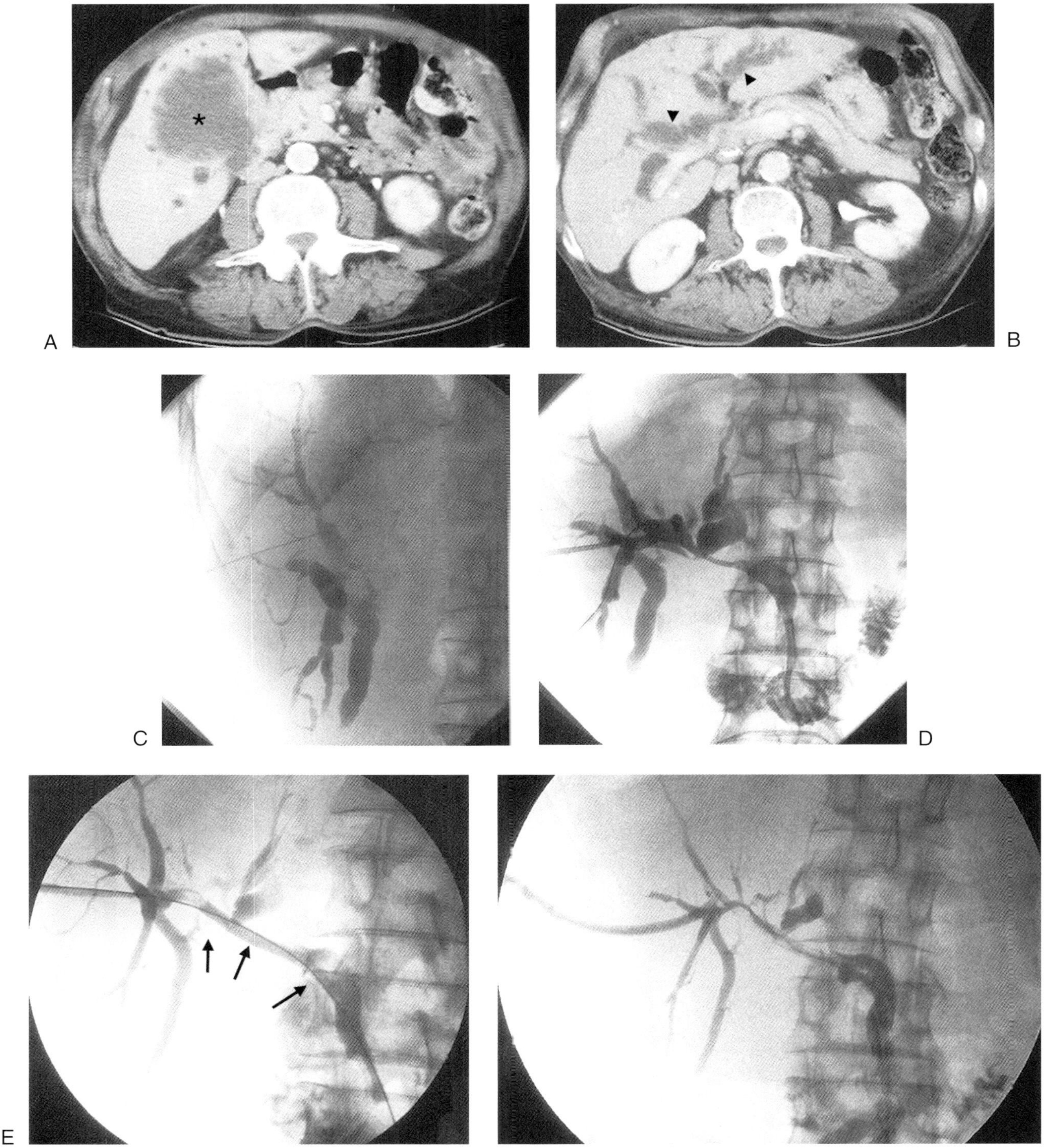

Figure 21-5. A 71-year-old man presented with a history of right upper quadrant pain and jaundice. (A and B) Computed tomography scans demonstrated a large mass centered in the gallbladder fossa (asterisk) with obstruction of the bile ducts (arrowheads). (C) Percutaneous transhepatic cholangiography confirmed intrahepatic biliary dilation. (D) An internal–external drain was placed. After a percutaneous biopsy, adenocarcinoma was diagnosed, the exact origin of which was believed, on the basis of imaging findings, to be the gallbladder. (E) Sixteen days after placement of the internal–external drain, internal metallic stents (arrow) were placed along the length of the common bile duct and main right hepatic duct. (F) A completion cholangiogram demonstrated patency of the newly placed stents with decompression of the intrahepatic ducts.

More recently, there have been claims of prolonged survival with this technique.[40,41]

REFERENCES

1. Klatskin G. Adenocarcinoma of the hepatic duct at its bifurcation within the porta hepatis: an unusual tumor with distinctive clinical and pathological features. *Am J Med* 1965;38:241–256.
2. Lai ECS, Tompkins RK, Roslyn JJ, Mann LL. Proximal bile duct cancer: quality of survival. *Ann Surg* 1987;205:111–118.
3. Baer HU, Stain SC, Dennison AR, Eggers B, Blumgart LH. Improvement in survival by aggressive resections of hilar cholangiocarcinoma. *Ann Surg* 1993;217:20–27.
4. Bismuth H, Nakache R, Diamond T. Management strategies in resection for hilar cholangiocarcinoma. *Ann Surg* 1992;215:31–38.
5. Stain SC, Baer HU, Dennison AR, Blumgart LH. Current management of hilar cholangiocarcinoma. *Surg Gynecol Obstet* 1992;175:579–588.
6. Mori K, Misumi A, Sugiyama M, et al. Percutaneous transhepatic bile drainage. *Ann Surg* 1977;185:111–115.
7. Pollock TW, Ring ER, Oleaga JA, et al. Percutaneous decompression of benign and malignant biliary obstruction. *Arch Surg* 1979;114:148–151.
8. Cameron JL, Gayler BW, Zuidema GD. The use of Silastic transhepatic stents in benign and malignant biliary strictures. *Ann Surg* 1978;188:552–559.
9. Molnar W, Stockum AE. Relief of obstructive jaundice through percutaneous transhepatic catheter—a new therapeutic method. *Am J Roentgenol* 1974;122:356–367.
10. Ring EJ, Oleaga JA, Freiman DB, Husted JW, Lunderquist A. Therapeutic applications of catheter cholangiography. *Radiology* 1978;128:333–338.
11. Bonnel D, Ferrucci JT, Mueller PR, Lacaine F, Peterson HF. Surgical and radiological decompression in malignant biliary obstruction: a retrospective study using multivariate risk factor analysis. *Radiology* 1984;152:347–351.
12. D'Agostino HB, vanSonnenberg E, Sanchez RB, Goodacre BW, Casola G. Imaging of the percutaneous cholecystostomy tract: observations and utility. *Radiology* 1991;181:675–678.
13. Mueller PR, Ferrucci JT, Teplick SK, et al. Biliary stent endoprosthesis: analysis of complications in 113 patients. *Radiology* 1985;156:637–639.
14. Dooley JS, Dick R, George P, et al. Percutaneous transhepatic endoprosthesis for bile duct obstruction; complications and results. *Gastroenterology* 1984;86:905–909.
15. Hamlin JA, Friedman M, Stein MG, Bray JF. Percutaneous biliary drainage: complications of 118 consecutive catheterizations. *Radiology* 1986;158:199–202.
16. Lammer J, Neumayer K. Biliary drainage endoprostheses: experience with 201 placements. *Radiology* 1986;159:625–629.
17. Ferrucci JT, Mueller PR, Harbin WP. Percutaneous transhepatic biliary drainage. *Radiology* 1980;135:1–13.
18. Carrasco CH, Zornoza J, Bechtel WJ. Malignant biliary obstruction: complications of percutaneous drainage. *Radiology* 1984;152:343–346.
19. Yee CAN, Ho CS. Complications of percutaneous drainage: benign vs. malignant diseases. *Am J Roentgenol* 1987;148:1207–1209.
20. Davids PHP, Groen AK, Rauws EAJ, Tytgat GNJ, Huibregtse K. Randomized trial of self-expanding metal stents versus polyethylene stents for distal malignant biliary obstruction. *Lancet* 1992;340:1488–1492.
21. Irving JD, Adam A, Dick R, et al. Gianturco expandable metallic biliary stents: results of a European clinical trial. *Radiology* 1989;172:321–326.
22. Lammer J. Biliary endoprostheses: plastic versus metal stents. *Radiol Clin North Am* 1990;28:1211–1222.
23. Berquist TH, May GR, Johnson CM, Adson MA, Thistle JL. Percutaneous biliary decompression: internal and external drainage in 50 patients. *Am J Roentgenol* 1981;136:901–906.
24. Dick BW, Gordon RL, LaBerge JM, Doherty MM, Ring EJ. Percutaneous transhepatic placement in 100 consecutive patients. *J Vasc Interv Radiol* 1990;1:97–100.
25. Gordon RL, Ring EJ, LaBerge JM, Doherty MM. Malignant biliary obstruction: treatment with expandable metallic stents—follow-up of 50 consecutive patients. *Radiology* 1992;182:697–701.
26. Lee MJ, Dawson SL, Mueller PR, et al. Percutaneous management of hilar biliary malignancies with metallic endoprostheses: results, technical problems, and causes of failure. *Radiographics* 1993;3:1249–1263.
27. Martin EC, Laffey KJ, Bixon R, Getrajdman GI. Gianturco-Rosch biliary stents: preliminary experience. *J Vasc Interv Radiol* 1990,1:101–105.
28. Bezzi M, Orsi F, Salvatori FM, Maccioni F, Rossi P. Self-expandable nitinol stent for the management of biliary obstruction: long-term clinical results. *J Vasc Interv Radiol* 1994;5:287–293.
29. Oikarinen H, Leinonen S, Karttunen A, et al. Patency and complications of percutaneously inserted metallic stents in malignant biliary obstruction. *J Vasc Interv Radiol* 1999;10:1387–1393.
30. Becker CD, Glattli A, Maibach R, Baer HU. Percutaneous palliation of malignant obstructive jaundice with the Wallstent endoprosthesis: follow-up and reintervention in patients with hilar and non-hilar obstruction. *J Vasc Interv Radiol* 1993;4:597–604.
31. Mathieson JR, McLoughlin RF, Cooperberg PL, et al. Malignant obstruction of the common bile duct: long-term results of Gianturco-Rosch metal stents used as initial treatment. *Radiology* 1994;192:663–667.
32. Boguth L, Tatalovic S, Antonucci F, et al. Malignant biliary obstruction: clinical and histopathologic correlation after treatment with self-expanding metal prostheses. *Radiology* 1994;192:669–674.
33. Lee MJ, Dawson SL, Mueller PR, et al. Failed metallic biliary stents: causes and management of delayed complications. *Clin Radiol* 1994;49:857–862.
34. Han Y, Hwang S, Lee J, Kim C. Metallic stents for the palliative treatment in malignant biliary obstruction: long-term clinical results in 84 patients. Poster presented at: SCVIR 2001 Annual Meeting; March 3–8, 2001; San Antonio, TX.
35. Rossi P, Bezzi M, Salvatorio FM, Maccioni F, Porcaro ML. Recurrent benign biliary strictures: management with self-expanding stents. *Radiology* 1990;175:661–665.
36. Savader SJ, Prescott CA, Lund GB, Osterman FA. Intraductal biopsy: comparison of three techniques. *J Vasc Interv Radiol* 1996;7:743–750.
37. Tamada K, Satoh Y, Tomiyama T, et al. Multiple bile duct biopsies using a sheath with a side port. *Am J Roentgenol* 2001;176:797–802.
38. Kuvshinoff BW, Armstrong JG, Fong Y, et al. Palliation of irresectable hilar cholangiocarcinoma with biliary drainage and radiotherapy. *Br J Surg* 1995;82:1522–1525.
39. Eschelman DJ, Shapiro MJ, Bonn J, et al. Malignant biliary duct obstruction: long-term experience with Gianturco stents and combined modality radiation therapy. *Radiology* 1996;200:717–724.
40. Golfieri R, Giampalma E, Muzzi C, et al. Unresectable hilar cholangiocarcinoma: combined percutaneous and radiotherapeutic treatment. *Radiol Med* 2001;101:495–502.
41. Shinchi H, Takao S, Nishida H, Aikou T. Length and quality of survival following external beam radiotherapy combined with expandable metallic stent for unresectable hilar cholangiocarcinoma. *J Surg Oncol* 2000;75:95–97.

CHAPTER 22

GENITOURINARY OBSTRUCTION

MICHAEL S. STECKER, MD
NILESH H. PATEL, MD
RICHARD BIHRLE, MD

INTRODUCTION

Intervention is commonly required for genitourinary (GU) obstruction due to pelvic neoplastic disease, such as bladder, prostate, or cervical carcinoma, as well as retroperitoneal malignancy. Genitourinary obstruction may also result as a complication of treatment for genitourinary neoplasm, including anastomotic strictures after cystectomy with creation of a neobladder and as a sequela of radiotherapy. These obstructions may result in decline in renal function, infection, and/or pain. The level of obstruction (proximal, mid-, or distal ureter; bladder outlet; urethra) and the cause influence both the immediate treatment and the long-term management of patients with GU obstruction. For example, in the setting of prior surgical resection, tumor recurrence must be excluded first before a patient is treated for a postoperative anastomotic stricture.

PERCUTANEOUS NEPHROSTOMY

The preferred treatment for ureteral obstruction is retrograde stenting performed via cystoscopy.[1] Although this approach may be more comfortable for the patient and obviates external drainage, it is not always successful. Percutaneous nephrostomy, commonly performed for GU obstruction, was introduced in 1955.[2] In more than half of patients referred for percutaneous nephrostomy, the indication is related to malignancy.[3] In these patients, ureteral obstruction may be due to primary GU malignancy (urothelial or prostatic carcinoma), extrinsic malignancy (cervical carcinoma, retroperitoneal malignancy or adenopathy), or prior treatment of malignant disease (obstructed ureteral stents and anastomotic strictures).

Percutaneous nephrostomy may also occasionally be helpful in the management of patients with obstruction distal to the ureter, particularly when the bladder does not function normally or is severely diseased, as in patients with advanced bladder or prostate malignancy. Also, percutaneous nephrostomy is particularly useful in the setting of GU obstruction resulting in severe infection, because it allows direct drainage of the infection without an internalized foreign body.

Several studies of the use of percutaneous nephrostomy in oncology patients have been reported. Chiou et al.[4] reviewed 37 patients with ureteral obstruction due to prostate cancer, 26 of whom had bilateral obstruction, who were treated with percutaneous nephrostomy. Overall, these researchers found a median survival time of 21 months with 57% survival at 1 year and 29% survival at 2 years. Of the 12 patients with severe renal failure before the procedure, 75% showed satisfactory return of renal function (defined as serum creatinine level less than 3 mg/dL).

Chapman and Reid[5] reported a series of 17 patients who underwent percutaneous nephrostomy because of renal failure due to malignant ureteral obstruction by a variety of primary neoplasms. They found that renal function improved in 88% of cases but that performance of bilateral nephrostomy was of no greater benefit than a unilateral procedure. The median survival time was only 18 weeks, and the tubes were well tolerated by the patients. At the other end of the spectrum, Hoe et al.[6] found that 15 of their 22 patients had a satisfactory quality of life after uroradiologic intervention. However, in all but 2 patients, only unilateral nephrostomy was performed, even if bilateral obstruction was present. Median survival time for the patients in this study was 19 weeks.

Watkinson et al.[1] reported their results in 50 patients who underwent percutaneous nephrostomy for renal failure resulting from advanced abdominopelvic malignancy. The patients were divided into the following four study groups: (1) those with renal obstruction caused by a nonmalignant complication as a result of previous surgery or radiotherapy (n = 8), (2) those with renal obstruction due to untreated primary malignancy (n = 16), (3) those with renal obstruction from relapsed disease for which there was a viable treatment option (n = 8), and (4) those with relapsed disease for which there was no viable treatment option (n = 18). No significant benefit was found when nephrostomy was used as a palliative measure without a definitive treatment plan for the relapsed disease; the median survival time in this subgroup of 18 patients was only 38 days, compared with 339 days for patients who had not previously received treatment for their malignancies and 334 days for those with disease recurrence for which there was a viable treatment option.

Lau et al.[7] studied 95 patients who underwent percutaneous nephrostomy for treatment of hydronephrosis with impaired renal function due to newly diagnosed or previously treated pelvic malignant disease. Only 1 patient did not experience return of serum creatinine level to normal within 2 weeks. Overall, median survival time was 26 weeks, with 30% of patients surviving at 2 years. As with previous studies, the median survival time in the group of patients with recurrent malignant disease for which no further treatment was available was only 6.5 weeks, and no patients survived beyond 1 year. The subgroup of patients with bladder cancer had a median survival time of 2 years with a 42% survival at 5 years.

In summary, percutaneous nephrostomy for treatment of malignant ureteral obstruction is very useful for infectious complications and for obstructive renal failure. However, its use in advanced disease remains somewhat controversial. Patients with ureteral obstruction due to recurrent disease for whom there is no viable treatment option for the underlying malignancy have poor prognosis, with median survival time on the order of 1.3–6.5 weeks.[1, 7] Some authorities advocate initial drainage of the more symptomatic or less hydronephrotic kidney, and performing drainage of the contralateral side only if renal function does not recover or if infection develops.[7] One must keep in mind, however, that all of the described studies were retrospective analyses of heterogeneous populations having various underlying malignancies. There have been no large, controlled studies to demonstrate which patients would derive the most benefit from percutaneous nephrostomy. Therefore, each patient must be evaluated and treated on an individual basis.

Technique

The percutaneous nephrostomy procedure has been detailed elsewhere in this series of syllabi (*SCVIR Syllabus: Thoracic and Visceral Nonvascular Interventions—Genitourinary Interventions*)[8]; our techniques are summarized here (**Fig. 22-1**). Most patients can undergo percutaneous nephrostomy place-

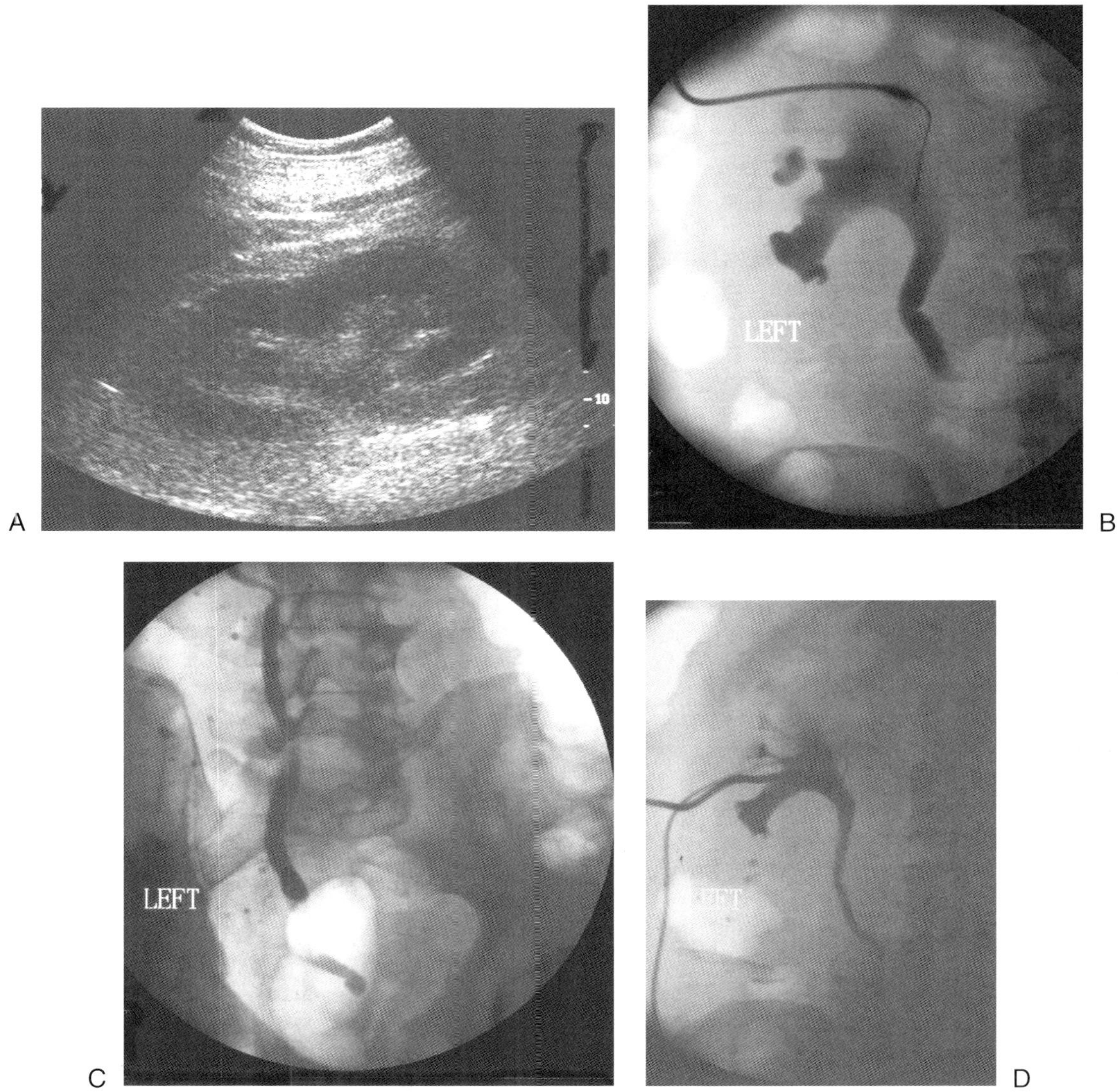

Figure 22-1. Percutaneous nephrostomy performed in a patient with obstructive uropathy due to metastatic prostate carcinoma. (A) Longitudinal ultrasound image demonstrates moderate hydronephrosis of left kidney. (B) Antegrade pyelogram also demonstrates moderate hydronephrosis and hydroureter. Calyces are easily visualized to facilitate definitive nephrostomy puncture. (C) Distal ureteral obstruction seen on pelvic image. (D) Nephrostomy tube placed via posterior interpolar calyx, with pigtail formed in renal pelvis.

ment under conscious sedation, generally with intravenous midazolam and fentanyl, and local anesthesia with lidocaine. However, patients who have difficulty lying prone, such as those with respiratory compromise or morbid obesity, may greatly benefit from the use of general anesthesia.

All patients undergoing percutaneous nephrostomy who are not already receiving therapeutic antibiotics should be given prophylactic antibiotics.[9] We use a combination of intravenous ampicillin and ceftriaxone. For patients known to have penicillin or cephalosporin allergy, levofloxacin is administered instead. Any coagulopathy should be corrected. If abnormal coagulation parameters cannot be successfully corrected, the procedure may be performed during the administration of fresh-frozen plasma or platelets.

Placement of percutaneous nephrostomy can generally be divided into two main steps, (1) visualization of the renal collecting system and (2) subsequent puncture of an appropriate calyx. The first step may be facilitated by the presence of residual contrast material in the renal collecting system in patients who have recently undergone intravenous pyelography or have recently been given intravenous contrast material for computed tomography (CT). Otherwise, an antegrade pyelogram is performed by puncture of the collecting system with a 21- or 22-gauge Chiba needle, with fluoroscopy or ultrasonography (US) used as guidance, to evaluate the anatomy, level of obstruction, and planning for access to a specific calyx. A posterior calyx is preferred. The posterior calyces can be highlighted by injection of small amounts of carbon dioxide through the pyelography needle. This procedure should be observed fluoroscopically as the gas bubble moves into the calyx, because gas in a calyx can sometimes be difficult to differentiate from overlying bowel gas. Injection of air instead of carbon dioxide should be avoided, because inadvertent air embolism may result in cardiopulmonary collapse.[10]

When a suitable calyx is identified, it is entered with either an 18-gauge trocar needle and 0.035-inch floppy-tipped guidewire or a 21-gauge needle and 0.018-inch mandril guidewire (Jeffrey set [Cook, Inc., Bloomington, Indiana], Neff set [Cook, Inc.], Accustick II introducer system [Boston Scientific Medi-Tech, Watertown, Massachusetts]). With the 21-gauge needle and 0.018-inch guidewire, a coaxial introducer is used to allow conversion to a 0.035-inch guidewire system.

In patients with coagulopathy and/or thrombocytopenia that does not respond to correction, direct puncture of a suitable calyx may be performed with high-resolution US guidance while appropriate blood products are administered concurrently.[11] Frequently, this procedure allows placement of the nephrostomy with a single puncture of the kidney, being successful on initial attempt in 96.3% of cases and after a second attempt in 98.5%.[11]

Barbaric et al.[12] have described CT guidance for puncture coupled with C-arm fluoroscopy for patients who cannot be positioned prone.[12] These authors report a 99% (100 of 101 attempts) success rate in native kidneys with patients positioned in a supine-oblique position. CT helps avoid the colon, spleen, and liver, which may be more vulnerable to injury in this more lateral approach.[12] No major complications were encountered, and minor complications (mild transient chills) occurred in only 3% of patients in this series. The use of CT-fluoroscopy has also been described for percutaneous nephrostomy tube placement.[13] The procedure was successful in 86.7% of patients, requiring a single puncture in 83.3% of cases and resulting in few complications.[13]

Once adequate access has been obtained, the tract is dilated over a stiff guidewire, and a locking pigtail drainage catheter is placed (**Fig. 22-2**). We prefer tubes at least 10F in size, as we have found them to drain better and to have a lower occlusion rate than smaller tubes. The catheter pigtail is formed in the renal pelvis and locked in place. Then the catheter is flushed, secured in place by affixing to the skin with suture material, and attached to a drainage bag.

After the procedure, patients should be observed for at least 6 hours. Many patients undergoing the procedure, however, have an underlying illness that would make outpatient nephrostomy less desirable,[14] such as hypertension, urinary tract infection, coagulopathy, or large staghorn calculi.[14, 15] We discharge some patients after the 6-hour observation period if they are comfortable and the urine is nearly clear. Additionally, another responsible adult should be at home with any patient who is discharged after this procedure. Occasionally, patients must be admitted to the hospital for delayed complications.[14] Patients in whom the urine continues to appear bloody, who have moderate to severe pain, or in whom infection is likely should be observed at least overnight and until clinically stable.

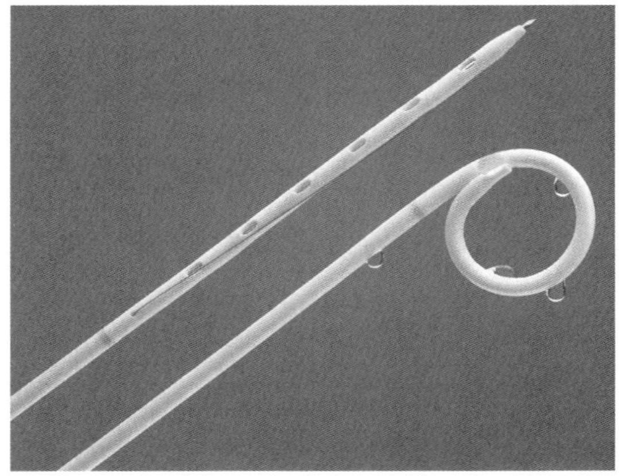

Figure 22-2. Percutaneous nephrostomy drainage catheter on its trocar-stylet delivery system and locked pigtail configuration.

Patients should be instructed in care of the tube, including twice daily flushes. Over-the-wire preventive maintenance changes of nephrostomy tubes should be performed every 3 months to avoid catheter dysfunction and deterioration. Some patients may require more frequent changes, and others may tolerate longer intervals between changes. All preventive maintenance tube changes can be performed on an outpatient basis with the use of mild conscious sedation and prophylactic antibiotics.

Once a ureteral obstruction is relieved by percutaneous nephrostomy, this access may be used for long-term urinary drainage, placement of a ureteral stent, stricture dilation, ureteral biopsy, and direct chemotherapy infusion. Infection and post-procedure bleeding must be resolved before additional interventions are performed via the nephrostomy access.[9]

URETERAL INTERVENTIONS

Ureteral obstruction due to malignancy may be caused by invasion or compression by an adjacent primary tumor, by local recurrence of a previously treated tumor, by compression due to malignant lymphadenopathy or retroperitoneal fibrosis, or as a complication of surgery or radiotherapy.

Internal Double-J Ureteral Stents

Patients with ureteral obstruction who wish to avoid an external drainage catheter may be candidates for double-J ureteral stents. These devices are completely internal, with a proximal J or pigtail in the renal pelvis and a distal J or pigtail in the bladder; each end contains multiple side-holes for urine flow. The pigtails keep the stent from migrating proximally or distally. One should keep in mind that if the bladder is extensively diseased and does not function normally (e.g., owing to extensive tumor involvement or radiation scarring), a patient may be better served by a percutaneous nephrostomy. In properly selected patients, however, ureteral stents may be better than percutaneous nephrostomy, because of easier home care, reduced risk of infection, and avoidance of accidental removal.[16]

In a study comparing 21 patients who had double-J ureteral stents with 13 patients who had percutaneous nephrostomies (although none for malignant obstruction), 62% of the nephrostomy patients had problems with leakage of the gravity drainage bags, and 33% had difficulty managing the drainage bags.[17] However, there were significantly higher rates of urinary symptoms (hematuria, dysuria, urgency, urinary frequency) in the stent group. Discomfort may result from stents that are too long, extending far into the bladder and causing trigonal irritation resulting in dysuria.[18] The discomfort may be less with stents made from newer, softer polymers.[19] Conversely, a stent that is that is too short may not function properly because of an insufficient number of side-holes in the renal pelvis or bladder. Complications of indwelling double-J ureteral stents include migration, reflux, infection, and erosion.[20]

There is some evidence that patients with malignancy should be treated with external drainage; a study reported by Docimo and Dewolf[21] suggests that the results of ureteral stenting in such patients are poor. In that study, the stents in 45% of patients who had extrinsic ureteral obstruction (not all due to malignancy) became occluded within 30 days; the stents in these patients, however, were only 6F–7F.[21] Harding[18] specifically studied antegrade ureteral stenting for malignant obstructions. Stent insertion was attempted in 37 ureters of 25 patients, with a 92% technical success rate.[18] Although the stents used were larger (8F) and made of a more urine-compatible material than those in Docimo and DeWolf's study,[21] the Harding study[18] involved no follow-up of the patients to assess patency rates. Using the same stents as Harding,[18] Lu et al.[22] attempted to place 37 stents for malignant ureteral obstruction and were successful in 95% of cases. Interestingly, they noted that retrograde placement of the stent via cystography had been attempted and had failed in 28 ureters. For the 44 total stents placed in their study (9 were for benign disease), the 3-month patency rate was 95%, and the 6-month rate was 54%, much better than the rates reported by Docimo and Dewolf.[21]

Watson and Patel[23] evaluated primary placement of ureteral stents (placement of a ureteral stent without an initial interval of decompression with a percutaneous nephrostomy) in hemodynamically stable patients in whom there was no suspicion of active infection. They achieved technical success in 84% of the 50 ureters so treated; 72% of the 38 patients studied had obstruction due to malignant disease. A subsequent attempt was successful in 7 of the 8 ureters in which the initial attempt at stent placement failed. It is noteworthy that although most of the 22 patients with preprocedure elevations in serum creatinine showed improvement after stent placement, the serum creatinine level returned completely to normal in only 10 patients.

Ureteral stents made of urine-compatible polymers have demonstrated improved patency, even beyond 6 months.[19, 24] Additionally, stent patency may be extended by encouraging greater oral fluid intake to increase urine flow, administration of prophylactic antibiotics, and avoiding placement of stents into ureters that are infected, contain blood clots, or have sanguineous output.[24]

Technique

Retrograde Double-J Ureteral Stenting. In most patients, double-J ureteral stent placement is most easily and expeditiously accomplished with the use of cystoscopic guidance and a retrograde, transurethral approach. This approach allows for a one-step procedure and obviates the risks associated with percutaneous puncture of the kidney. However, because rigid cystoscopy is used in most instances, general anesthesia is required. Furthermore, in patients with distal ureteral involvement that includes the bladder trigone, the ureteral orifice may be difficult or impossible to visualize. Similar technical challenge is present in patients with surgical urinary diversions. Difficulty may also be encountered if the stricture is very severe or the ureter is extremely tortuous.

Babel and Winterkorn[25] have described an alternative technique of fluoroscopically guided, transurethral

A, B 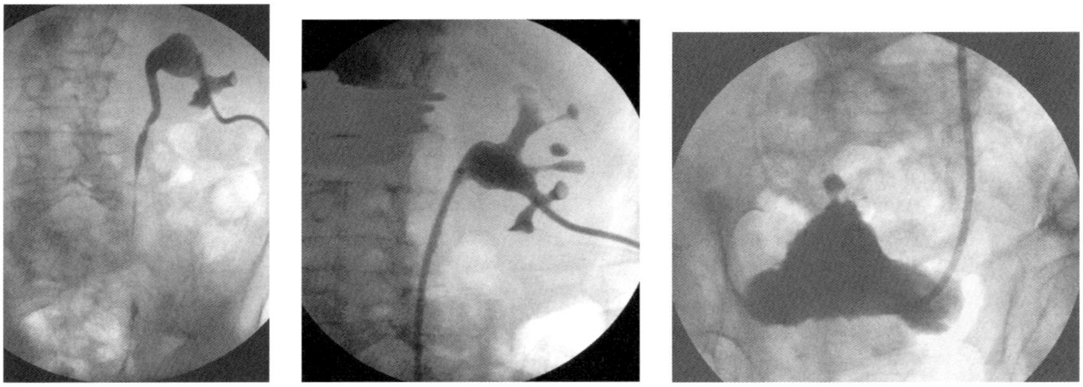 C

Figure 22-3. Antegrade double-J stent placement performed in a patient with obstructive uropathy due to metastatic prostatic carcinoma. (A) Nephrostogram demonstrates previously placed percutaneous nephrostomy tube. Irregular distal ureteral narrowing was persistent on multiple images and under fluoroscopy. (B) Proximal pigtail of a double-J stent is in the renal pelvis, and an Amplatz Anchor catheter maintains percutaneous access until function of the stent is confirmed. (C) Distal pigtail of double-J stent in mildly trabeculated bladder.

retrograde catheterization of the ureter. In their small series, the procedure was successful in five of seven patients, three of whom had malignant obstruction. In patients in whom ureteral catheterization was successful, fluoroscopy time was only about 3 minutes. Furthermore, ureteral stents were placed via this approach in three of the five patients.

Antegrade Double-J Ureteral Stenting. Percutaneous antegrade placement of ureteral stents was first described in 1979.[26] This technique is generally reserved for patients in whom cystoscopic placement is unsuccessful or is deemed to have a low likelihood of success because of patient characteristics (e.g., known tumor involvement of the bladder, surgical urinary diversion). Antegrade ureteral stenting is generally performed as a two-stage procedure, in which decompression and relief of obstruction are initially performed through the placement of a percutaneous nephrostomy, and a ureteral stent is subsequently placed to allow internal drainage. However, some authorities advocate primary placement of a ureteral stent at the time of the initial procedure.[23]

The antegrade double-J ureteral stent procedure has been detailed elsewhere in this series of syllabi (*SCVIR Syllabus*: *Thoracic and Visceral Nonvascular Interventions—Genitourinary Interventions*)[27]; our techniques are summarized here (**Fig. 22-3**). The existing nephrostomy tube is removed over a guidewire, and a percutaneous sheath is placed to maintain access. Leaving a safety wire in the renal collecting system is helpful. To avoid buckling in the renal pelvis, entry via a mid- or upper pole calyx is advantageous.[27] A directional catheter, such as a Berenstein catheter (Angiodynamics, Inc., Queensbury, New York), in conjunction with a hydrophilic guidewire, such as a Roadrunner (Cook, Inc., Bloomington, Indiana) or Glidewire Terumo Medical Corporation, Somerset, NJ (distributed by Boston Scientific/Medi-Tech), is used to navigate down the ureter and cross the stricture or obstruction. The torquable hydrophilic guidewire is particularly helpful for traversing very tortuous ureters. Intermittent injection of contrast material through the catheter may facilitate this procedure.

When the lesion is crossed, the catheter is advanced to the bladder, and its location is confirmed by injection of contrast material. The distance from the ureteropelvic junction (UPJ) to the ureterovesical junction (UVJ) should be measured, so that the correct length stent may be chosen. A stiffer guidewire is then placed, such as an Amplatz Super Stiff (Boston Scientific Corp.), which provides extra support, and the stent is advanced. A hydrophilic coating on the stent further aids in advancing it across the stricture. If necessary, use of a peel-away sheath may provide added support.

Occasionally, the ureteral narrowing may have to be dilated with an angioplasty balloon 5 or 6 mm in diameter. We generally place a 10F double-J ureteral stent, but if it will not pass despite ureteroplasty, we place an 8.5F double-J ureteral stent (**Fig. 22-4A**). The distal (bladder end), then proximal (renal pelvis end), pigtails are formed by withdrawing of the stent stiffener and guidewire (**Fig. 22-4B**). Over the safety wire, a nephrostomy tube is replaced, and stent patency is confirmed with injection of contrast material. We generally prefer to use a nonpigtail catheter, such as an Amplatz Anchor (Boston Scientific/Medi-Tech), so that it does not get caught on the ureteral stent pigtail and is therefore easier to remove.

The external drainage catheter is capped overnight and is not flushed. If the patient remains afebrile, with good urine output and no flank pain, the external drainage catheter is removed the next morning after injection of contrast material to verify patency of the ureteral stent. If blood clot is present in the renal pelvis,

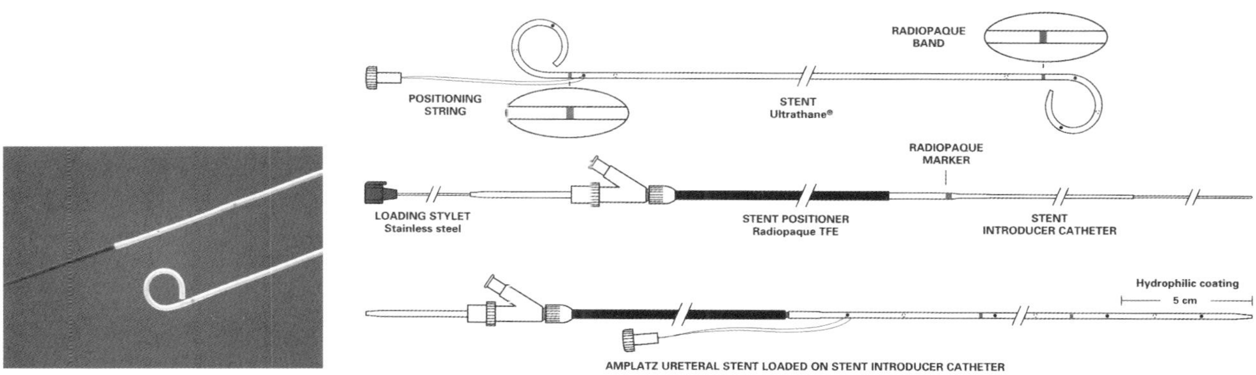

A B

Figure 22-4. Internal double-J ureteral stent. (A) Schematic drawing of stent, which has both a distal J and a proximal J (or pigtail). (B) Stent mounted on delivery system; when released, its proximal J or pigtail is formed.

as a result of a somewhat traumatic ureteral stent placement, the capped external drainage catheter is left in place. External drainage may be needed if the patient becomes symptomatic because of obstruction of the ureteral stent. The external drainage catheter may be removed after the blood clot has been naturally lysed by the patient's urine flow.

Double-J ureteral stents should be changed every 3–6 months to prevent occlusion. The exchange is generally accomplished via cystoscopy. However, an alternative technique using fluoroscopy has been described.[28, 29] This technique involves grasping the tip of the bladder end of the ureteral stent with an Amplatz Goose Neck snare (Microvena Corp., White Bear Lake, Minnesota) and withdrawing it out the urethra. The stent can then be changed over a guidewire. If the guidewire will not exit out the renal pelvis end of the ureteral stent, a long peel-away sheath can be applied over the stent and the exchange performed through it. This technique was successful in 97% of 161 patients in one study.[29] The procedure may be more technically challenging and may produce more discomfort in men, in whom the urethra is longer and prostatic enlargement may be present.[28, 29] However, this technique may be advantageous for patients in whom cystoscopy is difficult or fails or who are poor candidates for general anesthesia.[28]

Antegrade Nephroureteral Stents

Alternatives to double-J ureteral stents are antegrade nephroureteral stents. These devices allow for internal drainage while maintaining percutaneous access to the renal collecting system. The catheter traverses the skin and renal parenchyma into the renal collecting system, where there are proximal side-holes, then continues down the ureter and across the stricture or occlusion into the bladder, where there are distal side-holes. Antegrade nephroureteral stents are particularly useful for short-term stenting after performance of percutaneous ureteroplasty, because they hold open the ureteral lumen and maintain percutaneous access to the renal collecting system for subsequent procedures. They may also be advantageous in patients who cannot or do not wish to undergo repeated ureteral stent exchanges via cystoscopy.

Technique

Placement of nephroureteral stents is very similar to placement of antegrade double-J ureteral stents, with modifications as described here. After the lesion is crossed and the bladder is entered, the distance from the renal pelvis to the urinary bladder is measured. Subsequently, side-holes are created along the shaft of a nonlocking, pigtail, 10F–12F biliary-urinary drainage (BUD) catheter (Boston Scientific Corp.) to the measured pelvis-bladder distance. The nephroureteral stent is advanced over a stiff guidewire with the pigtail in the urinary bladder. Alternatively, one can use a nephroureteral stent with proximal and distal pigtails, which are formed in the renal pelvis and urinary bladder, respectively (**Fig. 22-5**). Then the catheter is capped to allow internal drainage.

The patient is instructed to flush the catheter twice daily with sterile water to help maintain stent patency. The catheters should undergo preventive maintenance changes every 3 months to avoid complications of tube clogging and deterioration. As with percutaneous nephrostomy tubes, catheter changes can be performed on an outpatient basis with local anesthetic and mild conscious sedation.

Retrograde Nephroureteral Stents

In patients who have undergone cystectomy for malignancy with creation of an ileal conduit, anas-

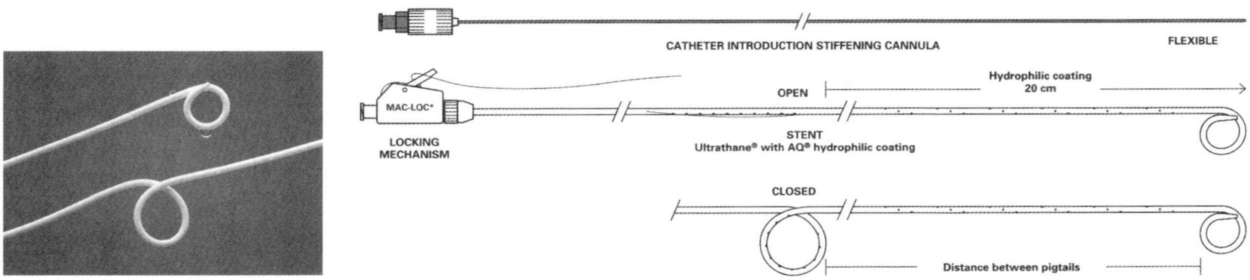

A B

Figure 22-5. Nephroureteral stent. (A) Schematic drawing of stent; note both a distal and a proximal pigtail. (B) The actual configuration of the distal and proximal pigtails.

tomotic strictures that develop and cause obstruction can frequently be treated with a retrograde nephroureteral stent. A nephroureteral stent can be placed in a retrograde fashion through the stoma, via the ileal conduit, up the ureter, and into the renal pelvis. The procedure, which can be performed under fluoroscopic guidance, was first described by Rosen et al.[30] in 1980. The technique involves catheterization of the ureter in a retrograde fashion, which completely avoids percutaneous puncture of the kidney.[31] However, some contrast material must reflux into the distal ureter; otherwise, the procedure can be extremely difficult, because the ureteral orifice is not identifiable for catheterization.[32]

We do not place nephroureteral stents in patients who have continent urostomies, because the tube may cause dysfunction of the continence mechanism, and stomal obstruction has been described in such patients.[31] Placement of retrograde nephroureteral stent has several benefits over other techniques. First, the stent drains into the existing urostomy bag and does not require an additional drainage bag. Also, the urostomy bag protects the stent from inadvertent removal. Second, no drainage tube protrudes out of the patient's back, which is cosmetically more appealing. Third, the patient may not require percutaneous puncture of the kidney and the risks associated with that procedure. Last but not least, retrograde nephroureteral stents tend not to become blocked by the mucus produced in the ileal conduit, as antegrade nephroureteral stents or double-J ureteral stents do.[32]

This last issue is of particular importance, because at least two deaths have been reported as a consequence of stent blockage.[33] In 9 of the 10 patients reported by Applbaum et al.,[32] carcinoma of pelvic organs was the primary indication for cystectomy with urinary diversion, and 5 of them required intervention for stricture or obstruction. Nineteen of 25 (76%) retrograde ureteral catheterizations were successful (some patients underwent more than one attempt), and there were no complications. Banner et al.[34] reported success with retrograde catheterization in 12 of 14 ureters (86%), but they did not attempt catheterization if the ureter did not show reflux on loopography. In their series of 14 patients, Zaleski et al.[31] reported 95% success (21 of 22 ureters) in placement of retrograde nephroureteral stents; however only 54% of the placements were successful from a "purely" retrograde approach.

Technique

The patient is placed supine on the fluoroscopy table, and the urostomy site is prepared and draped in a sterile fashion. A Foley catheter with the very tip cut off, to allow passage of a 5F diagnostic catheter, is placed into the conduit, and the balloon is inflated to prevent urinary leakage. Alternatively, a 10F or larger flexible percutaneous sheath (e.g., Arrow Percutaneous Sheath, Arrow International Corp., Reading, Pennsylvania) may be used if there is not much leakage around it. Contrast material is injected through the Foley catheter or percutaneous sheath to opacify the conduit and ureteroenteric anastomosis. The ureteroenteric anastomosis is catheterized with an angle-tip diagnostic catheter and hydrophilic guidewire combination. The catheter and guidewire are advanced up the ureter, across the stricture, and into the renal pelvis. We place a 10F–12F biliary-urinary drainage (BUD) catheter without extra sideholes, and we believe that a locking pigtail is not necessary. This catheter is advanced over a 0.035-inch stiff guidewire, the pigtail is positioned in the renal pelvis, and the distal end of the catheter is placed in the patient's urostomy bag.

If the ureter proximal to the severe stricture or occlusion cannot be visualized by reflux of contrast material, "blind" probing with the angle-tip catheter and hydrophilic guidewire can be performed. If probing is not successful, antegrade access to the renal collecting system for introduction of a guidewire may be attempted.[30, 31] For this procedure, the patient is rotated into a decubital position with the affected kidney up, and the flank is prepared and draped in a sterile fashion. With the use of US guidance and local anesthesia, the collecting system is punctured with a 21-gauge Chiba needle, and an antegrade pyelogram is performed (**Fig. 22-6**). Under fluoroscopic guidance, a 0.018-inch guidewire is advanced through the needle, down the ureter, across the stricture, and into the conduit. The guidewire is manipulated so that it exits the urostomy. In some instances, an Amplatz Goose Neck snare may be introduced through the urostomy so as to capture the distal tip of the wire and pull it out through the urostomy. A diagnostic catheter is then advanced over this wire in a retrograde fashion via the urostomy to the renal pelvis. The 0.018-inch guidewire is removed, and a 0.035-inch stiff guidewire is introduced through the catheter into the renal pelvis.

Alternatively, if the initial retrograde placement is unsuccessful, a percutaneous nephrostomy is placed to allow decompression of the collecting system and resolution of edema at the stricture. Another retrograde stent placement may be attempted, by introduction of an antegrade guidewire as discussed previously.

Retrograde nephroureteral stents may be flushed daily to preserve patency and should be exchanged every 3 months as a preventive maintenance measure.

Metallic Stenting Of Ureteral Narrowings

Plastic ureteral stents may fail as a result of obstruction from encrustation, debris, tumoral compression, and tumor ingrowth,[35] because of their small internal caliber, and from other complications, including infection, dislocation, and discomfort.[36] With the hope of circumventing some of these shortcomings, metallic stents have been evaluated for use in the upper urinary tract. Theoretically, metallic stents would become incorporated into the ureteral wall,[37] protecting them from encrustation. Metallic stents can be introduced into the ureter through a small-diameter antegrade percutaneous access or via a retrograde cystoscopic access. Furthermore, they can be expanded to diameters much larger than those of polyurethane and silicone ureteral stents, possibly improving patency. Because these stents treat the obstructing lesion itself, it is hoped that they might permit more physiologic urine flow.[37] Also, once expanded, they may serve not only as conduits but also as a buttress to open the ureter, a quality lacking with plastic stents.[38]

Wallstents (Boston Scientific Corp.) are the most described metallic stents used in the ureters. Their use was first reported by Lugmayr and Pauer[37] in 1992, in a series of 23 patients with 30 malignant ureteral obstructions. The technical success rate was 97%; however, 4 patients required additional metallic stents, and 5 patients needed subsequent placement of double-J ureteral stents. After a hyperplastic urothelial reaction to the Wallstents was noted to produce a temporary obstruction in the first 3 patients, polyurethane double-J ureteral stents were placed coaxially for 4 weeks in the remaining patients. The primary patency rate was 83% after 30 weeks, with a mean follow-up time of 31 weeks.

Flueckiger et al.[39] also reported the use of 7-mm-diameter Wallstents in 13 ureters in 10 patients with malignant ureteral obstruction, all of whom subsequently underwent chemotherapy or radiotherapy. Because of luminal encroachment due to urothelial reaction within 2 weeks of follow-up, double-J ureteral stents were subsequently placed in 4 ureters. Obstruction developed in a fifth ureter at 1 month, which was successfully treated by

A,B

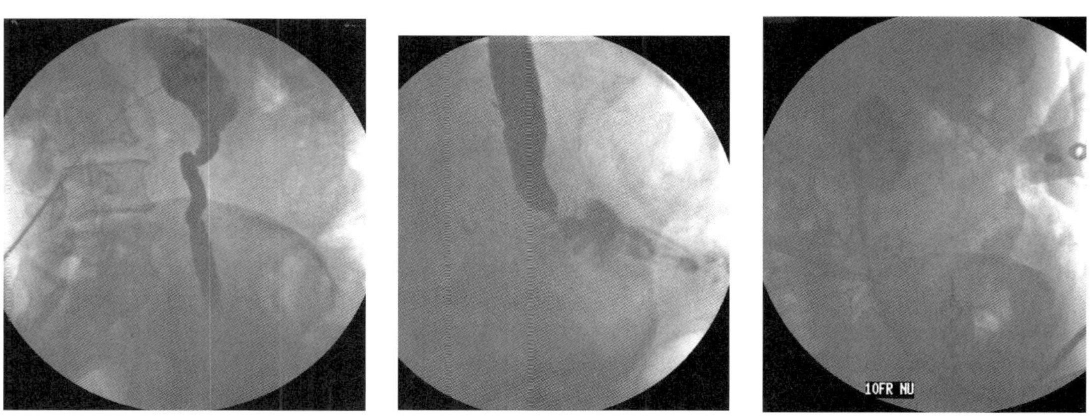

C

Figure 22-6. Retrograde nephroureteral stent placement performed in a patient with transitional cell carcinoma of the bladder, who had previously undergone cystoprostatectomy and ileal conduit creation. (A) Because there was no reflux of contrast material up the right ureter on prior loopogram, the kidney was punctured percutaneously, and antegrade pyelogram was performed. (B) Nearly occlusive ureteral anastomotic stenosis. A guidewire was then advanced antegrade through this access, across the stenosis, and into the conduit. Over the wire, a nephroureteral stent was inserted in a retrograde fashion. (C) Retrograde 10F stent in place with pigtail in renal pelvis.

placement of a retrograde double-J ureteral stent. Another ureter with a patent stent showed further narrowing due to lymphadenopathy proximal to the stent, requiring placement of a double-J ureteral stent. Although 1 ureter, including the distal end of the stented segment, was invaded by a local recurrence of tumor at 9 months, the stent lumen remained patent. Six ureters remained completely patent without additional stent placement at a mean of 5.5 months of follow-up. Flueckiger et al.[39] noted that ureteral peristalsis was no longer present in the stented segments but was preserved both above and below them.

Nine ureters with malignant obstruction in 6 patients who had incurable malignancies were treated with 10-mm-diameter Wallstents by vanSonnenberg et al.[38] Hydronephrosis and elevations of serum creatinine improved in all patients. Five patients underwent endoluminal US imaging during follow-up, which showed all stents to have intraluminal debris; the debris was better demonstrated with US imaging than with contrast pyelography. Two patients required placement of double-J ureteral stents through the metallic stents. Diaz-Lucas et al.[35] placed Wallstents in 14 ureters in 8 patients who had malignant ureteral obstruction. These researchers placed a Wallstent only after an 8F nephroureteral stent was successfully placed and then tolerated for at least 1 week. They used Wallstents ranging from 6 to 10 mm in diameter. Although specific survival rates are not given, 2 of the patents in this series lived for 4 years after stent placement.

One of the largest studies of Wallstents was conducted by Lugmayr and Pauer,[36] who treated 40 patients with 54 malignant ureteral obstructions. In all of these patients, the function of successfully placed double-J ureteral stents was unsatisfactory. Most of the ureters were stented in a retrograde fashion, and all patients received 7-mm-diameter Wallstents. To prevent temporary obstruction due to the initial mucosal hyperplasia that has been noted to occur after placement of metallic stents, Lugmayr and Pauer[36] placed 6F double-J ureteral stents coaxially for 4 weeks. Three ureters became occluded because of rapid tumor progression and were not treated further. The primary patency rates at 6 months and 12 months were 64% and 31%, respectively, with a median patency duration of 6 months. With additional interventions, the median patency duration was extended to 12.7 months. The median survival time for these patients after stent implantation was 8.8 months. Additional interventions were required in 26 ureters (48%), consisting of additional Wallstents in 11 patients and double-J ureteral stents in 12 patients because of tumor ingrowth. Tumor ingrowth in 5 other ureters was removed endoscopically. Encrustation was seen in 3 ureters, primarily at sites where the stent had not incorporated into the ureteral wall owing to poor apposition. The researchers observed that the early temporary mucosal reaction might be less pronounced in patients who have previously received radiation treatment to the area.

Barbalias et al.[40] evaluated the knitted tantalum balloon-expandable Strecker stent (Boston Scientific Corp.) and the nitinol self-expanding Accuflex stent (Medical Engineering Corp., New York, New York) each in six patients with malignant ureteral obstruction, which was bilateral in two patients. Four ureters required subsequent placement of another stent for various reasons. The other ureters remained patent during the follow-up period.

In a patient with proximal ureteral obstruction due to retroperitoneal lymphadenopathy from colonic carcinoma, Bosanac et al.[41] described the antegrade placement of a VascuCoil self-expanding metal spring stent (Medtronic, Minneapolis, MN) 4 weeks after initial percutaneous nephrostomy. They noted normal peristalsis across the stented segment with unimpeded flow of contrast material. No hydronephrosis was seen on US up to 12 months after the procedure.

Unfortunately, all of the preceding studies involved malignant obstruction with mixed causes. Lopez-Martinez et al.[42] reported their experience in 8 patients (12 ureters) with ureteral strictures due to prostate adenocarcinoma that were treated with Wallstents. Double-J ureteral stents were placed coaxially for 4 weeks and subsequently removed cystoscopically. Average duration of patency for the Wallstents was 19 months. All 6 patients who survived to 12 months had patent stents, compared with 3 of 5 at 24 months, 2 of 2 at 36 months, and 1 of 1 at 48 months. Three stents became occluded because of tumor extension, two of which underwent revision by placement of an additional stent.

In patients with distal ureteral obstruction, a metallic stent must be carefully placed so that the distal end is in the intramuscular section of the ureter and not in the bladder itself, to prevent reflux and dysuria.[35, 36, 39] However, intravesical extension of the stent is not always associated with bladder irritability.[40] The disproportion noted between the stented segment and adjacent normal ureter, with a "trumpet-like appearance," may mimic a stenosis but is generally found not to be urodynamically significant when evaluated further.[35, 36, 39]

Ureters treated with metallic stents nearly always demonstrate an early hyperplastic mucosal response that tends to resolve after about 4 weeks.[36, 39, 40] Overdistention of the ureter by a stent that is much larger in diameter may stimulate the hyperplasia.[43] In patients with more advanced malignancy, metallic stents may enable a better quality of life, without an external catheter and without complications due to double-J ureteral stents, such as bladder spasms and compression by malignant lesions. In such patients, long-term patency is less of a concern.

Metallic stents may have an adjunctive role, to provide radial force in order to allow easier passage of double-J ureteral stents. Use of metallic stents may also be limited by their higher cost. Overall, metallic stents should be used in the ureter with caution and only after the advantages have been weighed against the disadvantages.

Treatment Of Ureteroenteric Strictures

After surgical removal of the bladder for malignancy, a ureteral diversion is created, usually through anastomosis of the distal ureters to an isolated segment of bowel. Unfortunately, stricture develops at one or both ureteroenteric anastomoses in about 4%–8% of cases.[44] Patients may be asymptomatic or may present with pain, infection, renal insufficiency, or stone formation. Traditional treatment has consisted of surgical revision of the anastomosis, which may be technically difficult and carries surgical morbidity. Several investigators have searched for minimally invasive techniques for restoring patency to these strictured anastomoses. Malignant recurrence must be excluded, because patients with malignancy will fail non-surgical treatment and reobstruct quickly.[44, 45]

Dilation of ureteroenteric strictures with a balloon catheter was evaluated first and was generally combined with placement of a nephroureteral stent for 4–6 weeks (**Fig. 22-7**). Although the procedure was nearly always technically successful, the short-term clinical success rate was 30% and the 1-year patency rate was only

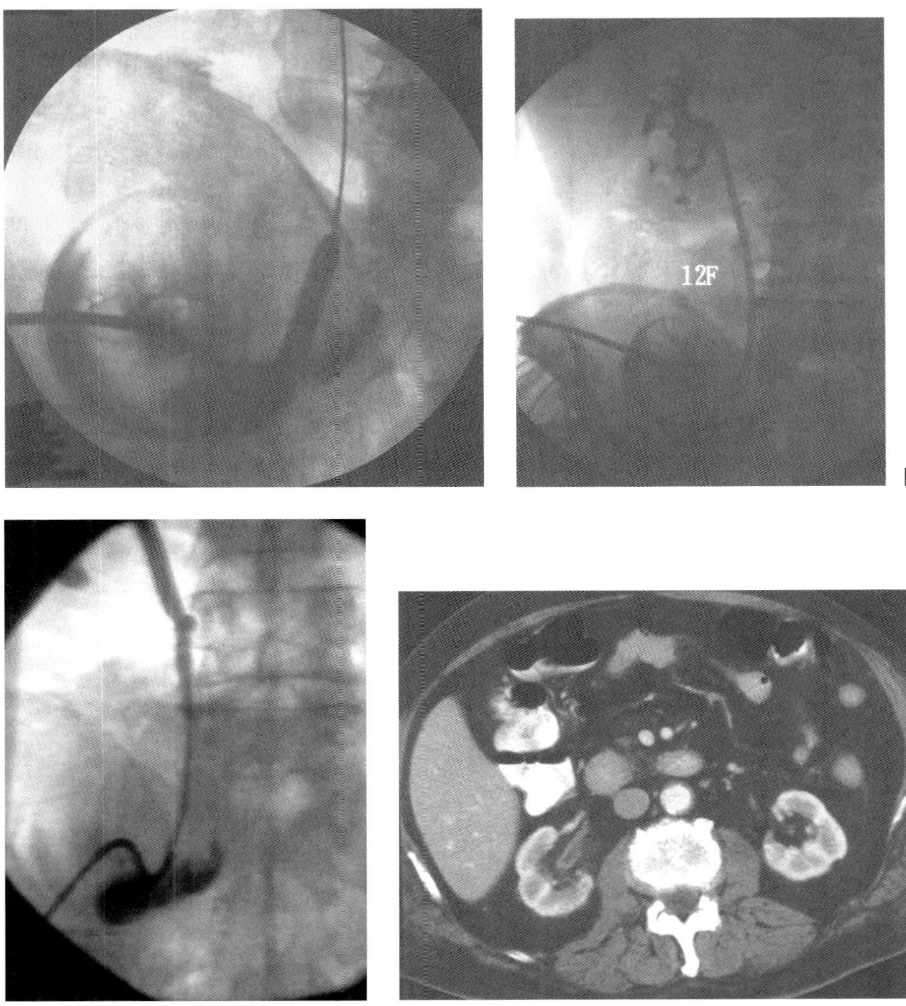

Figure 22-7. Ureteroplasty performed in same patient as shown in Figure 22-6. (A) Retrograde nephroureteral stent was removed over a stiff guidewire, and the stricture was dilated with a 6-mm balloon catheter. (B) New 12F retrograde nephroureteral stent was replaced. (C) Contrast injection near anastomosis demonstrated improved diameter, and the stent was removed. (D) On an abdominal CT scan obtained nearly 14 months later for unrelated indications, right kidney demonstrates no hydronephrosis and symmetric cortical enhancement.

16%.[46] Further dilation may be required after only a year, so it has been suggested that patients whose life expectancy exceeds 1 year may be best served by surgical revision. Addition of endoscopic incision of the stricture, with subsequent balloon dilation and stenting, improves patency somewhat, with 57% of ureters remaining patent at an average follow-up of 28.6 months in one study.[44] It has been theorized that dilation of strictures that are not ischemic in nature may have the best results.[44, 46]

The Acucise catheter (Applied Medical Resources, Laguna Hills, California) has also been introduced. It combines an 8-mm low-pressure balloon with a 3-cm-long noninsulated wire that connects to an electrocautery power supply. The initial report of the efficacy of this device, in conjunction with 6 weeks of stenting, was rather favorable. All four ureteroenteric strictures so treated remained patent for a mean follow-up of 22 months.[47] Other studies have shown patency rates similar to those for simple balloon dilation, with a 70% rate of recurrence and need for subsequent surgical revision.[45] Careful attention must be paid to avoid cutting with this device if blood vessels are near the anastomosis, and surgical techniques have been proposed for creation of anastomoses to minimize this risk in the event that a stricture later occurs.[47] Some researchers even employ endoluminal US prior to making an incision with the device.[45]

PERCUTANEOUS CYSTOSTOMY

Patients with bladder outlet or urethral obstruction require bladder decompression. A retrograde urethral catheter, such as a Foley catheter, is often the first-line treatment, because its placement is simple and inexpensive. Sometimes this technique is unsuccessful, however, and a suprapubic cystostomy must be performed. Additionally, suprapubic cystostomy is better for long-term treatment because of its advantages, which include decreased bacteriuria, greater patient comfort, and easier nursing care compared with indwelling or intermittent urethral catheters.[48] Suprapubic cystostomy can frequently be performed as a blind procedure, and only patients in whom the attempt was unsuccessful or the clinical scenario was more complex are referred for US or CT guidance. US is advantageous because it is simple, is readily available, and can be combined with fluoroscopy if necessary. CT is very useful, however, if there is concern about the location of bowel or other intervening organs.

In a series reported by Lee et al.,[48] 60 patients underwent large-bore percutaneous cystostomy with fluoroscopic or US guidance. Six of the patients had obstruction due to prostatic carcinoma and were unfit for surgical therapy; the remainder had benign obstructions. In 5 of the patients, prior surgical placement of cystostomy tubes had been unsuccessful, with failure due to small-capacity bladder, obesity and/or dense scar tissue. The latter two entities also prevented tract dilation at the time of the initial interventional radiologic procedure in 3 patients, requiring placement of a small-bore cystostomy tube and a second procedure to dilate the tract for placement of a large-bore tube. Complications included minor bleeding in two patients and urosepsis treated with antibiotics in one patient.

Mond and Lee[49] performed percutaneous suprapubic cystostomy under fluoroscopic guidance in 25 complex cases. Blind cystostomy placement had been unsuccessful or had resulted in malpositioning of the tube in these patients, who were obese or had fibrotic scars or decompressed bladders. One of the patients had obstruction due to malignancy.

Technique

The procedure is performed with the use of local anesthesia and conscious sedation. After sterile preparation and draping of the lower abdomen, an appropriate guidance technique (US or CT) and an 18-gauge needle are used to percutaneously puncture the bladder just above the symphysis pubis in the midline. Distention of the bladder with a urethral catheter can be helpful, particularly if iodinated contrast material is used. Alternatively, intravenously administered contrast material may opacify the bladder if transurethral catheterization is not possible. A drainage catheter, 10F or larger, is placed over a semistiff guidewire, such as a Rosen guidewire (Cook, Inc.), which has been coiled in the bladder (**Fig. 22-8**). For long-term drainage, the tract may be dilated with a balloon catheter and peel-

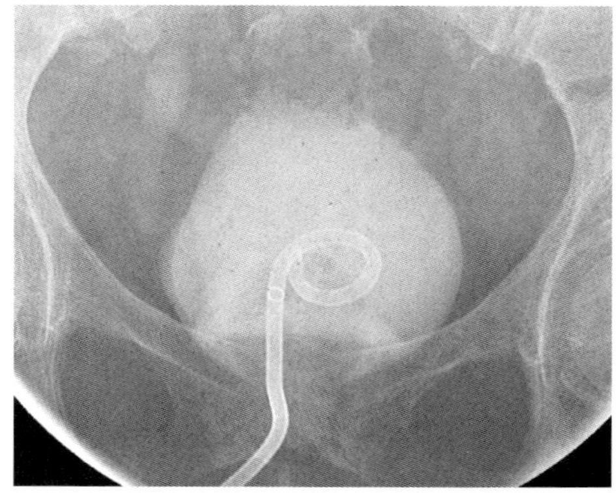

Figure 22-8. Percutaneous cystostomy. After ultrasonography to ensure that no intervening bowel was present, contrast material was injected through an indwelling Foley catheter. Fluoroscopic guidance was then used to place a pigtail cystostomy tube.

away sheath combination to allow placement of a larger 16F–20F, soft rubber, balloon-tipped catheter.[48]

This technique has the advantage of being a single-step dilation process with less discomfort than in conventional serial dilation.[48] The tubes are flushed twice daily with sterile water and changed over a guidewire every 3 months as a preventive maintenance measure to help maintain patency.

MANAGEMENT OF URETHRAL STRICTURES

Malignant bladder outlet obstruction is most commonly due to advanced prostatic carcinoma, and the mainstays of treatment are hormonal therapy with androgen blockade and indwelling bladder catheter, surgical resection, and percutaneous cystostomy. A few reports have been published describing the use of urethral stents for malignant obstruction, or of the sequelae of its treatment, as an alternative. Walsh and Keane first[50] employed this technique in the late 1980s using the UroLume self-expanding stainless steel mesh stent (American Medical Systems, Inc., Minnetonka, Minnesota) in patients who were not candidates for surgical treatment. The researchers noted, however, that because of tumor ingrowth, patients in whom this stent is placed require close follow-up.[50]

Guazzoni et al.[51] placed UroLume stents in the prostatic urethras of 11 patients with advanced prostate cancer and urinary retention for whom surgical treatment posed high risk and medical treatment with androgen blockade provided no relief. There were no major complications, and all patients voided spontaneously after stent placement. At 1-year follow-up, 9 of 10 patients were still free of urinary obstruction. These researchers' main criteria for eligibility for a UroLume stent were clear identification and noninvolvement of the bladder neck and verumontanum at urethroscopy.

Yachia and Aridogan[52] treated 27 patients who had advanced prostate cancer and urinary retention with placement of a ProstaCoil temporary self-expanding nitinol coil stent (Sulzer IntraTherapeutics, Inc., St. Paul, Minnesota) to relieve the obstruction. The patients subsequently underwent hormonal treatment, and the stents were removed in 22 patients. At a mean follow-up of 24.8 months after stent removal, 15 patients were voiding satisfactorily. Stent replacement was required in 3 patients because of inability to void, and surgical resection was needed in 2 patients because of poor response to hormone therapy. Additionally, the researchers believed that this technique was more economical than the use of indwelling bladder catheters, which require maintenance.

The self-expanding Memotherm nitinol knitted mesh stent (Bard Angiomed, Karlsruhe, Germany) was used for 35 patients with advanced prostatic carcinoma and urinary obstruction who were high-risk surgical candidates.[53] After stent insertion, 94% were able to void spontaneously; in those who could not, a second stent was placed, resulting in the ability to void. There were no major complications. Four patients experienced recurrent obstruction due to tumor growth; the recurrence occurred early in 2 patients, who were treated by cystostomy tube. The 2 patients with late recurrence of obstruction were treated by laser resection. Stents remained patent for more than 3 years in 4 patients.

Konety at al.[54] used the UroLume stent to relieve urinary outflow obstruction in 5 patients who had undergone transperineal brachytherapy for prostate cancer. In all 5 patients, treatment with alpha-blocker medications and intermittent catheterization either had failed or could not be tolerated. In some patients, urethral dilatation and suprapubic tube placement had also failed. All 5 patients were able to void spontaneously after stent placement. However, two stents had to be removed because of intolerable stent-related symptoms, which improved after stent removal.

REFERENCES

1. Watkinson AF, A'Hern RP, Jones A, King DM, Moskovic EC. The role of percutaneous nephrostomy in malignant urinary tract obstruction. *Clin Radiol* 1993; 47:32–35.
2. Goodwin WE, Casey WC, Woolf W. Percutaneous trocar (needle) nephrostomy in hydronephrosis. *JAMA* 1955;157:891–894.
3. Farrell TA, Hicks ME. A review of radiologically guided percutaneous nephrostomies in 303 patients. *J Vasc Interv Radiol* 1997; 8:769–774.
4. Chiou RK, Chang WY, Horan JJ. Ureteral obstruction associated with prostate cancer: the outcome after percutaneous nephrostomy. *J Urol* 1990;143:957–959.
5. Chapman ME, Reid JH. Use of percutaneous nephrostomy in malignant ureteric obstruction. *Br J Radiol* 1991;64:318–320.
6. Hoe JW, Tung KH, Tan EC. Re-evaluation of indications for percutaneous nephrostomy and interventional uroradiological procedures in pelvic malignancy. *Br J Urol* 1993;71:469–472.
7. Lau MW, Temperley DE, Mehta S, et al. Urinary tract obstruction and nephrostomy drainage in pelvic malignant disease. *Br J Urol* 1995;76:565–569.
8. Patel NH, Meglin AJ. Percutaneous nephrostomy. In: Trerotola SO, ed. *SCVIR Syllabus: Thoracic and Visceral Nonvascular Interventions Genitourinary Interventions*. Society of Cardiovascular and Interventional Radiology 1997:239–248.
9. Millward SF. Percutaneous nephrostomy: a practical approach. *J Vasc Interv Radiol* 2000;11:955–964.
10. Cadeddu JA, Arrindell D, Moore RG. Near fatal air embolism during percutaneous nephrostomy placement. *J Urol* 1997;158:1519.
11. Gupta S, Gulati M, Uday Shankar K, Rungta U, Suri S. Percutaneous nephrostomy with real-time sonographic guidance. *Acta Radiol* 1997;38:454–457.
12. Barbaric ZL, Hall T, Cochran ST, et al. Percutaneous nephrostomy: placement under CT and fluoroscopy guidance. *Am J Roentgenol* 1997;169:151–155.

13. LeMaitre L, Mestdagh P, Marecaux-Delomez J, et al. Percutaneous nephrostomy: placement under laser guidance and real-time CT fluoroscopy. *Eur Radiol* 2000;10:892–895.
14. Gray RR, So CB, McLoughlin RF, et al. Outpatient percutaneous nephrostomy. *Radiology* 1996;198:85–88.
15. Cochran ST, Barbaric ZL, Lee JJ, Kashfian P. Percutaneous nephrostomy tube placement: an outpatient procedure? *Radiology* 1991;179:843–847.
16. Sharma SD, Persad RA, Haq A, et al. A review of antegrade stenting in the management of the obstructed kidney. *Br J Urol* 1996;78:511–515.
17. Joshi HB, Adams S, Obadeyi OO, Rao PN. Nephrostomy tube or 'JJ' ureteric stent in ureteric obstruction: assessment of patient perspectives using quality-of-life survey and utility analysis. *Eur Urol* 2001;39:695–701.
18. Harding JR. Percutaneous antegrade ureteric stent insertion in malignant disease. *J R Soc Med* 1993;86:511–513.
19. Rackson ME, Mitty HA, Lossef SV, Dan SJ, Train JS. Biocompatible copolymer ureteral stent: maintenance of patency beyond 6 months. *Am J Roentgenol* 1989;153:783–784.
20. Saltzman B. Ureteral stents: indications, variations, and complications. *Urol Clin N Am* 1988;15:481–491.
21. Docimo SG, Dewolf WC. High failure rate of indwelling ureteral stents in patients with extrinsic obstruction: experience at two institutions. *J Urol* 1989;142:277–279.
22. Lu DS, Papanicolaou N, Girard M, Lee MJ, Yoder IC. Percutaneous internal ureteral stent placement: review of technical issues and solutions in 50 consecutive cases. *Clin Radiol* 1994;49:256–261.
23. Watson GMT, Patel U. Primary antegrade ureteric stenting: prospective experience and cost-effectiveness analysis in 50 ureters. *Clin Radiol* 2001;56:568–574.
24. Cardella JF, Castaneda-Zuniga WR, Hunter DW, Hulbert JC. Urine-compatible polymer for long-term ureteral stenting. *Radiology* 1986;161:313–318.
25. Babel SG, Winterkorn KG. Retrograde catheterization of the ureter without cystoscopic assistance: preliminary experience. *Radiology* 1993;187:547–549.
26. Mazer JM, LeVeen RF, Call JE, Wolf G, Baltaxe HA. Permanent percutaneous antegrade ureteral stent placement without transurethral assistance. *Urology* 1979;14:413–419.
27. Wilson MW. Percutaneous ureteral stents. In Trerotola SO, ed. *SCVIR Syllabus: Thoracic and Visceral Nonvascular Interventions—Genitourinary Interventions*. Society of Cardiovascular and Interventional Radiology 1997:255 –270.
28. Yedlicka JW, Aizpuru R, Hunter DW, Castaneda-Zuniga WR, Amplatz K. Retrograde replacement of internal double-J ureteral stents. *Am J Roentgenol* 1991;156:1007–1009.
29. de Baere T, Denys A, Pappas P, et al. Ureteral stents: exchange under fluoroscopic control as an effective alternative to cystoscopy. *Radiology* 1994;190:887–889.
30. Rosen RJ, McLean GK, Freiman DB, et al. Obstructed ureteroileal conduits: antegrade catheter drainage. *Am J Roentgenol* 1980;135:1201–1204.
31. Zaleski GX, Funaki B, Newmark G. Placement of retrograde nephroureteral stents through ileal conduits. *Am J Roentgenol* 1998;170:1275–1278.
32. Applbaum YN, Diamond AB, Rappoport AS. Retrograde ureteral catheterization via the ileal conduit. *Am J Roentgenol* 1986;146:61–63.
33. Walther PJ, Robertson CN, Paulson DF. Lethal complications of standard self-retaining ureteral stents in patients with ileal conduit urinary diversion. *J Urol* 1985;133:851–853.
34. Banner MP, Amendola MA, Pollack HM. Anastomosed ureters: fluoroscopically guided transconduit retrograde catheterization. *Radiology* 1989;170:45–49.
35. Diaz-Lucas EF, Martinez-Torres JL, Fernandez Mena J, et al. Self-expanding Wallstent endoprosthesis for malignant ureteral obstruction. *J Endourol* 1997;11:441–447.
36. Lugmayr HF, Pauer W. Wallstents for the treatment of extrinsic malignant ureteral obstruction: midterm results. *Radiology* 1996;198:105–108.
37. Lugmayr H, Pauer W. Self-expanding metal stents for palliative treatment of malignant ureteral obstruction. *Am J Roentgenol* 1992;159:1091–1094.
38. vanSonnenberg E, D'Agostino HB, O'Laoide R, et al. Malignant ureteral obstruction: treatment with metal stents–technique, results, and observations with percutaneous intraluminal US. *Radiology* 1994;191:765–768.
39. Flueckiger F, Lammer J, Klein GE, et al. Malignant ureteral obstruction: preliminary results of treatment with metallic self-expandable stents. *Radiology* 1993;186:169–173.
40. Barbalias GA, Siablis D, Liatsikos EN, et al. Metal stents: a new treatment of malignant ureteral obstruction. *J Urol* 1997;158:54–58.
41. Bosanac Z, Jain M, Monsour MJ. Treatment of malignant ureteric stricture with use of a Vascucoil spring stent. *J Vasc Interv Radiol* 1998;9:855–856.
42. Lopez-Martinez RA, Singireddy S, Lank EK. The use of metallic stents to bypass ureteral strictures secondary to metastatic prostate cancer: experience with 8 patients. *J Urol* 1997;158:50–53.
43. Pollak JS, Rosenblatt MM, Egglin TK, et al. Treatment of ureteral obstructions with the Wallstent endoprosthesis: preliminary results. *J Vasc Interv Radiol* 1995;6:417–425.
44. Meretyk S, Clayman RV, Kavoussi LR, Kramolowsky EV, Picus DD. Endourological treatment of ureteroenteric anastomotic strictures: long-term followup. *J Urol* 1991;145:723–727.
45. Lin DW, Bush WH, Mayo ME. Endourological treatment of ureteroenteric strictures: efficacy of Acucise endoureterotomy. *J Urol* 1999;162:696–698.
46. Shapiro MJ, Banner MP, Amendola MA, et al: Balloon catheter dilation of ureteroenteric strictures: long-term results. *Radiology* 1988;168:385–387.
47. Kabalin JN. Acucise incision of ureteroenteric strictures after urinary diversion. *J Endourol* 1997;11:37–40.
48. Lee MJ, Papanicolaou N, Nocks BN, Valdez JA, Yoder IC. Fluoroscopically guided percutaneous suprapubic cystostomy for long-term bladder drainage: an alternative to surgical cystostomy. *Radiology* 1993;188:787–789.
49. Mond DJ, Lee WJ. Fluoroscopically guided suprapubic cystostomy in complex urologic cases. *J Vasc Interv Radiol* 1994;5:911–914.
50. Walsh IK, Keane PF. Malignant sphincter stricture treated by a permanent indwelling stent. *Br J Urol* 1993;72:522.
51. Guazzoni G, Montorsi F, Bergamaschi F, Consonni P, Rigatti P. Prostatic UroLume Wallstent for urinary retention due to advanced prostate cancer: a 1-year followup study. *J Urol* 1994;152:1530–1532.
52. Yachia D, Aridogan IA. The use of a removable stent in patients with prostate cancer and obstruction. *J Urol* 1996;155:1956–1958.
53. Gottfried HW, Gnann R, Brandle E, et al. Treatment of high-risk patients with subvesical obstruction from advanced prostatic carcinoma using a thermosensitive mesh stent. *Br J Urol* 1997;80:623–627.
54. Konety BR, Phelan MW, O'Donnell WF, Antiles L, Chancellor MB. Urolume stent placement for the treatment of post-brachytherapy bladder outlet obstruction. *Urology* 2000;55:721–724.

CHAPTER 23

TRACHEOBRONCHIAL OBSTRUCTION

GORDON McLENNAN, MD
NILESH H. PATEL, MD
PRAVEEN N. MATHUR, MBBS

INTRODUCTION

Malignancies of the tracheobronchial tree may lead to obstruction and may cause acute respiratory distress or even asphyxia and death. An obstructive cancer may manifest as an endobronchial lesion, an extraluminal obstruction, or a combination of the two.

Multiple endoscopic techniques are available for palliation of nonresectable endobronchial malignancies. They include neodymium:yttrium-aluminum-garnet (Nd:YAG) laser therapy, cryotherapy, electrocautery, and brachytherapy. Palliation of extraluminal lesions is possible with bronchoscopic or balloon dilation, stent placement, and external-beam irradiation.

The patient with a tracheobronchial lesion usually presents with dyspnea, cough, chest discomfort, hemoptysis, stridor, or a localized wheeze. The patient's medical history may include known cancer, aspiration of a foreign body, prior airway surgery or intubation, recurrent pneumonia, or another underlying illness involving the airways, such as sarcoidosis or tuberculosis.

Although a tracheobronchial lesion may be detected on chest radiography or computed tomography (CT) scan, direct airway visualization with bronchoscopy is often needed to define the extent of the lesion and, if appropriate, to treat it—for example, by removing a foreign body or using a laser to resect a tracheal tumor. When treatment is not being given on an emergency basis, the type of therapy may be determined by the histology of an obstructing lesion, the existence of appropriate curative therapy, properties of the lesion (airway location, endobronchial mass with complete or partial

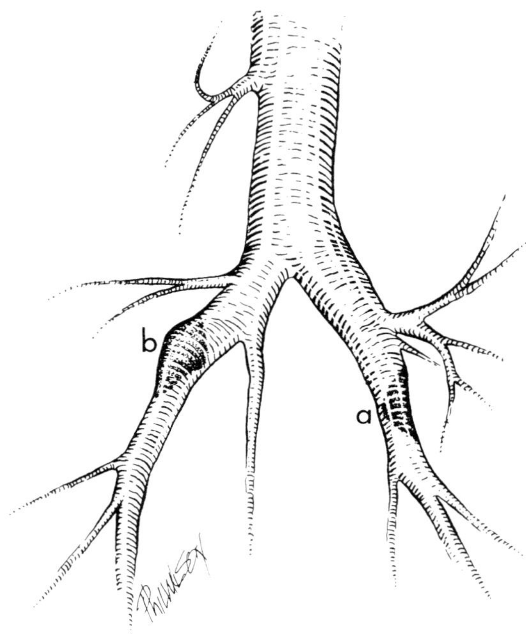

Figure 23-1. Endobronchial lesion (a) in the left main-stem bronchus is contained within the confines of the tracheal tree. The lumen is narrowed but the bronchus is not compressed. Such a lesion is easily treated bronchoscopically. In extrinsic compression (b), the lesion extends from outside the bronchus to intrude upon its lumen. Although the obstructing lesion may be partially treated endoscopically, the placement of a stent will buttress the force exerted by the lesion on the bronchus.

obstruction, extrinsic compression, stenosis, malacia), patient tolerance and acceptance, and the availability of appropriate equipment and experienced operators.

In this chapter, we summarize some of the salient features of Nd:YAG laser therapy, cryotherapy, electrocautery, and brachytherapy as local treatments for intraluminal tracheobronchial lesions (**Fig. 23-1A**). Also, we review the various forms of airway stents used to relieve extraluminal tracheobronchial obstruction (**Fig. 23-1B**).

ENDOLUMINAL LESIONS

The treatment of endoluminal lesions is primarily endoscopic. Techniques for the treatment of such lesions include laser therapy, cryotherapy, electrocautery, and brachytherapy.

Laser Therapy

With laser therapy, the goal is to deliver heat energy to initiate cell death. The CO_2 laser uses a wavelength of 10,600 nanometers to raise tissue temperatures to 100° Celsius and cause vaporization of water. The CO_2 laser has a relatively shallow depth of penetration, but its long wavelength requires an articulating arm and a series of mirrors to focus it. Therefore, it is most commonly used in the management of laryngeal or tracheal lesions involving the area around the glottic opening. The laser light most widely used for tracheobronchial lesions is the Nd:YAG laser; the light is produced by the stimulation of an yttrium-aluminum-garnet glass that has been coated with neodymium. The Nd:YAG laser has a wavelength of 1064 nanometers and is easily transmitted through pale tissues, with sizable scatter and a potential penetration of up to 5 to 10 mm from the focal point.[1] It can be delivered with the use of flexible, rigid, or flexible-through-rigid bronchoscopic technique.

Contraindications

Laser therapy of the tracheobronchial tree may be contraindicated because of the location of the lesion in relation to contiguous anatomy and the associated clinical condition of the patient (**Table 23-1**). Anatomic contraindications are relevant when the depth of injury causes destruction of tissue demarcating the boundaries between the target and such associated structures as the esophageal lumen, mediastinum, and vascular structures. Clinical contraindications are relevant in patients who may not tolerate conscious or general anesthesia because of severe cardiac or pulmonary disease or who have an uncorrectable coagulopathy. In addition, patients in whom atelectasis distal to the obstruction has been present for more than 4 to 6 weeks would probably not benefit from endoscopic laser resection because reexpansion of the involved lung is unlikely.

TABLE 23-1
Contraindications to Laser, Cryotherapy, and Electrocautery

Anatomic contraindications

- Extrinsic obstruction without endobronchial lesion
- Lesion incursion into bordering major vascular structure (e.g., pulmonary artery) with potential for fistula formation
- Lesion incursion into bordering esophagus with potential for fistula formation
- Lesion incursion into bordering mediastinum with potential for fistula formation

Clinical contraindications

- Patient a candidate for surgical resection
- Unfavorable short-term prognosis without hope for palliation of symptoms
- Inability of patient to undergo conscious sedation or general anesthesia
- Coagulation disorder
- Total obstruction for more than 4 to 6 weeks

Indications, Outcome, and Combined-Modality Therapy

Ramser and Beamis[2] provided an extensive report on the basic indications for endobronchial laser therapy. The indications depend on the anatomic characteristics of the obstructing lesion and the clinical conditions outlined in **Table 23-2**.

Patients with benign and malignant airway endobronchial lesions that have symptomatic or obstructive complications may benefit from endoscopic laser photoresection.[3–8] Laser photoablation of tracheal stenosis or stricture of multiple causes has been extensively documented. CO_2 laser therapy for subglottic and tracheal stenosis has been reported to be successful in 77% and 57% of treated patients, respectively, and decannulation has been possible in some patients. Laser therapy has also been performed for stenosis related to prolonged intubation,[9] stricture produced by inflammatory granulation tissue caused by mycobacterial infection or anastomotic granulation tissue after lung transplantation,[10] and suture granuloma[11] as well as in systemic inflammatory conditions caused by collagen vascular diseases such as Wegener's granulomatosis, Behçet syndrome, and relapsing polychondritis.[12, 13] Endobronchial laser therapy has also been effective in patients with symptomatic obstruction secondary to broncholithiasis.[14]

Patients with benign or low-grade tumors, such as hamartoma, spindle cell carcinoma, endobronchial Kaposi sarcoma, and even diffuse papillomatosis, have also benefited from Nd:YAG laser photoablation. Shah et al.[15] performed laser resection in 185 patients with benign tumors of the tracheobronchial tree; 317 procedures were performed, and the results of laser resection were thought to be very good in 62% of patients and good in 38%, with minimal complications.

Other larger series have documented operator and institution experience with laser resection of benign and malignant disease at multiple sites in the airway. Toty et al.,[9] in an early experience, were able to restore adequate respiratory function in 16 of 24 patients who presented in acute respiratory distress with recently detected tracheal carcinoma. Seventeen of 48 patients in the same series who had recurrent carcinoma received palliation from endobronchial therapy. Nine of these patients were alive a year later, and 8 survived for 6 months. Hetzel et al.[16] reported their experience in 100 patients referred for palliative treatment of tracheobronchial malignancy. These researchers noted objective improvement in peak flow and alleviation of hemoptysis in 63% of patients with airway obstruction and in 29% of patients with collapsed lung. They concluded that laser photoablation made a significant contribution to the management of tracheobronchial tumors.

Kavale et al.[6] reviewed their experience from 1982 to 1984 at Henry Ford Hospital. During this period, 55 patients received 82 treatments with laser therapy for obstructing lesions of the central airways, of whom 10 had benign lesions obstructing the subglottic larynx or trachea, and 45 had primary bronchogenic carcinoma or recurrent carcinoma of the lobar or main-stem bronchus or trachea. In 6 patients with malignancies, spirometry demonstrated postoperative improvement of FEV_1 (1-second forced expiratory volume) in 66% of patients and of FVC (forced vital capacity) in 83%. These researchers concluded, after an initial 18-month experience, that Nd:YAG laser therapy was successful in relieving central airway obstruction, alleviating dyspnea, and allowing drainage of affected areas of lung. Therapy also improved ventilation in some patients and may have prolonged their lives.

In 1986, Eichenhorn et al.[3] reported results of Nd:YAG laser photoablation in 19 patients with inoperable non–small-cell carcinoma and major symptomatic bronchial obstruction. The photoablation was performed with the goal of debulking the airways before conventional external-beam radiotherapy. The study was limited to patients with nearly complete exophytic obstruction of one major bronchus. Five of the successfully treated patients died in less than 3 months. However, the survival rate for the entire treated group was greater than that of historical controls receiving radiotherapy alone. Patients who underwent satisfactory debulking and subsequent radiotherapy had a significantly better outcome (mean survival 340 days, compared with less than 100 days; $P < 0.006$) than those in whom results of laser photoresection were unsatisfactory.

Desai et al.[17] also reported their experience treating 47 consecutive patients with inoperable primary bronchogenic carcinoma who underwent Nd:YAG photoresection between 1983 and 1986. The primary goal of this study was palliation, and laser therapy immediately relieved obstructive symptoms in all patients. While me-

TABLE 23-2
Indications for Laser, Cryotherapy, and Electrocautery

Benign or malignant airway lesion associated with dyspnea, uncontrolled cough, impending asphyxiation, or stridor
Inability to wean from ventilator owing to obstruction
Post-obstructive pneumonia
Symptomatic or unresolving atelectasis
Nearly complete (>50%) obstruction of one major bronchus
Recurrent hemoptysis
Closure of bronchopleural fistula not responsive to conventional therapy

dian survivor for patients who received radiation was longer than patients who received laser resection alone (304 days vs. 253 days), survival distribution was not significantly different. A significantly higher survival was noted among the subset of 15 patients who underwent emergency palliative photoresection as the initial therapeutic intervention compared with the subset of 11 patients who received palliative radiotherapy alone.

In the review of laser bronchoscopy by Ramser and Beamis,[2] 85% of 100 patients experienced relief of symptoms, and preoperative goals were achieved; 87% of the procedures were performed for lesions in mainstem bronchi, with no fatalities reported and an overall complication rate of 6.5%. Rare tumors of the tracheobronchial system have also been noted to benefit from laser resection. Although comparisons using survival as an end point have dealt largely with historical control groups, the palliation of symptoms and the ability to disconnect some patients from mechanical ventilation constitute evidence of the efficacy of laser therapy.

Combination therapy consisting of concurrent or sequential interventions, such as laser therapy, stent placement, brachytherapy, and more conventional adjuvant treatments, continues to be explored. In a review, Mehta et al.[18] outlined the use of lasers with the flexible bronchoscope in a group of patients who underwent Nd:YAG photoresection with subsequent external-beam radiotherapy or external-beam radiotherapy plus brachytherapy. Although the number of patients was small (17 of 300 patients), their survival rate was significantly greater than that of historical controls treated with radiotherapy only ($P = 0.022$). Cavaliere et al.[19] also supplemented earlier extensive case series with a report of their 13-year experience, outlining the treatment of 2008 patients who had malignant airway obstructions with combined therapy consisting of Nd:YAG laser resection, stent placement, and brachytherapy. Of the patients who underwent laser resection, 93% experienced immediate airway patency and consequent improvement in quality of life.

Complications

Complications of laser photoablation are related to the laser equipment or instruments, the anesthesia used, and perioperative causes. However, despite the possibility of severe, often fatal, complications, the overall risk is low for procedures performed by trained hands, with one series reporting only 60 complications and 12 deaths in association with Nd:YAG laser therapy in 2610 resections.[17]

Complications associated with the laser equipment may be caused by variation in the power setting, the mode, and the use of continuous or intermittent pulse delivery. A known complication of laser light is retinal damage; therefore, the laser must be in the standby mode whenever it is not inserted through the bronchoscope and aimed at the target.

Pulmonary complications of the anesthesia during laser therapy may be related to anoxia, hypercarbia, or fire. Patients selected for endobronchial therapy likely have compromised ventilation, which may be exacerbated by the insertion of the flexible bronchoscope or other equipment into the airway. Increased obstruction may also occur from hemorrhage or debris. Continuous pulse oximetry should be used for monitoring; however, hypercapnia and acidosis have also been reported in association with a reduction in PaO_2 in up to 93% of patients after endoscopic procedures.

A potential catastrophic intraoperative complication of laser therapy is endotracheal fire. Although the use of combustible anesthetic gases must be avoided, the use of supplemental oxygen is part of almost all bronchoscopic procedures, and the FIO_2 value should be less than 40%. The metal rigid bronchoscope cannot catch fire, but the use of the Nd:YAG laser through an endotracheal tube deserves special consideration. Because of the oxygen mixture, the possible additional fuel source provided by an endotracheal tube, and the potential for producing sparks when the laser light hits carbonized tissue, endotracheal fire is a serious concern. An immediate danger to the patient and operating room personnel is that of intratracheal explosion, in which the anesthetic gases or oxygen produce a "torch effect" with ignition of the endotracheal tube. Longer-term complications may result from the subsequent lower airway inhalation injury, with mucosal sloughing and airway obstruction caused by granulation tissue.

The most common perioperative complications occur in relation to perforation of an underlying or contiguous structure. Fatal hemorrhage is associated with perforation into an involved or contiguous vascular structure and requires careful preoperative assessment. Apart from creation of a fistula into the artery, which results in massive hemorrhage, perforation may also occur into adjacent structures with development of pneumothorax, pneumomediastinum, and tracheoesophageal fistula. In addition, pathologic changes may lead to distortion of usual relationships or appearance with subsequent laser application to vital structures. Systemic air embolism has been reported with laser therapy and is associated with the development of vascular communication with the tracheobronchial tree.

Summary

A primary goal of laser therapy is the safe, effective, and rapid palliation of symptoms due to tracheal or bronchial obstruction. Patient survival, as noted by Ramser and Beamis,[2] may not be the proper evaluative end point for the efficacy of therapy, which is meant to palliate airway obstruction from malignant causes. Laser therapy has proved to be beneficial in the therapy of benign and malignant obstructive lesions of the airway. Although future studies should prospectively examine survival, the current evidence firmly supports the use of laser therapy to provide palliative and potentially curative care to patients with lung disease.

TABLE 23-3
Cryosensitive and Cryoresistant Tissues

Cryosensitive	Cryoresistant
Skin	Fat
Mucous membrane	Cartilage
Nerve	Nerve sheath
Endothelium	Connective tissue
Granulation tissue	Fibrosis

Cryotherapy

The goal of cryotherapy is to destroy diseased tissue but spare normal tissue by lowering the tissue temperature to between −15° and −40° Celsius. Tissue damage is affected by the rates of freezing and thawing, the number of freeze-thaw cycles, the duration of freezing, and the mass of tissue frozen. Mazur[20] demonstrated that rapid freezing and slow warming result in maximum cell death. Repeating the cycle increases the amount of destruction. Sufficient time is required to reach and to sustain the critical temperature. A large contact area between the cryoprobe and the tissue enlarges the tissue mass exposed to freezing.

The effect of cryotherapy is a consequence of various cellular mechanisms. Intracellular dehydration leading to cell membrane disruption occurs when extracellular ice crystals form, thereby increasing the extracellular tonicity. Water is thus drawn from the intracellular to the extracellular space, causing greater intracellular tonicity, cell shrinkage, and membrane damage. Mechanical cellular damage from ice crystals occurs with rapid freezing and slow warming; intracellular ice crystals have been shown to damage various organelles, such as mitochondria and endoplasmic reticulum. Also, freezing affects the intracellular ionic strength and pH, leading to protein and enzyme damage. Lastly, freezing has been shown to cause vasoconstriction and the formation of microthrombi, primarily in the venules and capillaries, resulting in devascularization and subsequent cell death. This property may explain the success of cryotherapy in controlling hemoptysis.

Certain tissues are cryosensitive, whereas others are cryoresistant (**Table 23-3**). This fact may partially explain why some lesions respond to cryotherapy and why some complications, such as malacia, do not occur. Experimental evidence suggests that solid lung tumors may be more cryosensitive than normal lung tissue. Several investigators have used dog models to study the effects of cryotherapy on tracheal and bronchial mucosa. In general, these studies have shown that the microscopic epithelial and cartilaginous changes resolve over 4 to 6 weeks but that the airway mucosa appears macroscopically normal by 2 weeks. No stenoses, malacia, or airway perforations occurred in these studies, supporting the safety of cryotherapy in the airway. Finally, the effects of cryotherapy on the immune system—that is, any tumoricidal effects separate from direct injury—are not well elucidated. Some studies involving prostate carcinoma or melanoma have shown increases in numbers of activated peripheral blood lymphocytes with cryotherapy, whereas others have shown resolution of metastasis when cryotherapy was applied to the primary tumor.[20]

Indications and Patient Selection

Cryotherapy may be indicated if (1) the symptoms and signs are caused by an endobronchial lesion, (2) a histologic examination reveals that the lesion is not amenable to curative therapy, and (3) the lesion is accessible to the cryoprobe through the endoscope. In addition, the patient must be able and willing to undergo bronchoscopy. Cryotherapy is often ineffective in removing tissue rapidly, so laser ablation, surgery, or stent placement should be considered in a patient presenting in acute respiratory distress.

Patients whose lesions are polypoid, are short, have a large endobronchial component, and allow some visibility beyond them and in whom there is functioning lung distal to the lesion are prime candidates for cryotherapy. Lesions that are long and tapering or that involve the submucosa extensively are unsuited for this treatment. Similarly, if extrinsic airway compression is the cause of the problem, an alternative treatment must be considered.

Equipment and Technique

To effect cell death, the cryogen (or coolant) must be able to lower the tissue temperature to −15° to −40° Celsius. Liquid material is used so that, on vaporization, heat is removed and the probe and tissue are cooled (Joule-Thompson effect). Cryogenic material is usually stored under pressure in cylinders. The saturation temperature at atmospheric pressure is the temperature of interest. The cryogen passes through the probe, cooling the metal tip. Nitrous oxide and liquid nitrogen are most commonly used. Nitrous oxide is effective (saturation temperature –89° Celsius), inexpensive, and available. Selection of the cryoprobe depends on whether rigid bronchoscopy or fiberoptic bronchoscopy is used. Rigid bronchoscopy seems to be preferred in Europe. A flexible probe and a semirigid probe for use with the flexible bronchoscope are now available in the United States.

Nitrous oxide cools the probe tip to approximately –89° Celsius. The temperature increases approximately 10° Celsius with each millimeter of distance from the tip; therefore, the effective killing zone is approximately 5 to 8 mm. A flexible bronchoscope with a working channel diameter greater than the diameter of the probe is needed (the diameter of the flexible probe is 2.2 mm, and that of the semirigid, 2.6 mm).

The probe is attached to a console that regulates the coolant flow. After the airway is anesthetized, the patient is sedated (usually with a narcotic and a benzodiazepine), and the airway is intubated; then the tracheobronchial tree is inspected and the lesion localized. The cryoprobe is passed through the working channel until the tip protrudes from the bronchoscope approximately 2 cm, thus minimizing the risk of freezing the bronchoscope. Under direct visualization, the operator applies the tip of the probe to the lesion perpendicularly or tangentially and, by activating a foot pedal, begins the freezing.

An ice ball forms within 10 to 15 seconds. A freezing time of 30 to 60 seconds and multiple freeze-thaw cycles are applied. The probe is then retracted or removed. In addition, a forceps can be used to remove tissue and debris. Suctioning of blood or secretions between applications may be necessary. When an optimal amount of tissue or foreign body is removed, or if the patient's status becomes unstable, the procedure is terminated. The procedure may be repeated, if needed, in 1 to 2 weeks. Adjunctive treatment can be given simultaneously.

Outcomes

In most reports, endobronchial cryotherapy is used for palliation of either primary or metastatic malignancy. The literature on cryotherapy for benign tracheobronchial lesions and the documentation of objective improvement are limited.

Maiwand and Homasson[21] reported on 600 patients, most of whom had squamous cell carcinoma of the lung. Approximately one third of the patients received cryotherapy as either the initial or the only treatment. These investigators reported a 78% subjective improvement in patients' condition. Walsh et al.[22] evaluated 33 patients undergoing cryotherapy and reported improvement in respiratory function. Mathur et al.[23] stated that all tumors could be removed in 18 of their 20 patients and that 12 of 17 patients with dyspnea and all 5 patients with hemoptysis showed clinical improvement. There are too few case reports to make unequivocal conclusions, but cryotherapy seems to be successful for treatment of granulation tissue, carcinoid tumors, and cylindromas. The modality can be used to extract foreign bodies as well as blood clots and mucous plugs. Lastly, cryotherapy may be used in combination with other modalities. Vergnon et al.[24] reported better survival in patients who showed improvement in response to cryotherapy before undergoing external-beam radiotherapy than in patients who did not show improvement (which was defined as destruction of more than 50% of tumor with cryotherapy).

Complications

Complications of endobronchial cryotherapy are few and relatively minor. Maiwand and Homasson[21] reported one death from cardiorespiratory failure in 600 cases, the death occurring 5 hours after the procedure. Vergnon et al.[24] reported one death from catastrophic hemoptysis from tumor cryotherapy within 8 days of the procedure. Mathur et al.[23] reported one cardiopulmonary arrest; the patient survived the episode and left the hospital. Maiwand and Homasson[21] reported two cases of tracheoesophageal fistulas, one of which occurred in a patient who had also undergone irradiation. Rare episodes of pneumothorax, atrial fibrillation, bronchospasm, spillage from a postobstruction pneumonia, aggravation of cold-agglutinin anemia, mild fever, and bradycardia have also been reported.

Summary

Endobronchial cryotherapy seems to be a relatively effective palliative treatment for endobronchial obstruction caused by malignancy. More investigations of the use of endobronchial cryotherapy for benign lesions and in combination with other modalities are needed.

Electrocautery

Electrocautery uses alternating current at a high frequency (105–107 Hz) to generate heat that coagulates, vaporizes, or cuts tissue, depending on the power. The power applied to the electrocautery device (measured in watts) corresponds to the heat generated in the tissue, as related by the equation: power (watts) = current^2 (amperes) × resistance (ohms). Tissue resistance to the current generates the heat, and the resistance depends on the moisture and vascularity of the tissue. Low-frequency current (<105 Hz) stimulates nerve and muscle and thus should be avoided. Coagulation involves high amperage and low voltage, whereas vaporization uses high voltage and low amperage. Cutting tissue with the ability to coagulate blends these two settings.

Tissue coagulates at approximately 70° Celsius and carbonizes at more than 200° Celsius. The extent of destruction depends on the applied power, the electrical properties of the tissue, and both the time and the surface area of contact between the device and the tissue. Unlike cryotherapy, electrocautery causes greater tissue damage with a small contact area, which allows the current to be concentrated. When the device is in direct contact with the tissue, superficial coagulation occurs. If the probe is removed from contact and a higher power setting is chosen, an arc from the device to the tissue ensues, causing deeper coagulation.

When a tissue is heated sufficiently, cellular water evaporates, destroying the cell and then the tissue. Heating to higher temperatures leads to chemical breakdown of the cell and tissue constituents and eventual vaporization or carbonization. Most available electrocautery devices are monopolar; that is, they require that the bronchoscope, the generator, and the patient be grounded to complete the circuit, so as to prevent shocks and burns. The bronchoscope should be insulated. If the generator is not grounded, it should at least have an isolated power output to minimize current leakage and possible injury. Bipolar electrocautery devices limit the risks, but they are not available in the United States for use with the flexible bronchoscope.

Indications

The indications for electrocautery are similar to those for cryotherapy and Nd:YAG laser therapy.[25, 26] Like cryotherapy, electrocautery is usually a palliative treatment in patients with malignancy. Its role in bronchogenic dysplasia or carcinoma in situ has yet to be defined. For some benign lesions, electrocautery may be the only treatment necessary.

The patient must be medically able and willing to undergo this procedure; the lesion must be accessible and should have a large endobronchial component. Unlike cryotherapy, electrocautery can effect rapid debulking of tumor in some cases, and it may be a reasonable modality to relieve impending respiratory failure if laser therapy or surgery is unavailable or inappropriate. Lastly, unlike cryotherapy, electrocautery is not used to remove foreign bodies, mucous plugs, or blood clots.

Equipment and Technique

Insulated flexible bronchoscopes with working channels of 2.0 or 2.6 mm are now available in the United States. Additionally, an electrocautery blunt-tipped probe (1.9-mm diameter) and a snare (1.8-mm diameter) are available and are compatible with the flexible bronchoscopes. The generator should regulate the high-frequency current so that the operator can adjust the setting according to whether the procedure is intended to coagulate, cut, cut and coagulate, or vaporize. If a monopolar unit is used, the patient must be grounded with an electrode pad, which is placed close to the expected site of electrocautery, thus concentrating current for maximal effect. Also, the patient must not contact any metal while undergoing electrocautery.

Preoperative patient evaluation and patient monitoring procedures are the same as for fiberoptic bronchoscopy. If rigid bronchoscopy is used, general anesthesia is necessary; the procedure for electrocautery with fiberoptic bronchoscopy is similar to that described for cryotherapy. Intubation may be either oral or nasal, but use of an endotracheal tube is recommended.

After the patient has been intubated and the lesion located, the operator can use either a closed forceps or the blunt electrocautery probe to manipulate the lesion, and thus to assess its size, mobility, friability, and bleeding potential, and to locate any attachment to the airway. Elongated or flat lesions may be suited for the blunt probe, whereas polypoid lesions may be amenable to the snare. To apply the probe without an arc, the operator places the probe in contact with the tissue so that blanching occurs, and only then activates the generator. To create a probe-tissue arc for deeper coagulation, the operator holds the probe a few millimeters above the tissue, selects a higher power level, and activates the unit. Vaporization of tissue may require even higher power settings.

The snare is used to cut and remove tissue, and a blended current is used to cut and coagulate but not to vaporize. With the loop open, the snare is placed over the tissue as close to the base as possible. As the loop is tightened, a snugness is felt in the handgrip, which controls the snare. At this point, the unit is activated and the loop is slowly tightened. It is the heat that cuts and coagulates the tissue, not the mechanical effect of the wire. When the procedure is complete, the snugness is gone and the loop is retracted into the catheter. The severed tissue can be removed with the snare or a forceps. The patient will expectorate smaller debris. **Table 23-4** lists suggested power settings for electrocautery devices.

A relatively new device, the argon plasma coagulator (APC), is available for electrocautery coagulation. No tissue-probe contact occurs. Ionized argon gas serves as the current conductor between the probe and the tissue.

TABLE 23-4
Suggested Power Settings for the 1psd 20 Generator for Electrocautery

Treatment	Mode	Power setting (watts)
Polypectomy	Cut or blend	
Diameter <5 mm		10 to 20
Diameter >5 mm		15 to 30
Cauterization	Cut or blend	10 to 30
Coagulation for hemostasis	Coagulation	10 to 20

In a series of 60 patients, Morice et al. reported improvement in symptoms of hemoptysis and airway obstructive symptoms for a median of 53 days.[27]

Outcomes

In a study of 56 patients, Homasson[28] stated that hemoptysis was controlled in 75% of cases, dyspnea was alleviated in 67%, and cough or stridor was relieved in 55%. Petrou et al.[29] reported that 28 of 29 patients had symptomatic improvement after removal of a lesion with a snare. Sutedja et al.[30] found that 15 of 17 treated patients experienced immediate restoration of a patent airway (defined as greater than 75% of the normal airway), 8 had relief of dyspnea, and 4 had control of hemoptysis. Most series involve predominantly malignancies, and success is defined as removal of more than 50% of the tumor; success rates of 70% to 95% have been reported.[31–33]

Complications

Two endobronchial fires during electrocautery procedure have been reported[34]; both were associated with high concentrations of inspired oxygen, and in one case, a silicone stent ignited. Several investigators have reported hemorrhage, in most cases minor; one death secondary to hemorrhage has been reported. Operator and patient burns and electrical shocks are mentioned frequently as possible complications; however, published data are scant. Another concern is the use of electrocautery in patients with pacemakers or automatic implantable defibrillators, which may malfunction and cause dysrhythmia. Investigators have shown that airway stenosis and cartilage damage can occur when electrocautery is used in animal models.[28] This cartilage damage can lead to bronchomalacia. Systemic air embolism has also been reported in two cases and has been attributed to high-flow air cooling during laser use.[35]

Summary

Like cryotherapy, electrocautery seems to be an effective palliative treatment for an endobronchial lesion. It may be less expensive than laser therapy. With a grounded, flexible bronchoscope and accessories now available in the United States, use of this technique may increase. Complications seem to be limited in number and severity.

Brachytherapy

Endobronchial radiotherapy with the use of an implanted source of ionizing radiation (brachytherapy) was first used in the 1920s. Yankauer[34] reported on the implantation of radium into an endobronchial tumor with the use of a bronchoscope; the radium was in capsules attached to a string that exited through the mouth. Most patients who underwent this therapy required general anesthesia and either bronchoscopy or thoracotomy for direct implantation. In 1964, Henschke et al.[36] developed the remote afterloading device, thereby reducing radiation exposure for the health care staff. Almost 20 years later, the use of the flexible bronchoscope and a polyethylene catheter to hold the radioactive material for brachytherapy was described.[37, 38] Iridium 192, the radiation source currently used, was also first described then.[37]

In the mid-1980s, publications distinguishing low-dose-rate (LDR) from high-dose-rate (HDR) brachytherapy appeared. Schray et al.[39, 40] reported on LDR, and Seagren[41] on HDR. LDR brachytherapy is usually defined as less than 2 gray (Gy) per hour, with the total dose between 1500 and 5000 Gy, given over 3 days. HDR involves more than 10 Gy/h, in which the total dose and the dose per session (fraction) vary. Fractions have varied anywhere from approximately 300 to 1000 Gy, and the total dose from approximately 500 to 4000 Gy. Most later studies have described brachytherapy combined with either external-beam radiotherapy or laser therapy. The technique is applied frequently for palliation, and occasionally for cure.

Techniques and Dosage

Rigid bronchoscopy was initially used for permanent interstitial implantation of a source of low-energy ionizing radiation. This method has been supplanted by intraluminal brachytherapy, in which fiberoptic bronchoscopy is used to place an afterloading polyethylene catheter adjacent to the tumor. The placement of the catheter is verified by bronchoscopy and then by radiography of the chest. The catheter can be loaded with the radiation source manually or with a remote afterloader.

The dose rate of brachytherapy depends on the radioactivity of the radionuclide used. LDR is arbitrarily defined as a rate of 2 Gy/h at the point of reference. This modality, which was commonly used in the early years of endobronchial brachytherapy, required manual manipulation of the radionuclide, 30 to 70 hours of treatment, and cumbersome radiation protection measures.

HDR brachytherapy is defined as involving a dose rate of greater than 10 Gy/h. The apparatus designed to deliver HDR brachytherapy subsequently became commercially available, and iridium 192 became the radionuclide of choice; afterloading techniques and heavy shielded treatment rooms simplified the radiation protection practice. The major advantage of HDR over LDR brachytherapy has been a dramatic reduction in treatment time. HDR brachytherapy is usually delivered as fractionated doses to maximize its safety and effectiveness. Treatment schedules vary in clinical practice because the procedure requires bronchoscopy and placement of endobronchial catheters during each session.To minimize discomfort, most patients are treated once a week or once every 2 weeks rather than daily.

Indications and Contraindications

Endobronchial therapy has been used exclusively to treat patients with endobronchial tumors. Although the specific indications may vary among institutions, the general criteria for treatment are (1) biopsy-proven carcinoma of the lung or metastatic carcinoma, (2) ineligibility for or lack of response to potential curative therapies, (3) presence of symptoms due to malignant endobronchial lesions such as dyspnea, (4) occurrence of pneumonitis, hemoptysis, or intractable cough after debulking of the tumor with Nd:YAG laser therapy or cryotherapy, and (5) suitability of the site of lesions for placement of a brachytherapy catheter for the delivery of the radiation source.[42]

The usual goal of brachytherapy is palliation of symptoms due to airway obstruction by tumor. The modality can also be used, however, as an adjunct to external-beam radiotherapy for treatment in otherwise unresectable lung cancer. Sutedja et al.[43] have used brachytherapy in patients who have undergone tumor resection and in whom histology shows the surgical margins to be positive for tumor.

Two absolute contraindications to endobronchial brachytherapy are known fistulas to nonbronchial tissue areas and lesions that are not proven malignancies. Patients with endotracheal carcinoma causing high-grade obstruction should be treated with Nd:YAG laser therapy and possible placement of a stent before undergoing brachytherapy. This is because postradiation edema can lead to total airway obstruction. Brachytherapy should also be avoided in patients who cannot safely undergo bronchoscopy.

Efficacy

Most studies of brachytherapy have reported on its use in combination with external-beam radiotherapy or Nd:YAG laser therapy. The laser has been used for rapid symptom relief and canalization of the airway to place the catheter. The rate of subjective improvement after brachytherapy has ranged from 20% to 100%, depending on the symptom. Hemoptysis is reported to be relieved in more than 90% of treated patients. Relief of cough and dyspnea was moderate to minimal, probably owing to underlying chronic bronchitis or radiation fibrosis.[44–47]

Objective responses to brachytherapy have been evaluated by either chest radiography or bronchoscopy. These evaluations are semiquantitative at best, being based on visual assessment of the diameter of the airway lumen. An obstruction score has been designed by some investigators but is not widely used.[30] An extremely important factor that has affected the interpretations of these data is the variation in the selection of patients in the reported studies. A significant number of patients have had advanced disease and have refused subsequent bronchoscopy. In the studies reviewed, there was a greater than 50% improvement in patency of the airway. The positive response of most studies persisted for 6 months or longer.[39, 48]

Endobronchial Brachytherapy versus External-Beam Radiotherapy

Conventional external-beam radiotherapy relieves symptoms of hemoptysis, dyspnea, or chest pain in 50% to 80% of patients for 3 to 4 months.[49] Brachytherapy has been shown to be as effective as or even superior to external-beam radiotherapy for the relief of obstructive symptoms. In one study, after just one exposure to HDR brachytherapy, the tumor was debulked in approximately 88% of patients, and the hemoptysis was improved in 86%.[44] These responses were maintained for 4 months. In a smaller group of patients who had received external-beam radiotherapy, brachytherapy did not result in long-lasting relief of symptoms. There are no studies directly comparing external-beam radiotherapy with endobronchial brachytherapy. On the basis of existing data, however, endobronchial brachytherapy has been a first-line and second-line treatment option offering effective palliation.

Endobronchial Brachytherapy with Nd:YAG Laser Therapy

The Nd:YAG laser uses high energy to debulk tumor, resulting in rapid recanalization of the bronchial lumen.

Rapid regrowth of the tumor with renewed obstruction may require a second laser treatment, which carries risks for massive hemoptysis, fistula formation, bronchial perforation, and decreased efficacy.[40, 42] Schray et al.[39] reported response rates of 54% for combined laser therapy and LDR brachytherapy. In their retrospective review, Shea et al.[50] found significant differences in survival duration between patients who underwent combined LDR brachytherapy and laser and those who had laser therapy alone. The use of Nd:YAG with brachytherapy varies with the institution.

Brachytherapy as a Curative Therapy

Brachytherapy may have curative potential in selected patients who are not candidates for surgical resection. Sutedja et al. [43] have reported on two patients with poor cardiopulmonary function who were subsequently "cured" of intraluminal T1N0 squamous cell carcinoma after receiving three fractions of HDR brachytherapy. Nori et al.[48] described pathologically complete responses, which were documented 8 months after the last treatment. Saito et al.[51] conducted a prospective phase II study of external-beam radiation with LDR brachytherapy in patients with radiologically occult lung carcinoma. All of the 41 patients treated showed a complete response. These results are preliminary, however, and further studies are needed to evaluate this potential curative effect.

Complications

Brachytherapy has both early and late complications. In addition, the bronchoscopy procedure and the insertion of the catheter may cause pneumothorax, bleeding, infection, cough, catheter displacement, and bronchospasm. In experienced hands, however, the procedure has few and usually minor complications.

The two most serious complications of endobronchial brachytherapy are massive hemoptysis and formation of fistula with the mediastinum. Serious complications range from 0 to 42% in several large series.[42–54] The risk of massive pulmonary hemorrhage is likely related to the proximity of pulmonary arteries to the left upper lobe bronchus. Indeed, Bedwinek et al.[55] found a 32% rate of massive hemoptysis in patients undergoing brachytherapy for treatment of recurrent tumors in the right upper lobe, right main-stem bronchus, and left upper lobe bronchus. Khanavkar et al.[56] suggested that the risk for these life-threatening complications is high enough that (1) the procedure should not be used for tumors involving the major arteries and (2) the potential destruction in the bronchial wall and mediastinal invasion by tumors should be evaluated with CT, magnetic resonance imaging, or digital subtraction angiography before endobronchial therapy is instituted.

Summary

Since brachytherapy was first used 80 years ago, it has become an effective tool in the treatment of tracheobronchial malignancy, including primary and recurrent bronchogenic carcinoma and metastatic carcinoma. The technique has evolved from interstitial implantation of radiation sources directly to the tumor through the use of rigid bronchoscopy to intraluminal placement of a radiation source into a polyethylene catheter that is first inserted by fiberoptic bronchoscopy. Intraluminal brachytherapy is effective in palliating complications of malignant endobronchial tumors, such as dyspnea, hemoptysis, intractable cough, and pneumonia. Brachytherapy may be combined with external-beam radiotherapy or Nd:YAG laser therapy to enhance palliation. The risk of severe complications of brachytherapy may be related more to the location of the tumor being treated than to irradiation. Further investigations are necessary to determine the optimal dose scheme for brachytherapy and its efficacy when used in combination with external-beam radiotherapy or another endobronchial procedure, such as Nd:YAG laser therapy or cryotherapy.

AIRWAY STENTS

When an extraluminal malignancy compresses a large airway (**Fig. 23-2**), stents can play a major therapeutic role. The nature of the obstruction, the acuity of presentation, and the availability and the expertise of the bronchoscopist and interventional radiologist all affect the efficacy of the stenting procedure.[57] Over the past two decades, variously designed stents have been used in clinical practice. The ideal airway stent has characteristics that have never been achieved—ease of insertion and removal; availability in different sizes to match the obstruction; ability to maintain position without migration; resistance to compressive forces with sufficient elasticity to conform to the airway contours; construction with inert material that will not to irritate the airway, precipitate infection, or promote granulation tissue; and possession of characteristics of the normal airway so that mobilization of secretions is not impaired.

Indications

Stents may be used alone or with other techniques for palliation of dyspnea, cough, or respiratory insuffi-

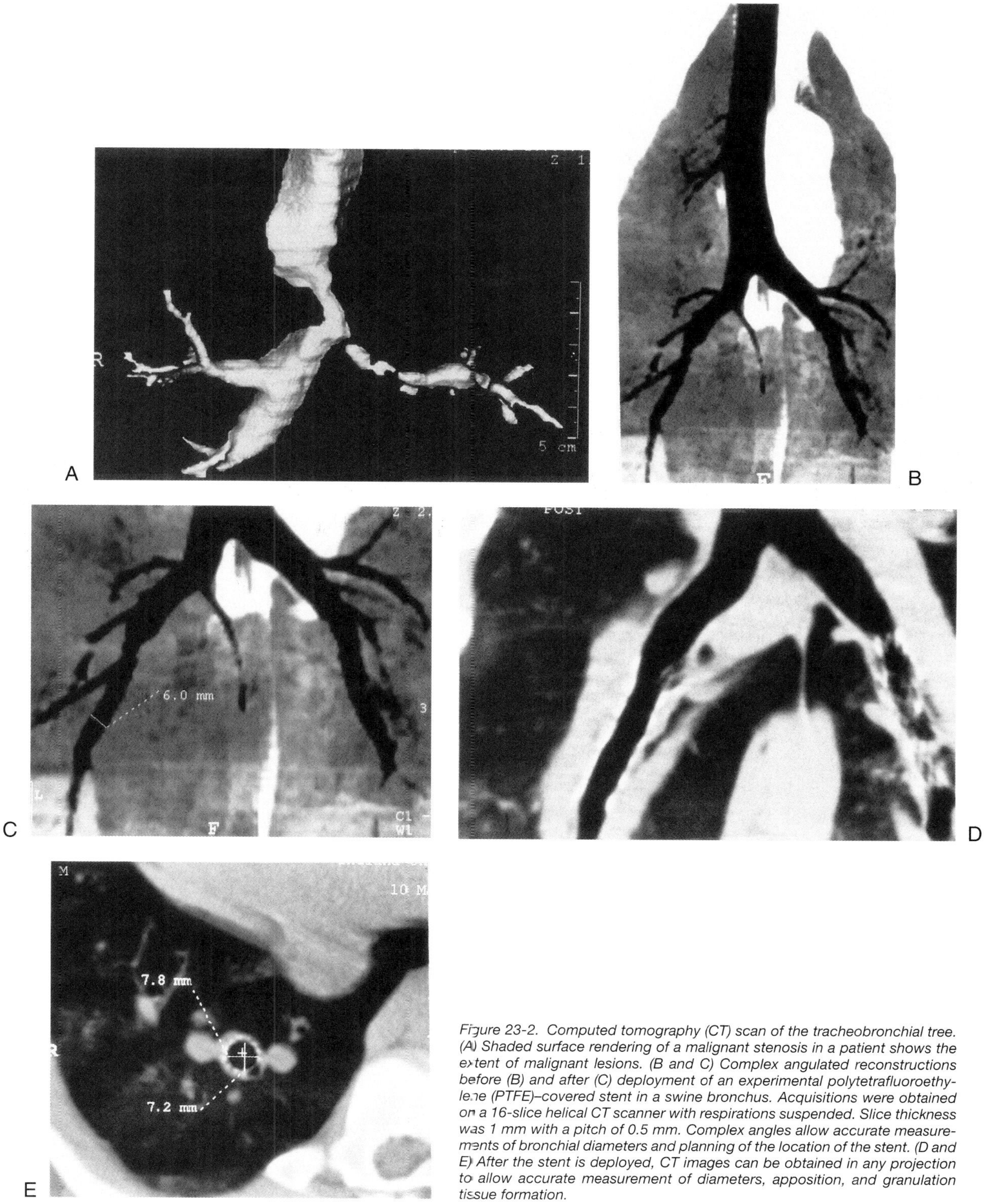

Figure 23-2. Computed tomography (CT) scan of the tracheobronchial tree. (A) Shaded surface rendering of a malignant stenosis in a patient shows the extent of malignant lesions. (B and C) Complex angulated reconstructions before (B) and after (C) deployment of an experimental polytetrafluoroethylene (PTFE)–covered stent in a swine bronchus. Acquisitions were obtained on a 16-slice helical CT scanner with respirations suspended. Slice thickness was 1 mm with a pitch of 0.5 mm. Complex angles allow accurate measurements of bronchial diameters and planning of the location of the stent. (D and E) After the stent is deployed, CT images can be obtained in any projection to allow accurate measurement of diameters, apposition, and granulation tissue formation.

TABLE 23-5
Indications for Stent Placement

Malignant conditions
- Malignant neoplasm with extrinsic compression of large airway
- Malignant tracheobronchial obstruction despite laser resection, cryotherapy, and dilation
- Malignant tracheobronchial obstruction in patients undergoing external-beam radiotherapy or chemotherapy
- Tracheobronchial esophageal fistula in conjunction with esophageal stent

Benign conditions
- Post-traumatic lesion after intubation
- Post-infectious stricture (endobronchial tuberculosis)
- Fibrosing mediastinitis
- Post-inflammatory (Wegener's granulomatosis)
- Complications after lung transplant (anastomotic stenosis, tracheobronchomalacia)
- Tracheobronchomalacia (after radiation, relapsing polychondritis)
- Benign tumors (amyloidosis)
- Congenital tracheoesophageal fistula
- Tracheal distortion due to kyphoscoliosis
- Extrinsic compression from esophageal stent

ciency due to central airway obstruction. Specific indications for their use are listed in **Table 23-5.**[58]

An airway stent supports the airway wall against collapse or external compression and can impede extension of tumor into the airway lumen. Stents can be safely used in patients undergoing external-beam radiotherapy or brachytherapy but can burn or break when subjected to Nd:YAG laser energy.

Types Of Stents

Tracheobronchial stents may be silicone, metal, or hybrid. The development of hybrid stents for tracheobronchial obstruction is an extension of the development of covered stents for use in the vascular system.

Silicone Stents

The most widely used type of stent for central airway obstruction is the silicone stent. Silicone rubber is a synthetic substance made of silicone elastomers; it is firm, is stable at high temperatures, and repels water. Silicone is easily molded and can be given various degrees of firmness or flexibility. Silicone stents are relatively inexpensive, are well tolerated, do not break down in place, and resist extrinsic compression from tumor, enlarged lymph nodes, and firm circumferential scars.

Placement of silicone stents usually requires rigid bronchoscopy and general anesthesia, although insertion of stents with flexible bronchoscopy has been described. Multiple stents can be inserted, if necessary, to palliate long areas of airway obstruction. Once placed, a silicone stent can be repositioned with rigid grasping forceps, and a stent of unsatisfactory size can be removed easily.

The first modern-day stent was the Montgomery silicone T tube, which was developed in 1965 for treatment of subglottic stenosis. Tracheotomy is required for placement of this stent.[59, 60] Complications include drying of secretions. The side tube can be closed to facilitate speech and humidification and can be opened for stent cleaning.

Silicone stents migrate more commonly than other prostheses (about 30% of the time), and may require several bronchoscopic procedures for repositioning. Obstruction by accumulated secretions occurs in most patients, and granulation tissue at the proximal or distal end of the stent may necessitate careful endoscopic laser therapy or cryotherapy for removal. Silicone stents of various lengths, shapes, and diameters are available. Custom prostheses can be ordered from several makers, and we commonly obtain them for patients who have benign, complex airway strictures due to Wegener's granulomatosis, tuberculosis, or tracheobronchomalacia. Various silicone devices are available, including the smooth-walled Hood stent, the studded Dumon stent, and the Reynders-Noppen tygon stent.

The smooth-walled Hood stent was one of the first silicone stents designed for use in the airway. It is a straight, smooth-walled silicone tube that can be ordered in varying lengths and diameters and in a Y-shape. Because the stent can be easily displaced within the airway by coughing, the design has been modified to include small flanges on its proximal and distal aspects. Nevertheless, stent migration still occurs.

The studded Dumon stent has become the most widely used airway stent in the world and is now regarded by many as the gold standard of tracheobronchial stents.[61, 62] The stent is manufactured in various diameters and lengths as well as in different shapes, including straight, L-shaped, and Y-shaped. The stent incorporates small studs on its external surface to help prevent migration. These studs embed themselves slightly within the airway wall mucosa, but do not cause damage. However, the migration rate for the Dumon stent is 30%. One of the shortcomings of the stent is its wall thickness, which offers a low internal to external diameter ratio, thus providing for a relatively smaller lumen.

Placement of the Dumon stent requires rigid bronchoscope with a special, expensive delivery system and the use of general anesthesia. Careful attention must be paid to size selection, and periodic bronchoscopy is needed for stent cleaning. Complications such as stent migration, obstruction from retained secretions, and granuloma are some of its important drawbacks. To circumvent the relatively small lumen of the thick-walled Dumon stent, an experimental self-expandable synthetic polyester wire mesh stent impregnated with a thin layer of silicone is being studied, and the initial results are encouraging.

The studded Hood Stent contains studs in a configuration similar to that in the Dumon stent. The performance and characteristics of the Hood stent appear to be equivalent to those of the Dumon stent.

The Reynders-Noppen tygon stent is not yet commercially available in the United States. It is a cylindrical tygon plastic tube molded into a screw-thread form. This stent is far more rigid than silicone stents. It must be pushed into place along the outside of a specific introducer; it cannot be folded into a bronchoscopic applicator for introduction. One study compared the outcome in 50 patients treated with either studded Dumon silicone stents or screw-thread stents. Stent migration occurred in more patients who received Dumon stents (24% versus 5%), although the difference was not statistically significant. Overall experience with screw-thread prostheses is limited.[62, 63]

Metallic Stents

Various metals, such as stainless steel, tantalum, and alloys incorporating cobalt, chromium, and molybdenum (Vitallium, Nobelium) are inherently inert and can be safely placed into living tissues. The clinical application of tube stents and the recognition that incorporation of metal adds to the rigidity of these stents, coupled with the successful use of metallic stents in animal models and in the esophagus, biliary tree, and vasculature, have led to the development of metallic tracheobronchial stents.

All metallic stents are radiopaque, exhibit varying degrees of dynamic expandability, are easy to insert, and maintain ventilation when placed across lobar orifices.[64–67] The stents can be further divided into fixed-diameter stents, which require balloon dilation, and self-expandable stents, which spring to a predetermined diameter once released. These stents are either made of bare metal or have a thin coating of silicone, polyethylene terephthalate (PET, Dacron®), polyurethane, or polytetrafluoroethylene (PTFE).

Uncovered stents that have been used in the tracheobronchial tree include balloon-expandable stents, such as the Palmaz stent (Cordis Endovascular, a Johnson & Johnson Co., Warren, New Jersey) and the Strecker Stent (Boston Scientific Corp., Natick, Massachusetts), and self-expandable stents, such as the Wallstent endoprosthesis (Boston Scientific Corp.) and the Gianturco Z-stent (Cook, Inc., Bloomington, Indiana).[68–74] Self-expandable stents are preferred for treatment of extrinsically compressible malignancies because they resist compressive forces such as breathing and coughing.

Metallic stents offer several advantages over silicone prostheses. They can be introduced with a fiberoptic bronchoscope and therefore need only topical airway anesthesia and conscious sedation for placement. These stents can also be inserted over fluoroscopically guided wires. Metallic stents rarely migrate within the tracheobronchial tree (<1%). If the airway cannot be dilated before stent insertion, self-expanding stents can be introduced and may generate sufficient force to distend the airway.

However, proper selection of stent size is essential, and there is a risk of airway perforation due to the expansile force of these devices. Metallic stents are more expensive then silicone prostheses. They are difficult, if not impossible, to remove. Granulation tissue or tumor can grow easily in the spaces between metal struts, leading to obstruction; this complication can be prevented by the covering on the newer stents.

The Gianturco Z-stent is made of a continuous loop of stainless steel wire and can be compressed into a narrow cylinder before bronchoscopic placement. The stent comes in varying diameters and in both single and double post-expansion lengths; multiple stents can be attached to bridge longer lesions. Once expanded, Gianturco Z-stents maintain an expansive force, and their small hooks embed in the airway mucosa to retard migration. Airway patency is maintained as long as tissue or tumor does not grow through the stainless steel wire. Complications of the Gianturco Z-stent include migration, tracheopharyngeal fistula, persistent cough, strut fracture, perforation, fatal erosion of pulmonary artery, and dislodgment and unraveling of the stent after entrapment of the suction catheter. The high pressures exerted by the stent over the airway mucosa at selected contact points may lead to mucosal ischemia and perforation.[74] Owing to the severity of reported complications, the Gianturco Z-stent is seldom used in the United States.

The Wallstent endoprosthesis is a self-expanding device made of cobalt alloy braided filaments in the form of a tubular mesh. It has a special feature of outward radial force provided by its integral design. It is inserted in a constrained form and, once deployed, expands to a preset diameter. The stent can be loaded into a delivery catheter for placement, after which it expands and shortens. Various lengths and diameters are available. This type of stent is becoming more widely used because it is placed with a fiberoptic bronchoscope and can therefore be placed by operators who do not perform rigid bronchoscopy (only 8% of U.S. bronchoscopists perform rigid bronchoscopy).[65] The covered metal stent prevents growth of tumor and granulation tissue through the spaces in the thin wire mesh.

Self-expandable stents made from nitinol have been used in clinical practice. The nickel-titanium alloy stent exhibits properties of "shape memory"; that is, the stent deforms plastically at cold temperatures and regains its original shape at higher or body temperatures.[75] Several series have reported successful treatment of endobronchial obstruction with nitinol stents.[76–78]

Stents incorporating both silicone and metal have been designed in an attempt to remedy some of the drawbacks of purely silicone or metal devices. These hybrid stents consist of expandable metal struts, which resist compression, covered by a silicone membrane or other material, which limits infiltration by tumor or granulation tissue. These devices are more expensive than stents made exclusively of silicone or metal but are designed to limit the granulation tissue formation that results in failure of metallic stents.

The covered Wallstent endoprosthesis is similar to the bare metal Wallstent endoprosthesis but is partially covered with a silicone membrane designed to prevent extension of tumor or granulation tissue through the spaces between the thin wire struts. It is available in various lengths and diameters, easily fits into a catheter for insertion, and is designed specifically for airway use. The stent is self-expanding and maintains its expansile force after insertion. Clinical experience with this stent is growing in the United States, and its utility remains hampered by the difficulty of repositioning or removing it. The Ultraflex stent (Boston Scientific Corp.) also comes with a silicone covering.

The Wallgraft endoprosthesis (Boston Scientific Corp.) is a PET (Dacron®)–covered stent. Currently in trial for vascular application, the Wallgraft is approved by the United States Food and Drug Administration (FDA) for use in the tracheobronchial tree. Newer stents under development include devices with PTFE covering. The hope is that these materials may be more durable than silicone while less prone to formatin of granulation tissue.

The Rusch Y-stent is a Y-shaped stent made of silicone with a firm anterior wall consisting of horseshoe-shaped metal struts that simulate the anterior tracheal wall; the posterior wall is made of soft silicone, simulating the pars membranosa of the trachea. The stent is quite long and comes in different diameters. The stent can be difficult to insert. It is placed during rigid laryngoscopy by means of a specially designed forceps, and the two distal limbs are inserted into the left and right main-stem bronchi. Experience with this stent is limited, but its use may be appropriate in the patient with significant tracheobronchomalacia or a long stricture involving the trachea and both main-stem bronchi.[79] However, the length of the Rusch Y-stent makes it difficult for patients to effectively clear airway secretions, and if it becomes obstructed, its removal can be difficult.

Stent Deployment

Bronchoscopy should be performed in all patients with symptoms or radiographic findings suggestive of tracheobronchial stenosis. When a stenosis is discovered, the distance from the vocal cords and the length and diameter of the lesion should be documented. A spiral CT scan with three-dimensional reconstruction is extremely helpful in the sizing of the stent. Exact measurements of the normal bronchial diameter and the length of the lesion are best obtained from the CT reconstructions. Imaging should be performed on a multidetector CT scanner if possible, to enable 1-mm slice thickness through the entire bronchial tree on a single breath-hold. This approach will limit the effects of motion artifact (see **Fig. 23-2**). The type of stent placed and the preference of the operator determine whether a rigid or flexible bronchoscopy is performed. The stent can be inserted as part of a bronchoscopic procedure, including cryotherapy, electrocautery, and Nd:YAG laser resection.[65]

If a lesion is not amenable to endoscopic removal, bronchial dilation should be performed so that the stent of greatest diameter can be inserted. When the rigidity of a lesion makes dilation unsafe or impractical, stents of increasing size can be inserted sequentially. This procedure is best accomplished with the use of silicone stents, which are easily removed and replaced. Alternatively, a self-expanding metal stent can be inserted and may restore airway patency. In such cases, proper selection of the caliber and length of the stent is essential.

Wallstents are exclusively inserted with the flexible bronchoscope. The operator measures the length of the obstructed segment by withdrawing the tip of the bronchoscope from the distal to the proximal end of the stenosis. CT of the chest, specifically three-dimensional reconstruction, allows for accurate measurement of the length and diameter of the stenosed segment as well as the diameter of the proximal normal airways and, particularly for tight stenosis, evaluation of the status of the distal airways.

The stent is placed with fluoroscopic guidance (**Fig. 23-3**). A team approach involving the interventional radiologist and pulmonologist is very helpful. The stent is delivered using a 7F–9F coaxial catheter system. It is mounted on an inner catheter whose central lumen allows a 0.035-inch guidewire to be passed easily. Radiopaque marker bands are placed on the inner catheter, marking either end of the stent. The initial step uses fiberoptic bronchoscopy and fluoroscopy to define the lesion and permit placement of skin markers corresponding to the distal and proximal ends of the ob-

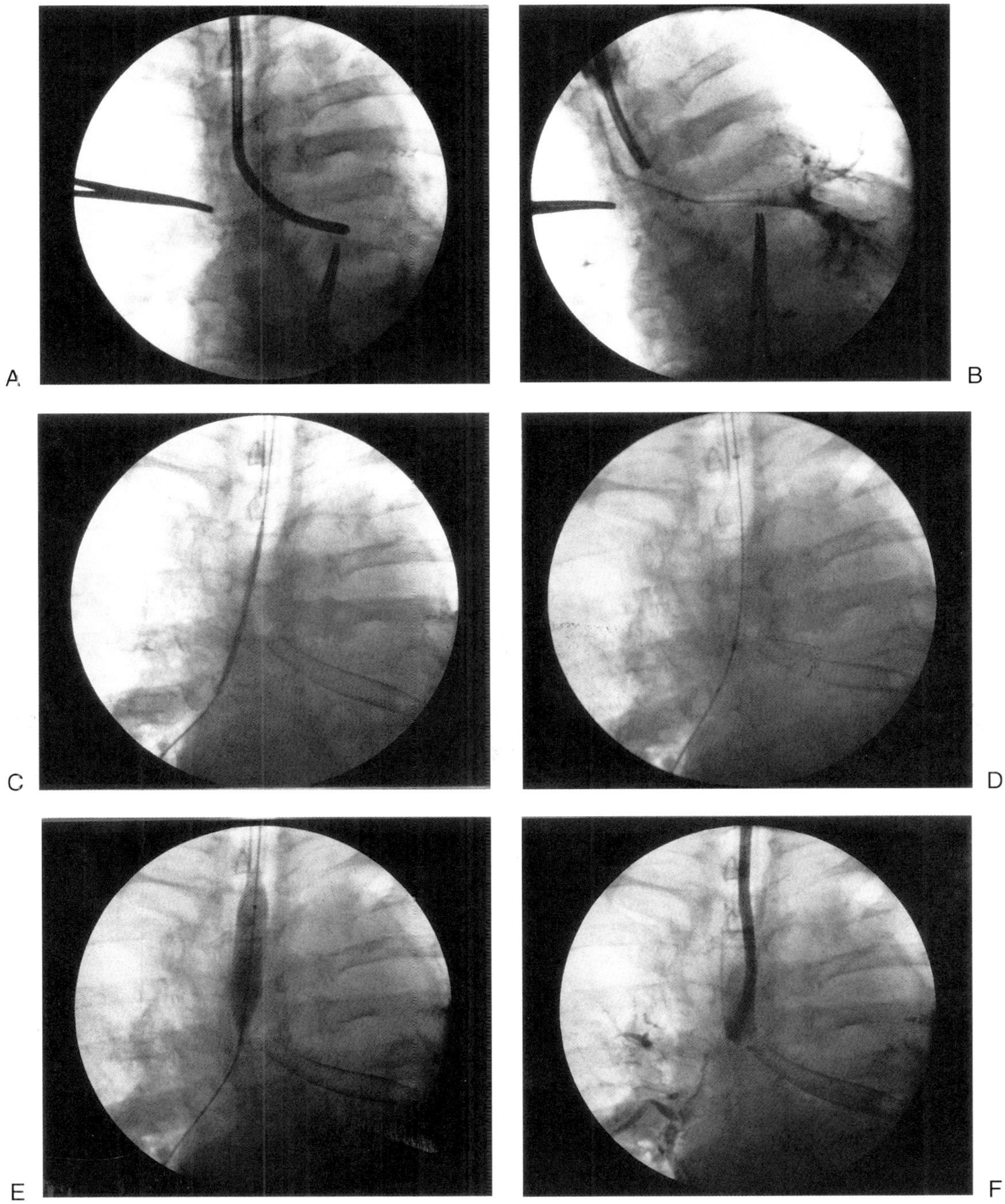

Figure 23-3. Deployment of tracheobronchial Wallstent endoprosthesis. On the basis of the CT scan shown in Figure 23-2A, treatment was undertaken. (A) With the use of endoscopy, the margins of the lesions were identified and hemostats were clipped to the drape. (B) A small amount of contrast material was injected to confirm the anatomy, and the Wallstent endoprosthesis was deployed in the left main-stem bronchus. (C and D) The endoscope was then used to direct a Rosen guidewire down the right main-stem bronchus, and a Wallstent endoprosthesis was positioned in the distal trachea and deployed. (E) A 16-mm balloon was used to post-dilate the tracheal stent. (F and G) The endoscope was then used to identify the lesion extending into the right main-stem bronchus, and another Wallstent endoprosthesis was deployed over a Rosen guidewire. (continued on next page)

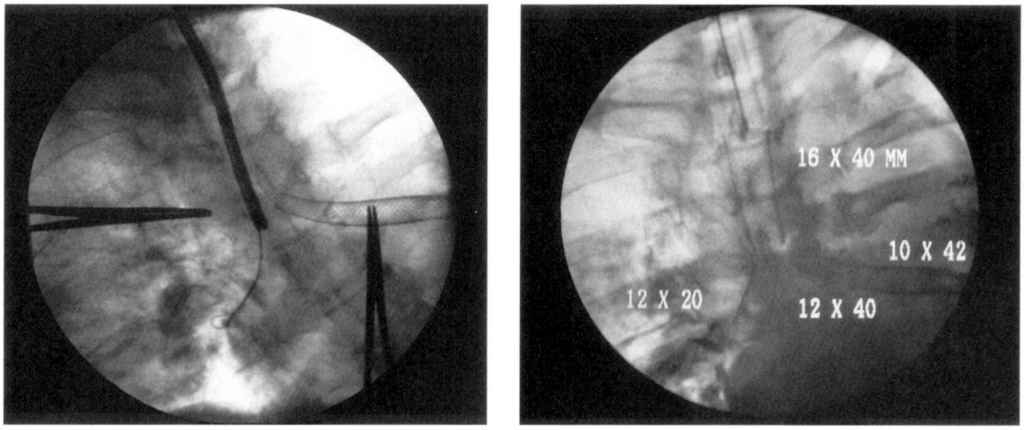

G H

Figure 23-3 (continued). (H) The final image shows a 16-mm tracheal Wallstent endoprosthesis, a 10-mm distal left main-stem Wallstent endoprosthesis, and a 12-mm Wallstent endoprosthesis in the proximal right and left main-stem bronchus.

struction. A 180-cm-long, 0.035-inch Rosen guidewire (Cook, Inc., Bloomington, Indiana) is then introduced past the obstructed segment through the use of bronchoscopic and fluoroscopic guidance. The scope is then carefully withdrawn, leaving the guidewire in place. The stent of a preselected size, with its delivery system, is inserted next over the guidewire, and the distal radiopaque marker band is aligned just beyond the distal skin marker. Gradual withdrawal of the outer catheter allows controlled deployment of the stent under continuous fluoroscopic monitoring. The delivery system is then easily removed through the expanded stent. The stent is dilated with a balloon catheter of appropriate size. This dilation step facilitates complete expansion of the stent; otherwise, compressive forces of the lesion operating against the stent may limit its full expansion.

In a study of 51 Wallstents placed in 37 patients, 18 of whom presented with acute symptoms,[65] symptomatic improvement occurred in 97% of patients, and bronchoscopic evidence of airway patency was seen in all. Granuloma formation was observed in 6 patients, and the inserted stents had to be withdrawn in 1 patient because of staphylococcal bronchitis. Technical problems related to inappropriate length of the stent occurred in 5 patients. Other investigators have reported results of Wallstent placement for a variety of indications. Common to many of these reports is the fact that stent placement is a palliative procedure, and symptomatic rather than objective improvement is the key. Their flexibility and elasticity permit the stents to mold to a tortuous or distorted airway. Patients can also be intubated through a Wallstent placed in the trachea; silicone stents must be removed to allow intubation.

Although insertion of a Wallstent is easy, there are certain technical limitations. To maintain integration of the stent, the individual alloy filaments must make a precise number of turns. Thus, for any given diameter, the stent must be of a particular length. The predetermined length may be either too short or too long for the stenosed segment. If the stent is shorter than the segment, coaxially overlapping a second stent within the first would be required. If the stent is longer, it may either protrude proximally or extend distally to cover lobar orifices. Although the latter situation does not interfere with ventilation initially, granuloma formation may obstruct the orifices, leading to lobar collapse. Careful selection of a stent of the appropriate size is important, so that only its body covers the stenosed segment, leaving the terminal ends free to become embedded in the airway mucosa.

Complications

Granulation tissue formation is the most vexing of all complications of tracheobronchial stents. It results from excessive reaction to the stent and resembles foreign body reaction. It is only when granulation tissue produces symptoms that interventions (laser therapy or cryotherapy) are required. Cough after stent placement is uncommon. Chest pain or discomfort, hemoptysis, and foreign body sensation have not been encountered.

Summary

Considerable progress has been made since the initial stents were manufactured. Despite their reported side effects, cumulative evidence suggests beneficial effects of stents when placed in properly selected patients. The technology is still in evolution, and design modifications continue to be made in a search for the perfect stent. The Dumon stent remains the standard against which the all other stents are measured.

REFERENCES

1. Dumon MC, Dumon JF. Laser bronchoscopy In: Feinsilver SH, Fein AM, eds. *Textbook of Bronchoscopy*. Baltimore: Williams & Wilkins; 1995;393–399.
2. Ramser ER, Beamis JF. Laser bronchoscopy. *Clin Chest Med* 1995;16:415–426.
3. Eichenhorn MS, Kvale PA, Miks VM, et al. Initial combination therapy with YAG laser photoresection and irradiation for inoperable non-small cell carcinoma of the lung. *Chest* 1986;89:782–785.
4. Gelb AF, Epstein JD. Neodymium-Yttrium-Aluminum-Garnet laser in lung cancer. *Ann Thorac Surg* 1987;43:164–167.
5. Macha HN, Becker KO, Kemmer HP. Pattern of failure and survival in endobronchial laser resection. *Chest* 1994;105:1668–1672.
6. Kvale PA, Eichenhorn MS, Radke JR, et al. YAG laser photoresection of lesions obstructing the central airways. *Chest* 1985;87:283–288.
7. Ross DJ, Mohsenifar Z, Koerner SK. Survival characteristics after neodymium:YAG laser photoresection in advanced stage lung cancer. *Chest* 1990;98:581–585.
8. Stanopoulos IT, Beamis JF, Martinez FJ, et al. Laser bronchoscopy in respiratory failure from malignant airway obstruction. *Crit Care Med* 1993;21:386–391.
9. Toty L, Personne C, Colchen A, et al. Bronchoscopic management of tracheal lesions using the neodymium yttrium aluminum garnet laser. *Thorax* 1981;36:175–178.
10. Madden BP, Kumar P, Sayer R, et al. Successful resection of obstructing airway granulation tissue following lung transplantation using endobronchial (Nd:YAG) therapy. *Eur J Cardiothorac Surg* 1997;12:480–485.
11. Brutinel WM, Cortese DA, Edell ES, et al. Complications of Nd:YAG laser therapy. *Chest* 1988;94:902–903.
12. Sacco O, Fregonese B, Oddone M, et al. Severe endobronchial obstruction in a girl with relapsing polychondritis: treatment with Nd YAG laser and endobronchial silicon stent. *Eur Respir J* 1997;10:494–496.
13. Witt C, John M, Martin H, et al. Behçet's syndrome with pulmonary involvement: combined therapy for endobronchial stenosis using neodymium-YAG laser, balloon dilation and immunosuppression. *Respiration* 1996;63:195–198.
14. Cahill BC, Harmon KR, Sumway SJ, et al. Tracheobronchial obstruction due to silicosis. *Am Rev Respir Dis* 1992;145:719–721.
15. Shah H, Garbe L, Nussbaum E, et al. Benign tumors of the tracheobronchial tree: endoscopic characteristics and role of laser resection. *Chest* 1995;107:1744–1751.
16. Hetzel MR, Nixon C, Edmondstone WM, et al. Laser therapy in 100 tracheobronchial tumors. *Thorax* 1985;40:341–345.
17. Desai SJ, Mehta AC, VanderBrug Medendorp S, et al. Survival experience following Nd:YAG laser photoresection for primary bronchogenic carcinoma. *Chest* 1988;94:939–944.
18. Mehta AC, Lee FY, DeBoer GE. Flexible bronchoscopy and the use of lasers. In: Wang KP, Mehta AC, eds. *Flexible Bronchoscopy*. Cambridge: Blackwell Science; 1995:247–274.
19. Cavaliere S, Venuta F, Foccoli P, et al. Endoscopic treatment of malignant airway obstructions in 2,008 patients. *Chest* 1996;110:1536–1542.
20. Mazur P. Cryobiology: the freezing of biologic systems. *Science* 1970;168:939–949.
21. Maiwand MO, Homasson JP. Cryotherapy for tracheal bronchial disorders. *Clin Chest Med* 1995;16:427–443.
22. Walsh DA, Maiwand MD, Nath AR, et al. Bronchoscopic cryotherapy for advanced bronchial carcinoma. *Thorax* 1990;45:509–513.
23. Mathur PN, Wolf K, Busk MF, et al. Fiberoptic bronchoscopic cryotherapy in the management of tracheobronchial disorder. *Chest* 1996;110:718–723.
24. Vergnon JM, Schmitt T, Alamartine E, et al. Initial combined cryotherapy and irradiation for unresectable non-small cell lung cancer. *Chest* 1992;102:1436–1440.
25. Hooper RG, Jackson FN. Endobronchial electrocautery. *Chest* 1985;87:712–714.
26. Hooper RG, Jackson FN. Endobronchial electrocautery. *Chest* 1988;94:595–598.
27. Morice RC, Ece T, Ece F, and Keus AL. Endobronchial argon plasma coagulation for treatment of hemoptysis and neoplastic airway obstruction. *Chest* 2001; 119:781–787.
28. Homasson JP. Endobronchial electrocautery. *Semin Respir Crit Care Med* 1997;18:535–543.
29. Petrou M, Kaplan D, Goldstraw P. Bronchoscopic diathermy resection and stent insertion: a cost effective treatment for tracheobronchial obstruction. *Thorax* 1993;48:1156–1159.
30. Sutedja G, van Kralingen K, Schramet FM, et al. Fiberoptic bronchoscopic electrosurgery under local anesthesia for rapid palliation in patients with central airway malignancies: a preliminary report. *Thorax* 1994;49:1243–1246.
31. Carpenter RJ, Neel T, Sanderson DR. Comparison of endoscopic cryosurgery and electrocoagulation of bronchi. *Trans Am Acad Ophthalmol Otolaryngol* 1977;84:313–323.
32. Sutedja G, Schramel FM, Smit EF, et al. Bronchoscopic electrocautery as an alternative for Nd:YAG laser in patients with intraluminal tumor. *Eur Respir* 1996;9(supp 23):S258–S259.
33. Lavandier M, Carre P, Rivoire B, et al. High frequency electrocautery in the management of tracheobronchial disorders [abstract]. *Respir Crit Care Med* 1996;75:A477.
34. Yankauer S. Two cases of lung tumor treated bronchoscopically. *N Y Med J* 1922;741–742.
35. Tellides G, Uguslu BS, Kim RW, and Hammond GL. Pathogenesis of systemic air embolism during bronchoscopic Nd:YAG laser operations. *Ann Thorac Surg* 1998;65:930–934.
36. Henschke UK, Hilaris BS, Mahan GD. Remote afterloading with intracavitary applicators. *Radiology* 1964;83:344–345.
37. Mendiondo OA, Dillon M, Beach JL. Endobronchial brachytherapy in the treatment of recurrent bronchogenic carcinoma. *Int J Radiat Oncol Biol Phys* 1983;9:579–582.
38. Moylan D, Strubler K, Unal A, et al. Work in progress. Transbronchial brachytherapy of recurrent bronchogenic carcinoma: a new approach using the flexible fiberoptic bronchoscope. *Radiology* 1983;147:253–254.
39. Schray MF, McDougall JC, Martinez A, et al. Management of malignant airway obstruction: clinical and dosimetric consideration using an iridium-192 afterloading technique in conjunction with the neodymium-YAG laser. *Int J Radiat Oncol Biol Phys* 1985;11:403–409.
40. Schray MF, McDougall JC, Martinez A, et al. Management of malignant airway compromise with laser and low dose rate brachytherapy: the Mayo Clinic experience. *Chest* 1988;93:264–269.
41. Seagren SL, Harrell JH, Horn RA. High dose rate intraluminal irradiation in recurrent endobronchial carcinoma. *Chest* 1985;88:810–814.
42. Allen MD, Baldwin JC, Fish VJ, et al. Combined laser therapy and endobronchial radiotherapy for unresectable lung cancer for bronchial obstruction. *Am J Surg* 1985;150:71–77.
43. Sutedja G, Baris G, Van Zandwijk N, et al. High-dose rate brachytherapy has a curative potential in patients with intraluminal squamous cell lung cancer. *Respiration* 1994;61:167–168.
44. Burt PA, O'Driscoll BR, Notley HM, et al. Intraluminal irradiation for the palliation of lung cancer with the high dose rate micro-Selectron. *Thorax* 1990;45:765–768.
45. Chang LF, Horvath J, Peyton W, et al. High dose rate after loading intraluminal brachytherapy in malignant airway obstructions of lung cancer. *Int J Radiat Oncol Biol Phys* 1994;28:589–596.
46. Gollins SW, Burt PA, Barber PV, et al. High dose rate intraluminal radiotherapy for carcinoma of the bronchus: outcome of treatment of 406 patients. *Radiother Oncol* 1994;33:31–40.
47. Speiser B, Spratling L. Remote afterloading brachytherapy for the local control of endobronchial carcinoma. *Int J Radiat Oncol Biol Phys* 1993;25:579–587.

48. Nori D, Allison R, Kaplan B, et al. High dose-rate intraluminal irradiation in bronchogenic carcinoma. *Chest* 1993;104:1006–1011.
49. Murren JR, Buzaid AC. Chemotherapy and radiation for the treatment of non-small cell lung cancer: a critical review. *Clin Chest Med* 1993;14:161–171.
50. Shea JM, Allen RP, Tharratt RS, et al. Survival of patients undergoing Nd:YAG laser therapy and compared with Nd:YAG laser therapy and brachytherapy for malignant airway diseases. *Chest* 1993;103:1028–1031.
51. Saito M, Yokoyama A, Kurito Y, et al. Treatment of roentgenographically occult endobronchial carcinoma with external beam radiotherapy and intraluminal low dose brachytherapy. *Int J Radiat Oncol Biol Phys* 1996;34:1029–1035.
52. Lo TC, Beamis JF Jr, Weinstein RS, et al. Intraluminal low-dose rate brachytherapy for malignant endobronchial obstruction. *Radiother Oncol* 1992;23:16–20.
53. Mehta MP, Shahabi S, Jarjour NN, et al. Endobronchial irradiation for malignant airway obstruction. *Int J Radiat Oncol Biol Phys* 1989;17:847–851.
54. Sutedja T, Baris G, Schaake-Koning C, et al. High dose rate brachytherapy in patients with local recurrences after radiotherapy of non-small cell lung cancer. *Int J Radiat Oncol Biol Phys* 1992;24:551–553.
55. Bedwinek J, Petty A, Bruton C, et al. The use of high dose rate endobronchial brachytherapy to palliate symptomatic endobronchial recurrence of previously irradiated bronchogenic carcinoma. *Int Radiat Oncol Biol Phys* 1992;22:23–30.
56. Khanavkar B, Stern P. Alberti W, et al. Complications associated with brachytherapy alone or with laser in lung cancer. *Chest* 1991;99:1062–1065.
57. Petrou M, Goldstraw P. The management of tracheobronchial obstruction: A review of endoscopic techniques. *Eur J Cardiothorac Surg* 1994;8:436–441.
58. Colt HG, Dumon JF. Airway stents. Present and future. *Clin Chest Med* 1995;16:465–478.
59. Westaby S, Jackson JW, Pearson FG. A bifurcated silicone rubber stent for relief of tracheobronchial obstruction. *J Thorac Cardiovasc Surg* 1982;83:414–417.
60. Dumon JF, Cavaliere S, Diaz-Jimenez JP, et al. Seven year experience with the Dumon prosthesis. *J Bronchol* 1996;3:6–10.
61. Dumon JF. A dedicated tracheobronchial stent. *Chest* 1990;97:328–332.
62. Noppen M, D'Haese J, Meysman M, et al. A new screw thread tracheal endoprosthesis. *J Bronchol* 1996;3:22–26.
63. Noppen M, Meysman M., Claes I, et al. Screw-thread vs Dumon endoprothesis in management of tracheal stenosis. *Chest* 1999;115:532–535.
64. Daniel RA Jr. The regeneration of defects of the trachea and bronchi. *J Thorac Surg* 1948;17:335–349.
65. Dasgupta A, Dolmatch BL, Abi-Saleh WJ, et al. Self-expandable metallic airway stent insertion employing flexible bronchoscopy: preliminary result. *Chest* 1998;114:106–109.
66. Nesbitt JC, Carrasco CH. Expandable stents. *Chest Surg Clinic N Am* 1996;6:305–328.
67. Nomori H, Kobayashi R, Kodera K, et al. Indications for an expandable metallic stent for tracheobronchial stenosis. *Ann Thorac Surg* 1993;56:1324–1328.
68. Filler RM, Forte V, Chait P. Tracheobronchial stenting for the treatment of airway obstruction. *J Pediatr Surg* 1998;33(2): 304–311.
69. Slonim SM, Razavi M, Kee S, et al.. Transbronchial Palmaz stent placement for tracheo-bronchial stenosis. *J Vasc Interv Radiol* 1998;9:153–160.
70. Bolliger CT, Heitz M, Hauser R, et al.. An airway Wallstent for the treatment of tracheobronchial malignancies. *Thorax* 1996;51:1127–1129.
71. Nakajima Y, Kurihara Y, Niimi H, et al. Efficacy and complications of the Gianturco-Z tracheobronchial stent for malignant airway stenosis. *Cardiovasc Intervent Radiol* 1999;22: 287–292.
72. Sawada S, Tanigawa N, Kobayashi M, et al. Malignant tracheobronchial obstructive lesions: treatment with Gianturco expandable metallic stents. *Radiology* 1993;188:205–208.
73. de Souza AC, Keal R, Hudson NM, et al. Use of expandable stents for malignant airway obstruction. *Ann Thorac Surg* 1994;57: 1573–1577.
74. Nashef SA, Dromer C, Velly JF, et al. Expanding wire stents in benign tracheobronchial disease: indications and complications. *Ann Thorac Surg* 1992;54:937–940.
75. Vinnograd I, Klin B, Brosh T, et al. A new intratracheal stent made from nitinol, an alloy with "shape memory effect." *J Thorac Cardiovasc Surg* 1994;107:1255–1261.
76. Ducic Y, Khalafi RS. Use of endoscopically placed expandable nitinol tracheal stents in the treatment of tracheal stenosis. *Laryngoscope* 1999;109:1130–1133.
77. Nakamura T, Shimizu Y, Matsui T, et al. Novel airway stent using a thermal shape-memory Ti-Ni alloy. *ASAIO Trans* 1991;37:M319–321.
78. Madden BP, Datta S, Charokopos N. Experience with Ultraflex expandable metallic stents in the management of endobronchial pathology. *Ann Thorac Surg* 2002;73:938–944.
79. Freitag L, Tekolf E, Stamatis G, et al. Clinical evaluation of a new bifurcated dynamic airway stent: a 5 year experience with 135 patients. *Thorac Cardivasc Surg* 1997; 45:6–12.

CHAPTER 24

GASTROINTESTINAL OBSTRUCTION

TIMOTHY W. I. CLARK, MD, MSC

ROBERT F. BERRY, MD

MUHAMMAD UMAR ISLAM, MD

STEVEN K. ARNASON, MD

ESOPHAGEAL OBSTRUCTION

It was estimated that in 2002, over 13,000 Americans would be found to have esophageal cancer[1] and that 40%–50% of these patients would have systemic metastases or locally advanced primary tumors precluding curative surgical resection.[2] For those undergoing complete resection of all locoregional disease, long-term survival is poor. One recent large, single-center study reported a median survival of 18 months for 454 patients who underwent esophagogastrectomy.[3]

Interest in esophageal cancer has recently heightened because of a dramatic rise in the disease's incidence since 1980 in North America and Europe, particularly among white, middle-aged men.[4] Primary esophageal adenocarcinomas almost always develop from a columnar epithelium–lined (Barrett's) esophagus. It is thought that gastroesophageal reflux results in acute mucosal injury (esophagitis) and induces columnar metaplasia of the normal squamous epithelium lining the esophagus. The resulting Barrett's esophagus appears predisposed to develop malignancy, at rates 40- to 50-fold greater than in the general population.

Conventional treatment approaches for patients with unresectable esophageal carcinoma have consisted of chemotherapy with concurrent or subsequent radiotherapy; most protocols are associated with significant local and systemic complications.[5–11]

Dysphagia is a leading—and often the most distressing—symptom of esophageal malignancy. The primary aim of palliation is therefore enabling the patient to consume a normal diet, thereby improving quality of life.

Leroy d'Étoiles was the first to insert an esophageal prosthesis in 1845.[12] Sir Charles Symonds manufactured a tube in 1885 that required external fixation to mustache or ears.[13] Gottstein in 1901 invented a rigid indwelling tube that did not require external fixation but was inserted blindly, with frequently fatal complications.[14] Sir Henry Souttar proposed the concept of an ideal esophageal prosthesis as "flexible, incompressible, non-traumatic and compact."[15] Most of these requirements are fulfilled by metallic self-expanding stents. Expandable esophageal prostheses were first employed by Domschke et al. in 1990.[16]

Table 24-1 outlines the main characteristics of currently available devices.[17–20] Several modifications of the Gianturco-Rösch Z stent (Cook, Inc., Bloomington, IN) and Wallstent (Boston Scientific Inc., Natick, MA) are available, but the Gianturco-Rösch Z stent is known for its inherent radial strength. The Ultraflex stent (Boston Scientific Inc.) is flexible in both the radial and longitudinal axes but requires some time to fully expand, because of its relatively low radial force. The Ultraflex and Esophacoil stents (Medtronic-Instent, Eden Prairie, MN) can be placed across sharply angled lesions.[20] The Wallstent is easy to reposition during deployment, provided that less than 50% of the stent has been released.[21] All stents embed to some degree into the esophageal wall.[19]

The Wallstent and Ultraflex stents exhibit significant shortening and therefore must be closely monitored during deployment. Covered stents are useful in sealing malignant tracheoesophageal and tracheopleural fistulae but are known for their high migration rate.[21] Compared to silicone, a polyurethane covering is more resistant to tearing.[22,23] Song et al. described a retrievable expandable metallic stent constructed of stainless-steel wire in a cylindrical zigzag fashion. The stent is polyurethane-covered and has a loop of nylon hooked inside the stent; this enables retrieval with a specific 10-F hook catheter within a 13-F sheath.[23]

Stent Placement Technique

Stents can be placed across an esophageal stricture irrespective of the tumor type. General indications for stent placement include unresectable malignant esophageal neoplasm or extrinsic neoplasm compressing the esophagus, contraindication to surgery or irradiation, recurrence causing dysphagia, or gastroesophageal anastomotic leak. Contraindications for esophageal stent placement include uncorrectable coagulopathy, esophageal varices, lesions less than 2–3 cm from the cricopharyngeus, or a life expectancy of less than 1 month. Sharply angulated lesions are technically very challenging and pose a relative contraindication.

All patients should be evaluated with contrast radiography and endoscopy prior to stent placement. Nonionic contrast should be used for esophagography in all patients with a suspected fistula. The degree of dysphagia should be graded to evaluate response to therapy during follow-up care. A commonly used grading system is provided in **Table 24-2**.[24] The procedure may be per-

TABLE 24-1

General Features of Common Esophageal Stents[17–20]

Stent	Type(s)	Length (cm)	Diameter (mm)	Delivery system(s) (F)	Covering	Radial force	Vendor	Material	Comments
Gianturco-Rösch Z	Covered	4.5–18	18; proximal end, 22.5	24, 28	Polyethylene	+++	Cook, Inc. (Bloomington, IN)	Stainless steel	Barbs on outer surface
Modified Gianturco-Rösch (Song)	Covered	4.5–18	18 and 20; flared ends	24, 28	Polyethylene	+++	Cook, Inc.	Stainless steel	No barbs
Wallstent	Both covered and bare	100, 105	20, 25	18, 22	Polyurethane	++	Boston Scientific Corp. (Natick, MA)	Elgiloy	30% shortening
Ultraflex	Both covered and bare	7, 10, 15	16, 18; flared upper ends	24	Gelatin	+	Boston Scientific Corp.	Nitinol	50% shortening
Esophacoil	Uncovered	10–15	16, 18	27	None	+++	Medtronic-Instent (Eden Prairie, MN)	Nitinol	

TABLE 24-2
Grades of Dysphagia

Grade	Description
0	No dysphagia
1	Ability to eat some solid food
2	Dysphagia to semisolids
3	Ability to swallow liquids only
4	Complete dysphagia

Adapted from Mellow and Pinkas,[24] with permission.

formed using fluoroscopy or fluoroscopy and endoscopy. Endoscopy is useful when placing stents within proximal esophageal lesions for marking the level of the cricopharyngeus muscle. Stents can usually be placed in lesions involving the middle and distal third of the esophagus with fluoroscopic guidance alone.

Although the patient can be placed in supine, prone oblique, or left or right lateral decubitus positions, most surgeons use a prone oblique position. The pharynx is anesthetized with lidocaine spray. Conscious sedation is provided using intravenous midazolam and fentanyl citrate. Prophylactic antibiotics are not indicated. An angled, 5-F to 7-F torquable catheter is inserted through a mouth guard. A hydrophilic guide wire may be needed when crossing a tight stenosis. Nonionic contrast material is injected while the catheter is slowly withdrawn, to outline the full extent of the stricture. Radiopaque markers may be placed on the patient's skin to delineate the lesion. If endoscopic guidance is also being used, submucosal injection of contrast may be performed to mark the distal and proximal limits of the stricture. The catheter is then readvanced past the stricture into the stomach, and a stiff exchange-length guide wire, such as an Amplatz superstiff wire, is introduced. Malignant lesions may be pre-dilated with a 12- to 15-mm diameter angioplasty balloon. Pre-dilation is avoided or limited to a smaller-caliber balloon in the case of a malignant fistula, because enlargement or perforation of the false tract may occur.[25–28]

Stent selection varies among interventional radiologists. It is recommended that the stent length extend at least 2 cm on either side of the lesion. Overlapping stents should be placed from the outset for longer (> 18 cm) stenoses. For midesophageal lesions, a disproportionate length of stent should be left above the stricture to reduce the risk of distal migration.[28] The lower end of the stent should be positioned in the lower esophagus for lesions above the cardia and in the gastric fundus for gastroesophageal junction malignancies. It should be kept in mind that a Wallstent or Ultraflex stent will shorten by one third to one half of its original length. The gelatin-covered Ultraflex stent will expand more slowly as the gelatin dissolves at body temperature.[20] All stents usually expand fully within 24–48 hrs (**Fig. 24-1**). Post-deployment balloon dilation may be carried out for the Ultraflex stent because of its low radial force or when the stent does not initially expand to at least 70% of its original diameter[17,26] (**Fig. 24-2**). Esophacoils expand within seconds and are good for tight, acutely angled stenoses. Polyurethane-covered stents effectively seal most malignant fistulae.

Percutaneous transgastric placement of esophageal stents has been described for patients unable to tolerate a peroral route or when the antegrade approach is technically difficult. The lower esophagus may be accessed through a preexisting or newly created gastrostomy using an angled catheter. Some operators recommend leaving the gastrostomy tube in place for 2 weeks even when it is created for access only; this may decrease the risk of intraperitoneal spill of gastric contents and enables easy reintervention should dysphagia symptoms fail to lessen in severity.[29] Most procedures can be successfully completed within 1 hour, and the majority of patients can leave the hospital on the same day.

Oral fluids are started 2–4 hours after stent placement. Oral fluids are delayed for 1 day when a fistula is present, until a follow-up esophagogram has been obtained to confirm fistula closure. Patients are advised to begin with low-residue food and chew it thoroughly. Small boluses are encouraged. Carbonated drinks or warm fluid at the end of the bolus may help to clear the stent of any entrapped food particles.[17,18,20,26,27,30]

Complications of Stent Placement

The overall complication rate secondary to esophageal stent placement ranges from 0% to 65%.[17,26,28,30,31] **Table 24-3** lists various complications and suggested management approaches. Migration is a frequent complication and has been reported with as many as 50% of covered Wallstents. Migration is more likely to occur when stenting gastroesophageal junction lesions or surgical anastomoses. Tumor shrinkage due to radiation may also induce stent migration. Covered stents and the gelatin-covered Ultraflex are more likely to show this complication. Migrated stents may cause gastrointestinal perforation, spontaneous passage from the rectum, or, more commonly, may remain within the stomach.[26]

Esophageal perforation is uncommon during stent placement and is more likely to arise with large stent delivery systems. Perforation is more likely in stent placement within acutely angled lesions or in the setting of prior radiotherapy or laser ablation. Radial strength may account for delayed perforations, especially with the Gianturco-Rösch Z stent and Esophacoil.[18]

Funnel phenomenon is the creation of a space between the proximal end of the stent and esophagus,

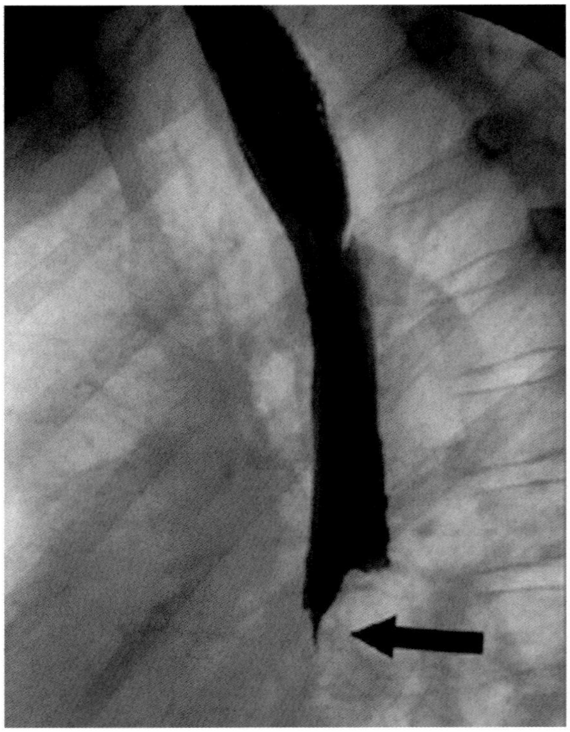

A

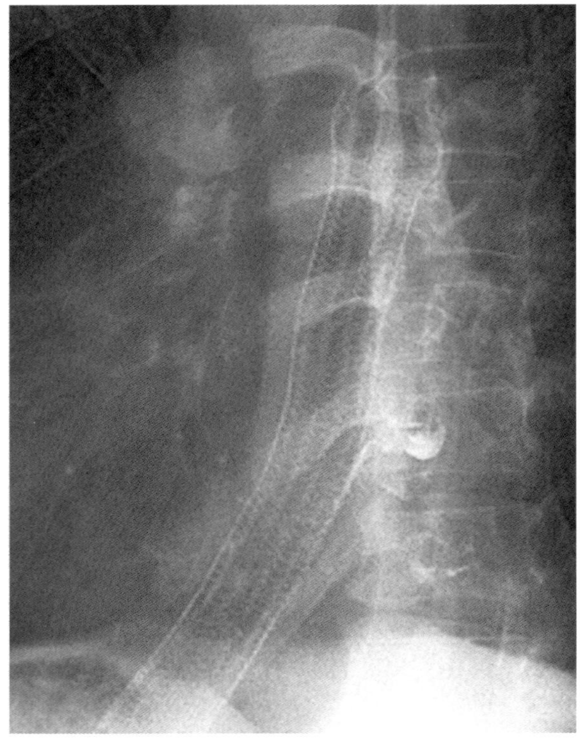

B

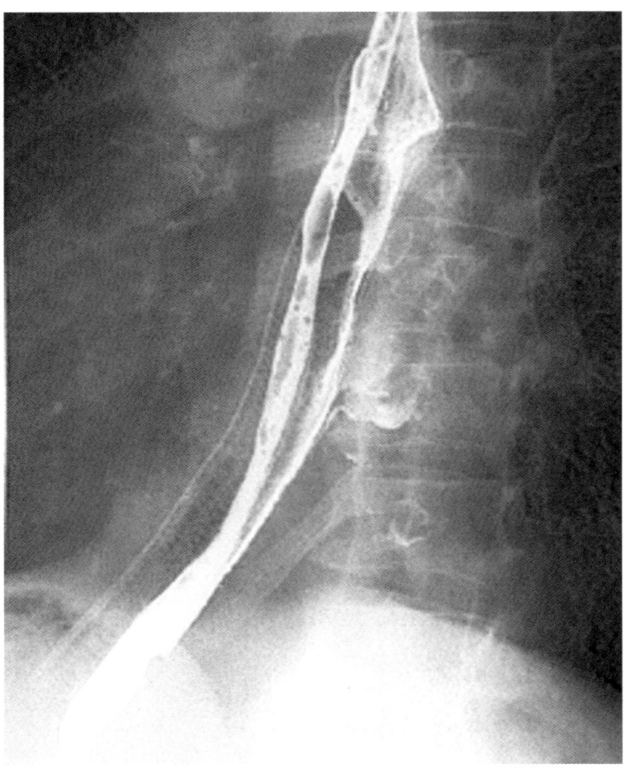

C

Figure 24-1. Esophageal stent placement in a 59-year-old man with biopsy-proven unresectable carcinoma of the esophagus. (A) The lateral view from an upper gastrointestinal series shows malignant distal esophageal stricture with abrupt tapering of the contrast column (arrow). (B) A lateral digital radiograph taken immediately after placement of a 23-mm × 150-mm Ultraflex esophageal stent. Note that the stent is fully expanded. (C) An oblique view from a barium swallow shows wide patency of stented esophagus.

A

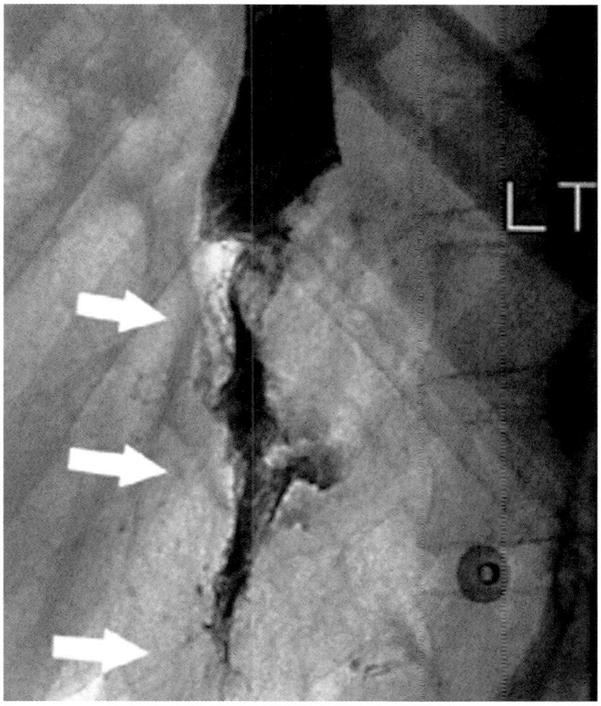

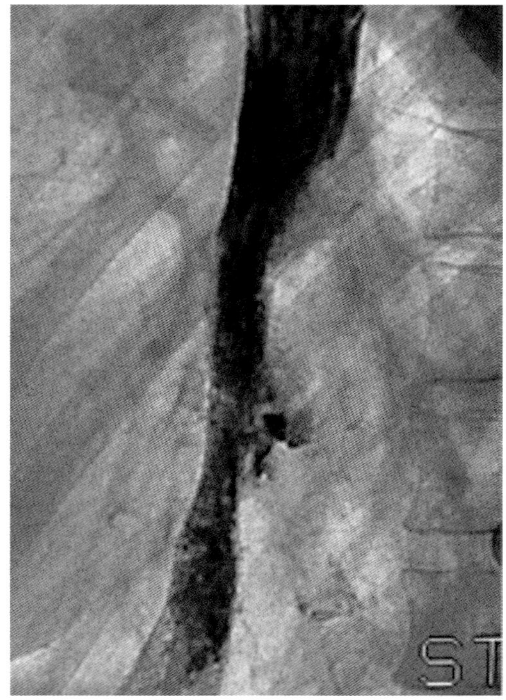

B

C

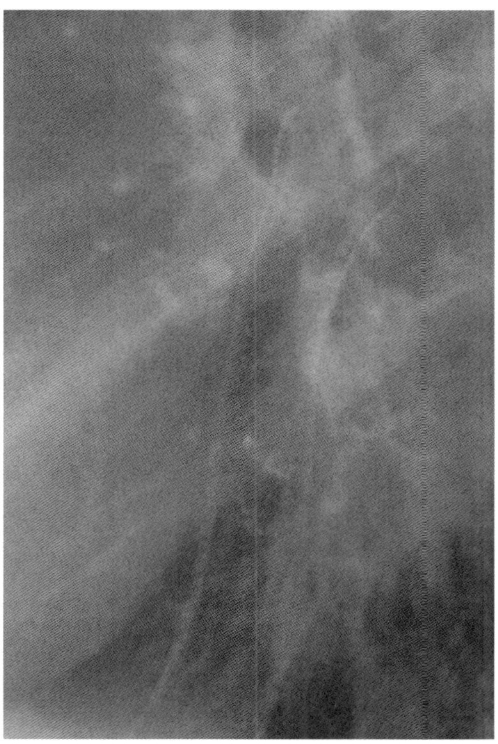

Figure 24-2. Esophageal stent placement in a 63-year-old man with biopsy-proven unresectable distal esophageal carcinoma. (A) An upper gastrointestinal image shows a long segment stricture secondary to carcincma (arrows). (B) A lateral fluoroscopic image taken immediately after deployment of a 23-mm × 150-mm Ultraflex esophageal stent across the lesion. (C) A lateral chest radiograph taken 1 day after the procedure shows the fully expanded stent.

TABLE 24-3
Complications of Esophageal Stent Placement and Their Management[12,21,28]

Complication	Management
Perforation	Overlapping covered stents Endoscopic closure with tissue glue
Fistula	Additional covered stents or tracheal stents
Hematemesis	Endoscopic local epinephrine injection
Tracheal compression	Tracheal stent Esophageal stent removal
Funnel phenomenon	Injection of tissue glue in persistent space endoscopically Conical Wallstent
Granulomatous tissue ingrowth or over-growth	Repeated balloon dilation Laser ablation
Tumor ingrowth or overgrowth	Laser ablation Stent within stent Balloon dilation
Stent covering disruption	Additional covered stents
Food impaction	Endoscopic removal of food; possible balloon dilation of stent
Persistent chest pain	Long term narcotics
Gastroesophageal reflux	Proton-pump inhibitor Elevation of head with pillows

caused by progressive dilation of the esophagus. It can result in the delayed opening of a malignant fistula.[26]

Recurrent dysphagia may be caused by granulation tissue or by tumor ingrowth or overgrowth. Tumor ingrowth occurs through the stent interstices and overgrowth occurs at the stent margins. The incidence is 26%–36%[14,27,28] and leads to progressive luminal narrowing.[20,32,33] Granulation tissue is most commonly found with Wallstents, whereas tumor ingrowth and overgrowth are unrelated to the stent type. Although covered stents would conceptually serve as a barrier to tumor ingrowth, tumor cells are capable of transgressing porous materials used as coverings of current stents. Therefore, the use of covered stents may simply delay inevitable tumor ingrowth.

Stents with greater radial strength may result in pressure necrosis, and a case of a resultant aorto-esophageal fistula has been described.[34] The same mechanism is responsible for tracheal compression that can present as a sudden emergency. Wang et al.[26] reported no hemorrhage with either Ultraflex stents or with any distal esophageal stents. In general, Ultraflex stents appear to be associated with the fewest complications, although no randomized studies have compared safety and efficacy between different esophageal stents.[17,26] Repeated interventions after initial stent placement may be required in approximately 50% of patients.[26,32]

Palliation of advanced esophageal tumor remains a challenge to clinicians. The ease of placement and lower complication rates with expandable metallic stents has virtually eliminated the role of plastic stents in palliative therapy for esophageal malignancies. The technical success rate is almost 100%, and relief from dysphagia is usually sustained until death from distant or locoregional disease. These metallic endoprostheses are substantially better than endoscopic laser therapy in terms of dysphagia amelioration and complications.[33] Despite the high cost of esophageal stents, the utility of this approach appears justified on the basis of shorter hospital stays, the lack of general anesthesia requirements, and the low incidence of complications.[35] Future directions in esophageal stent technology will likely include modified retention systems to prevent migration, and stents with one-way valves for avoiding gastroesophageal reflux when treating lesions involving the gastroesophageal junction.

GASTRODUODENAL OBSTRUCTION

Malignant gastric obstruction is most commonly associated with gastric, pancreatic, and gynecologic cancers. It was estimated that gastric carcinoma would account for nearly 13,000 cancer deaths in the United States in 2002, and pancreatic carcinoma, for over 29,000 deaths. Cervical, ovarian, and endometrial cancer were expected to account for 4,100, 13,900, and 6,600 deaths, respectively, in 2002.[36] As many as 40% of women with advanced gynecologic malignancies will develop some degree of gastrointestinal obstruction.[37] Patients who have received large doses of local external-beam radiotherapy can also develop gastroduodenal obstruction from radiation enteritis.

Management options for disease palliation in patients with unresectable malignant gastroduodenal obstruction includes nasogastric suction, surgical bypass, gastrostomy, and enteral stent placement. Prolonged nasogastric suction is a suboptimal means of palliation for these patients and incurs risks of aspiration, mucosal erosions, and perforation. Prolonged nasogastric intubation is also associated with a poor quality of life.

The conventional surgical bypass for gastric obstruction is gastrojejunostomy. Because many patients are too frail to undergo gastrojejunostomy by the time an obstruction develops, some surgeons advocate gastrojejunostomy at the time of initial staging laparotomy.

A prospective trial randomized 87 patients with unresectable periampullary carcinoma during exploratory laparotomy to prophylactic gastrojejunostomy or no gastrojejunostomy.[38] Although no difference was seen in survival, 19% of patients without gastrojejunostomy developed gastric outlet obstruction, whereas none of the patients who underwent gastrojejunostomy developed obstruction.

Surgical management of malignant gastric obstruction is limited by high morbidity and mortality rates. A single-center series of 20 patients undergoing palliative gastrojejunostomy had a 25% surgical mortality rate and a 20% complication rate; complications included anastomotic leak, hemorrhage, and early gastric obstruction.[39]

Percutaneous Gastrostomy and Transgastric Jejunostomy

Percutaneous gastrostomy provides a minimally invasive means of gastric decompression. In these situations, the gastrostomy tube does not function as a feeding tube; therefore, smaller tubes may provide adequate drainage. This concept is supported by a study by Cannizzaro et al., who randomized patients undergoing percutaneous gastrostomy for decompression to receive either 15-F or 20-F tubes; no difference in symptomatic relief was observed.[40]

Placement of a dual-lumen transgastric jejunostomy tube enables direct jejunal feeding and gastric decompression.

Patient Preparation

Large volumes of residual food and secretions may be present in gastroduodenal obstruction (**Fig. 24-3**). The risk of aspiration during percutaneous gastrostomy and spillage of gastroenteric contents into the peritoneal cavity can be minimized with nasogastric suction initiated the day before the procedure.

In cachectic patients, ultrasound (US) of the abdomen prior to fluoroscopically guided puncture can be useful to avoid injury caused by transgression of the left lobe of the liver. In some situations, transgression of the left lobe may be required as the only available percutaneous window for gastrostomy placement.[41] Some surgeons advocate routine US at the time of gastrostomy placement to avoid injury to the superior epigastric vessels.

Distention of the stomach with air is performed through the previously placed nasogastric tube. Insufflation may be poorly tolerated when there is intrinsic or extrinsic narrowing of the stomach. Use of intravenous antiperistaltic agents such as glucagon (0.5–1.0 mg intravenously) may assist in limiting egress of air into the small bowel.

Percutaneous gastrostomy can be performed in the presence of small amounts of ascites; however, this situation mandates the use of Cope T-fasteners (Cook, Bloomington, IN) or similar devices for gastropexy. Safe gastrostomy tube placement in the presence of larger amounts of ascites necessitates paracentesis. Placement of a paracentesis drainage catheter may be performed immediately prior to gastrostomy tube placement.

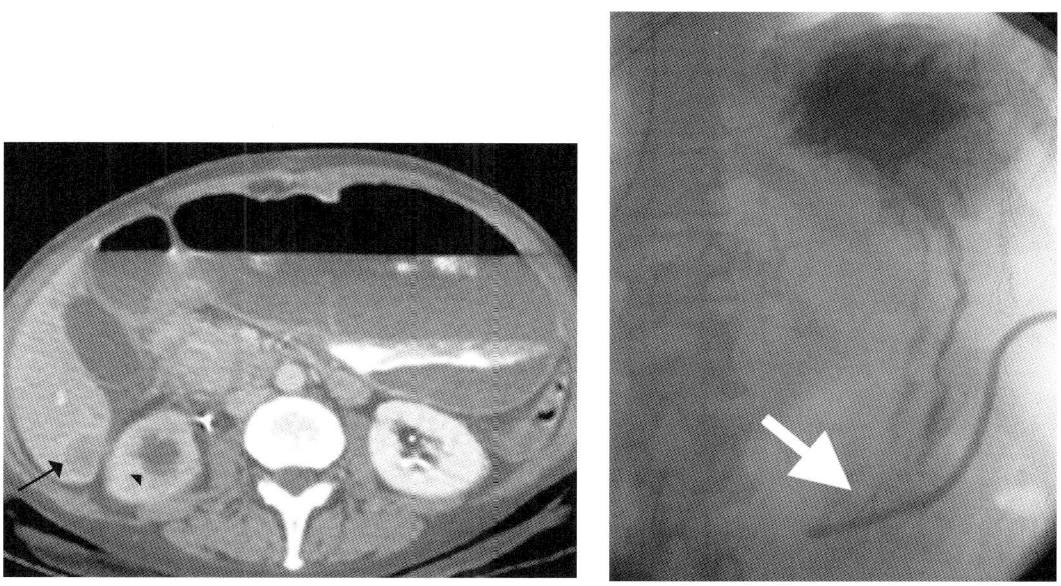

A B

Figure 24-3. Percutaneous gastrostomy for decompression in a 47-year-old woman with metastatic ovarian carcinoma and gastric outlet obstruction. (A) A computed tomography scan shows marked gastric distention prior to placement of percutaneous gastrostomy. Note the metastasis in the liver (arrow) and hydronephrosis of the previously stented right kidney (arrowhead). (B) A fluoroscopic image taken 1 week after placement of an 18-F percutaneous gastrostomy tube with a balloon retention system. Note the two T-fasteners placed for gastropexy (arrow). The stomach is no longer distended.

Technique

Individual surgeon and institution-specific preferences will dictate which type of gastrostomy tube is placed. At the University of Pennsylvania, we initially perform percutaneous gastrostomy for decompression using a 12- or 14-F Wills-Ogilsvy tube (Cook, Inc.). Gastric access is obtained using a Cope gastrostomy set (Cook, Inc.). Gastric puncture is performed under fluoroscopic guidance with a 16-gauge needle loaded with a Cope T-fastener. The tapered guide wire is passed through the needle into the stomach to deploy the T-fastener for gastropexy. The needle is removed with the guide wire in place, and firm traction on the T-fastener is maintained to secure the stomach to the anterior abdominal wall. A second T-fastener may be deployed through the needle or, more commonly, the needle is removed and the stomach is repunctured to enable placement of a second T-fastener. After placement of the second T-fastener, the needle is exchanged over a wire for a 5-F dilator. The initial entry guide wire is then exchanged for a stiff 0.035-in. guide wire, the tract is successively dilated to the desired French size, and then the gastrostomy catheter is placed. The guide wire is removed and the locking loop of the catheter is formed. The gastrostomy catheter is left to gravity drainage to enable gastric decompression. The patient is monitored clinically on a daily basis to ensure resolution of gastric obstruction. If after several days drainage through the catheter appears inadequate, with persistent clinical and/or radiographic signs of gastric distention, the existing gastrostomy tract may be serially dilated over a stiff guide wire to enable placement of a large-bore (18–24-F) gastrostomy tube.

Placement of a transgastric jejunostomy may be performed as the initial procedure or as a conversion procedure from a previously placed percutaneous gastrostomy. When it is performed as the initial procedure, we place a short 8-F working sheath over the stiff guide wire and position the tip of the sheath in the stomach. The pylorus and duodenum are then crossed with an angled-tip catheter and guide wire. In highly stenotic lesions, a Cope metal gastric guiding cannula (Cook, Inc.) may be invaluable in providing stable transpyloric access for guide wire manipulation beyond the obstruction. After this, an exchange-length guide wire is used for placement of a Carey–Alzate–Coons catheter (Cook, Inc.), the tip of which is positioned in the proximal jejunum. This tube is then secured in the stomach with its Malecot-type retention system. A separate gastric port enables gastric decompression. Because crossing a malignant gastroduodenal stricture may require several minutes of catheter manipulation, we prefer to place a percutaneous gastrostomy for initial decompression and then have the patient return later for transgastric jejunostomy when the gastrostomy tract is mature.

Results

Percutaneous gastrostomy for decompression in malignant obstruction has both a high technical success rate and a high clinical success rate (both > 90%). Malone et al. placed a percutaneous gastrostomy in 10 patients with terminal ovarian cancer for decompression and achieved resolution of obstructive symptoms in all patients.[42] Cunningham et al. performed percutaneous gastrostomy for decompression in 20 patients with advanced gynecologic malignancies and small bowel obstruction, including 8 patients with ascites.[43] All patients had symptomatic relief, and 12 patients (60%) were able to return home for palliative care.

Stenting of Malignant Gastroduodenal Obstruction

Stenting of malignant gastroduodenal obstruction can provide immediate and sustained relief of obstructive symptoms and enable return to a soft diet, eliminating the need for total parenteral nutrition or direct jejunal feedings.

The procedure may be performed using either fluoroscopic or combined endoscopic–fluoroscopic guidance. Endoscopic guidance alone may be used but is suboptimal because the proximal and distal ends of the stricture cannot be visualized simultaneously, meaning malpositioning of the stent may occur.

Patient preparation is similar to that for percutaneous gastrostomy, with nasogastric suction initiated the day before the procedure. After conscious sedation and local anesthesia spray to the oropharynx and hypopharynx, the existing nasogastric tube is exchanged over a guide wire for a directional catheter. We prefer to use a 7-F multipurpose angled (MPA) catheter (Cook, Inc.). Contrast is injected through the catheter to delineate the obstruction. This catheter is then manipulated with a steerable hydrophilic guide wire across the stenosis, and the distal aspect of the stricture is confirmed with an injection of contrast. With the proximal and distal edges of the stricture identified, radiopaque markers or stent tape may be placed on the patient. The catheter is removed over an exchange-length stiff guide wire, and an appropriately sized self-expanding stent is selected (typically 12–22 mm in diameter) with a sufficient length to provide at least 2 cm of stent coverage on either side of the stricture. Long strictures (7–10 cm) may therefore require placement of two overlapping stents. Balloon dilation is not performed before stent placement and is seldom required after stent placement, because gradual continued expansion of the stent can be anticipated for several days after initial placement. The stent deployment sheath is exchanged for a catheter, and a final contrast injection is performed.

When performed with endoscopic–fluoroscopic

guidance, the endoscope can function as a large guiding catheter to enable crossing of the stricture with an exchange-length guide wire. Contrast may be injected through the endoscope to fluoroscopically determine the proximal border of the lesion. However, if contrast does not pass through the obstruction to delineate the distal aspect of the stricture, the lesion may need to be crossed with the endoscope. This may prove to be difficult and time consuming, and therefore placement of an angiographic catheter alongside the endoscope to cross the lesion may be necessary. When the stricture margins are identified, the appropriate size stent is selected. Larger stents may not pass through the working channel of the endoscope and may therefore require peroral manipulation over a guide wire. In this instance, the endoscope may be removed over the guide wire across the stricture and exchanged for the stent deployment sheath. The endoscope is reintroduced alongside the stent system. After stent placement, a contrast injection is performed through the endoscope or a catheter to confirm patency of the stented segment.

After stent placement, patients are encouraged to gradually progress to a soft diet over the next several days. How quickly this can be achieved will vary greatly among patients and will depend in part on the degree of obstruction, the use of narcotic analgesics or other antimotility agents, and the baseline functional status of the patient.

Alternate Approaches

Highly stenotic, sharply angulated, or long strictures may prove difficult to cross from a peroral approach with either endoscopic or fluoroscopic guidance. Interventionalists should not hesitate to place a temporary percutaneous gastrostomy, because this procedure may be performed safely within a few minutes. Many surgeons prefer to leave the gastrostomy in place for 2 or 3 weeks to allow a tract to mature. Once the tract is mature, a working sheath is used through the gastrostomy tract for stent placement. This is then converted to a conventional decompression gastrostomy tube at the completion of the procedure and may be removed once the patient can tolerate a soft diet.

Patients with a previously established transhepatic biliary access may undergo enteral stent placement through the existing tract.[44] An example of this technique is shown in **Fig. 24-4**.

Patients with duodenal obstruction and coexisting biliary obstruction require biliary drainage before placement of a duodenal stent. If placement of a duodenal stent has occurred before biliary drainage or biliary obstruction develops after duodenal stent placement, transhepatic biliary drainage and stent placement can be performed (**Fig. 24-5**).

Use of an enterocutaneous fistula as a route for duodenal stent placement was described by Ernst et al. in a patient with pancreatic carcinoma.[45] This approach also enabled healing of the fistula after enteral decompression by stent placement.

Results

Published series using self-expanding stents such as the Wallstent have reported technical success rates of 70%–100%, with partial or complete relief of obstructive symptoms in almost all instances of technically successful placement.[46–51] In the series reported by de Baere et al., two patients with persistent obstructive symptoms after stent placement were later found to harbor tandem small bowel stenoses distal to the stented primary stricture.[48] This reinforces the need for preprocedural contrast radiography for all patients.

Complications

Stent migration was reported in one of 9 (11%) patients treated by Binkert et al.[46] and two of 12 (17%) patients reported by Soetikno et al.[50] A single case of delayed perforation after duodenal Wallstent placement has been described at 5 weeks after insertion.[52] Other potential complications include stent erosion and gastrointestinal bleeding. Although this has not yet been described in the gastroenteric stent literature, there have been several reported cases of duodenal erosion and hemorrhage after biliary Wallstent placement.[53–55]

The local tissue response of metal stents within malignant gastrointestinal strictures was studied by Bethge et al. in surgical or autopsy specimens of 12 patients who had undergone placement of biliary or duodenal Wallstents for malignant strictures.[56] In all cases, incorporation of the stent into the wall of the organ had occurred, accompanied by formation of a collagenous layer along the luminal surface and a fibrous reaction within the submucosa. No penetration of the stent struts beyond the submucosa occurred. On the basis of their observations and a review of the pathology literature, the authors postulated that the sequence of events that occur after enteral stent placement begins with initial stent expansion, which stretches the stenotic tumor and adjacent normal mucosa. As expansion of the stent continues, tissue beneath the stent undergoes pressure necrosis, with migration of the stent into the deeper layers of the mucosa and submucosa adjacent to the tumor. This produces a chronic inflammatory response with formation of collagen and fibrous tissue along the luminal surface. This smooth lining of reactive tissue prevents contact with enteral contents.

A B C

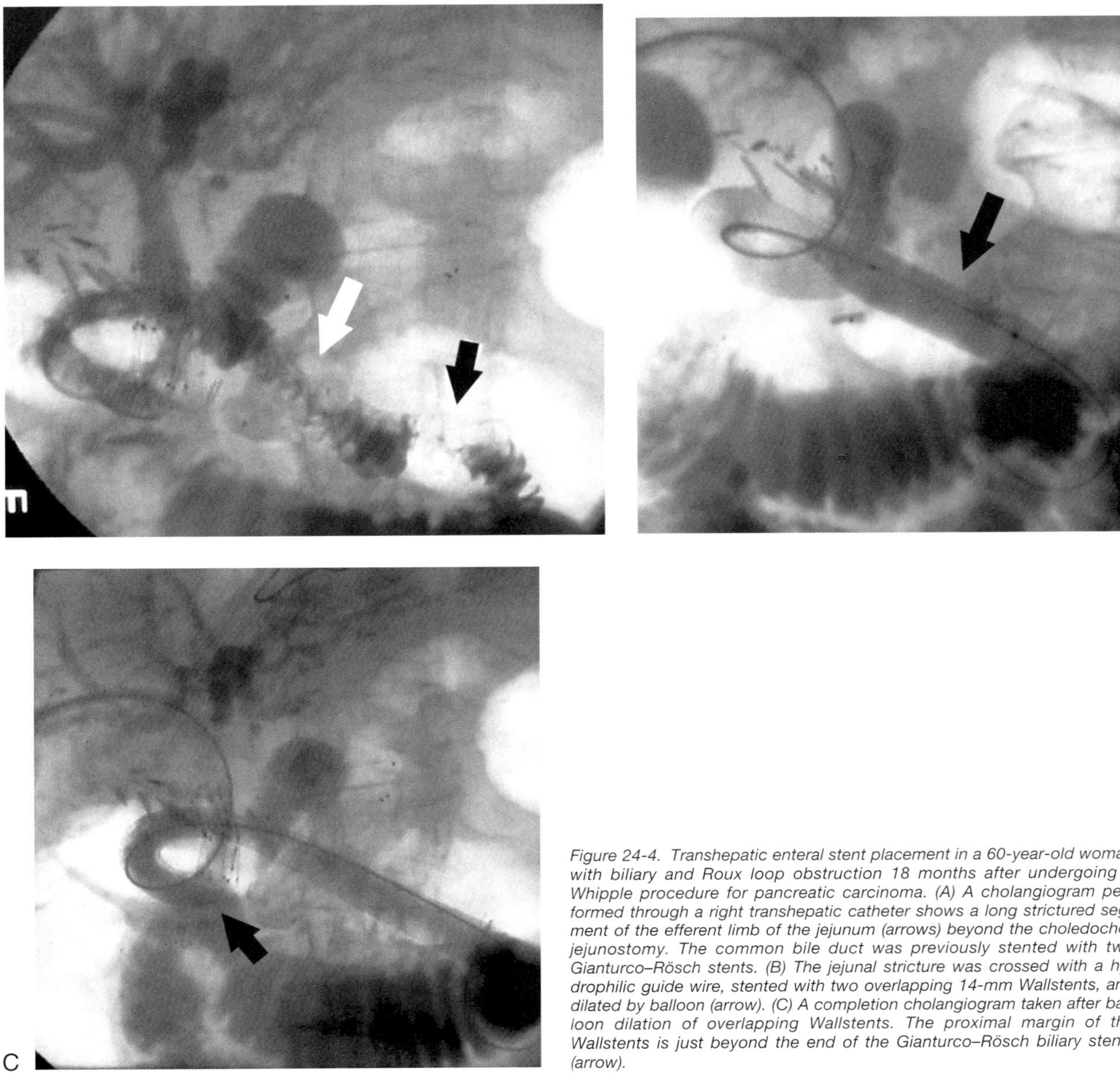

Figure 24-4. Transhepatic enteral stent placement in a 60-year-old woman with biliary and Roux loop obstruction 18 months after undergoing a Whipple procedure for pancreatic carcinoma. (A) A cholangiogram performed through a right transhepatic catheter shows a long strictured segment of the efferent limb of the jejunum (arrows) beyond the choledochojejunostomy. The common bile duct was previously stented with two Gianturco–Rösch stents. (B) The jejunal stricture was crossed with a hydrophilic guide wire, stented with two overlapping 14-mm Wallstents, and dilated by balloon (arrow). (C) A completion cholangiogram taken after balloon dilation of overlapping Wallstents. The proximal margin of the Wallstents is just beyond the end of the Gianturco–Rösch biliary stents (arrow).

Covered Stents

Recent interest has emerged in the use of covered stents for gastroduodenal obstruction, with the rationale of decreased or delayed tumor ingrowth. In malignant biliary obstruction, Hausegger et al. showed that polyurethane-covered Wallstents stents neither prevented tumor ingrowth nor prolong patency, when compared with noncovered stents.[57] Disadvantages of covered stents include larger-caliber delivery systems (and therefore greater potential difficulty in crossing tightly strictured segments) and the risk of covering the ampulla with resultant biliary obstruction. Covered stents may also have a higher rate of migration.

Park and colleagues constructed a modular Gianturco-type stainless-steel stent covered with polyurethane for palliative treatment of nine patients with advanced gastric or pancreatic cancer and enteral obstruction. The stent consisted of flared shoulders to prevent migration by anchoring the stent on either side of the stricture. A peroral approach was used with fluoroscopic guidance for delivery of the 18-F deployment system. Immediate technical success was achieved in six of 9 (67%) patients. In three patients, the stricture could not be crossed with either a guide wire or catheter. Median survival after stent placement (including initial failures) was 21 months.[58]

Jung et al. used a custom nitinol stent with a design

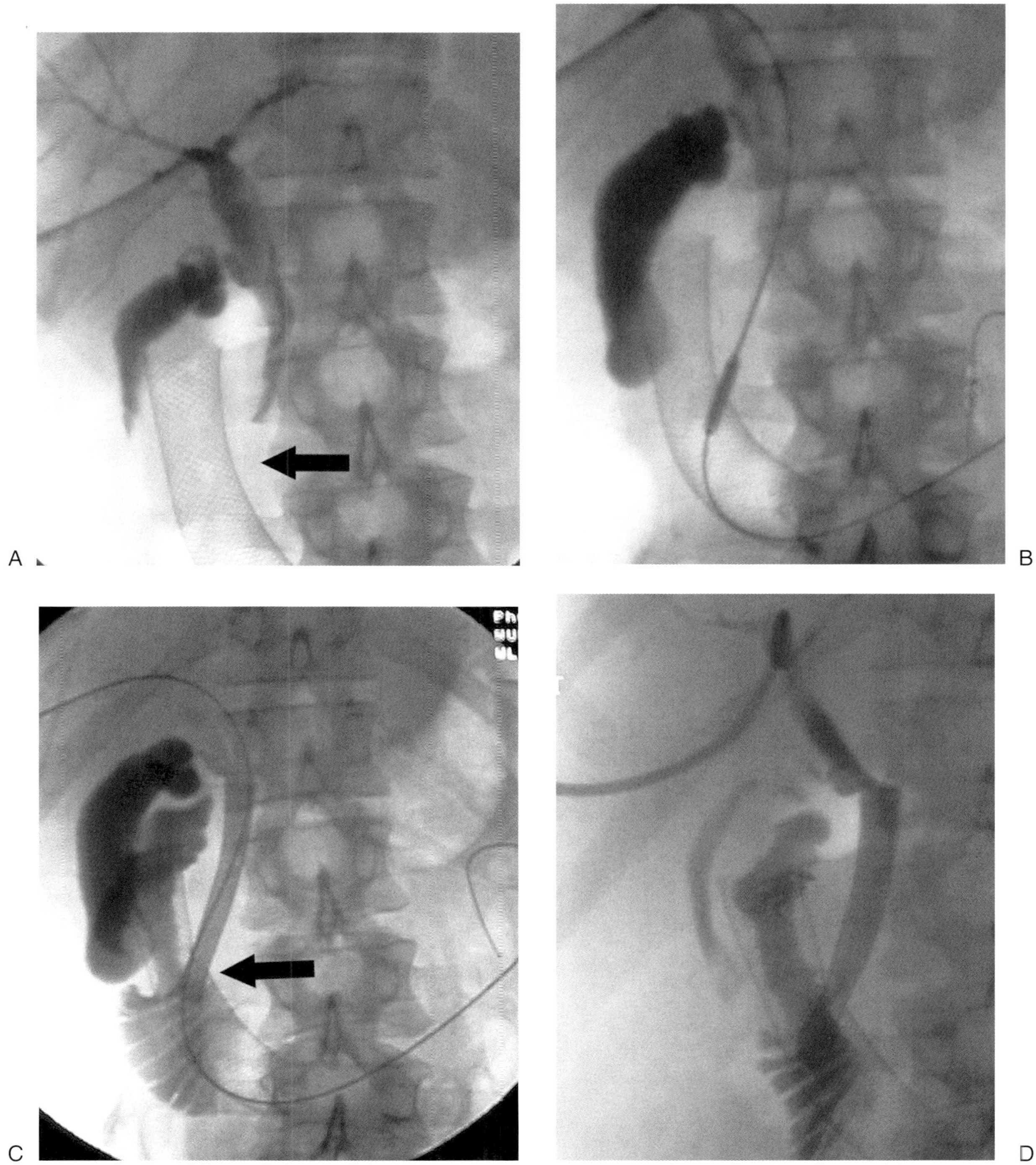

Figure 24-5. Combined duodenal and biliary stent placement in a 42-year-old woman with unresectable pancreatic carcinoma and jaundice. (A) A cholangiogram performed through a right transhepatic catheter shows that a previously placed duodenal 20-mm × 90-mm Wallstent (inserted perorally) covered the papilla (arrow). (B) The biliary obstruction and the interstices of the Wallstent were crossed with a hydrophilic guide wire and directional catheter, and serial dilation was performed from 4 mm to 10 mm through the duodenal Wallstent. (C) A cholangiogram performed immediately after placement and balloon dilation of two 10-mm × 68-mm overlapping Wallstents in the common bile duct. Note that the stents telescoped into the previously placed duodenal stent (arrow). (D) A cholangiogram performed 1 week after biliary stent placement showing patency of the duodenal and biliary Wallstents.

similar to that of the Wallstent and coated with polyurethane to treat 19 patients with malignant gastric outlet obstruction (n = 15) or duodenal obstruction (n = 4). Stent placement was technically successful in 18 of 19 (95%) patients, using a combination of fluoroscopic and endoscopic guidance from a peroral route. Stent migration occurred in 5 patients (26%) within 4 days of the procedure; these patients underwent repeat stent placement. No other procedure-related complications occurred. A decrease in symptoms occurred in 18 of 19 (95%) patients. Median survival was 11 months.[59]

Future Developments

A minimally invasive technique for creating gastroenteric anastomoses has been developed by Cope et al., using a magnetic compression technique.[60] A pair of rare-earth magnets is introduced from a peroral route using endoscopic and fluoroscopic guidance and positioned in the stomach and in the jejunum beyond the stricture. The distal magnet adheres to a conventional guide wire, allowing it to cross the duodenum. The pair is constructed with surfaces that gradually mate across the intervening bowel layers over several days, producing a leak-free anastomosis. A custom covered stent is then placed across the anastomosis, using a peroral route. In an animal model, these magnetic compression anastomoses have remained patent up to 5 months after placement. This technique is awaiting evaluation in a clinical setting.

Future efforts directed toward improving the long-term patency of gastroenteric stents will likely be directed toward the use of covered or coated stents.[61] Combining mechanical stenting with local delivery of antineoplastic agents or angiogenesis inhibitors may slow tumor ingrowth.

COLONIC OBSTRUCTION

Each year, an estimated 130,000 people in the United States are found to have colorectal cancer.[36] Of these patients, 10%–30% will initially present with an acute or subacute large bowel obstruction.[62–67] Acute large bowel obstruction is considered a surgical emergency because left untreated, the colonic distention will lead to intestinal ischemia, perforation, and septic shock, as well as dehydration with electrolyte and metabolic abnormalities.

The traditional surgical approach to the management of acute colonic obstruction is emergency diverting colostomy. This occurs in more than half of patients who undergo emergency surgery for colon cancer, with an associated 19% mortality rate.[68] These patients are then stabilized medically and undergo diagnostic studies for staging. If these tumors are resectable, they are removed in a second surgical procedure. Reversal of the colostomy may be undertaken at that time or may require a third operation. If the tumors are unresectable or the patients cannot tolerate the second procedure, the colostomy may be left as the definitive palliative procedure. Up to 25% of patients do not undergo reversal of their colostomy.[66]

Alternatively, management may consist of a two-stage Hartmann procedure of initial tumor resection and colostomy followed by a second procedure for colostomy reversal. More recently, there have been advocates for treatment with a single-stage procedure consisting of primary tumor resection, on-table lavage, and primary colonic reanastomosis. This generally requires use of an intracolonic bypass tube to prevent anastomotic breakdown and leakage.[69–71]

Several inherent difficulties are encountered during emergency surgery for acute large bowel obstruction. Patients are often elderly and debilitated, with dehydration and electrolyte and metabolic disturbances. Bowel distention presents difficulties with the creation of anastomoses, and the presence of fecal contents within the bowel lumen increases morbidity and mortality. In a retrospective literature review of reports of 2383 patients treated for malignant colorectal obstruction, Runkel et al. calculated a 22% surgical mortality in patients who underwent emergency surgery.[72] A later retrospective analysis by Deans et al. of treatment of 789 patients found a surgical mortality rate of 7.2%.[73] Interestingly, the overall mortality rates were similar for colostomy and for three-stage and single-stage procedures.

Compared with emergency surgery, elective colon resection after proper bowel preparation is associated with a surgical mortality rate of less than 6%.[74] Alternative therapies are therefore directed toward decompression of the acutely obstructed colon, to allow the patient to be medically stabilized, and bowel preparation, to be performed in the case of a surgically resectable lesion, thereby converting it to an elective resection. In the case of a surgically unresectable tumor, these alternative therapies may allow palliation without the need for colostomy and its associated surgical and psychological morbidity. Several nonsurgical modalities have been suggested for reestablishing luminal patency, including bougienage,[75] balloon dilation,[75] and endoscopic laser therapy.[76,77] These nonsurgical modalities have failed to gain widespread acceptance. Two techniques that have demonstrated effectiveness in treating colorectal obstruction are cecostomy and insertion of self-expanding metal stents.

Cecostomy

The role of catheter tube cecostomy as a method for colonic decompression remains controversial. Some authors have condemned catheter tube cecostomy, stating that it does not provide adequate colonic decompression or diversion of the fecal load.[78,79] Others strongly have advocated its use in acute malignant colonic obstruction.[80,81] They have stated the following advantages over proximal colostomy: the technique is easy to perform in an emergency; it is unaffected by abdominal wall obesity; the most dilated part of the colon is immediately decompressed; the peritoneal cavity is left intact; the second procedure (resection of the obstructing neoplastic lesion) can be performed after a short interval; the colonic anastomosis after tumor resection is protected by the cecostomy, which prevents distention; and the cecostomy should close spontaneously once the downstream obstruction has been removed.[81]

The indication for catheter tube cecostomy in malignant colonic obstruction is the need for temporary colonic decompression to allow bowel preparation and single-stage surgical resection. A secondary role of cecostomy is for palliation in patients with unresectable disease by allowing long-term colonic decompression.

Two fundamental techniques for the placement of catheter tube cecostomy exist—namely, surgical and percutaneous, analogous to gastrostomy tube placement. The surgical technique described by Perrier et al. is performed under local or general anesthesia.[81] A short incision is made over the cecum; the cecum is visualized directly and sutured intact to the anterior parietal peritoneum to exclude the peritoneum. A small incision is made in the cecum, a 38-F mushroom catheter is introduced, and the cecal wall is fixed to the catheter. The tube is secured to the skin and left for gravity-bag drainage, with frequent irrigation to ensure patency.

The percutaneous technique was first described by Casola et al. in 1986 using computed tomograph (CT) guidance and a trocar technique in a patient with colonic pseudo-obstruction.[82] Morrison et al., in 1990, published a case report of an elderly patient with malignant colonic obstruction who underwent percutaneous cecostomy using a technique previously described for percutaneous gastrostomy.[83]

With the patient under conscious sedation, the distended cecum is visualized under fluoroscopy, and with the patient under local anesthetic, four Cope-type T-fasteners are deployed, one at each corner of a 2-in square to affix the cecum to the anterior abdominal wall. T-fastener deployment is achieved by loading the fastener into an 18-gauge needle that is sharply inserted into the bowel. Once air is aspirated, the fastener is deployed by advancing a trocar or guide wire through the needle. The needle is removed, and the nylon thread is pulled against the anterior abdominal wall and secured. Catheter insertion is then carried out using the Seldinger technique in the center of the square created by the four T-fasteners, which should prevent fecal spillage into the peritoneum. Catheters up to 30 F can be placed using this technique. A modification of this technique by Chait et al. simplifies the placement of the T-fasteners; the entire procedure is carried out through a single needle puncture in the cecum.[84] In this described technique, initial access into the cecum is obtained with a 19-gauge needle loaded with a T-fastener. An 0.018-in guide wire is passed through the needle into the cecum to deploy the T-fastener. The needle is removed with the guide wire in place, and the T-fastener is pulled back to secure the cecum to the anterior abdominal wall. A coaxial sheath and dilator are then advanced over the guide wire. A second T-fastener is deployed through the sheath with a stiff 0.035 guide wire and is also secured to the anterior abdominal wall. Serial dilation can then be carried out to the desired French size, and the appropriate pigtail drainage catheter is placed. Once it is in place, bowel decompression and preparation for surgery can be achieved through the cecostomy tube. If during staging the tumor is found to be unresectable, the cecostomy tube can be left in place for palliation; in this case, depending on patient preference the initial catheter could be exchanged for a low-profile device, such as the Trapdoor device (Cook, Inc.), as described by Chait et al.[84]

To date, all reports of large series on tube cecostomy in malignant colonic obstruction have appeared in the surgical literature describing surgical cecostomy tube placement. In a series of 113 patients who underwent emergency cecostomy tube placement, Perier et al. reported a 13% perioperative mortality rate.[81] Ninety-eight patients (87%) went on to undergo elective definitive surgical procedures. Lethai et al. performed cecostomies on 11 patients with malignant colonic obstruction and reported a mortality rate of 14%.[85] They concluded that cecostomy was a reliable procedure and that it reduced the length of hospitalization. Hoffman and Jensen, in reporting on a series of 57 patients, concluded that catheter tube cecostomy is superior to loop colostomy in patients with acute left colon obstruction of neoplastic origin.[86] The percutaneous technique for cecostomy tube placement in malignant colonic obstruction should theoretically be valid but has not yet been proven so by a large series or a randomized clinical trial.

Colonic Stenting

The application of stents in the setting of acute malignant colonic obstruction was first described in 1986. In this report, a guide wire was placed per rectum across a malignant obstruction with the aid of a sigmoidoscope, over which a nasogastric tube was placed, resulting in decompression and allowing bowel preparation and single-stage surgery.[87] A similar technique has been described using a thoracostomy tube.[88] These types of tubes are limited by their relatively small caliber, stiffness, and difficulty being secured in position in the colon. They are not suited for long-term placement required in palliation. Self-expanding metal stents are ideally suited for placement of stents in malignant colonic strictures because of the high ratio of deployed diameter to diameter of the introducer system, high radial strength allowing gradual expansion of the stent, and flexibility for conforming to the tortuosity of the colon. Dohmoto et al., in 1991, were the first to describe colonic placement of self-expanding stents.[89] There is growing evidence in the literature for these stents' efficacy in relieving acute colonic obstruction, allowing elective surgical resection, palliation, or both.[90–109] The procedure has also been the topic of two excellent recent review articles.[110,111]

The indications for colonic stenting with self-expanding metallic stents are as follows: (1) for decompression in patients with acute large bowel obstruction, to allow bowel preparation and medical optimization, permitting one-stage surgical resection, and (2) for long-term decompression of the bowel in patients with unresectable malignant colorectal obstruction. The only absolute contraindication is bowel perforation, diagnosed clinically or by the presence of free intraperitoneal gas as shown on abdominal radiographs.

Technique

Once a patient is deemed a potential candidate for colonic stenting, a water-soluble contrast enema should be performed to confirm mechanical large bowel obstruction, determine the site of the obstruction and the length of the stricture, and determine the optimal patient position and fluoroscopy tube angle that best profiles the strictured segment. This information can be used to choose the appropriate guidance (fluoroscopic only versus endoscopic–fluoroscopic) system for stent delivery. In our experience, lesions in the descending colon and rectosigmoid region are typically amenable to the fluoroscopic technique, whereas more anatomically proximal lesions require a combined endoscopic–fluoroscopic technique.

Fluoroscopic Technique:

A rectal tube system may be fashioned by cutting a slit in the main channel of a 24-F Foley catheter. A 12-F vascular sheath is advanced through the slit to the tip of the Foley catheter (**Fig. 24-6**). This minimizes the loss of contrast material during the procedure and when the procedure is successfully completed, and it prevents the colonic fecal load from escaping during the procedure. The rectal tube system is introduced per rectum, and the balloon cuff is inflated to create a seal. The vascular sheath sidearm may then be used to inject water-soluble contrast material to opacify the colon. A stiff hydrophilic 0.035- or 0.038-in guide wire, in combination with a highly torquable catheter (typically a 7-F MPA catheter), is advanced through the sheath and manipulated through the colon and beyond the stricture. The guide wire is withdrawn, and contrast material is injected through the catheter to opacify the colon proximal to the stricture and to rule out perforation. The appropriate-size stent is chosen. A rigid 0.035- or 0.038-in exchange wire is advanced through the catheter beyond the stricture as far proximally as possible to straighten the bowel. The catheter is removed, and the appropriate-size stent (minimum diameter, 22 mm) is placed across the stricture and deployed such that there is at least 2 cm of overlap proximally and distally to the stricture (**Fig. 24-7**). Note that the Wallstent system can be deployed through the 12-F sheath–rectal tube but that other stents with larger delivery systems will necessitate the removal of the rectal tube at this point. The catheter is once again advanced over the guide wire proximal to

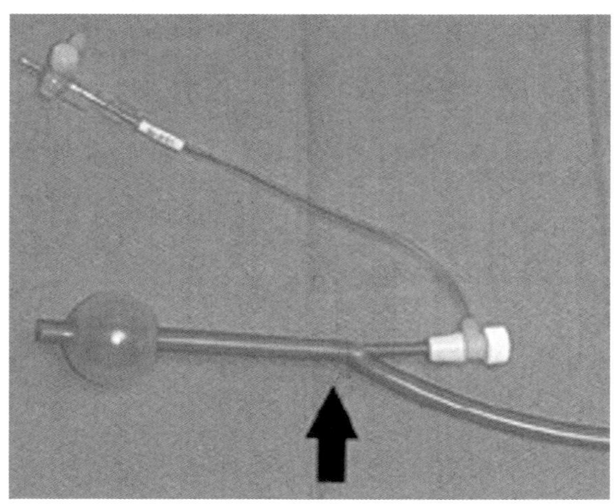

Figure 24-6. Modified rectal tube (D. Ferguson, MD, personal communication) for fluoroscopy-guided colonic stent placement. A 12-F vascular sheath has been inserted through a slit cut in the main lumen of a 24-F Foley catheter (arrow). With the Foley balloon inflated, loss of contrast material is prevented, as is escape of fecal material. During stent placement in completely obstructed patients, this amount may be considerable.

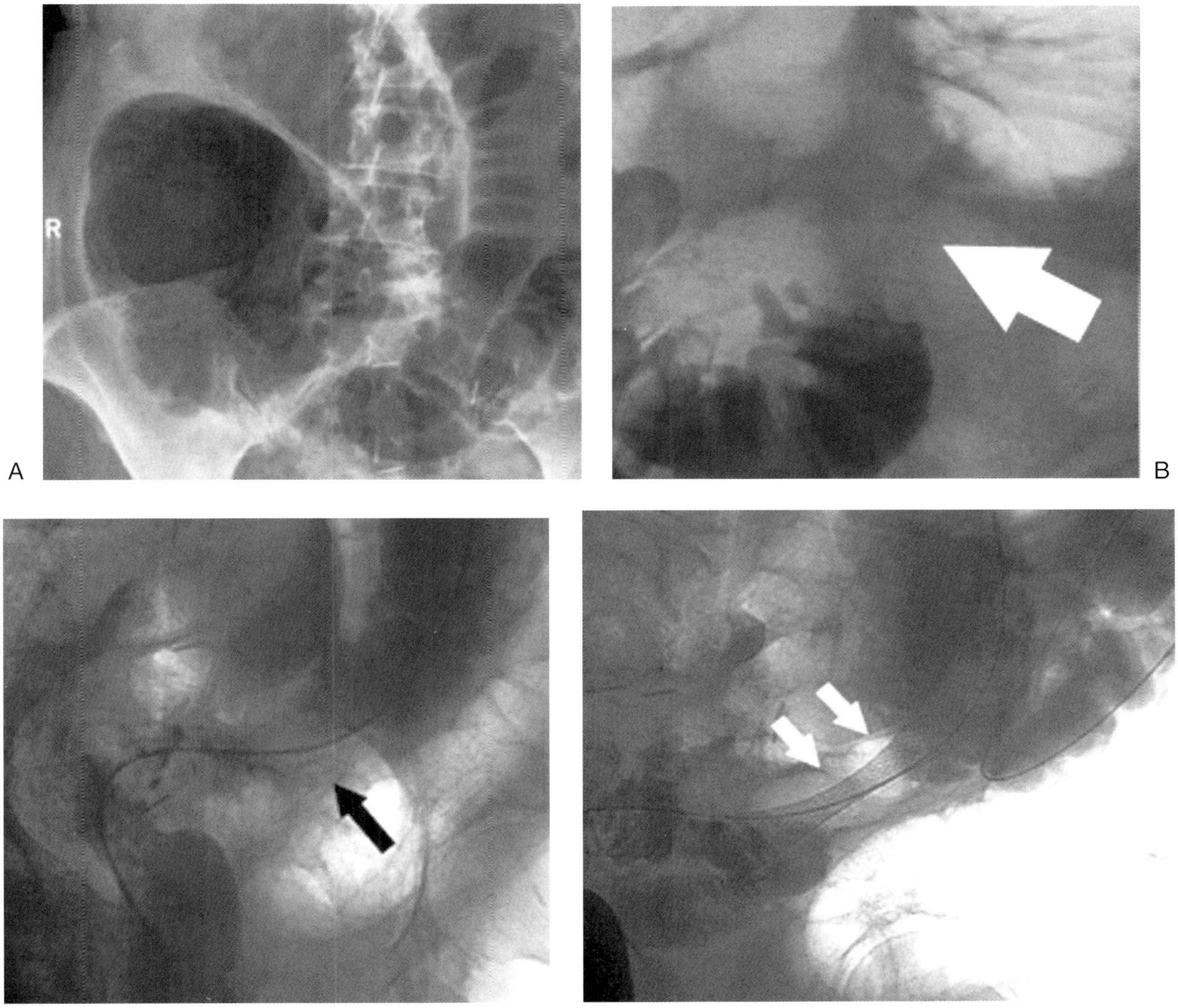

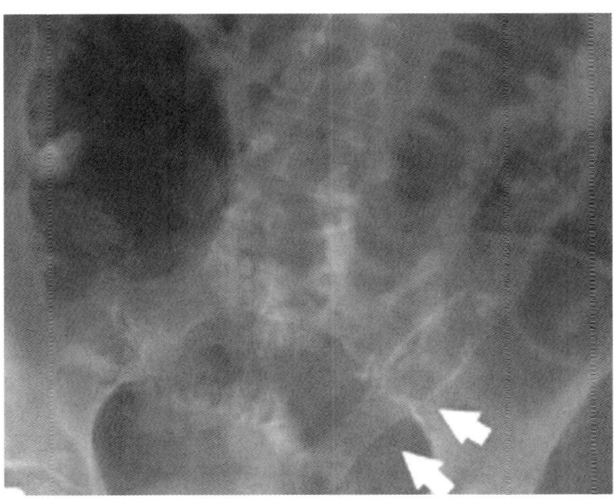

Figure 24-7. Colonic stent placement in a 78-year-old woman with a 2-day history of large bowel obstruction. (A) A frontal radiograph demonstrated dilated colon to the level of the distal descending colon (arrow). (B) A single water-soluble contrast enema done before stent placement shows sigmoid colon apple core lesion (arrow) with proximal air-filled distended colon. (C) An oblique fluoroscopic image shows the guide wire across malignant stricture (arrow). (D) A 24-mm × 70-mm Wallstent (arrows) was deployed across the lesion. (E) Frontal view of the abdomen 1 day after the procedure; the stent is in the left lower quadrant. The stent was then fully expanded, allowing complete bowel preparation and single-stage surgical resection. Note decompression of the colon proximal to the segment where the stent was placed.

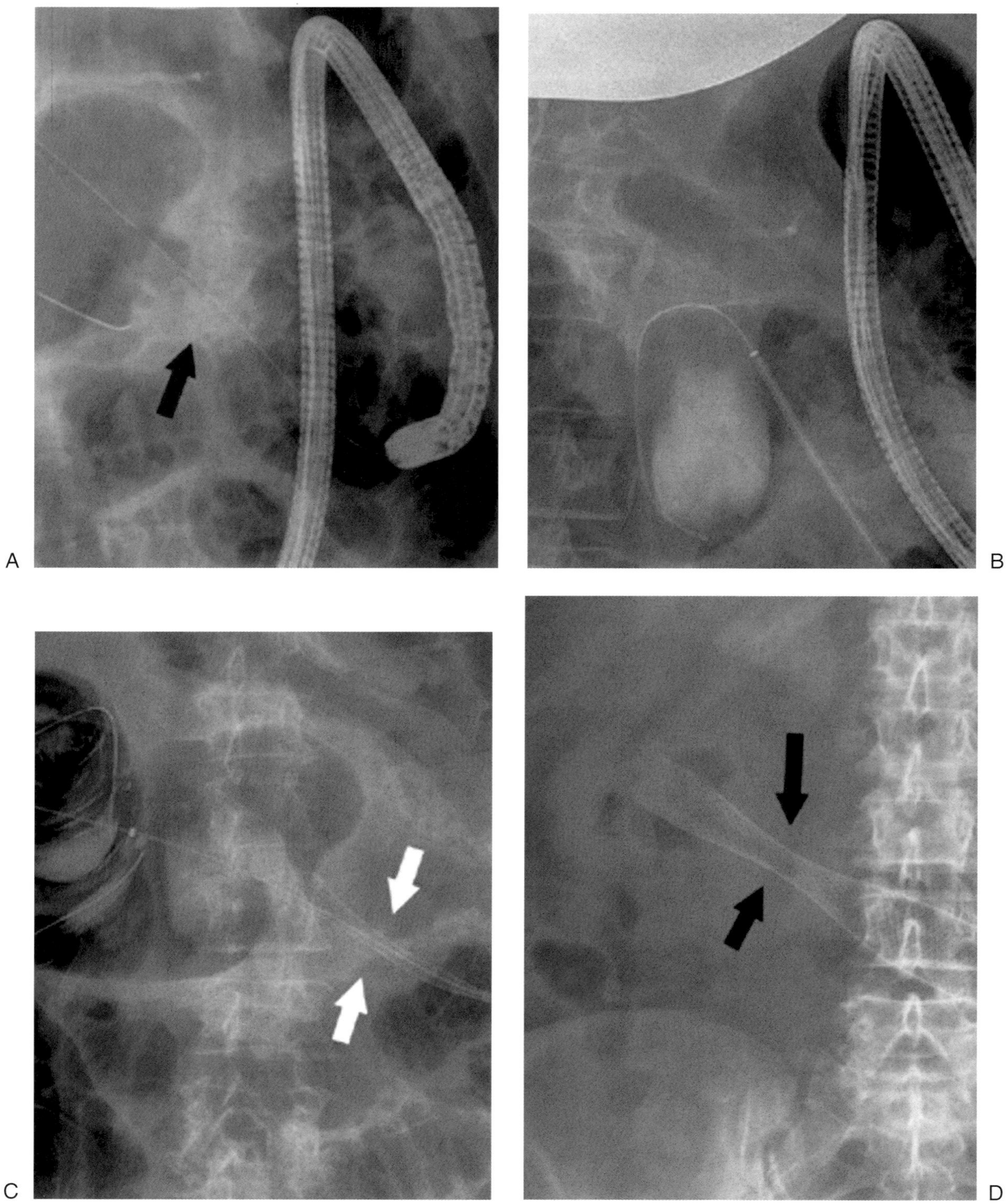

Figure 24-8. Colonic stent placement in a 67-year-old woman with acute large bowel obstruction secondary to a malignant stricture in the transverse colon. (A) The colonoscope was advanced to the distal end of stricture with a guide wire through the stricture (arrow) into the proximal dilated colon. (B) An undeployed 22-mm × 90-mm Wallstent across stricture via the working channel of endoscope. (C) An image of the partially deployed enteral Wallstent. Note the persistent waist (arrows) in the center of the stent. This was not dilated by balloon. (D) A frontal supine radiograph obtained 6 days after stent insertion shows marked reduction in caliber of dilated bowel loops, despite incomplete expansion of midstent (arrows).

the stent, and contrast material is injected to confirm stent position and patency and to rule out extravasation.

Endoscopic–Fluoroscopic Technique:

A colonoscope is advanced to the stricture, and a guide wire is passed through the stricture (**Fig. 24-8**). A catheter is advanced over the guide wire, and its tip positioned proximal to the stricture. Contrast material is injected to delineate the proximal aspect of the stricture. The appropriate-size stent is chosen, and a rigid guide wire is repositioned, again as far proximally as possible. Some stent delivery systems are narrow enough to fit through the working channel of the colonoscope. If not, the colonoscope is removed, leaving the guide wire in position, and readvanced next to the stent delivery system. The stent is deployed under fluoroscopic visualization to ensure proper positioning of the stent proximally, and under direct visualization through the colonoscope at the distal aspect of the stricture.

A waist will be seen in the center of a properly positioned stent. The temptation to use balloon dilation of this waist should be avoided because dilation of it is known to cause perforation. The inherent outward radial force of the stent will typically result in gradual but full expansion within 48 hours. A water-soluble contrast enema may be performed after the procedure or the following day to ensure stent patency and to rule out concurrent, more proximal lesions. The patient is monitored closely for signs of perforation, is medically stabilized, and may undergo diagnostic staging examinations. If the patient is deemed a candidate for surgery, full surgical bowel preparation will follow. Patients who are not surgical candidates but undergo stenting for palliation are instructed to maintain a low-residue diet and take stool softeners to minimize the risk of fecal impaction and or stent migration secondary to fecal load.

Results

In a retrospective literature review, Mauro et al. combined data for cases from 12 articles published between 1993 and 1999.[111] A total of 234 patients underwent colonic stent placement under fluoroscopic (136 patients), endoscopic (25 patients), and combined endoscopic–fluoroscopic guidance (73 patients). The technical success rate was 93%, with a clinical success rate (defined as relief of obstructive symptoms) of 90%. Since then, Camunez et al. have published a report on a series of 80 patients treated for acute malignant colonic obstruction with stent placement under fluoroscopic guidance.[108] The technical success rate was 88%, and the clinical success rate was 84%. Thirty-three patients underwent subsequent elective surgery, whereas stent placement was used for final palliative therapy in 35 patients. Tamin et al. reported on a series

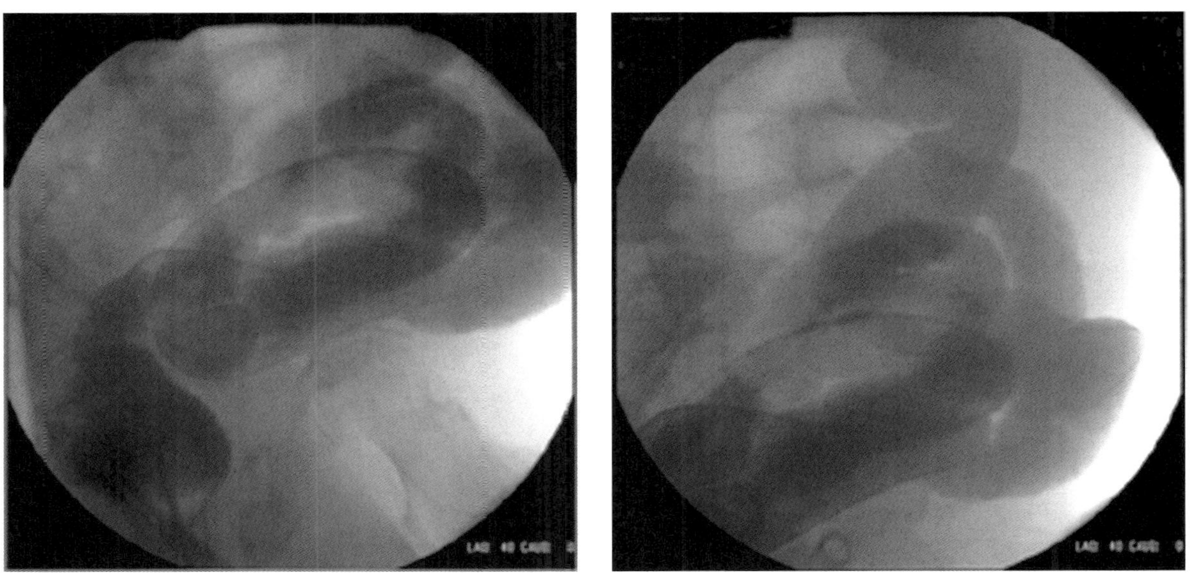

A B

Figure 24-9. Failure of colonic stent placement in a 74-year-old man with acute large bowel obstruction secondary to a malignant stricture at the splenic flexure. (A and B) Oblique fluoroscopic images of the left lower quadrant show the guide wire and catheter within a markedly redundant sigmoid colon. Redundancy could not be overcome even with the aid of a colonoscope, so the procedure was abandoned. The patient underwent a defunctioning colostomy.

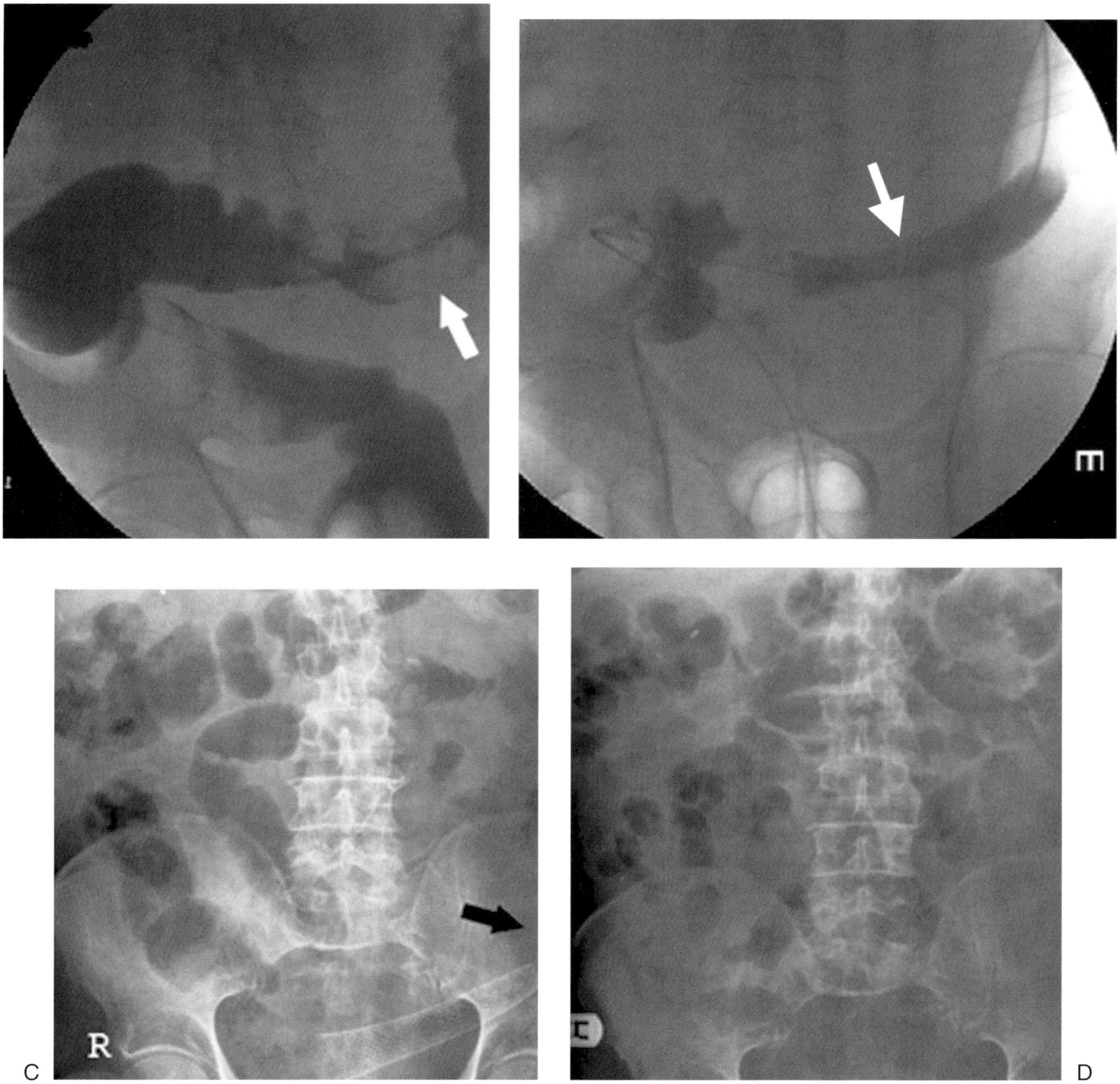

A B C D

Figure 24-10. Colon stent migration in a 66-year-old man with an obstructing sigmoid carcinoma. Stent placement was undertaken for palliation, as the patient was not a surgical candidate. (A) A fluoroscopic oblique image showing the guide wire and catheter across an apple-core sigmoid lesion (arrow). (B) A frontal fluoroscopic image taken immediately after placement of a 24-mm × 70-mm Wallstent shows the stent symmetrically positioned across the lesion (arrow). (C) A frontal radiograph taken 1 day after the procedure demonstrates the colonic stent in the lower left quadrant, with resolution of the large bowel obstruction. Early distal migration of the stent is evident in relation to the initial proximal margin after deployment (arrow). (D) A frontal radiograph obtained 6 months after stent placement. The patient has unknowingly passed the stent per rectum, although there has been no recurrence of the large bowel obstruction.

of 11 patients treated for acute colonic obstruction with stent placement using a combined endoscopic–fluoroscopic technique.[109] Technical and clinical success was achieved in 10 of 11 patients. Three patients underwent subsequent elective single-stage surgical resection, and 7 patients were treated palliatively. These two additional series yield a total of 325 patients reported in the literature to date, with the procedure having a technical success rate of 92% and a clinical success rate of 89%.

Technical Failures and Complications

In our experience, there are two principal causes for technical failure. The first is extreme tortuosity of the rectosigmoid colon (**Fig 24–9**). This may sometimes be overcome by converting from fluoroscopic guidance to combined endoscopic–fluoroscopic guidance. However, the distal colon is at times too tortuous even for the endoscope. The second cause is the inability to cross the stricture with a guide wire. Patience, persistence, and the routine use of stiff hydrophilic guide wires will usually result in successful passage of the guide wire.

Clinical failure can be divided into early and late causes. Early failure to achieve bowel decompression may be due to an unrecognized second obstructing lesion, incomplete stent placement across the entire lesion, poor stent positioning, fecal impaction, and stent migration. Late stent failure may also be due to stent migration (**Fig. 24-10**) and fecal impaction, but other causes include hyperplastic strictures induced by the stent, as well as tumor ingrowth or overgrowth. Most causes of late stent failure can be solved with additional stenting. Covered stents may delay tumor ingrowth but currently are still under development.

The most feared complication in colonic stent placement is perforation. Perforation may be retroperitoneal or intraperitoneal and has been reported to occur in up to 16% of cases,[111] but many perforations occurred with attempted balloon dilation of the stricture. Most surgeons agree that balloon dilation at the time of stenting should be avoided. Guide wire perforations can also occur but are seldom of any clinical significance. Post-procedure hemorrhage is usually minor and managed expectantly. Mild, transient pain is common and presumably related to the constant outward radial force exerted by the stent on the tumor. The exception to this is severe protracted tenesmus reported by patients who underwent stenting of low rectal lesions.[95] Stent placement across the squamocolumnar junction should therefore be avoided.

SUMMARY

The interventional radiologist now possesses a wide array of techniques and devices for minimally invasive palliation of disease in patients with malignant esophageal, gastroduodenal, and colorectal obstruction. A multidisciplinary approach, with close collaboration with the surgeon, oncologist, and gastroenterologist, will enable optimal patient selection and follow-up care. Further studies are needed to define the role of this technology through randomized trials, cost-effectiveness analyses, and quality of life assessments.

REFERENCES

1. 2002 Estimates of Cancer Statistics. American Cancer Society Web Site. Available at: http//www.cancer.org/eprise/main/docroot/stt/stt-O. Accessed 4/23/02.
2. Kelsen D. Multimodality therapy for adenocarcinoma of the esophagus. *Gastroenterol Clin North Am* 1997;26:635–645.
3. Ellis FH Jr., Heatley GJ, Krasna MJ, et al. Esophagogastrectomy for carcinoma of the esophagus and cardia: a comparison of findings and results after standard resection in three consecutive eight-year intervals with improved staging criteria. *J Thorac Cardiovasc Surg* 1997;113:836–848.
4. Devesa SS, Fraumeni JF Jr. The rising incidence of gastric cardia cancer. *J Natl Cancer Institute* 1999;91:747–749.
5. Herskovic A, Martz K, al-Sarraf M, et al. Combined chemotherapy and radiotherapy compared to radiotherapy alone in patients with cancer of esophagus. *N Engl J Med* 1992;326:1593–1598.
6. Hishikawa Y, Tanaka S, Miura T. Esophageal ulceration induced by intracavitary irradiation for esophageal carcinoma. *Am J Roentgenol* 1984;143:269–273.
7. Kelsen DP, Ginsberg R, Pajak TF, et al. Chemotherapy followed by surgery compared with surgery alone for localized esophageal cancer. *N Engl J Med* 1998;339:1979–1984.
8. Urba S, Orriger M, Turrisi A, et al. A randomized trial comparing transhiatal esophagogastrectomy to preoperative concurrent chemoradiation followed by esophagectomy in locoregional esophageal carcinoma [abstract]. *Proc Am Soc Clin Oncol* 1995;14:199.
9. Walsh TN, Noonan N, Hollywood D, et al. A comparison of multimodal therapy and surgery for esophageal adenocarcinoma. *N Engl J Med* 1996;335:462–467.
10. Bosset J-F, Gignoux M, Triboulet J-P, et al. Chemoradiotherapy followed by surgery compared with surgery alone in squamous-cell cancer of the esophagus. *N Engl J Med* 1997;337:161–167.
11. Minsky BD, Neuberg D, Kelsen DP, et al. Final report of Intergroup Trial 0122: Phase II trial of neoadjuvant chemotherapy plus concurrent chemotherapy and high-dose radiation for squamous cell carcinoma of the esophagus. *Int J Radiation Oncology Biol Phys* 1999;43(3):517–523.
12. d'Etoilles L. In: *De Lanacherie de l' Oesophaotomie*. Brussels, 1845.
13. Symonds CJ. A case of malignant stricture of esophagus illustration the use of the new form of esophageal catheter. *Trans Chir Soc Lond* 1885;18:155–158.
14. Guisez J. De l'intubation caoutchoutee esophagienne. *Presse Med* 1914;22:85–87.
15. Souttar HS. Cancer of the esophagus. *Br Med J* 1934;2:797–800.
16. Domschke W, Foerster EC, Matek W, Rodl W. Self-expanding mesh stent for esophageal cancer stenosis. *Endoscopy* 1990;22:134–136.
17. Tan BS, Mason RC, Adam A. Minimally invasive therapy for advanced esophageal malignancy. *Clin Radiol* 1996;51:828–836.
18. Gollub MJ, Gerdes H, Manjit B. Radiographic appearance of esophageal stents. *Radiographics* 1997;17:1169–1182.
19. Iwasaki Y, Nakjima Y, Ishikawa T, Wakabayashi M, Ashida H. CT appearance of implanted esophageal stents: pictorial essay. *J Comput Assist Tomogr* 2000;24(1):12–23.
20. Nevitt AW, Kozarek RA, Kidd R. Expandable esophageal prosthesis: Recognition, insertion technique and positioning. *Am J Roentgenol* 1996;167:1009–1013.
21. Watkinson AF, Mason RC, Adam A. Esophageal stent. In: Adam A, Doudelinger RF, Mueller PR, eds. *Textbook of Metallic Stents*. Oxford, England: Isis Medical Media; 1997:87–104.
22. Miyayama S, Matsui O, Kadoya M, et al. Malignant esophageal stricture with fistula: palliative treatment with covered Gianturco stent. *J Vasc Interv Radiol* 1995;6:243–248.
23. Song HY, Do YS, Han YM, et al. Covered expandable esophageal metallic stent tubes; experience in 119 patients. *Radiology* 1994;193:689–695.

24. Mellow MH, Pinkas H. Endoscopic laser therapy for malignancies affecting the esophagus and gastroesophageal junction: analysis of technical and functional efficacy. *Arch Intern Med* 1985;145:1442–1446.
25. Roy-Choudhury SH, Nocholson AA, Wedgwood KR, et al. Symptomatic malignant gastroesophageal anastomotic leak: management with covered metallic esophageal stents. *Am J Roentgenol* 2001;176:161–165.
26. Wang MQ, Sze DY, Wang ZP, et al. Delayed complications after esophageal stent placement for treatment of malignant esophageal obstruction and esophagorespiratory fistulas. *J Vasc Inter Radiol* 2001;12:465–474.
27. Saxon RR, Morrison KE, Lakin PC, et al. Malignant esophageal obstruction and esophagorespiratory fistula: palliation with polyethylene-covered Z-stent. *Radiology* 1997;202:349–354.
28. Watkinson AF, Ellul J, Entwisle K, Mason RC, Adam A. Esophageal carcinoma: Initial results of palliative treatment with covered self-expanding endoprostheses. *Radiology* 1995;195:821–827.
29. Novak Z Coldwell DM, Mitchell RD, Ryu RK, Kandarpa K. Percutaneous transgastric placement of esophageal stents. *J Vasc Interv Radiol* 1999;10:428–430.
30. O'Sullivan GJ, Grundy A. Palliation of malignant dysphagia with expanding metallic stents. *J Vasc Interv Radiol* 1999;10:346–351.
31. Knyrim K, Wagner HJ, Bethge N, Keymiling M, Vakil M. A controlled trial of an expansile metallic stent for palliation of esophageal obstruction due to inoperable cancer. *N Eng J Med* 1993;329;1302–1307.
32. Acunas B, Rozanes I, Akpinar S, et al. Palliation of malignant esophageal stricture with self-expanding nitinol stent; drawbacks and complications. *Radiology* 1996;199:648–652.
33. Adam A, Ellul J, Watkinson AF, et al. Palliation of inoperable esophageal carcinoma; a prospective randomized trial of laser therapy and stent placement. *Radiology* 1997;202:344–348.
34. Siersema PD, Tan TG, Sutorius FF, Dees J, Van Blankenstein M. Massive hemorrhage caused by a perforating Gianturco-Z stent resulting in an aorto-esophageal fistula. *Endoscopy* 1997;29:416–420.
35. Watson A. Self expanding metal esophageal endoprostheses; which is best? *Eur J Gastroenterol Hepatol* 1998;10:363–365.
36. 2002 Estimates of U.S. Cancer Statistics. American Cancer Society Web site. Available at: http://www.cancer.org. Accessed.
37. Ripamonti C, De Conno F, Ventafridda V, Rossi B, Baines MJ. Management of bowel obstruction in advanced and terminal cancer patients. *Ann Oncol* 1993;4:15–21.
38. Lillemoe KD, Cameron JL, Hardacre JM, et al. Is prophylactic gastrojejunostomy indicated for unresectable periampullary cancer? A prospective randomized trial. *Ann Surg* 1999;230:322–328.
39. Ekbom GA, Gleysteen JJ. Gastric malignancy: resection for palliation. *Surgery* 1980;88:476–81.
40. Cannizzaro R, Bortoluzzi F, Valentini M, et al. Percutaneous endoscopic gastrostomy as a decompressive technique in bowel obstruction due to abdominal carcinomatosis. *Endoscopy* 1995;27:317–320.
41. Picus D, Marx MV, Weyman PJ. Chronic intestinal obstruction: value of percutaneous gastrostomy tube placement. *Am J Roentgenol* 1988;150:295–297.
42. Malone JM Jr, Koonce T, Larson DM, et al. Palliation of small bowel obstruction by percutaneous gastrostomy in patients with progressive ovarian carcinoma. *Obstet Gynecol* 1986;68:431–433.
43. Cunningham MJ, Bromberg C, Kredentser DC, et al. Percutaneous gastrostomy for decompression in patients with advanced gynecologic malignancies. *Gynecol Oncol* 1995;59:273–276.
44. Davies NH, McCall J. Transhepatic placement of combined biliary and duodenal stents. *Am J Roentgenol* 1999;172:57–58.
45. Ernst S, Stippel D, Lackner K. Placement of Palmaz stents in malignant duodenal stenosis through a cutaneous fistula. *Eur Radiol* 1999;9:1142–1144.
46. Binkert CA, Jost R, Steiner A, Zollikofer CL. Benign and malignant stenoses of the stomach and duodenum: treatment with self-expanding metallic endoprostheses. *Radiology* 1996;199:335–338.
47. Feretis C, Benakis P, Dimopoulos C, et al. Palliation of malignant gastric outlet obstruction with self-expanding metal stents. *Endoscopy* 1996;28:225–228.
48. de Baere T, Harry G, Ducreux M, et al. Self-expanding metallic stents as palliative treatment of malignant gastroduodenal stenosis. *Am J Roentgenol* 1997;169:1079–1083.
49. Yates MR, Morgan DE, Baron TH. Palliation of malignant gastric and small intestinal strictures with self-expandable metal stents. *Endoscopy* 1998;30:266–272.
50. Soetikno RM, Lichtenstein DR, Vandervoort J, et al. Palliation of malignant gastric outlet obstruction using an endoscopically placed Wallstent. *Gastrointest Endosc* 1998;47:267–270.
51. Profili S, Meloni GB, Bifulco V, et al. Self-expandable metal stents in the treatment of antro-pyloric and/or duodenal strictures. *Acta Radiol* 2001;42:176–180.
52. Thumbe VK, Houghton AD, Smith MS. Duodenal perforation by a Wallstent. *Endoscopy* 2000;32:495–497.
53. Ee H, Laurence BH. Haemorrhage due to erosion of a metal biliary stent through the duodenal wall. *Endoscopy* 1992;24(5):431–432.
54. Gardiner MF, Long WB, Haskal ZJ, Lichtenstein GR. Upper gastrointestinal hemorrhage secondary to erosion of a biliary Wallstent in a woman with pancreatic cancer. *Endoscopy* 2000;32:661–663.
55. Roebuck DJ, Stanley P, Katz MD, Parry RL, Haight MA. Gastrointestinal hemorrhage due to duodenal erosion by a biliary Wallstent. *Cardiovasc Intervent Radiol* 1998;2:63–65.
56. Bethge N, Sommer A, Gross U, et al. Human tissue responses to metal stents implanted in vivo for the palliation of malignant stenoses. *Gastrointest Endosc* 1996;43:596–602.
57. Hausegger KA, Thurnher S, Bodendorfer G, et al. Treatment of malignant biliary obstruction with polyurethane-covered Wallstents. *Am J Roentgenol* 1998;170:403–408.
58. Park H, Do YS, Suh SW, et al. Upper gastrointestinal tract malignant obstruction: initial results of palliation with a flexible covered stent. *Radiology* 1999;210:865–870.
59. Jung GS, Song HY, Kang SG, et al. Malignant gastroduodenal obstructions: treatment by means of a covered expandable metallic stent—initial experience. *Radiology* 2000;216:758–763.
60. Cope C, Clark TW, Ginsberg G, Habecker P. Stent placement of gastroenteric anastomoses formed by magnetic compression. *J Vasc Interv Radiol* 1999;10:1379–1386.
61. Mezawa S, Homma H, Sato T, et al. A study of carboplatin-coated tube for the unresectable cholangiocarcinoma. *Hepatology* 2000;32:916–923.
62. Griffith R. Preoperative evaluation: medical obstacles to surgery. *Cancer* 1992;70(suppl):1333–1341.
63. Waldron RP, Donovan IA, Drumm J, Mottram SN, Tedman S. Emergency presentation and mortality from colorectal cancer in the elderly. *Br J Surg* 1986;73:214–216.
64. Ohman U. Prognosis in patients with obstructing colorectal carcinoma. *Am J Surg* 1982;143:742–747.
65. Kyllonen L. Obstruction and perforation complicating colorectal carcinoma. *Acta Chir Scand* 1987;153:607–614.
66. Deans GT, Krukowski ZH, Irwin ST. Malignant obstruction of the left colon. *Br J Surg* 1994;81:1270–1276.
67. MacKenzie S, Thomson SR, Baker LW. Management options in malignant obstruction of the left colon. *Surgery* 1992;174:337–345.
68. Scott NA, Jeacock J, Kingston RD. Risk factors in patients presenting as an emergency with colorectal cancer. *Br J Surg* 1995;82:321–323.
69. Stewart J, Diament RH, Brennan TG. Management of obstructing lesions of the left colon by resection, on-table lavage, and primary anastomosis. *Surgery* 1992;114:502–505.

70. Ruiz PL, Faccinto EM, Faccinto ME, et al. New intraluminal bypass tube for management of acutely obstructed left colon. *Dis Colon Rectum* 1995;38:1108–1109.
71. Rosati C, Smith L, Deitel M, et al. Primary colorectal anastomosis with the intracolonic bypass tube. *Surgery* 1992;112:618–622.
72. Runkel NS, Schlag P, Schnarz V, Herfarth C. Outcome after emergency surgery for cancer of the large intestine. *Br J Surg* 1991;78:183–188.
73. Deans GT, Krukowski ZH, Irwin ST. Malignant obstruction of the left colon. *Br J Surg* 1994;81:1270–1276.
74. Morel PH, Egeli RA Wachtl S, et al. Results of operative treatment of gastrointestinal tract tumours. *Arch Surg* 1989;124:662–664.
75. Oz MC, Forde KA. Endoscopic alternatives in the management of colonic strictures. *Surgery* 1990;108:513–519.
76. Daneker GW, Carlson GW, Hohn DC, et al. Endoscopic laser recanalization is effective for prevention and treatment of obstruction in sigmoid and rectal cancer. *Arch Surg* 1991;126:1348–1352.
77. Eckhauser ML, Mansour EG. Endoscopic laser therapy for obstructing and/or bleeding colorectal carcinoma *Am Surg*. 1992;55:358–363.
78. Goligher JC, Smiddy FG. The treatment of acute obstruction or perforation with carcinoma of the colon and rectum. *Br J Surg* 1957;45:270–274.
79. Rosenburg L, Gordon PH. Tube cecostomy revisited. *Can J Surg* 1986;29:38–40.
80. Benacci JC, Wolff BG. Cecostomy, therapeutic indications and results. *Dis Colon Rectum* 1995;38:530–534.
81. Perrier G, Peillon C, Liberge N, et al. Cecostomy is a useful surgical procedure. *Dis Colon Rectum* 2000;43:50–54.
82. Casola G, Withers C, vanSonnenberg E, et al. Percutaneous cecostomy for decompression of the massively distended cecum. *Radiology* 1986;158:793–794.
83. Morrison MC, Lee MJ, Stafford SA, Saini S, Mueller PR. Percutaneous cecostomy: controlled transperitoneal approach. *Radiology* 1990;176:574–576.
84. Chait PG, Shandling B, Richards HM, Connolly BL. Fecal incontinence in children: treatment with percutaneous cecostomy tube placement, a prospective study. *Radiology* 1997;203:621–624.
85. Lechai B, Gugenheim J, Bismuth H. Pour la rehabilitation de la caecostomie sur drain comme traitements initial des occlusions coliques tumorales. *J Chir* 1987;124:346–348.
86. Hoffmann J, Jensen HE. Tube cecostomy and staged resection for obstructing carcinoma of the left colon. *Dis Colon Rectum* 1984;27:24–32.
87. Lelcuk S, Ratan J, Klausner JM, et al. Endoscopic decompression of acute colonic obstruction avoiding staged surgery. *Ann Surg* 1986;203:292–294.
88. Keen RR, Orsay CP. Rectosigmoid stent for obstructing colonic neoplasms. *Dis Colon Rectum* 1992;35:912–913.
89. Dohmoto M, Rupp KD, Hohlbach G. Endoscopically implanted prosthesis in rectal carcinoma [German]. *Dtsch Med Wochenschr* 1990;115:915.
90. Saida Y, Sumiyama Y, Nagao J, Takase M. Stent endoprosthesis for obstructing colorectal cancers. *Dis Colon Rectum* 1996;39:552–555.
91. Campbell KL, Hussey JK, Eremin O. Expandable metal stent application in obstructing carcinoma of the proximal colon. *Dis Colon Rectum* 1997;40:1391–1393.
92. Lamah M, Mathur P, McKeown B, Blake H, Swift RI. The use of rectosigmoid stents in the management of acute large bowel obstruction. *J R Coll Surg Edinb* 1998;43:318–321.
93. Mainar A, Ariza MA, Tejeno E, et al. Acute colorectal obstruction: treatment with self-expandable metallic stents before scheduled surgery—results of a multicenter study. *Radiology* 1999;219:65–69.
94. Rey JF, Romanczyk T, Greff M. Metal stents for palliation of rectal carcinoma: a preliminary report on 12 patients. *Endoscopy* 1995;27:501–504.
95. Turegano-Fuentes F, Echenagusia-Belda A, Simo-Muerza G, et al. Transanal self-expanding metal stents as an alternative to palliative colostomy in selected patients with malignant obstruction of the left colon. *Br J Surg* 1998;85:232–235.
96. Diaz LP, Pabon IP, Lobato RF. Metallic stents as a palliative measure in obstructive colon cancer. *J Vasc Interv Radiol* 1998;13:24–30.
97. De Gregorio MA, Mainer A, Tefero E, et al. Acute colorectal obstruction: stent placement for palliative treatment—results of a multicenter study. *Radiology* 1998;209:117–120.
98. Velling TE, Hall LD, Brennan FJ. Colonic stent placement facilitated by percutaneous cecostomy and antegrade enema. *Am J Roentgenol* 2000;175:119–120.
99. Mainar A, Tejero E, Maynar M, Ferral H, Castaneda-Zuniga W. Colorectal obstruction: treatment with metallic stents. *Radiology* 1996;198:761–764.
100. Wallis F, Campell KL, Eremin O, Hussey JK. Self-expanding metal stents in the management of colorectal carcinoma—a preliminary report. *Clin Radiol* 1998;53:251–254.
101. Wholey MH, Levine EA, Ferral H, Castaneda-Zuniga W. Initial clinical experience with colonic stent placement. *Am J Surg* 1998;175:194–197.
102. Canon CL, Baron TH, Morgan DE, Dean PA, Koehler RE. Treatment of colonic obstruction with expandable metal stents: radiologic features. *Am J Roentgenol* 1997;168:199–205.
103. Binkert CA, Ledermann H, Just R, et al. Acute colonic obstruction: clinical aspects and cost effectiveness of preoperative and palliative treatment with self-expanding metallic stents—a preliminary report. *Radiology* 1998;206:199–204.
104. Choo IW, Do YS, Suh SW, et al. Malignant colorectal obstruction: treatment with a flexible covered stent. *Radiology* 1998;206:415–421.
105. Baron TH, Dean PA, Yates MR, Canon C, Koehler RE. Expandable metal stents for the treatment of colonic obstruction: techniques and outcomes. *Gastrointest Endosc* 1998;47:277–286.
106. Law WL, Chu KW, Ho JW, et al. Self-expanding metallic stent in the treatment of colonic obstruction caused by advanced malignancies. *Dis Colon Rectum* 2000;43:1522–1527.
107. Boorman P, Soonawalla Z, Sathananthan N, MacFarlane P, Parker MC. Endoluminal stenting of obstructed colorectal tumours. *Ann R Coll Surg Engl* 1999;81:251–254.
108. Camunez F, Echenagusia A, Simo G, et al. Malignant colorectal obstruction treated by means of self-expanding metallic stents: effectiveness before surgery and in palliation. *Radiology* 2000;216:492–497.
109. Tamim WZ, Ghellai A, Counihan TC, et al. Experience with endoluminal colonic wall stents for the management of large bowel obstruction for benign and malignant disease. *Arch Surg* 2000;135:434–438.
110. Lo SK. Metallic stenting for colorectal obstruction. *Gastroint Endosc Clin North Am* 1999;3:459–475.
111. Mauro MA, Koehler RE, Baron TH. Advances in gastrointestinal intervention: the treatment of gastroduodenal and colorectal obstructions with metallic stents. *Radiology* 2000;215:659–669.

INDEX

INDEX

Page numbers followed by f indicate figures. Page numbers followed by t indicate tables.

T

U

V

W

Z

CME Quizzes

CHAPTER 1: Radiological Interventions: Special Considerations in Cancer Patients

1. Assessment of performance status of cancer patients is important because it usually correlates well with:
   a. prognosis
   b. tumour histology
   c. end organ function
   d. age
   e. co-morbid conditions

2. Treatment with low molecular weight heparin (LMWH) would result in alteration of:
   a. INR (international normalized ratio)
   b. PT (prothrombin time)
   c. APTT (activated partial thromboplastin time)
   d. Bleeding time
   e. Anti-factor Xa activity

3. The strategy effective in preventing tumour lysis syndrome in a setting of interventional procedure includes:
   a. Reducing pH of urine
   b. Allopurinol
   c. Fasting
   d. Phosphate replacement
   e. Diuretics

4. Cytotoxic agent requiring dose adjustment in the setting of renal impairment includes:
   a. Methotrexate
   b. 5-fluorouracil
   c. vincristine
   d. Taxol
   e. Doxorubicin

5. Of the following, the tumour most likely to result in tumour lysis syndrome includes:
   a. breast cancer
   b. small cell lung cancer
   c. Burkitt's lymphoma
   d. Chronic lymphocytic leukemia
   e. Prostate cancer

6. Of the following, the factor most commonly associated with the risk of fungal infection in a cancer patient includes:
   a. Age
   b. Prolonged granulocytopenia
   c. Advanced solid tumour malignancy
   d. Presence of intravascular device
   e. Asplenia

7. Cytotoxic agent associated with risk of vasospasm includes:
   a. Bleomycin
   b. 5-fluorouracil
   c. anthracyclines
   d. vincristine
   e. cyclophosphamide

8. Neoadjuvant chemotherapy is usually administered:
   a. Prior to surgery
   b. After surgery
   c. Instead of surgery
   d. After radiotherapy
   e. Concurrently with radiotherapy

CHAPTER 2: Principles of Chemotherapy

1. True or false. Alkylating agents were the first agents used clinically to combat cancer.

2. True or false. Different drugs of the same class will always have the same effect on a particular tumor type.

3. True or false. Agents that damage cells only during DNA synthesis are considered G-specific.

4. The Gompertzian model of tumor growth states all of the following except:
   a. Tumor growth is exponential
   b. The growth fraction decreases exponentially as the tumor size increases
   c. Multiple treatment cycles are required with sufficient dose intensity.
   d. A single surviving cell will lead to treatment failure

5. True or false. Pharmacodynamics refers to the absorption, distribution, metabolism, and excretion of drugs.

6. All of the following classes of agents affect DNA and/or RNA synthesis except:
   a. Alkylating agents
   b. Antimetabolites
   c. Plant alkyloids
   d. Platimum salts

7. True or false. When the procedure is completed, all contaminated needles, syringes, and protective garb should be placed in an appropriate container labeled as toxic waste.

8. True or false. Multidrug regimens use agents from the same class.

CHAPTER 3: Embolization—Principles, Agents, and Techniques

1. Gelfoam is all of the following EXCEPT:
- a. Readily available
- b. Cheap
- c. Permanent
- d. Easy to use

2. True or false? Digital subtraction technique saves time and contrast load?

3. Particulate embolization:
- a. Always causes permanent occlusions
- b. Causes ischemia when large particles are used
- c. Cannot be used through a microcatheter
- d. Should not be used when embolizing an arteriovenous fistula

4. True or false? Coils cause permanent vessel occlusions by inducing superimposed thrombosis?

5. Lipiodol:
- a. Has been used in the vascular system for 80 years
- b. Should never be mixed with chemotherapeutic agents
- c. Does not cause vascular occlusion, but rather is just used as a contrast agent
- d. Is made from poppyseed oil

6. Which of the following is a patient-specific issue regarding cancer patients?
- a. Coagulation
- b. Pain control
- c. Immunosuppression
- d. Renal failure
- e. All of the above

7. True or false? Regional chemotherapy infusion, without accompanying embolization therapy, has no efficacy.

8. Accepted complication rates may be 5% or greater for all of the following EXCEPT:
- a. Nontarget embolization
- b. Access-site hematoma
- c. Post-embolization syndrome
- d. Tumor lysis syndrome

CHAPTER 4: Principles Of Gene Therapy

1. The gene therapy strategy that aims to block existing gene function by interfering with processing of the primary transcript is _______.
- a. transcription factor decoy oligonucleotides
- b. suicide gene transfer
- c. antisense oligonucleotides
- d. replication selective viral oncolytic therapy

2. Which of the following are vectors used in gene therapy?
- a. replication-deficient adenovirus
- b. replication-deficient retrovirus
- c. cationic liposomes
- d. plasmids
- e. all of the above

3. An example of suicide gene therapy is ________.
- a. gene transfer of TP53 followed by radiation therapy
- b. gene transfer of interleukin-2 followed by chemotherapy
- c. gene transfer of herpes virus thymidine kinase followed by ganciclovir
- d. gene transfer of adenoviral E1a followed by endostatin therapy

4. Characteristics of adenoviral vectors include all of the following except ______.
- a. ability to integrate into host genomes, ensuring long-term expression
- b. ability to transfect a wide variety of cell types
- c. ability to cause cytotoxicity when given in high titers
- d. ability of first-generation vectors to produce small amounts of viral proteins and therefore activate the immune system.

5. Which of the following statements about viral oncolytic therapy is false?
- a. The virus is the therapeutic agent.
- b. The virus is rendered replication-deficient so that each viral particle can infect only one cell.
- c. The adenovirus ONYX-015 has been safely administered by intravenous, intra-arterial, and intraperitoneal routes.
- d. ONYX-015 cannot be therapeutic against p53-competent cells.

6. **The largest hurdle facing gene therapy today is ________.**
   a. vector design
   b. public fear
   c. delivery
   d. regulation of transgene expression

7. **Which vector can transduce only a replicating cell?**
   a. adenovirus
   b. retrovirus
   c. cationic liposome
   d. plasmid

8. **Which adenoviral vector has the largest transgene carrying capacity?**
   a. first-generation adenoviral vector
   b. second-generation adenoviral vector
   c. gutless adenoviral vector
   d. helper-dependent adenoviral vector
   e. C & D

CHAPTER 5: Regional Pain in the Cancer Patient: Interventional Image-Guided Pain Treatment Modalities

1. **Celiac Plexus Block**
   a. Should not be performed bilaterally
   b. Causes postural hypotension
   c. Is performed laterally at T10 interspace
   d. Controls pain associated with pancreatic cancer

2. **Landmarks of stellate ganglion block include the**
   a. Cricoid cartilage
   b. Hyoid bone
   c. Transverse process of C6
   d. Mastoid process

3. **A 55-year-old man with pancreatic carcinoma undergoes a celiac plexus block for pain relief. Thirty minutes later he falls to the floor when attempting to walk. The causes include**
   a. Total spinal anesthesia
   b. Block of vasoconstrictor fibers to the viscera
   c. Intravascular injection of local anesthetic
   d. Spread of anesthetic to the upper lumber nerves

4. **Which of the following statements regarding the superior hypogastric plexus is not true?**
   a. It is most appropriate for pelvic pain of visceral origin
   b. It is associated with few side effects
   c. It may or may not be performed under fluoroscopy
   d. It is most appropriate for upper abdominal pain

5. **The most common side effect of a celiac plexus block is**
   a. Hypotension
   b. Seizure
   c. Subarachnoid infection
   d. Retroperitoneal hematoma
   e. Constipation

6. **In performing a celiac plexus block, the final resting point of the needle is**
   a. Anterior to the aorta
   b. Posterior to the aorta
   c. In the intervertebral disc
   d. Inside paravertebral muscle

7. **The structure lying in close proximity to the trigeminal ganglion is the**
   a. Internal carotid artery
   b. Posterior cavernous sinus
   c. Temporal lobe
   d. Arch of zygoma
   e. All of the above

8. **The glossopharyngeal nerve exits from the skull through the**
   a. Foramen ovale
   b. Foramen rotundum
   c. Jugular foramen
   d. Foramen magnum

9. **The most commonly used neurolytic agent for celiac plexus block**
   a. 100% alcohol
   b. 6% phenol in glycerin
   c. Hypertonic saline
   d. 50% alcohol
   e. All of the above

10. **Indications for ganglion limpar block**
    a. Cancer of the pancreas
    b. Cancer of the liver
    c. Cancer of the stomach
    d. Complex regional pain syndrome of the lower extremity
    e. Pelvic cancer

CHAPTER 6: Pertinent Patient Management Issues

1. True or false? Ondansetron is a selective type 3 serotonin receptor antagonist.

true
false

2. A complication encountered specifically with left internal jugular vein venous access is _______.

a. pneumothorax
b. venous rupture
c. chylothorax
d. catheter malposition

3. The agents that are implicated in tumor fever are ______.

a. cytokine
b. tumor necrosis factor
c. interleukins 1 and 6
d. interferon
e. all of the above

4. The malignancy that is NOT known to be associated with tumor fever is ________.

a. renal cell carcinoma
b. lymphoma
c. lung cancer
d. acute and chronic myelogenous leukemias

5. The role of psycho-oncology is to understand the psychological reaction of patients at all stages of the disease as well as those of the family and healthcare staff, and to explore the psychological, social, and behavioral factors that may affect cancer incidence and survival.

true
false

CHAPTER 7: Diagnostic Dilemmas: Algorithms for Non-Invasive Imaging of Hepatic Masses

1. Hemangioblastoma is the most common liver tumor in infants $<$6 months old.

a. True
b. False

2. Biphasic CT scans of the liver are particularly helpful with hypervascular tumors.

a. True
b. False

3. All of the following represent hypervascular tumors of the liver EXCEPT:

a. Hepatoma
b. Hemangiomas
c. Hemangioendothelioma
d. Lymphoma

4. Target lesions (hyperechoic center and hypoechoic rim) tend to be benign.

a. True
b. False

5. Which of the following lesions is most likely to enhance following administration of the superparamagnetic iron oxide (SPIO) agent?

a. Hepatoma
b. Focal nodular hyperplasia
c. Hemangioma
d. Hepatic cyst

6. At what time should lesions displaying typically benign appearances on CT or US be re-imaged?

a. 1 month
b. 3 months
c. 6 months
d. No need to re-image

CHAPTER 8: Percutaneous Image-Guided Biopsy: Review of and Emphasis on Special Approaches

1. Needles designed to obtain cores of tissue for histologic analysis are known as ________.
  a. aspirating needles
  b. liver needles
  c. cutting needles
  d. spinal needles
  e. large-bore needles

2. Approaches to the biopsy of deep pelvic masses include all of the following except ________.
  a. transgluteal
  b. transvaginal
  c. transrectal
  d. transthoracic

3. Approaches or techniques available to the radiologist for percutaneous biopsy of thoracic, abdominal, or pelvic masses that are not readily accessible via simple percutaneous approaches include all of the following except ________.
  a. transsternal
  b. transvaginal
  c. use of curved needles
  d. transsphenoidal
  e. transgluteal

4. Which of the following statements is correct regarding biopsy of cystic pancreatic masses?
  a. Percutaneous biopsy of cystic pancreatic masses using an access route that traverses colon is recommended if no other safe access is available.
  b. Biopsy of all pancreatic masses, solid or cystic, should be performed using endoscopic ultrasound only.
  c. Fluid should be sent for measurement of tumor markers such as CA 19-9.
  d. If the fluid cannot be completely removed with a needle, a drainage catheter should be placed.
  e. Masses near the bile duct should not undergo biopsy.

5. Approaches or techniques to biopsy mediastinal lesions with limited percutaneous access include all of the following except ________.
  a. transsternal
  b. creation of an extrapleural percutaneous path by saline injection
  c. transaortic
  d. use of curved needles

6. In a patient with a known lung cancer and all of the following computed tomography findings, which of the following is the most appropriate lesion to biopsy for staging purposes?
  a. 1.5-cm adrenal mass measuring 1 HU
  b. 3-cm solid liver lesion representing the largest of multiple solid liver lesions that do not have characteristics of hemangiomas
  c. One of two solid spleen lesions measuring 2 cm and 3 cm, respectively
  d. 9-mm retroperitoneal lymph node
  e. 1-cm groin node with fatty center

7. Percutaneous biopsy should never be performed with an access path that goes through bowel.
  a. True
  b. False

8. Biopsy of bowel masses should be performed only with the endoscopic approach.
  a. True
  b. False

9. All hepatic hemangiomas require percutaneous biopsy.
  a. True
  b. False

10. Percutaneous biopsy of solid renal masses may change disease management for patients who have malignancies of the lung, breast, or gastrointestinal tract.
  a. True
  b. False

CHAPTER 9: Angiographic Diagnosis of Abdominal Neoplasms

1. The spectrum of angiographic findings of malignancy typically includes all of the following *except* ________.
  a. arteriovenous shunting
  b. aortic dissection
  c. irregular luminal narrowing
  d. venous invasion.

2. Drugs used to enhance the portal phase of visceral arterial injections during digital subtraction angiography include which of the following? ________
  a. glucagon
  b. epinephrine
  c. acetylcysteine
  d. nitroglycerin

1. **The spectrum of angiographic findings of malignancy typically includes all of the following *except* _______.**
   a. arteriovenous shunting
   b. aortic dissection
   c. irregular luminal narrowing
   d. venous invasion.

2. **Drugs used to enhance the portal phase of visceral arterial injections during digital subtraction angiography include which of the following? _______**
   a. glucagon
   b. epinephrine
   c. acetylcysteine
   d. nitroglycerin

3. **True or False? Narrowing of an artery or vein in the absence of atherosclerosis or spasm is diagnostic of malignancy.**

4. **True or False? Serpinginous encasement of an artery is conclusive of malignancy.**

5. **Circumferential spoke wheel appearance of arteries in a renal mass is typical of _______.**
   a. oncocytoma
   b. renal cell carcinoma
   c. transitional cell carcinoma
   d. lymphoma

6. **The angiographic appearance of hepatoma includes all of the following *except* _______.**
   a. portal venous invasion
   b. hepatic venous invasion
   c. neovascularity
   d. contraction of the mesenteric arteries

7. **The incidence of portal vein thrombus in association with hepatoma has been reported to be in the range of _______.**
   a. 15%
   b. 30%
   c. 45%
   d. 55%

8. **The incidence of invasion of the inferior vena cava by renal cell carcinoma has been reported to be in the range of _______.**
   a. 2%
   b. 10%
   c. 20%
   d. 30%

CHAPTER 10: Interventional Radiology Techniques for Localization of Endocrine Tumors

1. **In patients with endocrine disorders, arteriography and venous sampling are best used**
   a. As the first localization techniques
   b. To establish the diagnosis of endocrine disease
   c. To confirm the diagnosis of endocrine disease
   d. To identify the location of a source of hormone overproduction

2. **Regarding venous sampling:**
   a. Sensitivity is independent of tumor size
   b. Precise localization is provided
   c. It is generally less demanding technically than arteriography
   d. It yields normal results in patients without endocrine disease

3. **Which of the following statements is false?**
   a. Adrenocorticotropic hormone (ACTH)-independent Cushing syndrome is usually caused by an adrenal tumor
   b. A pituitary adenoma is the ACTH source in 85% - 90% of patients with ACTH-dependent Cushing syndrome
   c. Identification of a pituitary adenoma on MRI excludes the ectopic ACTH syndrome
   d. Alcoholism, obesity, or major depression can sometimes mimic Cushing syndrome

4. **In patients with ACTH-dependent Cushing syndrome**
   a. Jugular venous sampling is more difficult than petrosal sinus sampling
   b. Jugular venous sampling is less accurate than petrosal sinus sampling
   c. Cavernous sinus sampling is superior to both jugular venous sampling and petrosal sinus sampling
   d. A patient with negative jugular sinus sampling requires no further evaluation

5. **Which of the following statements regarding primary hyperparathyroidism is false?**
   a. Invasive localization studies are frequently required prior to initial neck exploration
   b. Approximately 80% of cases are due to a solitary adenoma
   c. Approximately 15% of cases are due to hyperplasia
   d. It is a common disorder

6. **Regarding patients with persistent or recurrent hyperparathyroidism**
   a. Invasive localization studies should be performed first, since they are more sensitive
   b. An abnormal parathyroid gland should be demonstrated by at least three different imaging modalities to avoid false-positive localizations
   c. Parathyroid arteriography should be performed before parathyroid venous sampling
   d. Parathyroid arteriography will demonstrate an abnormal parathyroid gland in one third of patients

7. **Regarding parathyroid arteriography, which of the following statements is false?**
   a. Each parathyroid is usually supplied by a single artery
   b. Most individuals have 4 parathyroid glands
   c. Anterior mediastinal glands are usually supplied by the inferior thyroid artery
   d. Superselective catheterization of both thyrocervical trunks, both internal mammary arteries, and both common carotid arteries is usually required

8. **Adrenal venous sampling is usually performed for**
   a. Primary hyperaldosteronism
   b. Cushing syndrome
   c. Pheochromocytoma
   d. Virilizing disorders
   e. All of the above

9. **Regarding adrenal venous sampling:**
   a. The right adrenal vein is constant in location
   b. The right adrenal vein bifurcates approximately 2 cm from the inferior vena cava
   c. The left adrenal vein empties directly into the inferior vena cava
   d. The sampling catheter should have a small hole punched in the side of the catheter near the tip

10. **Regarding interpretation of adrenal venous sampling results:**
   a. ACTH stimulates cortisol production but not aldosterone production
   b. The aldosterone/cortisol (A/C) ratio is used to correct for the presence of multiple adrenal veins
   c. The purpose of the test is to determine if one adrenal gland is not producing aldosterone
   d. To establish a diagnosis, the A/C ratios for each adrenal gland are compared

CHAPTER 11: Hepatic Arterial Interventions

1. **True or False? Both hepatic neoplasms and normal liver receive their dominant blood supply from the hepatic artery.**

2. **Hepatic arterial intervention is indicated for selected unresectable metastases from all of the following neoplasms *except* _______.**
   a. colorectal carcinoma
   b. ocular melanoma
   c. gastrointestinal leiomyosarcoma
   d. gastric adenocarcinoma

3. **An absolute contraindication to hepatic arterial interventions for hepatic malignancy is _______.**
   a. hepatic encephalopathy
   b. marked AV shunting
   c. immediate contact of large HCC to liver capsule
   d. main portal vein obstruction

4. **True or False? Regarding the technique of hepatic artery chemoembolization, right and left lobes are treated during the same procedure.**

5. **Advantages of Lipiodol use in hepatic artery chemoembolization are: _______.**
   a. greater tumor necrosis of infiltrative lesions and daughter nodules
   b. lipiodol visibility within lesion on CT
   c. a and b
   d. none of the above

6. **True or False? Hepatic arterial infusion produces up to 400-fold greater concentration levels of chemotherapy than systemic infusion.**

7. **True or False? The most commonly used radiomicrospheres are ^{131}I-Lipiodol and yttrium^{90}.**

8. **The rate of major complications following hepatic artery chemoembolization is approximately _______.**
   a. 1%
   b. 5%
   c. 10%
   d. 15%

9. **The tumor that shows the most dramatic symptomatic response to TOCE is:**
   a. neuroendocrine metastases
   b. HCC
   c. ocular melanoma
   d. colorectal carcinoma

10. **True or False? Post-embolization syndrome is the most common major complication following hepatic arterial embolization procedures.**

CHAPTER 12: Preoperative Portal Vein Embolization to Increase Safety of Major Hepatectomies for Hepatobiliary Malignancies

1. The overall incidence of portal venous variants is:
   a. <1%
   b. 10%–15%
   c. 25%–30%
   d. 35%–40%

2. Which of the following statements is true of PVE:
   a. PVE is similar to transarterial embolization (TAE) in that it is used as "definitive treatment" for hepatobiliary malignancy
   b. PVE is an adjunctive procedure that reduces the risk of post-resection liver failure
   c. PVE helps to add to the pool of surgical candidates by decreasing FLR mass
   d. PVE usually has no effect on the length of hospital stay

3. Which of the following statement best defines Makuuchi's rationale for performing PVE prior to major hepatic resection:
   a. PVE redistributes hepatotrophic factors so that they are carried by hepatic arteries
   b. PVE decreases portal venous blood flow to the embolized liver to promote atrophy
   c. PVE minimizes the sudden elevation in portal pressure that may lead to post-resection congestion and hepatic dysfunction
   d. PVE leads to large metabolic changes in the liver after resection

4. Following PVE, fastest rate of hypertrophy occurs:
   a. Within 12 hours
   b. Within 3 days
   c. Within 2 weeks
   d. After 1 month

5. Which of the following statements is true about PVE:
   a. Pathologically, PVE results in apoptosis, not necrosis
   b. Synthetic function is almost always affected
   c. Large changes in liver function tests are seen
   d. PVE is considered to be more toxic than transarterial embolization (TAE)

6. Which of the following is *true* about the ipsilateral approach for PVE:
   a. General anesthesia is required
   b. It is performed only in procedure rooms that are operating-room compatible
   c. It is used in an attempt to avoid injury to the FLR
   d. It is used primarily when the portal veins are thrombosed

7. To avoid post-resection liver failure in patients with otherwise normal livers (metastatic disease), the estimated FLR liver volume should be at least:
   a. 10%
   b. 25%
   c. 40%
   d. 65%

8. To avoid post-resection liver failure in cirrhotic patients (injured liver), the estimated FLR liver volume should be at least:
   a. 10%
   b. 25%
   c. 40%
   d. 65%

9. Similar to patients with cirrhosis, which systemic disease has been shown to have slower rates of hepatic hypertrophy:
   a. Systemic lupus erythematosus
   b. Atherosclerosis
   c. Rheumatoid arthritis
   d. Diabetes mellitus

10. When comparing embolic agents for PVE, the agent found to be most efficacious is:
   a. Cyanoacrylate
   b. Fibrin glue/Lipiodol®
   c. Polyvinyl alcohol particles with coils
   d. No embolic agent has been found to have superior effectiveness

CHAPTER 13: Multimodality Therapy for Hepatic Malignancies

1. Most studies have shown that adjuvant (postoperative) hepatic artery infusion chemotherapy decreases hepatic recurrence after resection of hepatoma.
   a. True
   b. False

2. Randomized controlled trials demonstrate improved survival with adjuvant (postoperative) hepatic artery chemotherapy after resection of hepatoma.
   a. True
   b. False

3. Chemoembolization causes complete necrosis in 20%–25% of hepatomas.

a. True
b. False

4. Combining chemoembolization with percutaneous tumor ablation increases the rate of complete necrosis to 90%–100%.

a. True
b. False

5. Neoadjuvant (preoperative) treatment of hepatoma can be used as a bridge to transplantation.

a. True
b. False

6. Neoadjuvant therapy of hepatoma improves survival after transplantation.

a. True
b. False

7. Chemoembolization prior to transplantation complicates subsequent transplant surgery.

a. True
b. False

8. Neoadjuvant image-guided therapy can be used to downstage liver tumors to make them resectable.

a. True
b. False

9. Adjuvant (postoperative) hepatic artery chemotherapy improves recurrence rates and survival after resection of colorectal metastases.

a. True
b. False

CHAPTER 14: Vascular Interventions in Nonhepatic Malignancies

1. Which of the following statements regarding the use of embolic agents for renal artery embolization of renal cell carcinoma is true?

a. Coils are placed in the distal main renal artery or its branches to allow easy clamping and transection during surgery.
b. Proximal embolization of the main renal artery is the best way to achieve complete tumor necrosis.
c. Small (50–100 μ) PVA particles are preferred over larger particles in presence of large arteriovenous shunting.
d. Temporary agents like Gelfoam should not be used for preoperative embolization.

2. All of the following statements regarding the use of ethanol for arterial embolization of renal cell carcinoma are true *except:*

a. Balloon occlusion catheter can be used to prevent reflux during embolization.
b. Intra-arterial lidocaine can be used to decrease the pain during the procedure.
c. Embolization with ethanol primarily results in proximal vessel occlusion.
d. The occlusion balloon should be placed in the midportion of the renal artery distal to the origin of the adrenal and gonadal arteries.

3. All of the following statements regarding renal artery embolization for renal cell carcinoma are true *except:*

a. Ideally, nephrectomy should be performed within 24 to 48 hours of embolization.
b. Postembolization syndrome is typically seen 1 to 3 days after the procedure.
c. Presence of gas in the embolized tumor is pathognomonic for renal abscess.
d. Patients with unresectable tumors and persistent hematuria may benefit from renal artery embolization.

4. All of the following statements regarding transcatheter arterial embolization of bone metastases are true *except:*

a. Embolization for hypervascular bone metastases is generally performed preoperatively to reduce blood loss during surgery.
b. Surgery should ideally be performed 7 to 10 days after embolization.
c. Embolization can also be used for palliation of pain and/or bleeding in unresectable tumors.
d. Both particulate materials and liquid agents can be used for embolization of bone metastases.

5. Intra-arterial chemotherapy for extremity osteosarcomas is primarily used:

a. For control of metastatic disease.
b. Postoperatively for treatment of residual tumor.
c. Preoperatively for inducing local tumor regression.
d. For palliation of local symptoms.

6. All of the following statements regarding intraarterial infusion of chemotherapy for extremity sarcomas are true *except:*

a. A pulsatile pump can be used to allow better mixing and a more homogenous distribution of chemotherapeutic agents.
b. Curved or angled catheter tip configurations are preferred over straight catheter tips to decrease the chances that the tip will migrate into a side branch.

c. Multiple–side-hole infusion catheters or wires placed coaxially through 5F or 4F guide catheters may be used to achieve adequate distribution of chemotherapeutic agent into the multiple branches feeding a tumor.
d. A nuclear flow study may be performed after catheter placement to ensure adequate distribution of the drug to the tumor.

7. All of the following statements regarding chemotherapy infusion for pelvic tumors are true *except:*

a. Superselective uterine or vesical artery infusion is generally preferred over internal iliac artery infusion.
b. Proximal portions of the superior and inferior gluteal arteries can be embolized with coils to reduce the risk of muscle or skin necrosis and neurotoxic side effects.
c. Use of balloon-occluded arterial infusion chemotherapy can achieve higher local concentration of drug.
d. Regional infusion can result in complications like transient rash, buttock pain and ulceration, and transient neuropathies involving the sacral or femoral nerves.

8. All of the following statements regarding regional intra-arterial infusion for head and neck cancers are true *except*:

a. Cisplatin is the most commonly used chemotherapeutic agent for intra-arterial infusion to treat head and neck cancers.
b. Nonselective infusion into the external carotid artery is preferred over superselective arterial infusions.
c. Intravenous thiosulfate can be given simultaneously with intra-arterial cisplatin for systemic drug neutralization.
d. Arterial infusion of indigocarmine dye can be used to identify the feeding vessels for head and neck tumors that are located at a visible site.

CHAPTER 15: Management of Dysfunctional Central Venous Catheters in the Patient with Cancer

1. The first approach to the management of a patient with a nonfunctioning central venous catheter should be _____.

a. a trial of continuous infusion of thrombolytics through the dysfunctional catheter
b. a diagnostic chest radiograph
c. intravenous ultrasound
d. removal of the old catheter and placement of a new central venous catheter from another venous site

2. The preferred site of central venous access, from most to least desirable, would be _____.

a. right internal jugular → right subclavian → left internal jugular → left subclavian
b. left internal jugular → right internal jugular → left subclavian → right subclavian
c. right internal jugular → left internal jugular → left subclavian → right subclavian
d. right internal jugular → left internal jugular → right subclavian → left subclavian

3. Superior vena cava syndrome can present with signs and symptoms of all of the following except _____.

a. cerebral edema
b. dysphagia
c. dyspnea
d. uphill varices
e. arm swelling

4. As of 2001, the most widely used thrombolytic agent to treat dysfunctional central venous catheters in the United States is _____.

a. streptokinase
b. urokinase
c. tissue plasminogen activator
d. heparin

5. Alternative venous access, for the placement of central venous catheters, may include all of the following except _____.

a. the inferior vena cava (translumbar)
b. the external jugular vein
c. the hepatic vein (transhepatic)
d. the intercostal vein
e. the internal thoracic vein

6. Indications for the use of mechanical thrombectomy devices, in the treatment of venous occlusions, include all of the following except _____.

a. patients with borderline renal dysfunction
b. patients who are not surgery candidates
c. patients with contraindications to anticoagulation
d. patients who require immediate recanalization of the occluded vein segment

7. Exchanging a tunneled catheter over a wire has all of the advantages except _____.

a. a lower infection rate
b. a high technical success rate
c. sparing venous access sites
d. a short procedural time

8. Catheter thrombosis has been associated with all of the following except _____.

a. patient hypercoagulability
b. underlying malignancy
c. thrombocytopenia
d. catheter duration
e. catheter infection
f. infusate

9. Central venous access has been associated with _____.

a. superior vena cava syndrome
b. sepsis
c. paresthesia
d. pulmonary embolism
e. all of the above

10. The routine prophylactic use of low-dose thrombolytics has been shown to decrease catheter-related infections and thrombosis.

true
false

CHAPTER 16: Radiofrequency Tumor Ablation

1. Which of the following statements regarding the operational principles of radiofrequency ablation is/are true?

a. Radiofrequency ablation is a type of interstitial therapy.
b. The RF electrode probe itself heats and incites cell death.
c. Cytotoxic injury results in diminished capacity to conduct electrical current.
d. a and b
e. a and c

2. Strategies to increase the size of ablated tissue include _____.

a. multiple-array probe configurations
b. saline-cooled probes
c. increasing the power wattage
d. a and b
e. all of the above

3. Thermal energy–induced irreversible cellular death occurs at 5–6 minutes with temperatures of _____.

a. 42° C
b. 45° C
c. 50°–55° C
d. 60°–100° C
e. 100°

4. Strategies for track management post-ablation include _____.

a. hypertonic saline injection
b. probe activation and "burning the track"
c. Gelfoam occlusion
d. a and c
e. b and c

5. The most common complication of hepatic radiofrequency tumor ablation is _____.

a. biliary duct damage
b. track seeding
c. abscess
d. pain
e. thermal injury to adjacent bowel

6. Which of the following statements regarding radiofrequency ablation of lung lesions is/are true?

a. RF lung ablation can be used for both primary and secondary tumors.
b. The most common primary lung cancer is non–small cell cancer.
c. Pleural effusions and brown-colored sputum are reported post-procedure.
d. RF lung ablation should be avoided in patients with cardiac pacers.
e. all of the above

7. Which of the following statements regarding radiofrequency for osteoid osteoma is/are true?

a. RF for osteoid osteoma should be considered a neoadjuvant procedure for definitive surgical resection.
b. The clinical success rate is > 90%.
c. Clinical success can be achieved by placement of the probe in the thickened cortex adjacent to nidus.
d. all of the above
e. none of the above

8. Regarding radiofrequency ablation in the breast, which of the following is/are true?

a. Breast radiofrequency ablation is considered investigational.
b. RF ablation of breast carcinoma is indicated for stage III disease.
c. There may be a role for RF ablation in early-stage breast cancer.
d. a and b
e. a and c

CHAPTER 17: Interstitial Tumor Ablation

1. Bile duct injury requiring percutaneous intervention is more common following peripherally treated HCC.
a. True
b. False

2. The concentration of acetic acid required to cause the same degree of necrosis as absolute ethanol is the same for an equally delivered volume.
a. True
b. False

3. At what concentration of acetic acid does the degree of necrosis plateau? ________.
a. 15%
b. 25%
c. 50%
d. 99.5%

4. Immediately following treatment of tumors with percutaneous ethanol injection or acetic acid, imaging characteristics of the treated lesion on ultrasound/CT are ________.
a. hypoechoic/hyperattenuating
b. hypoechoic/hypoattenuating
c. hyperechoic/hypoattenuating
d. hyperechoic/hyperattenuating

5. No special equipment is required for the injection of absolute ethanol.
a. True
b. False

6. What maximum volume of absolute ethanol is recommended in one treatment session?
a. 1 cc
b. 100 cc
c. 60 cc
d. 20 cc

7. Based on current studies, percutaneous microwave coagulation therapy is more effective than PEI for HCC > 3 cm.
a. True
b. False

8. With cryotherapy, tumoricidal temperatures are typically reached in what range?
a. zero Kelvin
b. zero Celsius
c. 0 to −10 Celcius
d. −20 to −50 Celcius

9. Are there any randomized controlled trials that demonstrate a statistically significant difference in survival between different ITA therapies?
a. Yes
b. No

10. What is maximum diameter of coagulation necrosis that can be achieved with a single Nd: YAG laser fiber?
a. 1 cm
b. 1.6 cm
c. 3.1 cm
d. 5 cm

CHAPTER 18: Intratumoral Gene Therapy

1. Existing gene therapy strategies include all of the following *except:*
a. Tumor suppression.
b. Anti-angiogenesis.
c. Increased immune response.
d. Promotion of oncogene expression.

2. An advantage of image-guided direct intratumoral vector delivery over non–image-guided therapy is:
a. Improved efficiency of tumor therapy.
b. Ability to repeat therapy.
c. Reduction of allergic reactions.
d. Ability to treat patients with larger tumor burden.

3. General principles of gene therapy include alteration of all of the following *except:*
a. Regulatory pathways.
b. Normal cell replication.
c. Immune response.
d. Response to other therapies.

4. Which of the following statements about p53 genes is true?
a. They are required for normal cell cycle kinetics.
b. They cause a cytotoxic effect when added to cells deficient in p53 genes.
c. Their deficiency has not been correlated with prognosis.
d. They cannot be given by a direct intratumoral injection.

5. All of the following are specific examples of intratumoral gene therapy *except:*

a. p53 gene transfer.
b. Replication-selective oncolytic adenovirus.
c. Magnetic activation of tumor antigenicity.
d. Proactivating enzymes.

6. Which of the following statements about regulatory and safety issues with gene therapy is true?

a. All gene transfer therapies in humans are investigational.
b. The Office of Protocol Research at the National Institutes of Health has oversight over all gene therapy trials.
c. Oversight for gene therapy trials is provided only at the federal level.
d. No specific respiratory precautions are necessary because gene therapy has no proven adverse effects.

CHAPTER 19: Intracavitary Therapy

1. In the setting of underlying malignancy, cytologic evaluation of the ascitic fluid is generally diagnostic in what percentage of patients? _______.

a. 5%
b. 25%
c. 60%
d. 90%

2. The volume of ascites produced and reabsorbed by the peritoneum under normal physiologic circumstances is about _______.

a. 4–5 ml/hr
b. 40–50 ml/hr
c. 400–500 ml/hr
d. 4–5 l/hr

3. Contributing factors to the accumulation of malignant ascites includes all of the following *except* _______.

a. increased levels of vascular endothelial growth factor (VEGF)
b. albumin leakage from tumor endothelium
c. diaphragmatic lymphatic drainage obstruction
d. tumor angiogenesis

4. Le Veen, or peritoneovenous, shunts are associated with all of the following complications *except* _______.

a. catheter occlusion/obstruction
b. heart failure
c. coagulopathy
d. epidural abscess
e. infection

5. High pH (>7.4) and high glucose (>60mg/dL) in pleural fluid samples portend a poor response to pleurodesis.

a. True
b. False

6. Sclerosant agents for pleurodesis include all of the following *except* _______.

a. bleomycin
b. doxycycline
c. urokinase
d. talc

7. Pericardial tamponade is most likely clinically manifested by which of the following constellation of symptoms?

a. dyspnea, rales, and pitting edema
b. chest pain, left arm pain, and dyspnea
c. jugular distention, dyspnea, and pericardial friction rub
d. altered mental status, dysarthria, and facial droop
e. cough, fever, and dyspnea

8. External beam irradiation can be effective treatment for malignant pericardial effusion, but myocarditis may be an unwanted side effect.

a. True
b. False

CHAPTER 20: Image-Guided Brachytherapy: "Interventional Brachytherapy"

1. **Modern brachytherapy makes use of the following imaging modality(ies):**
   a. Computed tomography
   b. Magnetic resonance imaging
   c. Ultrasound imaging
   d. All of the above

2. **Temporary implant brachytherapy may make use of the following radionuclides:**
   a. Cesium 137
   b. Iridium 192
   c. Palladium 103
   d. a and b
   e. b and c

3. **Permanent seed brachytherapy is possible because of the following property(ies) of radionuclides:**
   a. Half-life
   b. Emitted photon energy
   c. Specific activity
   d. Inverse square law

4. **Image-guided brachytherapy is an advance over conventional brachytherapy because _____.**
   a. visualization of bony landmarks are made possible.
   b. placement of radioactive sources is accomplished.
   c. the patient's own anatomy is presented.
   d. All of the above

5. **Interventional brachytherapy makes use of the following technology that is different from other forms of brachytherapy:**
   a. CT scanner
   b. Fluoroscopy
   c. Stereotactic arm
   d. Stealth technology

6. **The following anatomic areas are now approachable for brachytherapy because image guidance is available:**
   a. Head and neck regions
   b. Thoracic targets
   c. Paraspinal targets
   d. Pelvic tumors
   e. All of the above

7. **The following tumor types are amenable to treatment with image-guided brachytherapy:**
   a. Leukemia
   b. Lymphoma
   c. Sarcoma
   d. Solitary pulmonary nodules
   e. a and b
   f. c and d

8. **The following data are necessary to accurately calculate dose distributions from point-source seed brachytherapy:**
   a. Soft-tissue anatomic details
   b. Seed coordinates
   c. Distance between seeds and anatomy
   d. Interapplicator distances

CHAPTER 21: Malignant Biliary Obstruction

1. **At what level of the biliary tract does metastatic lymphadenopathy cause obstruction?**
   a. Intrahepatic
   b. At the confluence of the main right and left ducts
   c. At the porta hepatis
   d. In the common bile duct
   e. At the ampulla

2. **The main therapeutic goal of percutaneous biliary drainage in the majority of patients with malignant biliary obstruction is the prolongation of life.**
   a. True
   b. False

3. **Metallic stents are used in patients with a life expectancy exceeding 6 to 8 months.**
   a. True
   b. False

4. **What is first line therapy for benign biliary strictures?**
   a. Internal metallic stents
   b. Internal/external plastic stents
   c. Surgical resection
   d. Observation

5. **For the initial puncture into the left hepatic ducts, segment II is better than segment III.**
   a. True
   b. False

6. During the initial percutaneous cholangiogram, if the obstruction is identified but cannot be passed with a wire or catheter, the next step should be to ________.

a. leave the patient to external drainage
b. call surgery for surgical placement of a drainage tube
c. abandon the procedure completely
d. leave the patient to external drainage and try again in 24 hours

7. Which of the following methods has the highest sensitivity for establishing the diagnosis of malignancy?

a. Bile cytology
b. Brush biopsies
c. Imaging
d. Serum markers
e. Forceps biopsy during percutaneous drainage

8. A patient underwent a percutaneous drainage procedure 24 hours ago. She developed copious bleeding into her drainage bag, which has continued despite upsizing of her tube. What is the next step?

a. Call surgery to perform a hepatic segmentectomy.
b. Call endoscopy to perform endoscopic cholangiography to identify the source of bleeding.
c. Hold pressure.
d. Check the patient's coagulation profile, and if it is normal, perform hepatic arteriography.
e. Administer cryoprecipitate

9. Brachytherapy is an important adjunct in the treatment of hepatocellular carcinoma.

a. True
b. False

CHAPTER 22: Genitourinary Obstruction

1. With regard to percutaneous nephrostomy:

a. It is the preferred method for treatment of malignant ureteral obstruction.
b. It is the preferred method for treatment of ureteral obstruction when associated with severe infection.
c. Obstruction due to adenopathy is a contraindication.
d. It is the treatment of choice for malignant bladder outlet obstruction.

2. Patients with malignant ureteral obstruction:

a. Should always undergo bilateral drainage procedures when both kidneys are obstructed.
b. Are not candidates for percutaneous nephrostomy when due to relapsed disease because of their overall poor prognosis.
c. Will have at least partial return of renal function a majority of the time.
d. Do not need prophylactic antibiotics prior to percutaneous nephrostomy.

3. The technique for placement of a percutaneous nephrostomy:

a. Requires CT guidance to gain access into the collecting system.
b. Should initially be done with only a small bore (6 or 8 French) tube.
c. Is absolutely contraindicated in patients with coagulopathy and/or thrombocytopenia, even when clinically unstable (i.e., septic).
d. May be performed with a single percutaneous puncture of the kidney.

4. Patients with the following characteristic may be considered for outpatient percutaneous nephrostomy:

a. Hypertension.
b. Bilateral obstruction.
c. Coagulopathy.
d. Active urinary tract infection.

5. Concerning post-procedural care:

a. Once a urinary drainage tube is placed it should have preventive maintenance care, generally every three months.
b. Patients do not need any follow-up care unless they develop a problem.
c. Urinary drainage tubes should never be flushed because of risk of introducing infection.
d. The percutaneous tract cannot be used for subsequent procedures; these procedures require an additional percutaneous access.

6. Regarding double-J ureteral stents:

a. They may be beneficial even in patients with an extensively diseased bladder.
b. Antegrade placement is always preferable to retrograde placement.
c. They allow easier home care, decreased risk of infection, and lower rate of accidental removal.
d. Placement at the time of initial renal drainage is always preferable and more successful.

7. **Patients who have undergone cystectomy for malignancy:**
   a. Always have ureteral obstruction due to benign strictures.
   b. Are excellent candidates for retrograde nephroureteral stent placement when the stricutured ureter does not reflux on loopography.
   c. Should undergo retrograde nephroureteral stent placement when a continent neobladder has been created.
   d. Can generally be treated with retrograde nephroureteral stents when an ileal conduit has been created.

8. **Regarding metallic stents in the genitourinary system:**
   a. They appear to be useful in malignant prostatic urethral strictures in patients who are poor surgical candidates.
   b. They offer much improved ureteral patency over plastic double-J stents.
   c. When properly placed in the ureter, they rarely require additional interventions.
   d. The typical hyperplastic mucosal response when implanted in a ureter resolves in 7–10 days.

CHAPTER 23: Tracheobronchial Obstruction

1. **Treatment choices for endoluminal malignant lesions include all except ________.**
   a. laser therapy.
   b. electrocautery.
   c. cryotherapy.
   d. brachytherapy.
   e. metallic stent placement.

2. **Complications of laser photoablation include ________.**
   a. retinal damage to operator or patient.
   b. endotracheal fire.
   c. intratracheal explosion.
   d. perforation.
   e. all of the above.

3. **What percentage of patients can expect symptomatic relief from laser bronchoscopy of a main-stem bronchus endoluminal malignant lesion?**
   a. 10%–20%
   b. 20%–30%
   c. 30%–50%
   d. 50%–70%
   e. 70%–90%

4. **Regarding the tissue sensitivity of cryotherapy, the maximum cell death is seen with ________.**
   a. rapid freeze.
   b. slow freeze.
   c. rapid thaw.
   d. slow thaw.
   e. both a and d.

5. **Indications for endoluminal brachytherapy are _______.**
   a. biopsy-proven carcinoma involving the bronchial tree.
   b. unavailability of curative therapy.
   c. symptoms of dyspnea or hemoptysis after laser debulking.
   d. suitable site for delivery of radiation source.
   e. all of the above.

6. **Ideal characteristics of an airway stent for malignant obstruction are _______.**
   a. is easy to insert.
   b. is easy to retrieve.
   c. resists compressive forces.
   d. is made of an inert material that does not promote granulation tissue formation.
   e. all of the above.

7. **The advantages of the Dumon studded silicone stent over a metallic stent are ________.**
   a. promotes formation of less granulation tissue.
   b. is easier to retrieve.
   c. is less likely to migrate.
   d. both a and c.
   e. both a and b.

8. **The disadvantage of the silicone stents in comparison with metallic stents is _______.**
   a. granulation tissue formation.
   b. migration.
   c. extrinsic compression.
   d. allergic reaction to silicone.
   e. none of the above.

9. **Which of the following airway stents are covered with silicone?**
   a. Dumon.
   b. Wallgraft.
   c. Permalune.
   d. Gianturco Z-stent.
   e. both a and c.

10. **The complication of self-expandable stents that limits their long-term efficacy is:**
   a. perforation.
   b. granulation tissue formation.
   c. migration.
   d. metal allergy.
   e. extrinsic compression.

CHAPTER 24: Gastrointestinal Obstruction

1. **Most primary esophageal adenocarcinomas arise from _____.**
   a. tobacco use
   b. p53 mutation
   c. habitual ingestion of hot liquids
   d. lye injury
   e. columnar metaplasia (Barrett's esophagus)

2. **Patients with a suspected fistula should undergo the following prior to esophageal stent placement:**
   a. esophageal pH monitoring
   b. double-contrast barium esophagography
   c. single-contrast barium esophagography
   d. esophagography with nonionic contrast
   e. CT scan with barium paste

3. **The initial approach to an entrapped food bolus following esophageal stent placement is _____.**
   a. guide wire manipulation
   b. nasogastric tube insertion
   c. administration of intravenous glucagon
   d. carbonated drink ingestion

4. **The most common complication of esophageal stent placement is _____.**
   a. distal migration
   b. proximal migration
   c. perforation
   d. gastrointestinal hemorrhage
   e. fistula

5. **Management options for malignant gastric outlet obstruction include the following:**
   a. prolonged nasogastric suction
   b. surgical gastrojejunostomy
   c. decompression gastrostomy
   d. endoluminal stent placement
   e. all of the above

6. **The use of covered stents, compared with bare stents, for malignant gastrointestinal obstruction prevents tumor ingrowth.**
   a. true
   b. false

7. **The following approaches may be used for gastroduodenal stenting:**
   a. peroral
   b. transgastric
   c. transbiliary
   d. all of the above

8. **The following are contraindications to colonic stent placement:**
   a. involvement of the squamocolumnar junction
   b. acute large bowel obstruction
   c. bowel perforation
   d. perforation by guide wire during crossing of the stricture
   e. all of the above
   f. (a) and (c) only

9. **Balloon dilation is recommended after placement of a self-expanding stent for malignant colonic obstruction:**
   a. true
   b. false

SOCIETY OF INTERVENTIONAL RADIOLOGY
Enhanced care through advanced technology℠

SIR Syllabus #12
Interventions in Oncology
Application for CME

Last Name First Name MI Degree

Hospital or Group Affiliation

Address City State Zip

Daytime Phone Fax E-mail Address

Are you a member of SIR? ☐ yes ☐ no

TO BECOME ELIGIBLE FOR CME CREDIT AS OUTLINED IN YOUR BOOK, THE USER MUST SUBMIT

1) APPLICATION FORM
2) COMPLETED EVALUATION SURVEY, and
3) COMPLETED QUIZ ANSWER SHEET, along with
4) $20 ADMINISTRATIVE FEE TO:

Society of Interventional Radiology
ATTENTION: CME Office
10201 Lee Highway, Suite 500
Fairfax, VA 22030

SIR will provide 24 Category 1 CME credits for *Interventions in Oncology*

PLEASE NOTE:

Only the individual who purchased this volume is eligible for the $20 CME fee upon completion. Should the purchaser wish to share this volume with others, duplicate copies of the CME examination materials can be obtained from the SIR office.

Please direct questions to CME@SIRweb.org

The Society of Interventional Radiology designates this educational activity for a maximum of 24 category 1 credits toward the AMA Physician's Recognition Award. Each physician should claim only those credits that he/she actually spent in the activity.

SOCIETY OF INTERVENTIONAL RADIOLOGY
Enhanced care through advanced technology℠

Society of Interventional Radiology
Syllabus #12: *Interventions in Oncology*

Evaluation Form

1. **What is your present level of training?**
   - ☐ Radiology resident
   - ☐ Interventional Fellow
   - ☐ Post-graduate SIR member
   - ☐ Post-graduate SIR non-member
   - ☐ Other (please specify) ______________________________

2. **Which learning mode do you prefer?**
   - ☐ Printed book
   - ☐ Computerized on Macintosh platform
   - ☐ Computerized on PC platform

3. **Please rank on a scale of 1 to 10 each of the following formats for overall educational value:**

	1 = Useless							10 = Very Useful		
Tutorials / Chapters	1	2	3	4	5	6	7	8	9	10
Quizzes	1	2	3	4	5	6	7	8	9	10

4. **Please comment on how each section could be improved.**

   Tutorials / Chapters:

   ____

   ____

   Quizzes:

   ____

   ____

5. **What topics would you like to see covered in future syllabi?**

____

____

The Society of Interventional Radiology designates this educational activity for a maximum of 24 category 1 credits toward the AMA Physician's Recognition Award. Each physician should claim only those credits that he/she actually spent in the activity.

Society of Interventional Radiology
Syllabus #12: *Interventions in Oncology*

Quiz Form

Chapter 1 1. ____ 2. ____ 3. ____ 4. ____ 5. ____ 6. ____ 7. ____ 8. ____	Chapter 5 1. ____ 2. ____ 3. ____ 4. ____ 5. ____ 6. ____ 7. ____ 8. ____ 9. ____ 10. ____	Chapter 9 1. ____ 2. ____ 3. ____ 4. ____ 5. ____ 6. ____ 7. ____ 8. ____	Chapter 13 1. ____ 2. ____ 3. ____ 4. ____ 5. ____ 6. ____ 7. ____ 8. ____ 9. ____	Chapter 17 1. ____ 2. ____ 3. ____ 4. ____ 5. ____ 6. ____ 7. ____ 8. ____ 9. ____ 10. ____	Chapter 21 1. ____ 2. ____ 3. ____ 4. ____ 5. ____ 6. ____ 7. ____ 8. ____ 9. ____
Chapter 2 1. ____ 2. ____ 3. ____ 4. ____ 5. ____ 6. ____ 7. ____ 8. ____	Chapter 6 1. ____ 2. ____ 3. ____ 4. ____ 5. ____	Chapter 10 1. ____ 2. ____ 3. ____ 4. ____ 5. ____ 6. ____ 7. ____ 8. ____ 9. ____ 10. ____	Chapter 14 1. ____ 2. ____ 3. ____ 4. ____ 5. ____ 6. ____ 7. ____ 8. ____	Chapter 18 1. ____ 2. ____ 3. ____ 4. ____ 5. ____ 6. ____	Chapter 22 1. ____ 2. ____ 3. ____ 4. ____ 5. ____ 6. ____ 7. ____ 8. ____
Chapter 3 1. ____ 2. ____ 3. ____ 4. ____ 5. ____ 6. ____ 7. ____ 8. ____	Chapter 7 1. ____ 2. ____ 3. ____ 4. ____ 5. ____ 6. ____	Chapter 11 1. ____ 2. ____ 3. ____ 4. ____ 5. ____ 6. ____ 7. ____ 8. ____ 9. ____ 10. ____	Chapter 15 1. ____ 2. ____ 3. ____ 4. ____ 5. ____ 6. ____ 7. ____ 8. ____ 9. ____ 10. ____	Chapter 19 1. ____ 2. ____ 3. ____ 4. ____ 5. ____ 6. ____ 7. ____ 8. ____	Chapter 23 1. ____ 2. ____ 3. ____ 4. ____ 5. ____ 6. ____ 7. ____ 8. ____ 9. ____ 10. ____
Chapter 4 1. ____ 2. ____ 3. ____ 4. ____ 5. ____ 6. ____ 7. ____ 8. ____	Chapter 8 1. ____ 2. ____ 3. ____ 4. ____ 5. ____ 6. ____ 7. ____ 8. ____ 9. ____ 10. ____	Chapter 12 1. ____ 2. ____ 3. ____ 4. ____ 5. ____ 6. ____ 7. ____ 8. ____ 9. ____ 10. ____	Chapter 16 1. ____ 2. ____ 3. ____ 4. ____ 5. ____ 6. ____ 7. ____ 8. ____	Chapter 20 1. ____ 2. ____ 3. ____ 4. ____ 5. ____ 6. ____ 7. ____ 8. ____	Chapter 24 1. ____ 2. ____ 3. ____ 4. ____ 5. ____ 6. ____ 7. ____ 8. ____ 9. ____

The Society of Interventional Radiology designates this educational activity for a maximum of 24 category 1 credits toward the AMA Physician's Recognition Award. Each physician should claim only those credits that he/she actually spent in the activity.